ESSENTIAL RADIOLOGY

ESSENTIAL RADIOLOGY

Clinical Presentation • Pathophysiology • Imaging

RICHARD B. GUNDERMAN, M.D., Ph.D.*

Departments of Radiology and Medicine
The University of Chicago
Chicago, Illinois

Currently Assistant Professor of Radiology and Medical Education
Indiana University School of Medicine
Indianapolis, Indiana

1998
Thieme
New York   •   Stuttgart

Thieme Medical Publishers, Inc.
333 Seventh Avenue
New York, NY 10001

Essential Radiology
Richard B. Gunderman, M.D., Ph.D.

Library of Congress Cataloging-in-Publication Data

Gunderman, Richard B.
    Esstential radiology : clinical presentation, pathophysiology,
  imaging / Richard B. Gunderman.
        p.   cm.
    Includes bibliographical references and index.
    ISBN 0-86577-684-9 (TNY). — ISBN 3-13-110471-6 (GTV)
    1. Radiography, Medical.   I. Title.
    [DNLM: 1. Radiography—handbooks.   WN 39 G975 1998]
  RC78.G85   1998
  616.07′572—DC21
  DNLM/DLC
  for Library of Congress   97-31577
                                                              CIP

Copyright © 1998 by Thieme Medical Publishers, Inc. This book, including all parts thereof, is legally protected by copyright. Any use, exploitation or commercialization outside the narrow limits set by copyright legislation, without the publisher's consent, is illegal and liable to prosecution. This applies in particular to photostat reproduction, copying, mimeographing or duplication of any kind, translating, preparation of microfilms, and electronic data processing and storage,

Important note: Medical knowledge is ever-changing. As new research and clinical experience broaden our knowledge, changes in treatment and drug therapy may be required. The authors and editors of the materials herein have consulted sources believed to be reliable in their efforts to provide information that is complete and in accord with the standards accepted at the time of publication. However, in view of the possibility of human error by the authors, editors, or publisher of the work herein, or changes in medical knowledge, neither the authors, editors, publisher, nor any other party who has been involved in the preparation of this work, warrants that the information contained herein is in every respect accurate or complete, and they are not responsible for any errors or omissions or the results obtained from use of such information. Readers are encouraged to confirm the information contained herein with other sources. For example, readers are advised to check the product information sheet included in the package of each drug they plan to administer to be certain that the information contained in this publication is accurate and that changes have not been made in the recommended dose or in the contraindications for administration. This recommendation is of particular importance in connection with new or infrequently used drugs.

Some of the product names, patents, and registered designs referred to in this book are in fact registered trademarks of proprietary names even though specific reference to this fact is not always made in the text. Therefore, the appearance of a name without designation as proprietary is not to be construed as a representation by the publisher that it is in the public domain.

Printed in the United States of America

5 4 3 2

TNY ISBN 0-86577-684-9
GTV ISBN 3-13-110471-6

Table of Contents

Preface

When he discovered the X ray just over a century ago, Wilhelm Roentgen transformed medical vision to a degree unrivaled by any scientific breakthrough since the invention of the microscope. Just as the microscope revealed the world of such fundamental biological entities as cells, so Roentgen's discovery of the "invisible light" enabled us to peer inside the body of a living, breathing patient without the use of a scalpel.

Since Roentgen's epochal discovery, medicine's imaging armamentarium has grown dramatically to encompass new modalities such as computed tomography, ultrasound, nuclear medicine, and magnetic resonance imaging. Today we are able to observe human anatomy and physiology dynamically, in real time; for example, we use ultrasound in obstetrics to assess fetal morphology and well being, magnetic resonance angiography to evaluate blood flow within arteries and veins, and positron emission tomography to observe regional changes in cerebral metabolism associated with different cognitive tasks. Through the dedicated efforts of many investigators, radiology has opened up magnificent new vistas on human health and disease, ranging from many ground-breaking discoveries in the basic medical sciences to countless critical diagnostic insights in the care of individual patients. Today, diagnostic imaging remains one of medicine's most dynamic and exciting fields.

It is impossible to practice medicine anywhere in the industrialized world and not face on a regular basis practical questions about how to make optimal use of diagnostic imaging. Virtually every medical specialty uses radiology daily to care for its patients. This interdisciplinary style of practice is one of the traits that makes radiology such a challenging and enjoyable field.

However, despite its vital role in biomedical science and clinical medicine, radiology's pedagogical potential has often been less than fully realized. Only a small minority of U.S. medical schools have incorporated formal radiology course work into their required curricula, and many medical students emerge from medical school with a limited understanding of the science of imaging, the radiologic manifestations of disease, and the optimal use of radiology's resources in the care of their patients. Moreover, radiology's potential to enrich students' understanding of such basic medical sciences as anatomy, physiology, and pathology has often gone untapped, with continued overreliance on cadaver dissection, dog labs, and autopsies at a time when new radiologic techniques can dramatically illustrate the structure and function of the living human patient, using the very same imaging studies that students will soon rely on to care for their own patients.

In part, the blame for this underutilization of radiology in medical education lies at the feet of academic radiologists themselves, who have often let other medical fields such as pathology and internal medicine shoulder the lion's share of the teaching load. Today the incentive is growing for radiologists to assume an increasing role in medical education, in part because changes in the way health care is organized and financed are stimulating academic radiology's ambition to excel at its distinctively academic missions, research and teaching. In addition, because radiology's inherently interdisciplinary character spans the basic medical sciences and clinical practice, recent pedagogical initiatives to make these traditional poles of the curriculum a more seamless web will naturally invite an increased contribution from radiology.

This book represents one answer to the call for an increased radiologic presence within the medical school curriculum. Having accepted the challenge at my own medical school to develop a larger role for radiology within the medical school curriculum, I sought to create a text that would fruitfully combine basic medical science and clinical medical practice in a way that students would find engaging and valuable. For the author of a basic radiology text, the temptation can be great to create a compendium of imaging techniques, signs, and differential diagnoses, as though the goal were to produce a "junior radiologist." By contrast, the overarching goal of this book is to use radiology as a lens through which to study medicine and to highlight with images some of the essential principles one must grasp in order to excel as a physician.

The discussions are organized, where appropriate, around categories of disease: congenital, infectious, tumorous, inflammatory, metabolic, iatrogenic, traumatic, and vascular. These categories provide students with a theoretical scaffold around which to build cogent case presentations that will enable them to shine on rounds, and more importantly, to provide better care for their patients. Traditionally "non-radiologic" data—epidemiology, pathophysiology, and clinical presentation—are regularly presented along with the imaging findings of particular diseases, in order to provide constant integration of imaging and the care of the patient. Finally, the text is organized largely by anatomic and physiologic systems, not by imaging modalities, because the structure and function of the human organism provide the most logical blueprint for learning medical imaging.

These organizational characteristics stem from my convictions that imaging is best understood—and in fact truly comprehensible—only in light of essential principles of anatomy, pathophysiology, and clinical medicine, and that building on and reinforcing those principles represents one of the central and enduring missions of the medical educator in any course. If students are to understand the essential role that radiology plays in contemporary medical care, as well as to appreciate the essence of radiology as a way of looking at human health and disease, then it is on the foundation of these principles that our teaching must be based.

Acknowledgments

This book grew largely from the fertile soil of two courses in medical imaging at the University of Chicago, designed primarily for second- and fourth-year medical students. I would like to thank Drs. John Fennessy, Martin Lipton, Lawrence Wood, and Norma Wagoner at Chicago for their support and encouragement in the creation of these courses. Early on, a two-year Spencer Fellowship from the national Academy of Education was critical in stimulating my own pedagogical pursuits, and an inaugural course development award from Dr. Wood's office of the Faculty Dean for Medical Education at Chicago provided additional support. The idea to build the courses into a book came from Dr. Ruth Ramsey, and Jane Pennington, Ph.D., of Thieme, was instrumental in bringing that suggestion to fruition at every stage of the process. The hundreds of wonderful students who enrolled in the courses provided perhaps the greatest stimulus and direction of all, through their unflagging interest and enthusiasm for learning.

The text itself was written largely during my tenure as chief resident in diagnostic radiology at the University of Chicago. Balancing my responsibilities in clinical practice and administration with the work of teaching and writing was often challenging, and I would like to thank my colleagues on the faculty and house staff at Chicago for their patience and support during that time. In addition, I would like to thank my colleagues at Indiana University, who enabled me to bring the manuscript to completion and have laid the groundwork for new teaching initiatives through which this work will continue. In particular, Drs. Mervyn Cohen, John Smith, and Aslam Siddiqui have made vital contributions in this regard.

Numerous individuals deserve thanks for their contributions to the manuscript. Chapters were reviewed by Drs. Ellen Benya, Abraham Dachman, Larry Dixon, John Fennessy, Craig Hackworth, Martin Lipton, Heber MacMahon, Geraldine Newmark, and Ruth Ramsey. Key images were provided by Drs. John Fennessy, Daniel Huddle, Ruth Ramsey, Richard Reba, James Ryan, Robert Schmidt, Douglas Seeb, George Szymski, Fred Winsberg, and in particular Arunas Gasparaitis. Additional individuals who made important indirect contributions through their teaching included Drs. Tamar Ben-Ami, David Levin, Charles Metz, and David Yousefzadeh. Able secretarial support was provided by Sherri Sachs, Debbie Cop, Barbara Dodds, and Ruth Patterson. Most of the photographs used in the text were prepared by Harold Tyler and I would like to thank Audrey Kuang for her assistance in cataloging the images. I also must thank Craig Gosling and his colleagues in the Department of Illustration at the Indiana University who provided the line illustrations. Throughout the phases of manuscript preparation and production, Kathy Lyons at Thieme provided critical editorial assistance.

Finally, I would like to express my deepest gratitude and affection to my wife Laura and to my children Rebecca, Peter, and David.

Foreword

Radiology may be defined as that specialty of medicine that is dedicated to imaging and utilizes X rays for patient diagnosis and therapy. Compared with many other specialties, such as pathology and internal medicine, which were practiced by the ancient civilizations, radiology is a very new field. Radiology began with the discovery of X rays just over 100 years ago by W.C. Roentgen. Since that time, it has grown into a major specialty, and during the past two decades has become one of the fastest growing and most exciting areas in medicine.

There are a number of reasons why medical students should be familiar with radiology. Perhaps the most urgent and compelling reason is that all general practitioners, as well as subspecialized physicians, rely on diagnostic imaging procedures for the management of almost every patient. It is very helpful, therefore, for students to have a grasp of radiology techniques, know what they offer, and understand their limitations. Not only are many noninvasive and invasive techniques used for diagnosis, but also new subspecialties have emerged, such as interventional radiology, which encompasses procedures such as balloon angioplasty and the deployment of an increasing number of devices, replacing surgical procedures and reducing long hospital stays and costs. Radiology is a widely expanding imaging-based field. The medical student is expected to be sufficiently familiar and knowledgeable in this area so that as physicians they can utilize this technology appropriately and optimally.

The medical school curriculum continues to escalate in complexity, with expansion of new services such as organ transplantation and molecular biology. These increasing demands, along with the advent of "managed care," are reducing the number of patient days in hospital and more procedures are being performed in an outpatient setting. In addition, students and physicians must be sensitive to medical-legal issues and increasing regulatory agency rules as these apply to diagnosis. Radiology issues are a part of this broader knowledge base to which medical students are exposed.

Essential Radiology: Clinical Presentation, Pathophysiology, Imaging provides a sound introduction to the specialty of radiodiagnosis and imaging. It is written by an outstanding teacher who trained at the University of Chicago. Dr. Gunderman obtained a Doctor of Philosophy (PhD) degree in Social Thought, in which he subsequently lectured and for which he received awards recognizing him as an outstanding teacher at the University of Chicago. Subsequently, Richard attended medical school at the University of Chicago, graduating at the top of his class. Dr. Gunderman commenced his Radiology Residency Training Program four years ago, also at the University of Chicago; this book, based on the radiology courses he taught, was begun during his second year of residency training. The text benefits from the author's perspective of having so recently been a medical student. The chapters are arranged by organ system and the text is easy to read and understand. The imaging aspects are intelligently integrated with the principles of general medicine using case based studies in the overall context of patient care. The text is generously illustrated with radiographs and images from multiple modalities. These images are elegantly and concisely described in the legends.

The first chapter of the text enables the reader to experience the excitement accompanying the discovery of X rays, and provides a thorough discussion of the development of the basic concepts of interpreting images with a description of the principles underlying the clinical practice of modern radiology. Subsequent chapters describe not only how to interpret images but relate this to clinical presentation and to the pathophysiology of the disorder. This continuity helps to make the text interesting and enjoyable yet incorporates the critical fundamentals of radiodiagnosis. A final chapter for self assessment has been included at the end of the book; this should be of great assistance in testing the effectiveness of the text.

All of the chapters have been reviewed by senior University of Chicago faculty to ensure accuracy and appropriate emphasis. Therefore, the book reflects and embodies much of the Department of Radiology's principles and practices. The department is proud of Dr. Gunderman's efforts and believes that this book fills an important need.

Very few radiology textbooks have been written specifically with the medical student's special needs primarily in mind. This book is an excellent introduction to what all medical students should know. It does not, however, masquerade as a comprehensive, all inclusive compendium of radiology practice. It will be of educational and practical value to residents and educators in other medical specialties. Dr. Gunderman has produced a soundly written text in a very user friendly and enjoyable style. It should assist the student in developing good judgment as well as knowledge, commodities that are so crucial for every physician in this day and age.

Martin J. Lipton, MD
Professor of Radiology and Medicine
Chairman, Department of Radiology
University of Chicago

Foreword

The practice of radiology has changed dramatically over the past decade. With the addition of new imaging methods and capability has come a level of uncertainty about the appropriate studies or procedures for a particular clinical situation. For those clinicians who do not actually enter the field of radiology, this uncertainty persists well into their years of practice. In general, a medical student's introduction to radiology is limited at best, and this lack of an adequate introduction compounds the problem of appropriate utilization.

Good textbooks, designed to introduce medical students to the field of radiology (diagnostic imaging in all of its modern aspects), are not easy to find. A good text will describe the imaging options, illustrate instructive cases, and relate the pathophysiology to the morphologic changes shown by the appropriate imaging study. This textbook, by Dr. Richard Gunderman, I am delighted to say, is an excellent one for medical students and postgraduate house staff for a number of reasons. Remarkably, Dr. Gunderman is only recently out of his residency training and, therefore, still remembers the questions, needs, and expectations of medical students and house staff. His consistent discussion of the pathophysiologic processes occurring in each of the organ systems relates the morphologic abnormalities (so well illustrated in his careful selection of cases) to the clinical presentation, which is so meaningful to medical students and house staff.

Dr. Gunderman's appreciation for the rich language of medicine is apparent in his frequent referral to the Latin and Greek roots of our most commonly used anatomy and pathology terms. Additionally, the writing style is well suited to the purpose of this textbook: it is clinically oriented, interesting, and enjoyable reading.

Essentially all of the relevant imaging methods are well shown and explained in clear language. The underlying physical principles of computed tomography, magnetic resonance imaging, ultrasonography, radionuclide imaging, as well as conventional and digital radiography are easily understood, thanks to the optimal mix of text, drawings, and instructive photographs. The section on vascular and interventional radiology introduces the student and trainee to the expanding field of therapeutic interventions, some of which were considered beyond the realm of possibility as recently as a decade ago.

This textbook falls into the continuum of educational programs Dr. Gunderman first initiated at the University of Chicago while still a resident, and, I am confident, will be followed by many more ventures aimed at enlightening, motivating, and improving the quality of medical students and physicians of the future. I deeply appreciate the opportunity to comment on this outstanding scholarly effort and extend my congratulations to Dr. Gunderman for his accomplishment.

Robert J. Stanley, MD
Professor and Chairman, Department of Radiology
University of Alabama at Birmingham

ESSENTIAL RADIOLOGY

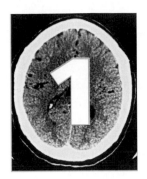

Introduction to Radiology

(continued)

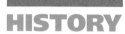

HISTORY

The foundations of the medical specialty of radiology were laid when German physics professor Wilhelm Roentgen presented his preliminary report, "On a New Kind of Rays," to the secretary of the Wurzburg Physico-Medical Society in Germany on December 28, 1895, announcing the discovery of X rays for which he would 6 years later receive the first Nobel Prize in physics. Within weeks, newspapers around the world trumpeted the story of his "marvelous triumph of science," noting that Roentgen was "already using his discovery to photograph broken limbs and bullets in human bodies." A new age was dawning, in which humans would for the first time peer into the hidden reaches of the body without the use of a scalpel (Fig. 1–1).

Roentgen had achieved his great discovery 7 weeks earlier, late on the Friday afternoon of November 8, 1895. While experimenting with cathode ray tubes in his darkened laboratory, Roentgen discovered quite by accident that its discharges produced shimmers of light on a nearby fluorescent screen. Repeating the experiment multiple times, he proved to himself that the emissions were invisible to his own eyes, yet able to penetrate the walls of the cardboard box in which the tube was enclosed. After investigating the phenomenon further, he concluded that only one explanation was possible: the cathode ray tube was producing a new kind of ray.

So revolutionary was Roentgen's discovery that, rather than accept that the great physicists of the day had repeatedly failed to detect such a momentous new phenomenon throughout 10 years of experimentation with cathode rays, Lord Kelvin initially speculated that X rays were a hoax. Yet the phenomenon was undeniable. The Prussian Academy of Sciences later wrote to Roentgen: "Probably never has a new truth from the quiet laboratory of a scientist made triumphal progress so quickly and universally as has your epoch-making discovery of those wonderful rays." In the history of medicine, only the microscope could boast of a comparable technological contribution to medical vision.

Figure 1–1. How many lumbar vertebral bodies are visible in this abdominal radiograph of a 28-year-old woman? Despite the fact that the lumbar spine contains five vertebral bodies, the answer is not five, but ten. Why? Superimposed over the mother's lumbosacral spine and pelvis are the bones of another person, her unborn fetus. Note the fetal cranium, spine, and femurs. The fetus is turned to its mother's right. Moreover, it lies in breech position, meaning that the buttocks and not the head lie in the mother's pelvis, against her cervix. The hips are flexed and the knees are extended. This information was critical to the obstetrician who delivered the fetus by cesarean section soon after this film was exposed.

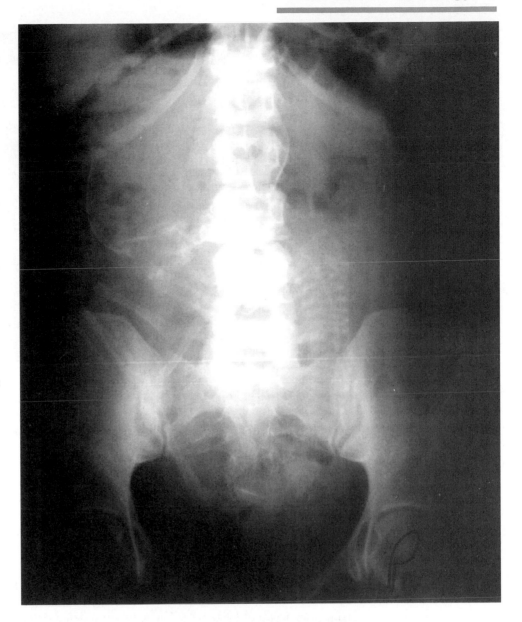

Roentgen himself was a remarkable man (Fig. 1–2). Although he lived another 27 years after his discovery, which he made at the age of 50 years, he declined nearly all of the great honors and invitations to speak accorded him, and donated the entire sum of his Nobel Prize money (50,000 Swedish kroner) to the University of Wurzburg, to be used for scientific research. He resisted all suggestions that he profit by his discovery, saying "I am of the opinion that . . . discoveries and inventions belong to humanity," thereby establishing a tradition of altruism that continues among radiologists down to the present day. Sadly, despite his extraordinary eminence, Roentgen's last years were difficult. Shortly after the death of his wife following a long and painful illness, Roentgen's personal property was consumed by postwar inflation. He died in 1923.

Roentgen saw himself as a physicist, and devoted his attention to the investigation of the physical properties of the new rays. In view of this fact, it is fitting that a discussion of medical imaging should begin with a discussion of the physics of imaging.

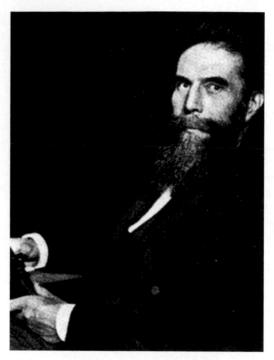

Figure 1–2. Wilhelm Roentgen.

VISUAL CHARACTERISTICS OF IMAGES

Contrast and Detail

From a physical point of view, an image exhibits two critical characteristics, contrast and detail. The level of contrast between a structure and its background must be at least several percent if it is to be detected by the human eye. Through image postprocessing, rendered possible by digital radiography, it is often possible to adjust and optimize the level of contrast in an image, and to perform such manipulations as edge enhancement (Fig. 1–3). The maximum detail detectable by the unaided human eye is approximately 10 line pairs per millimeter. Each radiologic modality has a characteristic range of detail or spatial resolution. In decreasing order, they are plain radiography, fluoroscopy, computed tomography (CT), magnetic resonance imaging (MRI), ultrasound, and nuclear medicine. Under ideal conditions, the detail captured by plain radiography is so high that magnification enhances detail, as in the detection of microcalcifications in mammography.

Noise

"Noise" refers to a variety of factors that detract from the information contained in an image. Some amount of noise is inherent in every modality, but additional noise may be added by the techniques used to generate or view the image. For example, ambient light in the viewing room decreases the signal-to-noise ratio; when the overhead lights in the viewing room are turned on, many of the photons striking the observer's retina no

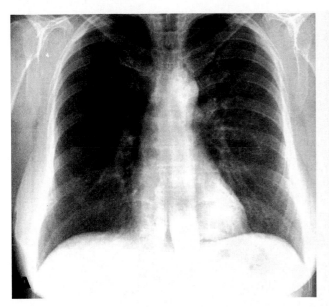 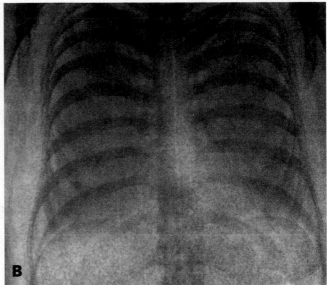

Figure 1–3. **(A)** Note the apparent solitary pulmonary nodule in the mid-base of this patient's right lung. Normally, the patient might need to be called back for further imaging evaluation, to determine if the finding truly represents an intrapulmonary lesion. However, dual-energy subtraction technique makes it possible to selectively accentuate the bones, at the expense of lung tissue. **(B)** Using this technique the lesion is clearly seen to lie within the anterior aspect of the right fifth rib, making further evaluation unnecessary. This is but one example of the extra capabilities provided by digital radiography.

longer carry diagnostic information. In contrast, when the overhead lights are dimmed and the only source of light is the viewbox on which a film is mounted, the signal-to-noise ratio is maximized. Radiologists work in darkened rooms not because they fear the sun, but because they are attempting to maximize the signal-to-noise ratio.

THREE MODES OF IMAGE PRODUCTION

There are three basic means by which radiologic images are produced: transmission of energy, reflection of energy, and emission of energy.

Transmission Imaging

The so-called X ray or radiograph is produced by the transmission of energy. A beam of high-energy photons is passed through the body, some of which are attenuated or blocked when they strike subatomic particles. The higher the atomic weight of the substance through which the photons are passing, the "denser" it appears to photons, and the more likely they are to be attenuated. In decreasing order of density, the principal densities in a radiograph are metal, bone, water (including soft tissues such as muscle), fat, and air (Fig. 1–4). Of course, even though muscle is denser than fat, the X-ray beam would be more attenuated by passing through a meter of fat than a centimeter of muscle. Both density and thickness, then, are factors to take into account in assessing the degree of opacification noted on a radiograph (Fig. 1–5).

Figure 1–4. This plain abdominal radiograph reveals an unexpected structure within the rectum of this patient. Can you determine from its shape and density what it might represent? The answer, of course, is that it is a chicken egg. Aside from the characteristic ovoid shape, the mineralized matrix of the egg shell, which gives it a density roughly approximating that of bone, provides a broad hint as to the object's nature.

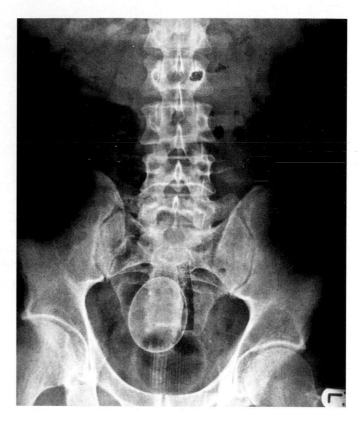

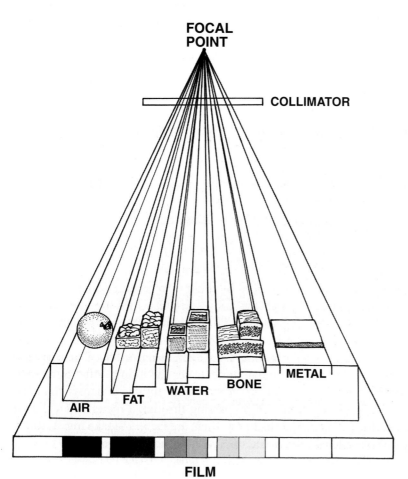

Figure 1–5. The effects of density and thickness on the exposure of X-ray film, using commonly imaged substances. Note that air blocks virtually none of the beam, while metal blocks virtually all of it.

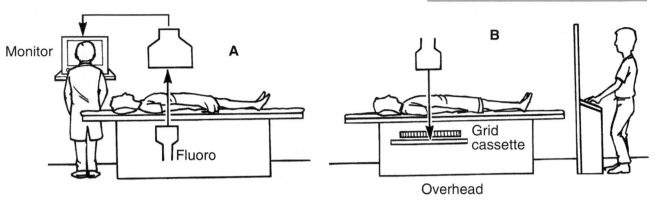

Figure 1–6. The contrast between (**A**) fluoroscopy and (**B**) plain radiography. In fluoroscopy, the X-ray tube sends X rays up through the patient from below, where the transmitted photons are captured by an image intensifier and projected onto a television screen in "real time." In plain film radiography, on the other hand, the beam passes from the tube above through the patient and exposes the film below. The exposure cannot be obtained at a precise moment based on the position of contrast material because its position is not known.

The principal transmission modalities include plain radiography, such as chest radiographs and abdominal radiographs, fluoroscopy, and CT. Plain radiography may be conceptualized as a snapshot: it provides a static view of anatomic structure obtained in a fraction of a second. Fluoroscopy represents a kind of "movie," or moving picture, in which continuous detection and display of the pattern of photon transmission enables the visualization of dynamic processes in real time (Fig. 1–6). CT gathers transmission data from multiple perspectives and employs a mathematical algorithm (the Fourier transform) to reconstruct an image of the slice of tissue through which the X-ray beams passed (Fig. 1–7). In each case, the contrast in the image is a reflection of the attenuation of the X-ray beam by the tissues through which it passes.

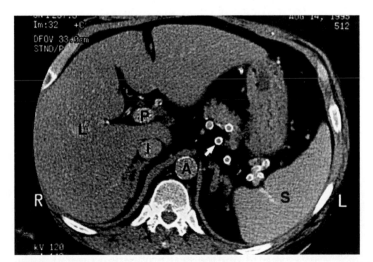

Figure 1–7. This axial image from a contrast-enhanced computed tomography (CT) scan of the abdomen reveals many high-density circles within the left upper quadrant, some of which are surrounded by very low-density tissue. These represent calcifications within the intima of the splenic artery, surrounded by abdominal fat. Although the splenic artery, a branch of the celiac artery, normally courses in a nearly axial plane, long-standing hypertension and diabetes have produced a very tortuous configuration, with the serpentine artery passing into and out (above and below) of the plane of this section. The excellent contrast resolution of CT enables us to visualize the interface between the very dense calcium deposits in the artery and the low-density abdominal fat immediately surrounding it. A = aorta, I = inferior vena cava, L = liver, P = partal vein, S = spleen.

Figure 1–8. Digital subtraction angiography. (A) Scout radiograph. (B) A few seconds later, radiographic contrast is obscured by unwanted shadows. (C) Image (B) is made into a negative. (D) Image (A) (scout) and image (C) (negative with contrast) are superimposed together and transilluminated on a final film. All unwanted shadows have cancelled each other out, but there is nothing to cancel the injected contrast, which is thus clearly visible against a uniform background.

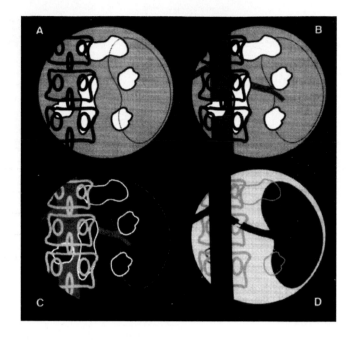

Another important difference between plain radiography and digital modalities such as CT (as well as MRI and ultrasound) is the fact that plain radiography combines detection and display in a single step: the film. The X-ray film both detects the X ray and displays the image. The digital modalities enable separation of these two functions, permitting the optimization of each. Moreover, the display function can be further subdivided into image production and image processing (Fig. 1–8). For example, when a CT examination is performed, the initial data acquired bear no resemblance whatsoever to a medical image. The image acquired with CT results from the ability of a powerful computer to perform countless computations necessary to assemble the data into a CT image. Once an image is produced, however, further processing is possible to optimize desired image characteristics, such as the contrast between soft tissue structures. It is also possible to "reconstruct" the data acquired in an axial plane to produce sagittal or coronal images.

PENETRATING LIGHT

X rays are a form of electromagnetic radiation (Fig. 1–9). In medicine, they are produced when electrons boiled off from a tungsten cathode filament are accelerated by a potential difference into a tungsten anode, with which they collide. These collisions result in the production of a considerable amount of heat, but a small percentage of the electronic energy is converted into X-ray radiation (generally about 1%). Hence the cathode functions in electron production, and the rotating anode functions in converting electron energy into X rays. The anode rotates to spread out the heat production over its surface, so that it is less likely to melt. The quantity of X rays produced is proportional to the current flowing through the cathode (in milliamperes), while the energy of the X rays produced is proportional to the kinetic energy with which the electrons strike the anode (in kilovolts potential) (Fig. 1–10).

What enables the X ray to penetrate the entire human body? The answer lies in the

Figure 1–9. The position of X rays within the electromagnetic spectrum that includes visible light. Note that ultrasound does not appear on this spectrum, because it is not a form of electromagnetic radiation.

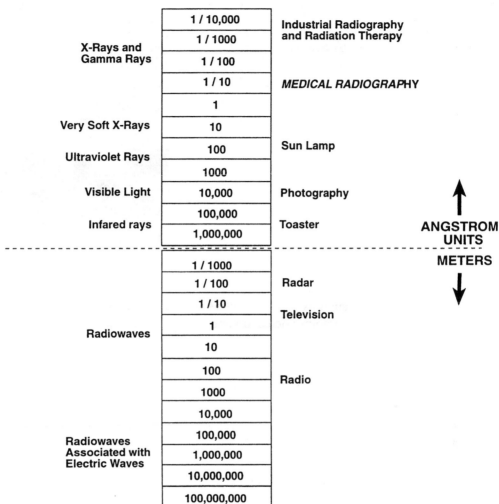

ELECTROMAGNETIC RADIATION

FORMS		APPLICATIONS
X-Rays and Gamma Rays	1 / 10,000	Industrial Radiography and Radiation Therapy
	1 / 1000	
	1 / 100	
	1 / 10	*MEDICAL RADIOGRAPHY*
	1	
Very Soft X-Rays	10	
Ultraviolet Rays	100	Sun Lamp
	1000	
Visible Light	10,000	Photography
Infared rays	100,000	Toaster
	1,000,000	

ANGSTROM UNITS

METERS

	1 / 1000	
	1 / 100	Radar
	1 / 10	Television
Radiowaves	1	
	10	
	100	Radio
	1000	
	10,000	
Radiowaves Associated with Electric Waves	100,000	
	1,000,000	
	10,000,000	
	100,000,000	

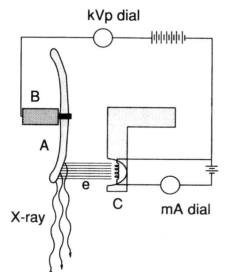

Figure 1–10. X-ray tube. **(A)** Rotating anode. **(B)** Rotor. **(C)** Cathode filament. "Boiled off" electrons (e) are accelerated in a vacuum and collide with anode.

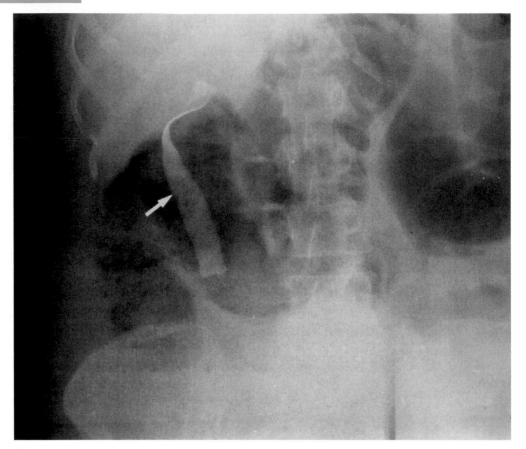

Figure 1–11. This abdominal radiograph was obtained in the operating room as the surgeons were closing the patient's laparotomy incision. The surgical nurse had noticed that the "sponge count" was off by one, and the possibility arose that a sponge had been inadvertently left in the patient's abdomen. The radiograph confirms the presence of the sponge's radiopaque marker in the right upper quadrant (arrow). While metallic instruments such as forceps and scalpels require no special treatment to be visible on radiographs, surgical sponges and other devices with physical densities less than or equal to normal tissues have radiopaque material sewn into them. It is much easier to obtain an abdominal radiograph than to reexplore the abdomen looking for a sponge.

fact that the photon, which can be thought of as a mobile electromagnetic field with no mass and no charge, is incredibly small. Moreover, the atoms of which we are composed are, relatively speaking, incredibly big and have an incredibly low density, meaning that their volume is almost entirely composed of "empty space." For example, the diameter of an atom is about one million times the diameter of its nucleus, where almost all of its "matter" is found. If the nucleus were 1 mm in diameter, the atom would be 1000 m wide, or about the length of ten football fields. Hence, the chance that a photon would strike any particular atom in the body is very low. Even so, however, only about one in 100 photons in a medical X ray actually passes completely through the patient and strikes the film (Fig. 1–11).

As photons pass through the patient, they may be scattered. In the case of a scattered photon, the place on the film that is exposed does not correspond to an anatomic structure in the patient. Hence scattered photons degrade the signal-to-noise ratio. Grids are commonly employed to screen out scattered photons, although at the cost of some increase in patient radiation exposure (Fig. 1–12).

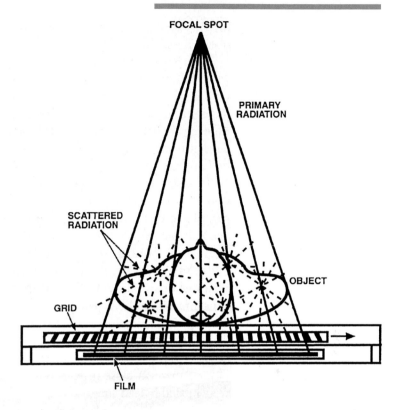

Figure 1–12. Illustration of how grids help to prevent radiation scattered within the patient from reaching the X-ray film and degrading the signal-to-noise ratio.

HAZARDS OF IONIZING RADIATION

Each of the transmission imaging modalities utilizes X rays, and therefore subjects the patient to ionizing radiation. Ionizing radiation refers to electromagnetic emissions of sufficient energy that, when they strike molecules in the human body such as hydrocarbons, they tend to disrupt their structure. They do so by colliding with atoms and causing the removal of one of their electrons, which causes the atom to become positively charged and highly reactive. Because most of the human body is water, most of the photons absorbed ionize water, resulting in the formation of highly reactive free radical molecules, which may in turn react chemically with such molecules as DNA and proteins, damaging them. Happily, sophisticated protective and reparative physiologic systems are in place that are capable of softening the blow. However, these repair mechanisms are not 100% effective.

The hazards of ionizing radiation were recognized soon after the discovery of the X ray by Roentgen in 1895. A famous example is that of Antoine-Henri Becquerel, the professor of eventual two-time Nobel laureate Marie Curie, one of the discoverers (along with her husband, Pierre) of radium. In 1902, she had painstakingly extracted a tenth of a gram of the new metal from large quantities of pitchblend, in which it was contained at a concentration of one part per million. The professor was so proud of his pupil's discovery that he carried a vial containing the first sample of radium ever produced in his vest pocket. Soon he noticed that he had developed a severe burn on the skin of his abdomen underneath the vial. The causative role of the radium in the production of the burn was verified when other researchers intentionally taped pieces of the new metal to their skin, producing similar burns. Experiments on animals by the Curies and others led to the development of therapeutic uses of radium emissions, known at the time as Curie therapy. That the same invisible rays used to diagnose diseases such as cancer could also both cause and cure the disease puzzled early X-ray researchers.

Another notable example of the potential harm associated with the new radiation was that of Clarence Dally, assistant to inventor Thomas Alva Edison. Soon after the X ray's discovery, Edison began to devote considerable time and energy to developing the commercial potential of the new rays. As Edison's assistant, Daly's hand and face were exposed to X rays for many hours every day. As a result, he developed progressive dermatitis and hair loss, and in 1904 died from a radiation-induced cancer, becoming perhaps the first X-ray martyr.

In 1925, another well-known case of excessive radiation exposure was reported, that of the watch dial painters at the Radium Watch Company. It was common practice to paint the watch dials with radium, which rendered them luminescent and enabled the proud watch owner to read his or her dial in the dark. Unfortunately, many of the women employed as watch dial painters adopted the habit of using their lips to put a fine point on their brush tips, and as a result over months ingested considerable quantities of radium. Radium behaves much like calcium in the body and is concentrated in the skeleton. The watch dial painters subsequently experienced a huge increase in the incidence of necrosis of the jaw, severe anemia, and primary bone sarcomas. In some cases, the rates of radioactive emission from these patients at autopsy was high enough to allow exposure of photographic plates simply by positioning them in close proximity to one of the patient's bones. A number of patients were buried in lead-lined coffins.

DOSIMETRY

The unit of biologic dose employed in radiology is the rem, which is based on another unit, the rad, which is the energy absorbed per gram of absorbing substance, which is in turn based on another unit, the roentgen (R), which is equivalent to a certain number of ionizations per kilogram of air. The rem is a biologic dose equivalent and is used to estimate the amount of biologic damage associated with various radiation exposures.

The exposures involved in various medical imaging procedures vary widely. The highest routinely encountered exposures are seen in cardiac catheterization and vascular radiology laboratories, where patients receive exposures of 2 to 3 R/min, and may undergo tens of minutes or even hours of near-continuous fluoroscopy, particularly in the performance of therapeutic procedures such as angioplasty and endovascular stent placement. By comparison, a single posteroanterior (PA) chest radiograph usually involves an exposure of approximately 10 mR. The whole body exposure during a plain radiograph of the abdomen is approximately 300 mR, and that of a lumbar spine radiograph is approximately 700 mR. Higher exposures are seen in CT scanning, where a typical abdominal CT examination would involve a dose of approximately 5 R.

"NATURAL" RADIATION

Everyone receives a daily dose of ionizing radiation, whether or not they are exposed to medical X rays. There are three sources of so-called background radiation (Fig. 1–13): cosmic radiation is emitted by the sun and other celestial bodies; radioisotopes are found in soil and building materials, and include radon, which has been found in the basements of homes in certain areas of the United States and is thought to be an important causative agent in lung cancer; and intrinsic isotopes (e.g., potassium-40, carbon-14), which are found in small amounts in the human body, meaning that everyone is

Figure 1–13. The common sources of background radiation, as well as the contribution of medical X rays.

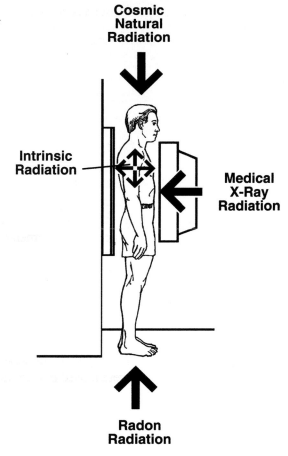

"naturally" radioactive to a small degree. Knowing the decay rates of such isotopes makes possible accurate dating of specimens in geologic and archaeological research.

In most parts of the United States, individuals living at sea level experience a total annual background dose of approximately 150 mR. The figure for the mile-high city of Denver is approximately twice that. There are areas in South America where the background radiation is approximately 100 times that level (due to high levels of radium and uranium in the soil), yet no increased incidence of cancer or birth defects has been documented.

RADIATION PROTECTION

The hazards of ionizing radiation have sparked physicists and physicians to seek means of minimizing the health risks of medical imaging. The current concept governing radiation exposure for both health care workers and patients is ALARA, which stands for "as low as reasonably achievable." The patient's exposure to ionizing radiation often can be dramatically decreased by following a few relatively simple steps. First, examinations should be performed only when they are truly indicated. It was once thought that nearly every patient scheduled for surgery should receive a preoperative chest radiograph, but we now know that most young, otherwise healthy patients will derive no significant benefit from the examination, because the pretest probability of significant pathology is quite low. Hence, one means of reducing the patient's radiation exposure is to avoid unnecessary examinations.

A second maneuver is to limit the dose received by the patient during the examination. Even in such routine examinations as chest and abdominal radiography, it

Figure 1–14. Scatter distribution during fluoroscopy. A leaded glass shield between operator and patient, and a leaded shield strategically placed at patient's side and at top of the table, will dramatically reduce radiation dose to the operator.

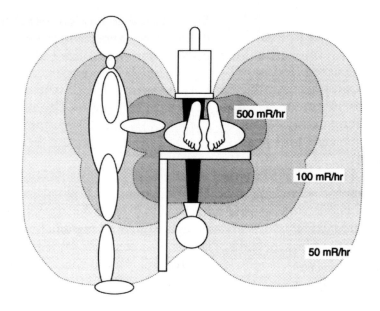

500 mR/hr

100 mR/hr

50 mR/hr

may be possible to reduce the patient's dose by several times merely by optimizing the X-ray source, collimation, and the detector (usually film). Another commonsense step is to reduce as much as possible the number of repeat exposures that are made. Every time a second exposure must be made, as when a portion of the chest is "off the film," the patient's dose is doubled. When fluoroscopy is involved, limiting the amount of time required to perform the examination can produce large gains. For example, if the length of time required to perform an upper gastrointestinal (GI) contrast study can be reduced from 6 to 2 minutes of fluoroscopy time, the patient's dose is reduced by two-thirds.

Both of these steps reduce exposure not only to the patient, but to the health care worker as well. However, many routine examinations involve essentially no exposure to anyone but the patient. Chest and abdominal radiographs, for example, are usually exposed with the technologist outside of the examination room, which is shielded with lead.

In the case of portable radiography, however, such shielding is not available. In that case, the single most effective protection is distance—the farther away from the patient a person is positioned, the lower their dose (Fig. 1–14). In fact, dose varies inversely with the square of the distance, meaning that the dose at a distance of 1 m from the patient is reduced by three-quarters at a distance of 2 m. In fluoroscopy, the dose may be further reduced by the use of personal lead shielding, such as lead aprons, gloves, and lead-impregnated eye glasses. By far the greatest exposure occurs in the direct path of the X-ray beam, and the operator's limbs should be kept out of the path between the X-ray source and detector. Thereafter, the greatest exposure is from X rays that are deflected or scattered during their course through the patient, and upon emerging from the patient strike the operator. Hence, lead shields and drapes are usually interposed between the patient and operator during fluoroscopy.

COMPUTED TOMOGRAPHY

The first clinical CT scanners were introduced in 1972. They drew upon the work of two investigators who shared the Nobel Prize for their work in this area in 1979. The first was the South African Allen McCormack, who devised a means of displaying the varying attenuation coefficients found in the various portions of a section of body tissue as a gray-scale image. The second was Godfrey Hounsfield, who worked in the 1960s and 1970s at Electronic Music Industries (EMI) in London, England. EMI, known throughout the world for its contributions to the recording industry through such groups as the Beatles, was able to devote a portion of its ample financial resources to fruitful use in support of Hounsfield's work.

EARLY HURDLES

When Hounsfield initially suggested that CT scanning held major promise for medical imaging, his audience was skeptical to say the least. In the early 1970s, Hounsfield was up against four strong disadvantages: (1) CT was at least two orders of magnitude slower than conventional radiography. In fact, the computers then available usually labored overnight before the images were available for inspection. (2) The spatial resolution of CT was two orders of magnitude poorer than that of plain radiography. Critics of the new modality, who had been struggling for decades to squeeze ever greater degrees of spatial resolution out of plain X rays by refining the X-ray source, collimation, and film emulsions, were not favorably disposed to a technology that seemed to abandon at the outset their hard-won gains. (3) CT involved higher radiation doses, perhaps as much as 50 times higher. (4) CT was at least 10 times as expensive as plain radiography.

CT'S STRENGTH

Despite these apparently overwhelming weaknesses, CT had one tremendous advantage—it could markedly increase the radiologist's sensitivity to differences in tissue contrast. Because many lesions exhibit a degree of X-ray attenuation different from that of normal tissues, even a slight increase in contrast sensitivity might pay huge dividends in lesion detection. In fact, whereas plain radiography requires about a 10% difference in X-ray attenuation to detect an abnormality, CT can detect differences as small as 0.5%.

To understand how this huge increase in contrast resolution is achieved, it is necessary to explore further the differences between plain radiography and CT. The conventional X-ray beam, though in many respects virtually miraculous, exhibited several imaging shortcomings. First, the information contained in a radiograph is presented in two dimensions, such that the information contained in the depth dimension is presented in collapsed form, or superimposed. Obtaining a second radiograph in the orthogonal projection only compensates for this to a minor degree. Second, soft tissue resolution by conventional radiography is very poor. We can distinguish to some degree between air, fat, water (or soft tissue), bone, iodinated contrast agents, and metal, but further differentiation is very difficult or impossible. Third, the conventional radiograph is unable to distinguish between the differing densities of the tissues through which it has passed. Once it passes through a very dense substance, the conventional radiograph will make the entire thickness through which a particular X-ray "beam" has passed appear quite dense, or white, regardless of the density of the tissue on either side of the dense structure.

CT, on the other hand, is able to measure and display the varying X-ray attenuations of the tissues in a section of the body, by passing X rays through the section from many different angles, and then utilizing reconstruction algorithms and the computational capacities of a computer to display the differing densities in a gray-scale image (Fig. 1–15). In contemporary CT scanners, a circular array of detectors around the patient acquires data as the X-ray tube rotates around the patient (Fig. 1–16). Sufficient data to image a single "slice" of the body can be acquired in 1 to 2 seconds, or even faster by so-called ultrafast scanners. Not only have generations of CT scanners subsequent to Hounsfield's been able to accentuate the innate strengths of CT, but many of its shortcomings in speed, spatial resolution, radiation dose, and expense have been dramatically improved. It should be noted, however, that CT will never rival plain radiography in terms of sheer spatial resolution.

Hounsfield's contributions are memorialized in the Hounsfield scale, which is used to measure the X-ray attenuation values in CT scanning. Water is arbitrarily assigned a value of 0 Hounsfield units (HU), air is –1000 HU, and dense cortical bone is 1000 HU. Also known as CT numbers, the respective attenuation values of many volume units within the patient are measured and used to construct the two-dimensional image. Measurements of attenuation values can also be used to

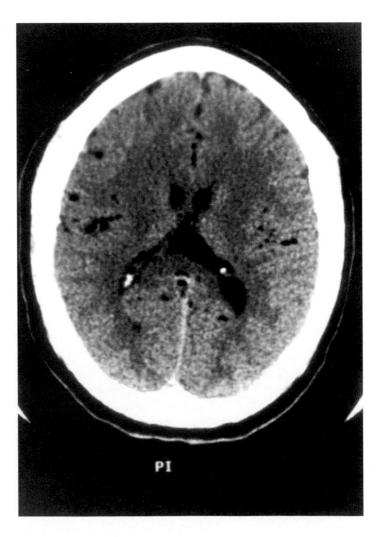

Figure 1–15. This axial image from a computed tomography (CT) scan of the head demonstrates the extraordinary ability of CT to characterize the differing densities of tissues in a tomographic "slice" of the body, which often proves critical in arriving at a diagnosis. In this case of a patient who presented with sudden onset of meningitic symptoms, multiple focal areas of fat density (dark) are visualized within the subarachnoid space, diagnostic of a ruptured dermoid. A dermoid is a benign congenital tumor of ectodermal origin that often contains fat; when such a tumor ruptures, it allows fat-density material to disseminate throughout the subarachnoid space, producing chemical meningitis. Note also the high-density (bright) calcifications within the choroid plexus of the lateral ventricle, a normal finding.

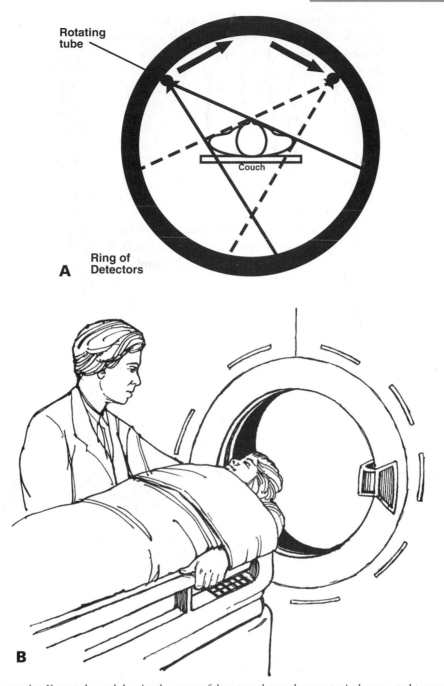

Figure 1–16. (**A**) The rotating X-ray tube and the circular array of detectors that make up a typical computed tomography scanner. (**B**) The patient is placed on a table that moves through the donut-shaped gantry as shown.

determine the density of a lesion. For example, a cystic structure with a homogenous attenuation value of 0 HU represents a simple water-filled cyst. A solid lesion with an attenuation value of –100 HU represents a fat-containing lesion such as a lipoma or dermoid. In both cases, such lesions could be dismissed as benign and would not require biopsy. Furthermore, we can optimize contrast in a density area of interest by altering the window width and window level settings at which the image data are displayed (Fig. 1–17). Typically, the window level is set at 35 HU when examining the abdomen, above 100 when examining bone, and at –700 when examining the air-filled lungs. In each case, a window width is then selected that optimizes contrast resolution of the type of structures being examined (Fig. 1–18).

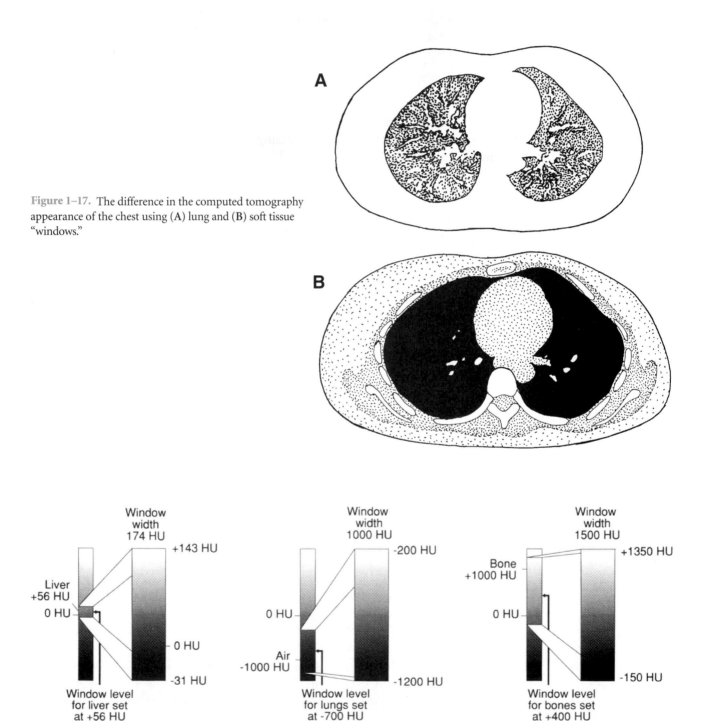

Figure 1–17. The difference in the computed tomography appearance of the chest using (**A**) lung and (**B**) soft tissue "windows."

Figure 1–18. Window level and window width are chosen for viewing and printing of an already acquired digital image, depending on which area of the body is viewed and on the amount of contrast needed to best display pathologic processes.

Reflection Imaging

The radiologic modality that exemplifies reflection imaging is ultrasound. As we shall see, ultrasound creates images not according to the density differences between various tissues, but by their acoustic differences. A very low density structure such as fat, which appears black on an radiograph, may be very "echogenic" acoustically, and hence appear bright on a sonogram.

ULTRASOUND

AUDITORY DIAGNOSIS

The use of sound as a means of "visualization" far predated the evolution of the human species, its most widely known example being the highly developed ultrasonic system of airborne navigation employed by bats, which enables them to maneuver with precision even in the dark. The use of sound waves as a medium of medical diagnosis extends at least back to the time of the ancient Hippocratics, who recognized the importance of the sound of air and fluid sloshing about in the thorax, which we today call the "succussion splash." The medical production of sound for diagnostic purposes began in earnest when the eighteenth-century German physician Leopold Auenbrugger, the son of a brewer, realized that the percussion used to assess the amount of beer remaining within barrels could also be applied to patients, with various disease processes producing characteristic percussive findings (compare the tympanitic sound of a gas-distended abdomen to the dullness of percussion of the chest overlying a consolidated lung).

TECHNICAL DEVELOPMENTS

From a medical point of view, the use of sound as a means of visualizing human structures required a dramatic technological innovation; specifically, some means of producing sounds and receiving echoes that would permit the construction of a two- or three-dimensional picture. The first crucial development occurred in the nineteenth century, when Pierre and Jacques Curie discovered the piezoelectric effect, by which passing an alternating electric current through certain ceramics causes them to contract and expand, producing sound waves (sound production). The process also works in reverse, meaning that sound waves striking the crystal produces electrical currents (echo detection).

During World War II, naval powers made extensive use of ultrasound, then known as SONAR (*so*und *na*vigation and *r*anging), to track the movements of enemy submarines. Ultrasound is widely used today in industry, where echoes are used to detect a variety of flaws in materials and construction. One of the best known examples occurs in the airline industry, where tiny, imperceptible cracks in the wings of an airplane can be identified and corrected prior to catastrophic failure.

While ultrasound now enjoys many medical applications, its most common uses include the evaluation of the structure and function of the heart via echocardiography, obstetrical ultrasound, and abdominal imaging (such as the detection of gallstones) (Fig. 1–19).

The so-called Doppler effect, named after Johann Doppler, the Austrian physicist who described it, refers to the change in frequency of sound waves as their source

Figure 1–19. How the ultrasound probe can be positioned to obtain images of the gallbladder in both (A) longitudinal and (B) transverse planes. The orientation of the transducer can be varied with instant image feedback to determine which position provides the best images.

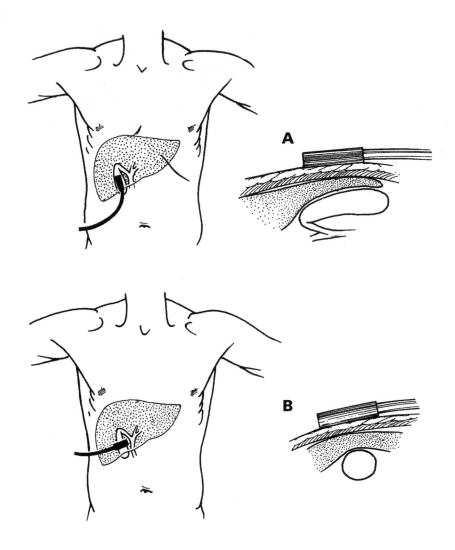

moves toward or away from the observer. The whistle of an approaching train seems relatively high in frequency as it approaches, and shifts to a lower frequency once it has passed. This principle is exploited in vascular imaging, where the change in the frequency of echoes produced by the motion of red blood cells allows a dynamic estimation of their velocity.

PHYSICS

Sound waves can be thought of as alternating bands of compression and rarefaction within the medium through which they are transmitted. A critical element in the preceding sentence is the fact that sound waves require a medium for their transmission; unlike visible light and X rays, there is no sound in a vacuum. This stems from the fact that the pressure waves of sound require interaction between molecules, with the vibrations being passed from one molecule to another. Because some media are denser than others, meaning that molecules are more tightly packed together, the speed of sound transmission varies by medium. Sound travels through air at a velocity of approximately 330 m/s, while sound in the soft tissues of the body travels at approximately 1540 m/s. Hence the distance between the ultrasound transducer and a structure within tissue can be computed by multiplying 1540 m/s by the time it takes for the sound wave to return to the transducer, then dividing by

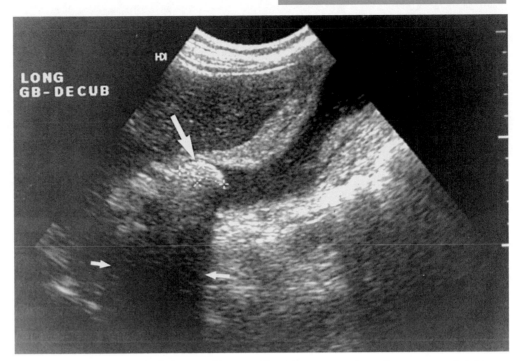

Figure 1–20. This longitudinal ultrasound image of the right upper quadrant demonstrates a bright, echogenic structure in the neck of the gallbladder (large arrow) that is casting a prominent acoustic shadow (small arrows). This represents a gallstone. The acoustic interface between the gallstone and the surrounding structures is characterized by such a large difference in acoustic impedance that virtually all of the sound is either reflected back to the transducer (producing many echoes and appearing bright) or being absorbed by the stone.

two (because the sound wave first travels out from and then back to the transducer) (Fig. 1–20).

Frequency

The frequency (often called pitch) of sound is measured in hertz (Hz) or cycles per second. The range of frequencies audible to the human ear extends from approximately 20 to 20,000 Hz, with the greatest hearing acuity in the area of 4000 Hz, the approximate frequency of the human voice. Medical ultrasonic frequencies, by contrast, are measured in millions of hertz or MHz. The higher the frequency, the shorter the wavelength and the higher the energy of the sound.

Attenuation

The sound beam is not transmitted with 100% efficiency through tissues. Factors that cause the beam to be attenuated include reflection, scattering, and absorption. Reflection is the critical factor, because it allows us to create images by collecting the echoes that return to the transducer. The reflections themselves result from differences in acoustic impedance between tissues (Fig. 1–21). In some cases, the difference in acoustic impedance between two tissues is so great that the entire ultrasound beam is reflected from their interface, rendering it impossible to image structures deep to that interface. Examples of such interfaces include the interface between the chest wall and

Figure 1–21. An ultrasound examination of the bladder shows how a stone within the urine-filled bladder may reflect nearly all of the beam, which would produce the appearance of a highly echogenic, shadowing interface.

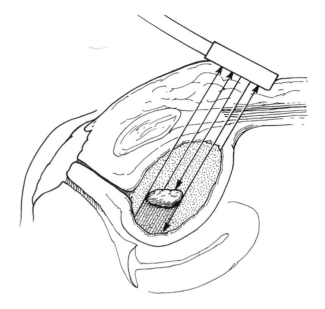

the lung (air) and the interface between muscle and bone cortex, which explains why ultrasound cannot be used to image aerated lung and bone. On the other hand, the difference in acoustic impedance between most soft tissue structures is very small, causing only approximately 1% of the beam to be reflected (which causes enough echoes to form an image), but allowing most of the beam to be transmitted to deeper structures, where additional echoes can produce an image of structures 10 to 20 cm deep, or even deeper. The tiny differences in acoustic impedance within the parenchyma of an organ such as the liver are responsible for its gray-scale echotexture, or characteristic parenchymal appearance.

Frequency and attenuation

The frequency of sound used affects both the resolution and penetrating power of the beam. The higher the frequency, the better the resolution, meaning that finer details in the structure being inspected can be imaged. On the other hand, higher frequency also entails less penetration power, meaning that only superficial structures can be imaged. These principles are exemplified in the clinical selection of ultrasound transducers, the "probes" that the ultrasonologist holds in his or her hand when performing an examination. (Recall that a transducer is a device that converts energy from one form to another, just as the inner ear converts sound energy to electrical energy.) Clinically, this means that when imaging superficial structures such as the carotid arteries or the testes, a high frequency transducer should be used, in the range of 7 or even 10 MHz. On the other hand, when imaging deep structures such as the liver or the kidneys, especially in large patients, lower frequency transducers must be used, such as 3 or 5 MHz.

IMAGING

As we have seen, the critical scientific breakthrough that made the development of clinical ultrasound instruments possible was the discovery of the piezoelectric crystal, which can be made to vibrate by an electric current and will generate an electric current in response to mechanical vibrations to which it is subjected. By first passing

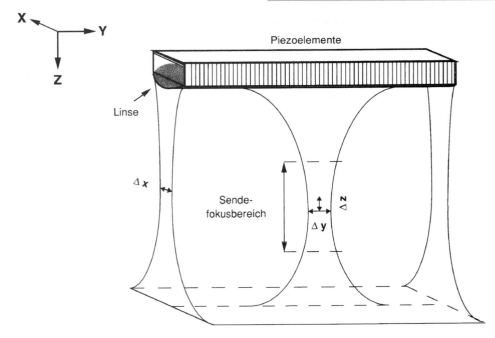

Figure 1–22. How the array of piezoelectric crystals that make up a transducer can be used to produce a focused beam, thereby optimizing spatial resolution.

a current through the crystal, we can send out sound waves into tissue, and then by turning off the current and allowing the crystal to receive echoes generated by the tissues, thereby generating electrical impulses, we can create a "picture" of the tissues. Most contemporary scanners are composed of arrays of 64 to 200 transducers, which create an equal number of separate beam components that can be used to focus and steer the beam as a whole (Fig. 1–22). In real time ultrasound, the piezoelectric crystals can be alternated back and forth between the transmit and receive modes with sufficient frequency to generate 10 to 15 images per second, enabling almost instant feedback as the examiner adjusts the direction and other characteristics of the beam.

DOPPLER ULTRASOUND

Doppler ultrasound exploits the fact that the frequency of a reflected sound wave is affected by the velocity of the object generating the echo, producing a frequency shift (Fig. 1–23). An object moving toward the transducer will cause an increase in the frequency of the reflected sound, while an object moving away from the transducer will produce a decrease in the received frequency. This is familiar to anyone who has ever stood on a passenger platform as a train whistled past; just as the train passes by, the pitch of its whistle drops, due to the Doppler effect. In the case of medical Doppler imaging, the most important moving reflector of sound is the red blood cell, which enables us to determine the velocity of flow of blood within a vessel. Of course, the frequency shift also depends on the angle at which the beam strikes its moving target. At an angle of 90 degrees, no shift will occur, because the blood is moving neither toward nor away from the transducer. A good angle of incidence is somewhere between 0 and 60 degrees, which allows a reasonably accurate assessment of velocity.

Several refinements of the Doppler technique are widely used in clinical imaging.

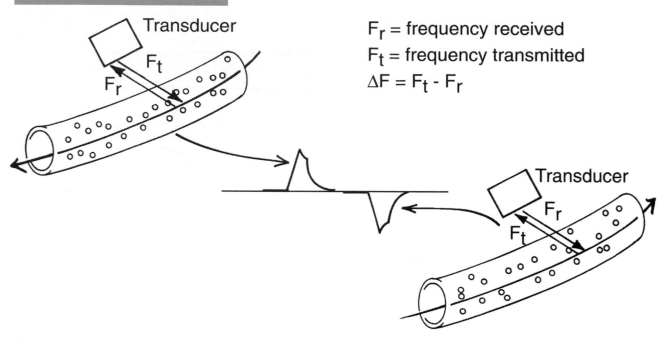

Transducer

F_r = frequency received
F_t = frequency transmitted
$\Delta F = F_t - F_r$

Figure 1–23. The Doppler frequency shift, in which the frequency of echoes returning from reflectors moving toward the transducer is increased (and above the baseline), while the frequency of echoes returning from reflectors moving away from the transducer is decreased (and below the baseline).

Duplex Doppler ultrasound employs a combination of gray-scale and Doppler imaging by using two different transducers within the probe, which usually operate at different frequencies. Using duplex, one can simultaneously view a gray-scale image of a vessel and a waveform being generated by flow within it (Fig. 1–24). In color flow Doppler, velocity measurements are assigned color values, with red used to represent blood flowing toward the transducer, and blue, blood flowing away. In contrast to duplex Doppler, which measures the maximal velocity of reflected sound, color flow Doppler measures the mean velocity. Color Doppler allows the assessment of flow within larger fields of view, although it is associated with poorer temporal resolution (due to the lower associated rate of sampling). One way of minimizing the latter drawback is to limit the area of Doppler sampling.

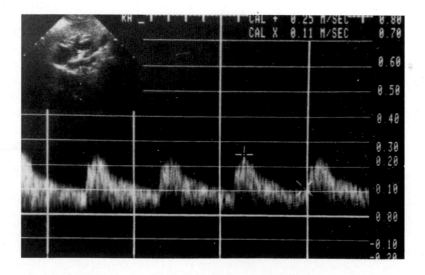

Figure 1–24. This duplex Doppler image provides a spectral display of the frequency shift produced by the motion of red blood cells in an artery over time. Peak systolic (+) and diastolic (x) velocities are displayed in m/s. The shape of the resultant curve is influenced by factors such as the resistance to flow in the vessel being interrogated, as well as resistance in the distal vascular bed.

Figure 1–25. (A) A duplex sonogram of the brachial artery in a normal subject at rest demonstrates a high-resistance, triphasic waveform. This is characterized by a sharp systolic velocity increase (A,B), a rapid drop in velocity late in systole (C,D), diastolic flow reversal (E,F), and late diastolic forward flow (G). (B) After exercise consisting of ten fist clenchings, the waveform shifts to a low-resistance pattern, with a pronounced forward flow in diastole (arrow). (C) An image of the normal internal carotid artery, which supplies the brain, demonstrates a very low resistance waveform, with less pulsatility and very high forward flow in diastole.

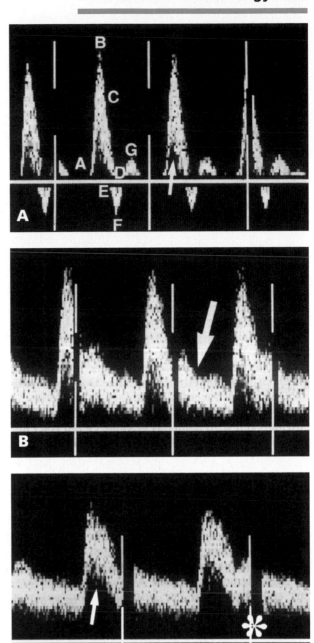

As expected, different organs in the body exhibit varying normal flow resistance patterns, producing varying characteristic duplex Doppler waveforms. For example, the brain and kidneys are low-resistance vascular beds, which demonstrate forward flow throughout the cardiac cycle. On the other hand, arteries supplying resting skeletal muscles typically demonstrate a high-resistance flow pattern, with a reversal of flow during diastole. In disease states, organs may exhibit alterations in their normal flow patterns; for example, the finding of reversed diastolic flow in the renal artery of a transplant kidney would suggest rejection of vascular obstruction. Of course, these resistance patterns are not always static, and may vary under normal circumstances. For example, a muscle at rest will exhibit a high-resistance flow pattern but convert to a low-resistance pattern at exercise (Fig. 1–25).

Emission Imaging

The emission modalities include MRI and nuclear medicine. MRI creates images by distinguishing between the nuclear magnetic properties of various tissues, a property very different from simple atomic density. This ability is crucial to MRI's greater soft tissue differentiation capabilities, as compared to transmission modalities. MRI also utilizes no ionizing radiation, and constructs images using a magnetic field and radiowaves.

The other emission modality, nuclear medicine, creates images by introducing radioisotopes into the human body and then detecting their emission of gamma rays or X rays. Nuclear medicine introduces an additional dimension to medical imaging, by depicting not only static or dynamic anatomy, but physiology. This is accomplished by attaching the radioisotope to molecules that enter into a physiologic pathway, which causes them to localize in particular locations, from which their photon emissions can then be detected. Like the transmission modalities, nuclear medicine also involves the use of ionizing radiation.

MAGNETIC RESONANCE IMAGING

Although MRI only came into wide clinical use in the 1980s, most of the physics behind it had been worked out in the 1940s, by two independent researchers, Felix Bloch at Stanford and Edward Purcell at Harvard. Both knew that many atomic nuclei behave like tiny bar magnets, tending to align their axes with an externally applied magnetic field, around which they precess, or spin like a top. The frequency of a proton's precession, which depends in part on the strength of the magnetic field it is in, is called the Larmor frequency, and is measured in MHz (millions of cycles per second). They discovered that this axis of precession could be displaced by electromagnetic radiation in the radiofrequency range, and that once the radio signal was withdrawn, the nuclei would gradually return to their previous orientation, during which time they would become radiofrequency emitters (Fig. 1–26). The phenomenon was called nuclear magnetic resonance (NMR), and Bloch and Purcell shared the Nobel Prize in physics for their discovery in 1952.

APPLICATIONS IN CHEMISTRY

During the first few decades after this discovery, NMR was employed primarily by chemists, who could exploit a phenomenon called the chemical shift artifact to characterize different chemical compounds. The chemical shift referred to the fact that the resonant frequency (the frequency at which the nuclear magnetic moments precess) varies according to the chemical environment in which the nuclei find themselves. NMR spectroscopy remains today an invaluable tool in chemical research. For some time, NMR was regarded as a strictly chemical tool, and its potential in biological and medical research was largely unrecognized. This had to do with the fact that a key characteristic of NMR from an imaging point of view was regarded by chemists largely as a flaw or impurity; this characteristic was the inhomogeneity of the magnetic field. Because of field nonuniformity, protons in different locations tended to process at slightly different frequencies, which "contaminated" the purity of the received radiofrequency signal. The larger the specimen, the greater the potential effect of these nonuniformities.

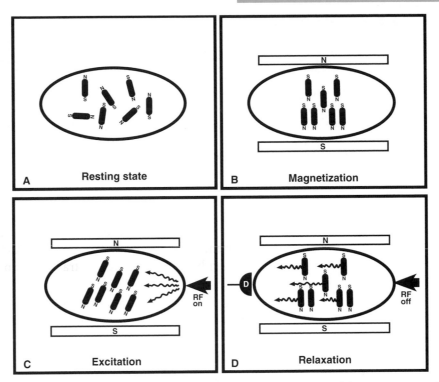

Figure 1–26. The basic principles behind MRI. (**A**) The magnetic moments of the protons are randomly oriented. (**B**) The protons have acquired a net magnetic moment due to their presence in the powerful magnet of the magnetic resonance unit. (**C**) A radiofrequency (RF) pulse has tipped the protons' axis, around which they precess like a top. (**D**) The radio pulse emitter has been turned off, and the radio-frequency signals emitted by the protons as they return to their state in (B) is measured and used to produce an image.

MEDICAL IMAGING

In the 1970s, Paul Lauterbur at State University of New York realized that these nonuniformities in the magnetic field could be exploited for imaging purposes. The nonuniformities could be regarded not as a contaminant, but as a means of encoding the spatial location of the protons whose radiofrequency emissions are being received. This could be accomplished by intentionally superimposing a spatially graded magnetic field over the specimen (a portion of a patient's body). Because this external magnetic field varies in strength across a specimen, the Larmor frequency will also vary, and these variations in the frequency of radiofrequency emissions will "encode" the location from which they emanate. In combination with the phase-encoding gradient (which causes some protons to be at 1 PM in their precession, others at 2 PM, and so on), frequency encoding permits the determination of the point of origin within a slice of the patient of a particular radiofrequency emission in both the X and Y axes.

The first two-dimensional image of a section of the human body was produced in 1977, and in the early 1980s, researchers were demonstrating the superior sensitivity of NMR as compared to CT in the differentiation of benign and malignant tissues, and in the detection of lesions in disorders such as multiple sclerosis (Fig. 1–27). More powerful magnets were introduced, exploiting the phenomenon of superconductivity

Figure 1–27. These axial computed tomography (CT) and magnetic resonance imaging (MRI) images in a 48-year-old multiple sclerosis patient dramatize the superior sensitivity of MRI in a variety of neurologic disorders. (A) The nonenhanced CT image at the level of the lateral ventricles demonstrates a mild degree of ventriculomegaly, but no suspicious lesions. Incidentally noted are a cavum septum pellucidum and cavum vergae, which are seen in 15% of adults, and represent cerebrospinal fluid spaces between the lateral ventricles. The proton density (B) and T2-weighted (C) MR images at the same level demonstrate areas of increased intensity around the anterior and posterior aspects of both lateral ventricles, representing multiple sclerosis plaques (arrows). Contrast administration is not necessary to demonstrate these lesions by MRI, although it may be helpful in differentiating between acute and chronic demyelination.

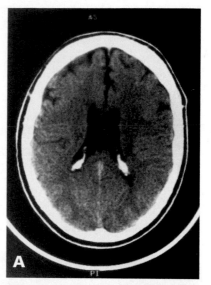

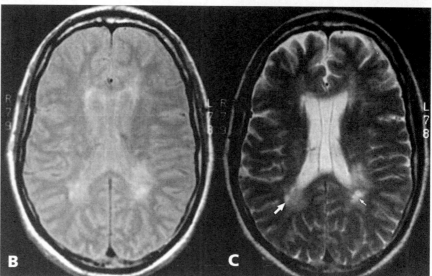

(using liquid helium at a temperature of −269°C), which enabled the commercial production of magnets with strengths of several tesla (by comparison, the earth's magnetic field is less than 1/10,000th of a tesla). By the early 1980s, NMR was rapidly gaining wide acceptance, and it soon became the imaging modality of choice for the central nervous system (CNS). In the mid-1980s, however, concern was voiced about the public's reaction to the term *nuclear* in the modality's name, and a decision was reached that the modality would be designated *magnetic resonance imaging*.

STRENGTHS OF MRI

The advantages of MRI over the other cross-sectional imaging modalities—CT, ultrasound, and positron emission tomography—are numerous. First, like ultrasound, it employs no ionizing radiation, and poses no known human health risks. Unlike ultrasound, it can produce images through an entire section of the body, and the images are not degraded by the presence of bone or air in the imaging plane. MRI provides soft-tissue contrast superior to that of the other modalities, and is able to

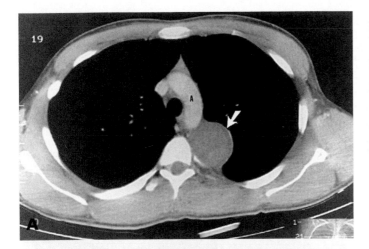

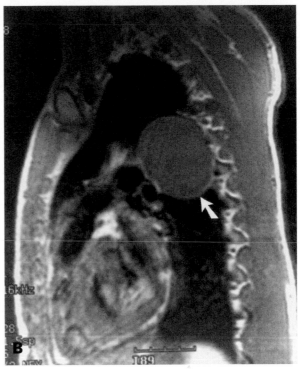

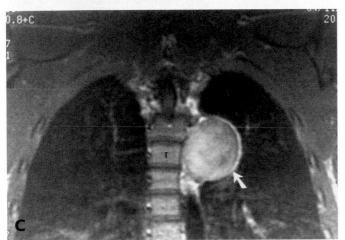

Figure 1–28. Three images from this 19-year-old male with a posterior mediastinal mass detected on chest radiography demonstrate the multiplanar imaging capabilities of magnetic resonance imaging (MRI). (A) The first image, taken from a contrast-enhanced thoracic computed tomograph (CT), demonstrates the axial plane of imaging almost invariably employed in CT. In order to "see" structures in other planes, it is usually necessary to "reconstruct" the axially acquired data. The image reveals a nonenhancing, well-circumscribed, round left paraspinal mass (arrow). In MRI, however, it is easy to image directly in other planes. (B) A nonenhanced T1-weighted image in the sagittal plane better demonstrates the continuity of the low-signal intensity lesion (arrow) with the spine and great vessels and shows that it extends over 2.5 vertebral body lengths. (C) The third image, obtained in the coronal plane after contrast infusion, demonstrates homogeneous enhancement of the mass and no evidence of invasion of the spine (arrow). At surgery, the mass proved to be a glanglioneuroma, a neural tumor derived from the sympathetic ganglia.

image in multiple planes, including the sagittal, coronal, axial, and various obliquities (Fig. 1–28). Its sensitivity to motion enables the visualization of vascular structures with or without the administration of contrast material. MRI spectroscopy, which is still under development, may provide important clinical benefits through the in vivo characterization of chemical composition and metabolic activity.

WEAKNESSES OF MRI

MRI has certain weaknesses as well. As compared to the other imaging modalities, it is relatively expensive and often not as widely available. Some patients cannot undergo MRI evaluation, including those who are too large to fit in the bore of the

Figure 1–29. This T1-weighted coronal image of the shoulder demonstrates torn and retracted fibers of the supraspinatus muscle (large arrow), as well as atrophy of the supraspinatus tendon near its insertion on the humerus (small white arrow). Along with the subscapularis, infraspinatus, and teres minor, the supraspinatus muscle makes up the rotator cuff, which is relatively frequently torn, as in this case.

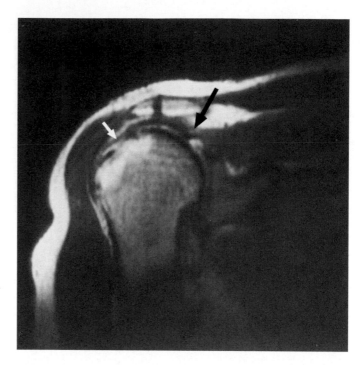

magnet (although this is not an issue with the newer "open bore" scanners), those who are too claustrophobic (although this problem can often be alleviated with sedation), patients with cardiac pacemakers or other electrical devices in which the magnet would create currents, and patients with certain ferromagnetic foreign bodies, such as certain cerebral aneurysm clips. Surgical staples and prosthetic joints create imaging artifact, but do not generally constitute contraindications to MRI.

T1- AND T2-WEIGHTING

What is the meaning of *T1-weighted* and *T2-weighted* images? These two most common types of MR images provide different assessments of the molecular environment surrounding the protons of the tissues imaged. T1 measures the ability of protons within a tissue to exchange energy with the surrounding environment, or how quickly the tissue can become magnetized, while T2 measures how quickly it loses its magnetization. So-called proton density images are neither T1- nor T2-weighted and measure exactly what one would expect; namely, the density of protons within the tissue. In broadest terms, T1 images are best for viewing anatomy, and T2 images are best for detecting pathology (Fig. 1–29).

NUCLEAR MEDICINE

Nuclear medicine relies on the use of radioactive materials to evaluate the functional status of various organs and tissues. As such, it differs from the X-ray imaging modalities, whose strength lies in the imaging of anatomy, from which function can often be inferred. By contrast, nuclear medicine typically produces an image of functional activity, from which anatomy can be inferred. The spatial resolution of nuclear medicine images is relatively poor, but the opportunity to directly visualize function more than makes up for this deficiency in numerous clinical and research contexts. Nuclear medicine studies are employed as part of the diagnostic workup of up to 15% of patients admitted to hospitals in the United States, where approximately 12 million examinations are performed each year (Fig. 1–30).

NUCLEAR RADIATION

The ionizing radiation employed in most diagnostic nuclear medicine imaging is no different from that employed in X-ray imaging, in the sense that both types of imaging involve the detection of photons emerging from the patient's body. However, the photons employed are of two types. X rays are high-energy photons that originate in an extranuclear source, most often produced by bombarding an atom (e.g., tungsten) with electrons. By contrast, the gamma rays used in nuclear medicine are produced by the decay of unstable nuclei.

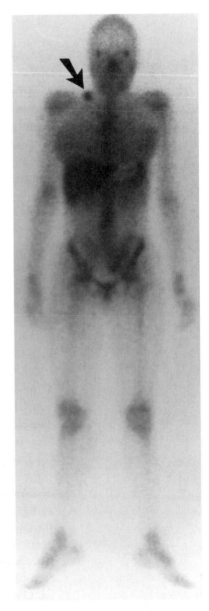

Figure 1–30. A 30-year-old woman presented with a palpable supraclavicular mass. Biopsy of the supraclavicular node showed Reed-Sternberg cells, leading to a diagnosis of Hodgkin's lymphoma, a non-B, non-T cell lymphoma with an incidence of 1:50,000 and a biomodal age distribution with peaks at 30 and 70 years. A nuclear medicine gallium scan was requested for staging. The radioisotope is gallium-67 citrate, which is bound to iron transport proteins such as transferrin and lactoferrin, and localizes in areas of infection and tumor due to leukocyte uptake and binding of these proteins in areas of inflammation. Uptake in the lacrimal glands, liver, spleen, and bone marrow is normal. This whole-body image at 24 hours after injection demonstrates an intense focus of activity in the right supraclavicular region (arrow), site of the known lymphadenopathy, but no other abnormal areas of uptake. This indicates stage I disease, which enjoys an excellent prognosis.

SCINTILLATIONS

The foundations of nuclear medicine were laid in the first decades of the twentieth century, when chemist Ernest Rutherford discovered that the emissions of certain radioactive elements could be detected using a zinc sulfide screen, producing tiny flashes of light called *scintillations*. Over the ensuing decades, a number of researchers pursued the medical connotations of this observation and soon were able to demonstrate that various isotopes could be introduced into the body of a patient, the photons emitted could be identified by newer scintillation detectors, and an image could be produced of the distribution of the isotope within the body. When isotopes were coupled to other chemical compounds that are handled by the body in various stereotypical ways, the radiopharmaceutical (or radiotracer) was born.

DIAGNOSIS AND THERAPY

Radiopharmaceuticals fall into one of two fundamental categories, diagnostic or therapeutic. The ideal diagnostic radiopharmaceutical is a pure gamma emitter, has an energy in the range of 100 to 250 keV and a half-life in the body of one to two times the duration of the test, exhibits a high target:nontarget ratio (meaning that it is especially concentrated by the organ or tissue of interest), involves a minimal radiation dose to the patient, and can be inexpensively and safely produced and handled. Far and away the most commonly employed radiolabel in diagnostic nuclear medicine studies is technetium (Tc)-99m, which has a half-life of 6 hours, has principal imaging photons with an energy of 140 keV, and is inexpensive, safe, and easy to produce on site from commercially available generators.

The ideal therapeutic radiopharmaceutical should be a pure beta particle (electron) emitter, because beta particles, in contrast to gamma rays, transfer a considerable amount of energy to tissue as they pass through it, leading to greater tissue destruction. In addition, it should have a moderately long half-life (days), a high target:nontarget ratio (decreasing the dose to nontarget organs), and, like diagnostic agents, should be inexpensive and safe.

MECHANISMS OF LOCALIZATION

Radiopharmaceuticals localize in the body by a variety of mechanisms. The most important example of the mechanism of localization, called capillary blockade, is pulmonary perfusion imaging, in which tiny particles of Tc-99m-labeled macroaggregated human albumin injected into a systemic vein embolize to the pulmonary capillary bed. This produces an image of the perfusion of each lung, with more radiopharmaceutical accumulating in more heavily perfused areas, and none accumulating in lung tissue devoid of perfusion (as in pulmonary embolus).

The phagocytic activity of Kupffer cells in the reticuloendothelial system can be exploited to image the reticuloendothelial system, with phagocytosis the mechanism of localization. For example, micron-sized particles of Tc-99m-sulfur colloid are avidly phagocytized by the reticuloendothelial system, with the biodistribution of the radiopharmaceutical providing an image of normal tissue in the liver, spleen, and bone marrow. In scans of the liver for metastatic disease, a metastasis from colon carcinoma, which contains no Kupffer cells, would appear as a photopenic ("cold") area surrounded by normal "hot" hepatic tissue.

Compartmental localization is the mechanism used in such studies as pulmonary ventilation imaging, GI bleeding scans, and voiding cystograms. In these studies, a radiopharmaceutical is injected into a fluid space, into which it quickly diffuses (Fig. 1–31). Images are then obtained of the compartment in question. In the case of lung scans, inhaled xenon-133 gas provides an image of ventilated portions of the lung. In the GI bleeding study, Tc-99m-labeled erythrocytes accumulate within the bowel lumen at the point where bleeding is occurring. In the voiding cystogram, vesicoureteral reflux is detected as scintillations extending retrograde up into the ureter.

Thyroid scans use the mechanism of active transport, in which the radiopharmaceutical substitutes for iodine in the energy-requiring process of thyroxin synthesis within the thyroid gland. Thyroid tumors, which often carry out this process less efficiently, tend to appear as "cold" areas within the normally "hot" tissue of the thyroid gland. In Grave's disease, however, the entire overstimulated gland tends to appear diffusely enlarged and "hot." Another example of active transport is the use of thallium-201 in myocardial perfusion studies, where the radiopharmaceutical is

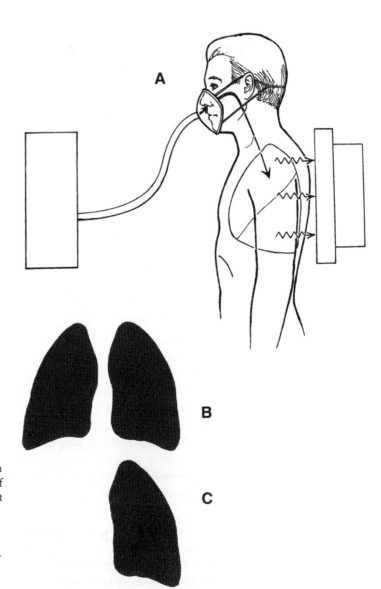

Figure 1–31. (A) How radioactive xenon-133 gas can be administered to a patient through a mask. (B) There is normal radiotracer activity in both lungs, producing images of each lung when the patient is placed in front of a scintillation detector. (C) One lung is blocked by a mucus plug, and no radiotracer activity is detected in it.

transported across the myocardial cell membrane as though it were a potassium ion. Active transport of Tc-99m-MAG-3 is used in renal imaging, where it is actively secreted by the renal tubules.

The localization of Tc-99m-HDP in skeletal imaging occurs by the process of physicochemical adsorption. The phosphate groups in the bone agent are avidly bound to the hydroxyapatite element of bone mineral. Areas of active bone metabolism, such as the epiphyseal growth plate, most metastatic bone lesions, and osteomyelitis, are imaged as "hot" spots. Conversely, multiple myeloma and certain other tumors that replace bone without exciting a metabolic response from it may appear as "cold" areas against the normally "warm" surrounding bone.

Certain recently introduced radiopharmaceuticals exploit other mechanisms of localization, such as binding to specific hormone receptors (e.g., the receptors for somatostatin in several endocrine tumors) and antigen-antibody binding, as in the use of monoclonal antibodies to image recurrent or metastatic colorectal and ovarian carcinomas.

CONTRAST AGENTS

Enhancement

Enhancement is a term frequently used by radiologists to describe the effect of contrast agents on the conspicuity of anatomic or pathologic structures.

BARIUM

One of the most common types of enhancement seen in radiology is that produced by introducing radiopaque substances into body cavities or vessels. In GI radiology, barium is frequently employed to opacify portions of the GI tract. For example, the colon is normally visible on plain radiographs only if it contains air, and even then, the ability to discern structural details of colonic anatomy and pathology is severely limited. However, by filling the colon with barium, many of its structural features, including pathologic lesions, become apparent, because of the impression they make on the barium column. The so-called single-contrast examination is excellent for discerning large masses or extrinsic pressure effects, but is somewhat limited in the detection of smaller mucosal lesions. For this purpose, the double-contrast technique is superior, which involves coating the wall of the colon with a relatively small amount of barium and then insufflating air, which distends its walls (Fig. 1–32). In fact, a properly performed double-contrast examination is superior to the single-contrast examination in virtually every imaging respect, and it is only in patients whose colons are not well-prepped or whose physical limitations prevent the turning necessary for a good double-contrast examination that the single-contrast examination is preferable.

IODINATED COMPOUNDS

A similar rationale underlies the use of iodine-containing contrast agents in angiography. While the aorta is normally visible on PA and lateral chest radiographs,

Figure 1–32. This overhead radiograph from a double-contrast barium enema demonstrates the exquisite mucosal detail that can be obtained by coating the colonic mucosa with barium and then filling its lumen with air. By comparison, the colon is nearly invisible on plain radiographs of the abdomen.

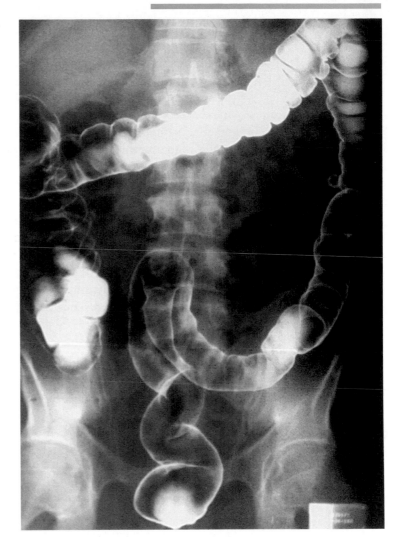

only portions of its outline are typically seen. With the exception of portions of the aorta and the superior and inferior vena cavae, the arteries and veins of the body are not normally visible on plain films at all, the exception being patients whose arteries are calcified, most often secondary to atherosclerosis. When contrast is injected into a vessel, however, its lumen is outlined in the same way that barium outlines the mucosa of the colon. Of course, when contrast is injected into a blood vessel, it moves with the blood, and imaging of any vessel is possible only during the fraction of a minute that the contrast is injected. When contrast is injected into an organ such as the lung, both arterial and venous phases can be distinguished, the arterial phase beginning as soon as the injection into the pulmonary artery commences. Once contrast passes through the capillary bed, it begins to appear in the pulmonary veins, which is the venous phase. Similar principles apply to the angiographic examination of any organ.

Radiologists inject iodinated contrast media into many other spaces as well. In a cystogram, for example, contrast is usually injected through a urethral catheter into the bladder, and multiple X-ray pictures are taken in different projections to outline the shape of the bladder mucosa. A cystourethrogram extends the examination to include views of the ureters, bladder, and urethra, which are useful to assess for vesicoureteral reflux, urethral morphology, and the dynamic character of the voiding process. Contrast is often injected into the subarachnoid space (utilizing a technique similar to that employed for routine lumbar puncture) to assess for a variety of CNS and spinal pathologies, such as a herniated intervertebral disk pressing on the thecal sac. With the advent of CT and MRI, a variety of other contrast examinations have become rare. For example, high-resolution CT and bronchoscopy have virtually eliminated bronchography, which was performed by introducing contrast into the tracheobronchial tree. Pneumoencephalography, which utilized air as a contrast medium to examine the cerebral ventricles, has likewise become a thing of the past.

ENHANCEMENT IN CT AND MRI

The term *enhancement* is most often employed in the context of CT and MRI studies, and an understanding of its meaning is vital to understanding these two types of examinations. A crucial point to be made about the difference between the enhancement that takes place with contrast administration in CT and MRI is the fact that they rely on completely different physical principles. The enhancement of vessels or tissues in CT is due to the presence of iodine-containing molecules within them, which attenuate the X-ray beam. The more iodine present, the more the beam is attenuated. In MRI, by contrast, the enhancement is due to the shortening effect of gadolinium on the T1-relaxation times of protons within its local magnetic field.

The contrast material used in CT is the same as that employed in angiography and urography; namely, iodinated molecules based on a benzene ring. These agents diffuse rapidly into the extracellular space and are excreted primarily via glomerular filtration. These come in two broad varieties, often referred to as ionic and nonionic agents, although high- and low-osmolality agents are more accurate terms.

Contrast Reactions

The use of iodinated contrast agents is associated with a small but important risk of adverse reactions. It is common for patients and even some physicians to speak of "iodine allergies," although such reactions are neither iodine mediated nor true allergies. Another popular misconception is that such reactions are associated with allergies to shellfish. The widespread use of iodinated contrast materials in contemporary medicine means that every physician should possess a general understanding of their risks and benefits, in order to maximize the benefit-to-risk ratio of medical imaging. In addition, it is important to be prepared to manage adverse reactions when they occur.

HIGH- AND LOW-OSMOLALITY AGENTS

High-osmolality agents have been in use for decades, provide good contrast, and cost relatively little. Their disadvantages relate to their high osmolality (up to six times that of serum). They produce mild adverse reactions in approximately 1 in 20 patients, severe reactions in approximately 1 in 1000 patients, and death in approximately 1 in 40,000 patients. The newer low-osmolar contrast agents have an osmolality only about twice that of serum, and exhibit a lower rate of adverse reactions. Often erroneously referred to as "nonionic" agents, they are associated with an 80% reduction in mild and severe adverse reactions, but have not been demonstrated to reduce the risk of death.

GADOLINIUM

The contrast agent utilized in MRI, often referred to as gadolinium, is actually gadolinium-labeled diethylenetriamine pentaacetic acid. Gadolinium is a rare-earth paramagnetic substance that shortens the relaxation times of hydrogen nuclei, particularly T1. Like the iodinated contrast agents used in X-ray imaging, gadolinium diffuses rapidly into the extracellular space and is excreted primarily via glomerular filtration. While the rate of adverse reactions to gadolinium is much lower than that of the iodinated agents and tends to be minor (approximately 1 in 750 administrations), pregnancy and lactation are considered contraindications.

RISK FACTORS

One might suppose that patients could be screened for liability to contrast reactions via the administration of small test doses of contrast material. However, this strategy is not effective, as the patient who will suffer a severe contrast reaction such as an anaphylactoid response will do so whether the contrast dose is 1 or 150 mL. In other words, the most severe forms of contrast sensitivity are not dose-related, and there is no means of testing whether a particular patient is a "contrast reactor." On the other hand, the first response to a presumed contrast reaction is to terminate the contrast injection, thereby limiting as much as possible the patient's exposure to the noxious agent.

HISTORY

While there is no means to determine before injection whether a particular patient will suffer an adverse reaction, there are risk factors. Before a contrast examination is requested, the referring physician should ascertain that the patient exhibits no risk factors for an adverse reaction. One of the most important risk factors is a history of previous adverse reactions, ranging from mild symptoms such as nausea to potentially lethal anaphylactoid responses. Others at increased risk include patients with multiple drug allergies or asthma, and patients with certain chronic medical conditions, such as diabetes or sickle cell disease, particularly when compounded by cardiac or renal disease. The history of a prior reaction is critical, as the risk of repeat reactions is about 1 in 3 if high-osmolar contrast is used, but can be reduced to 1 in 20 by the use of low-osmolar contrast. Because of the importance of obtaining a history in assessing the risk of contrast reaction, patients unable to provide a history (as in trauma or dementia) should probably receive low-osmolar contrast.

PREMEDICATION

By combining a premedication regimen with the use of low-osmolar contrast, the risk of repeat reaction can be further reduced almost to nil. A common premedication regimen includes the administration of prednisone 50 mg orally 13, 7, and 1 hour prior to the study, accompanied by one 50 mg dose of diphenhydramine 1 hour prior to the study. In many cases, it may be possible to avoid the use of contrast agents altogether, for example, by performing an ultrasound examination or helical CT instead of an intravenous (IV) urogram in suspected acute urinary tract obstruction, or by performing MRI instead of myelography in suspected spinal cord compression.

TREATMENT

The vast majority of contrast reactions are mild, and include nausea, vomiting, and hives. Many patients experience a feeling of heat as they are injected. While no treatment is generally required to manage such reactions, agents such as diphenhydramine 50 mg PO may be employed to minimize urticaria, and ice packs are sometimes used to reduce the swelling associated with hives. Histamine$_2$ (H$_2$)-blockers such as cimetidine may also be of benefit.

More serious reactions include bronchospasm, hypotension, bradycardia, and shock (Fig. 1–33). Bronchospasm is best managed with the metered dose inhalers commonly used in the treatment of asthma, such as metaproterenol, which possess the advantage of providing effective bronchodilation without the systemic side effects of tachycardia and anxiety associated with the systemic administration of epinephrine. Whenever respiratory compromise is encountered, oxygen is also administered. If wheezing persists despite the proper administration of an inhaler, 0.1 to 0.3 mL of a 1:1000 epinephrine solution may be administered subcutaneously.

Vagal reactions are not caused by iodinated contrast and may also be seen in other studies that involve no IV injection, such as barium enemas. They are characterized by bradycardia and hypotension and are often heralded by patient complaints of lightheadedness, dizziness, or syncope. Usual management principles apply, including the use of the Trendelenberg position to increase intravascular volume in the thorax and head, as well as the administration of IV fluids. The ever-present possibility of a contrast reaction is one reason that IV access should be maintained throughout the study, even after the actual injection has ceased. Patients who do not respond to fluids and positioning may require anticholinergic therapy to counteract bradycardia, such as atropine 0.75 mg intravenously, which may be repeated up to two times as necessary.

The most feared reaction is cardiovascular collapse, the so-called anaphylactoid response. While such reactions are exceedingly rare, they demand immediate attention to rescue the patient's life. IV fluids should be aggressively administered, and should consist of normal saline or colloids, as hypotonic solutions are not as effective at supplementing intravascular volume and may tend to exacerbate problems such as pulmonary edema. Epinephrine is the other mainstay of management, and should be administered intravenously, as subcutaneous absorption may be severely impaired. The dose employed is 1 to 3 mL of a 1:10,000 solution over several minutes. Needless to say, a positive inotropic and chronotropic agent such as epinephrine should be avoided in patients whose symptoms are secondary to cardiac ischemia, and the physician should be confident that the patient is not suffering a myocardial infarction before administering epinephrine.

COST

Low-osmolar agents are much more expensive than the higher-osmolar agents, costing 10 times as much or more. In an era of health care cost containment, the fact that utilizing 150 cc of low-osmolar contrast agent may add $300 to the charge for an abdominal CT examination is one that few institutions can afford to ignore. While some institutions use the low-osmolar contrast agents in most or all patients, many restrict their use to patients with known risk factors, patients unable to provide a history (as in trauma or intoxication), and very young patients.

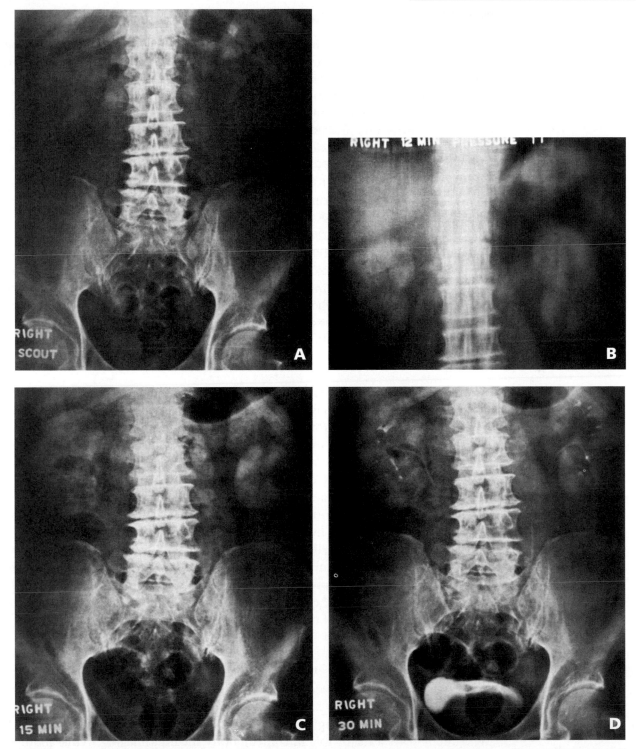

Figure 1–33. This sequence of films illustrates a serious contrast reaction that occurred during an intravenous urogram. (A) The scout film demonstrates some degenerative changes in the lumbar spine, but is otherwise unremarkable. (B) A renal tomogram obtained at 12 minutes after injection demonstrates bilaterally symmetrical nephrograms, but no excretion into the renal collecting systems. This is a highly abnormal finding, as contrast should appear in the renal pelvis and ureters within several minutes. In a previously healthy patient, it strongly suggests systemic hypotension due to a contrast reaction. (C) A film obtained at 15 minutes still demonstrates no contrast excretion. When showed this film, the radiologist monitoring the examination made the diagnosis and started treatment. The patient's systolic blood pressure was 80 mm Hg. (D) A radiograph after treatment demonstrates contrast in the renal collecting systems and bladder.

CONTRAST NEPHROTOXICITY

Iodinated contrast media also pose a risk of contrast-mediated renal failure, which is believed to result from a combination of direct toxic effect of the contrast on the renal tubules and arteriolar vasoconstriction. Generally, increases in serum creatinine after contrast administration are transient and mild, resolving within several days. Such transient impairment in renal function is seen in approximately 1 in 50 patients. In some cases, however, more severe and intractable renal damage may occur. The risk of renal failure is increased in patients with preexisting renal failure, particularly patients with serum creatinines above 2 mg/100 mL. Additional risk factors include diabetes, sickle cell disease, severe heart failure, severe hypertension, severe peripheral vascular disease, and dehydration. Recent reports suggest that the risk in multiple myeloma patients has been overstated, and multiple myeloma is no longer regarded as a contraindication to contrast administration.

Unlike contrast reactions, contrast nephrotoxicity is dose-related. When contrast examinations are deemed medically indicated in patients at increased risk, the contrast load should be kept to a minimum. A patient who has already undergone a high-dose contrast examination within the last 48 to 72 hours is at increased risk for renal injury, and the examination should be postponed wherever possible.

RISK MANAGEMENT

What is the appropriate management of a patient in severe, chronic renal failure in whom a contrast examination is indicated? In that case, the damage to the kidneys has already been done, and nephrotoxicity is not as great an issue. So long as the patient will undergo dialysis within the next 24 hours, such patients can generally receive contrast, although low-osmolar contrast is generally preferred. While there is no definitive evidence that low-osmolar agents pose a lower risk in well-hydrated patients, many centers tend to employ them when risk factors for nephrotoxicity are present. In general, hydration is felt to reduce the risk of an adverse reaction in all patients, although aggressive hydration prior to and at the time of the procedure is somewhat counterproductive, because it decreases the serum and urine concentration of contrast, thereby compromising opacification. This is of less concern in imaging outside the urinary tract, but aggressive hydration can significantly compromise contrast urography, because the degree of opacification of the urinary tract is directly related to the concentration of the agent.

ANGIOGRAPHY

Though not a distinct imaging modality in the sense of ultrasound or MRI, angiography plays a major role in contemporary medical imaging. While multiple angiographic imaging procedures are discussed in detail in the following chapters, it is helpful to undertake a brief systematic overview of angiography at this point, in order to cover some of the general principles that apply in every angiographic context. Broadly speaking, angiography employs intravascular injection of contrast agents to characterize both vascular and parenchymal pathologic processes, using fluoroscopic monitoring and digital or conventional radiographic recording. Common examples include the diagnosis of vascular disorders such as atherosclerosis and vasculitis, evaluation of trauma, characterization of tumor vascularity, and preoperative assessment in organ transplantation (where the vascular supply of the transplanted organ is critical). Moreover, various therapeutic endovascular procedures may be undertaken, as described later.

Preprocedure Assessment

The preprocedure assessment of the patient is vital to good angiographic practice. Aside from the risk factors for contrast reaction, additional points to be assessed are the patient's bleeding profile, the patient's ability to lie still on the angiographic table, and the presence of residual contrast material from a previous examination such as a barium enema. Generally, a prothrombin time (PT) of below 15 seconds, a partial thromboplastin time (PTT) within 1.2 times control, and a platelet count greater than 75,000/mL will be acceptable, although these parameters vary depending on individual circumstances. Warfarin, the most common cause of an elevated PT, should be discontinued several days prior to the procedure. A high PT can often be reversed acutely by the administration of fresh frozen plasma or with vitamin K 4 to 6 hours prior to the procedure. Heparin therapy is the most common cause of an elevated PTT and should be discontinued 4 hours prior to the procedure. Heparin reversal is accomplished with protamine sulfate.

INFORMED CONSENT

Because angiographic procedures involve puncture of an artery or vein, with attendant risks of bleeding and infection, contrast injection with risks of adverse reaction, and risks inherent to each particular procedure, informed consent must be obtained. The goal of informed consent is not to obtain the patient's signature as quickly and effortlessly as possible, but to explain the procedure and its risks, as well as any alternatives, in terms that the patient can understand. Although medicolegal risk was the driving consideration in the evolution of the informed consent forms found in every hospital, in reality physician–patient communication and the partnership that it implies simply represents good medical practice. Informed consent is not required by law in an emergency, if the patient is incompetent, or if the patient wishes not to be informed (although this should be documented).

VASCULAR ACCESS

The most common technique for obtaining vascular access is the Seldinger technique, most often employed at the common femoral artery or common femoral vein, both of which are located at the level of the femoral head, just below the inguinal ligament (Fig. 1–34). Position can be verified fluoroscopically using an radiopaque marker. Puncture is performed at this level because the femoral head provides a firm structure against which to compress the artery or vein postprocedure, when hemostasis is critical. The arterial pulse is palpated, recalling that the vein is located approximately 1 cm medial to the artery. Lidocaine is infiltrated at the planned puncture site, the 18-gauge needle is advanced through the vessel to the bone at a 45 degree angle to the skin, the center stylet is withdrawn, and the needle gradually pulled back until blood flow is seen. In the case of the artery, there is pulsatile flow of bright blood, while the vein generally produces a trickle of dark blood. A guidewire is then inserted into the vessel through the needle, the needle withdrawn, and a catheter passed over the guidewire. When the procedure is

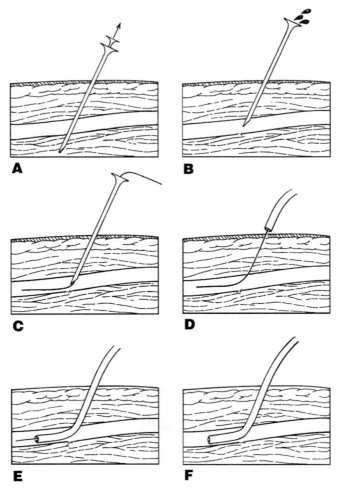

Figure 1–34. The normal Seldinger technique of obtaining intravascular access. **(A)** A needle is advanced at an angle through the vessel. **(B)** The needle is withdrawn until blood return is seen, which indicates that the needle tip is in the lumen. **(C)** A wire is advanced through the needle. **(D)** The needle is withdrawn and the wire left in place. **(E)** A catheter is advanced over the wire into the vessel. **(F)** The wire is withdrawn, and the catheter is left in place in the vessel.

finished, pressure is held at the puncture site for 10 to 15 minutes, and the patient is given strict instructions not to move at the hip for 6 to 8 hours, to ensure hemostasis.

Specific diagnostic angiographic procedures, such as coronary angiography, pulmonary angiography, and cerebral angiography, are discussed in subsequent chapters. In addition to diagnosis, angiographic techniques may also be applied to therapy. Following are brief discussions of several interventional angiographic procedures.

Angioplasty

Transluminal angioplasty is commonly used to treat stenosis of the coronary and iliofemoral arteries, and has applications elsewhere as well. A balloon catheter is placed into a stenotic region of vessel under fluoroscopic guidance, and the balloon is

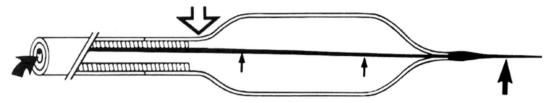

Figure 1–35. A balloon catheter in both its deflated and inflated states. Inflation of the balloon within an area of vessel stenosis expands the vessel walls outward and creates a larger lumen for blood flow.

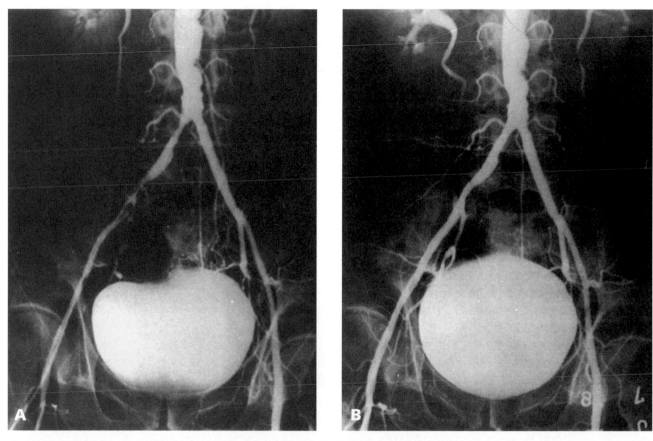

Figure 1–36. These frontal radiographs from an angiogram were obtained by introducing a catheter through the femoral artery up into the aorta and injecting contrast. (**A**) Note thrombi manifesting as filling defects in both the right internal and external iliac arteries. The large contrast-filled viscus in the pelvis is the bladder, in which renally excreted contrast material has collected. (**B**) Later, after the intraarterial administration of the thrombolytic agent urokinase and balloon dilatation of the areas of stenosis, the right iliac arteries are now patent.

then inflated (Fig. 1–35). Circumferential increased intraluminal pressure fractures the intima and media of the vessel, stretching the adventitia, and expanding the luminal orifice. The atherosclerotic plaques themselves are resistant to cracking and generally remain intact. Examples of indications for angioplasty include angina pectoris in coronary disease and claudication, rest pain, and tissue loss in the lower extremities (Fig. 1–36). Angioplasty may be augmented by the placement of intravascular stents, which help to prevent restenosis. The stents are usually composed of a metallic mesh, which expands when released from the catheter sheath and can be further dilated using a balloon catheter.

Embolization

Transcatheter embolization is used primarily to halt uncontrolled bleeding, to destroy arteriovenous malformations or tumors, and in the presurgical setting to decrease operative blood loss, as in nephrectomy. A variety of techniques are employed. Vasopressin may be selectively infused into an artery supplying a bleeding lesion, almost always in the GI tract, relying on its potent arteriolar vasoconstrictive activity to stop the hemorrhage. Of course, another name for vasopressin is antidiuretic hormone, and when it is administered in continuous infusions, the patient's fluid and electrolyte status must be monitored. So-called gelfoam may be placed into the arteries supplying a bleeding lesion, which causes temporary occlusion that will become recanalized in a period of weeks. Permanent occlusive agents include alcohol, glue, coils, and balloons (Fig. 1–37). The more proximal to the site of bleeding the vessel is occluded, the less likely infarction will result, due to the presence of collaterals; on the other hand, the presence of collaterals also decreases the probability of completely halting bleeding.

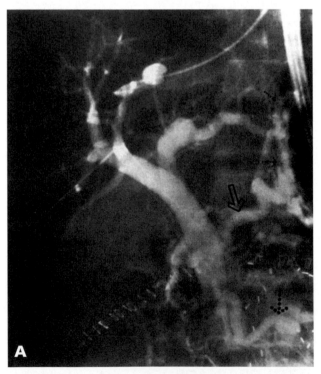
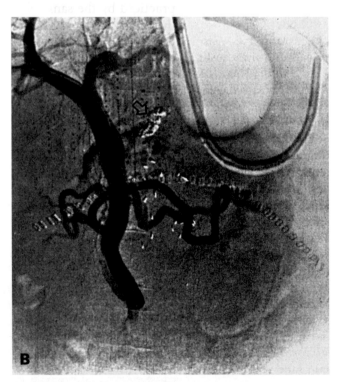

Figure 1–37. In patients with portal hypertension, complications such as upper gastrointestinal bleeding from gastroesophageal varices and ascites are common. In this patient with portal hypertension, a percutaneous transhepatic portogram was performed by introducing a catheter through the liver into the portal vein and injecting contrast. (**A**) A preembolization image demonstrates multiple gastric varices (small dotted arrow) arising from the left coronary vein (open arrow), as well as mesenteric collaterals (large dotted arrow). (**B**) This digital subtraction image obtained after embolization with metallic coils (arrow) demonstrates obliteration of the varices.

Thrombolysis

The most commonly employed thrombolytic agent is urokinase, a naturally occurring urinary enzyme that directly converts plasminogen to plasmin, which in turn degrades the insoluble fibrin in blood clots. Thrombolytics are commonly used to declot dialysis grafts, and may develop a role in the treatment of acute myocardial and cerebral ischemia. Contraindications include active bleeding, recent CNS surgery or cerebrovascular accident, and intracranial neoplasms. Potential complications include bleeding and the formation of emboli, due to the distal migration of a partially lysed clot.

INTERVENTIONAL RADIOLOGY

Like angiography, interventional radiology is not a distinct imaging modality, but it too plays a major role in contemporary medical and surgical therapeutics. Interventional radiology involves the use of the various imaging modalities, including fluoroscopy, CT, ultrasound, and even MRI, in conjunction with equipment such as wires, catheters, needles, and vascular endoluminal stents, to perform a variety of diagnostic and therapeutic procedures that were formerly either impossible or required more laborious, hazardous, and costly techniques. It should be noted that angiography and interventional radiology are closely related fields, and both are often practiced by the same subspecialists. In order to develop a general sense of what interventional radiology does, let us briefly review two interventional procedures, percutaneous abscess drainage and transjugular intrahepatic portosystemic shunting (TIPS). Other interventional procedures, such as percutaneous thoracic biopsy and the placement of nephrostomy tubes, are reviewed in the appropriate chapters.

Abscess Drainage

Along with herniorrhaphy, incision and drainage of abscesses constitutes one of the most commonly performed surgical procedures in the world. For millennia, surgeons have recognized that drainage of pus is critical to the treatment of localized infection. In the days prior to bacteriology and aseptic technique, the flow of pus from a traumatic or surgical wound was greeted by physicians with rejoicing, as it meant that the wound was beginning to heal. Absent the flow of pus, a loculus of infection had most likely developed, which in many cases would prove fatal, if not adequately drained. In contemporary medicine, abdominal abscesses and fluid collections remain a major clinical challenge. Untreated, many abscesses continue to result in fatality, and even in this era of effective antibiosis, drainage of such collections remains a critical component of therapy.

SURGICAL VERSUS CATHETER DRAINAGE

Before such abdominal collections could be reached percutaneously, open laparotomy was the mainstay of surgical treatment, and was often necessary not only for treatment but for diagnosis. With the advent of CT scanning and ultrasound, it became possible to accurately localize and characterize such collections. By "characterize" I mean that we could determine with a high degree of confidence whether a mass represented a solid tumor or a fluid collection, and further ascertain whether fluid collections were simple (more likely to be a simple cyst) or complex (more likely to represent an area of hemorrhage or infection).

Soon it became apparent that these imaging modalities could be used not only to find the lesions, but to guide aspiration of them as well. Percutaneous aspiration is considerably simpler, less invasive, less hazardous, and less costly than open laparotomy for diagnostic purposes. A patient undergoing laparotomy for drainage of an abdominal abscess requires general anesthesia, hospitalization, a relatively long period of postoperative recovery, and a general course of care that typically costs in the tens of thousands of dollars. On the other hand, percutaneous aspiration can be performed on an outpatient basis, with only local anesthesia, and the patient is often ambulatory the next day, at a total cost in the hundreds or thousands of dollars. If the aspiration yields pus, a percutaneous drainage catheter may be left in place to prevent or treat sepsis and allow the infectious process to resolve.

RISKS OF PERCUTANEOUS DRAINAGE

The principal contraindication to percutaneous drainage is the lack of a safe route, such as the presence of major blood vessels, solid organs such as the spleen, or bowel between the skin and the abscess. Transgressing the bowel and potentially seeding the abdomen with enteric contents is associated with an increased risk of peritonitis, while puncturing a major blood vessel or a vascular organ increases the risk of hemorrhage. Fortunately, the risks of both are decreased when a skinny biopsy needle, such as a 21-gauge, can be used. As with angiographic procedures, coagulopathies must be corrected, and the usual preangiographic considerations obtain.

PROCEDURE

The procedure is performed by positioning the patient, setting up a sterile field, using real-time ultrasound or CT guidance to mark the skin entry point, administering local anesthesia, and then advancing the appropriate needle into the collection, using imaging to verify position. Fluid is withdrawn for Gram stain, culture and sensitivity, and special chemistry tests (such as amylase in a pancreatic pseudocyst). Often, the fluid is frankly purulent, and the interventionalist may proceed directly to therapeutic drainage. Using the diagnostic needle already in place, a wire is advanced through the needle, which can then be used to guide the placement of a suitable catheter, typically a 10 to 14 French catheter with multiple side holes for adequate drainage. The cavity is then aspirated, followed by irrigation with normal saline until the return is clear. It is usually desirable to evacuate the cavity completely, but the catheter is typically left to gravity drainage for routine irrigation (Fig. 1–38). Typically, drainage produces resolution of sepsis and fevers within a day or two, and the persistence or recurrence of fevers within this period suggests inadequate drainage or the presence of another source of infection.

Transjugular Intrahepatic Portosystemic Shunting

TIPS represents a relatively new technique for the treatment of patients with portal hypertension resulting in bleeding from gastroesophageal varices or intractable ascites.

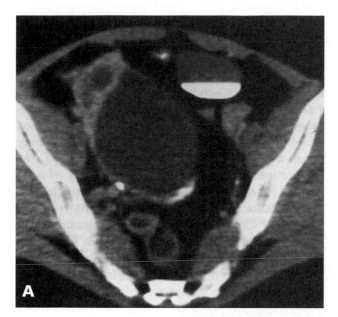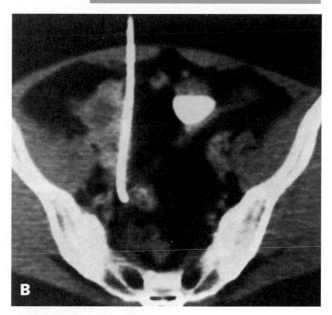

Figure 1–38. A 32-year-old woman with Crohn's disease and persistent fevers underwent a computed tomography (CT) scan for abscess detection and localization. (**A**) An axial image at the level of the iliac bones demonstrates a large pelvic fluid collection, representing an abscess. (**B**) Under CT guidance, a catheter was placed in the abscess, and 230 mL of pus was aspirated, leading to obliteration of the fluid collection. After 18 days of percutaneous drainage, the catheter was removed, and the abscess did not recur.

Portal hypertension is defined as a portal venous pressure in excess of 10 mm Hg. The portal vein receives drainage from the inferior mesenteric, superior mesenteric, and splenic veins, thus providing the liver "first crack" at substances absorbed into the bloodstream through the GI tract. This represents one of two major portal systems within the body, the other being the portal system that connects the hypothalamus with the anterior lobe of the pituitary gland, and provides the pituitary gland "first crack" at hypothalamic tropic hormones. The causes of portal hypertension are numerous, and include presinusoidal types of obstruction (e.g., compression of the portal vein by tumor), sinusoidal obstruction (e.g., alcoholic or postinfectious cirrhosis), and postsinusoidal obstruction (e.g., Budd-Chiari syndrome, due to occlusion of the hepatic veins, or obstruction of the inferior vena cava).

SURGERY VERSUS TIPS

The TIPS procedure partially replaces a number of complex surgical procedures that are associated with significant morbidity, mortality, and cost, such as portocaval and splenorenal shunts. Like TIPS, each of these procedures aims to decompress the portal vein by creating a shunt between it and the systemic veins (Fig. 1–39). Increased portal venous pressure is associated with a variety of complications, comprised of ascites (due to alteration of the Starling forces that normally tend to keep the peritoneal cavity relatively "dry" [see the discussion of these forces in Chapter 2]), and autonomous efforts to decompress the portal system, such as recanalization of the umbilical vein, the recruitment of the coronary vein to drain through "upward" esophageal varices into the azygous system, and a number of additional possible routes. By pro-

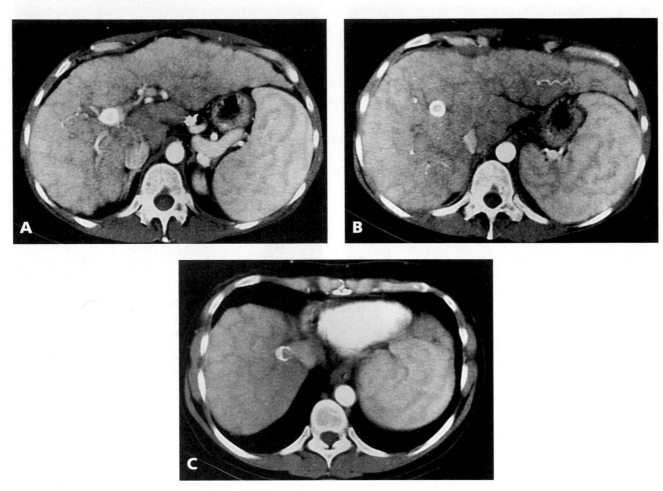

Figure 1–39. These three contrast-enhanced axial computed tomography (CT) images demonstrate the most common etiology and appearance of transjugular intrahepatic portosystemic shunting placement. Each of the images demonstrates a nodular, mottled-appearing liver, representing a combination of hepatic fibrosis and regenerative nodules in cirrhosis. (A) The caudal tip of the shunt can be seen inserting into the portal vein. (B) In a slightly more cephalad image, the shunt (the white, round structure in the center of the left-hand side of the image) can be seen passing through the hepatic parenchyma on its way to the hepatic vein. (C) At the most cephalad aspect of the liver, the shunt can be seen inserting into the hepatic vein, into which the previously hypertensive portal vein is now decompressed. Note also the splenomegaly.

viding intrahepatic decompression of the portal system, TIPS allows other shunts to regress, reducing hemorrhage from esophageal varices, and allowing the increased hydrostatic pressure that causes ascites to resolve.

PROCEDURE

The TIPS procedure is performed via a right internal jugular vein approach. After the usual preparation, a needle is placed into the vein, a wire is introduced through the needle, and a catheter is advanced under fluoroscopic guidance into the superior vena cava, past the right atrium, into the inferior vena cava, and into a hepatic vein. A needle is then advanced through the hepatic vein into the portal vein, and a stent is placed into the tract, which forms a permanent route of portal vein decompression (Fig. 1–40). Measurement of pressures before and after the tract is dilated confirms the

Figure 1–40. In this digital spot film from a transjugular intrahepatic portosystemic shunt procedure, a guidewire extends down the inferior vena cava, into the hepatic vein, and across a portion of liver into the portal vein. Two metallic stents have been placed into the newly created portosystemic shunt tract, connecting the right hepatic vein and one of the main branches of the right portal vein.

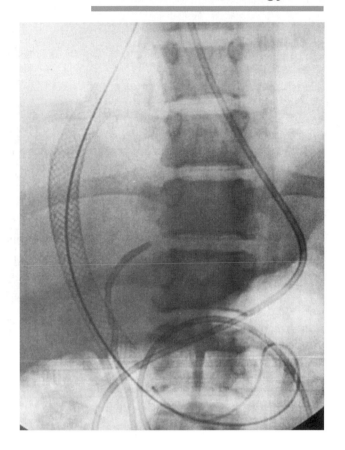

absence of a significant pressure gradient between the two veins, providing assurance that decompression has been achieved. If necessary, varices in the coronary vein may be embolized at the time of the TIPS placement. The patient is left with no external scars, and only a relatively minor postprocedure recovery, as compared to an open shunt procedure. The procedure is not without complications, however, one of the most common (15%) being new or worsening encephalopathy, presumably stemming from the fact that less blood is flowing into the liver through the portal veins for detoxification.

PRINCIPLES OF MEDICAL IMAGING

Clinical Context of Medical Imaging

UNCERTAIN OR LOW PROBABILITY OF PATHOLOGY

Medical imaging studies are obtained for a variety of reasons. One common reason is the search for unspecified pathology. In this case, the clinician is unable to formulate a solid diagnostic hypothesis, and the imaging study is obtained in the hopes that it will uncover a morphologic or functional explanation for the patient's symptoms and

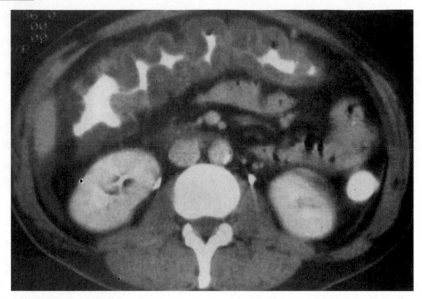

Figure 1–41. In an adult patient with nonspecific abdominal pathology, computed tomography (CT) is generally preferred to ultrasound because of its ability to quickly and thoroughly image the entire abdomen. This axial image from an infused CT scan of the abdomen in a patient with acquired immunodeficiency syndrome demonstrates marked thickening of the transverse colon (which lies in the anterior abdomen across the top of the image) due to cytomegalovirus colitis.

signs. On occasion, such studies may amount to "fishing expeditions," the yield of which is often relatively low. A similar situation is that of trauma, in which the clinical suspicion of significant injury is often low, but the adverse consequences of a missed diagnosis are so grave that an imaging study is obtained "just in case." Certain types of studies are less suited to this role than others. For example, ultrasound performs better as a means of testing specific diagnostic hypotheses regarding specific anatomic areas or organs, such as the right upper quadrant or the kidneys, than as a general screening test for abdominal pathology. This is true in part because the ultrasound beam can only be directed at a relatively small portion of the patient's anatomy at a time, and surveying the entire abdomen is a time-consuming and laborious process. CT, on the other hand, which naturally images the entire abdomen in a relatively short period of time, is usually better suited to the search for unspecified abdominal pathology (Fig. 1–41).

KNOWN DIAGNOSIS

Imaging studies play an important role even in cases where the diagnosis is known. From a surgeon's point of view, imaging studies may prove immensely useful in surgical planning. For example, the surgeon planning to perform laparoscopic cholecystectomy may wish to obtain a CT, ultrasound, or MRI in order to visualize the anatomy of the biliary tree and rule out anomalies, such as aberrant ductal anatomy, that could produce postoperative complications. Similarly, angiographic studies are often obtained as part of a routine presurgical workup in patients being evaluated as potential organ donors, to assess such factors as vascular and ductal anatomy.

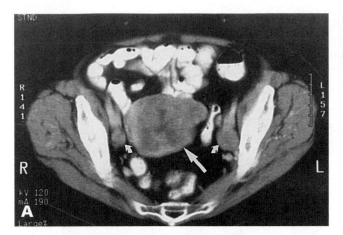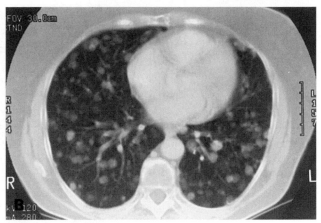

Figure 1–42. A 64-year-old woman with a history of vaginal bleeding was referred to the radiology department for computed tomography evaluation and staging of a biopsy-proven endometrial carcinoma. (**A**) An axial image through the pelvis demonstrates an 8 × 6 cm irregular, heterogeneously enhancing mass (large arrow) in the expected location of the uterus, with bilateral adenopathy in the external iliac region, greater on the left than on the right (small arrows). (**B**) An axial image through the lungs at the level of the heart (using lung "windows") demonstrates innumerable bilateral pulmonary nodules, indicative of stage IV metastatic disease. The advanced stage of the disease carries important prognostic implications, and indicates that surgery cannot be performed with curative intent.

Another important role of imaging is in the staging of malignant neoplasms (Fig. 1–42). Prognosis and therapy are often powerfully affected by radiologic staging of such neoplasms as lung cancer and Hodgkin's disease. Imaging also plays a major role in evaluating response to therapy. A chemotherapy protocol may be abandoned if imaging studies demonstrate continued growth of a patient's tumor; on the other hand, a significant reduction in tumor burden represents an indication to continue with the current regimen. In the case of interventional radiology, imaging studies are obtained as an integral part of therapy, as when ultrasound is utilized to guide percutaneous abscess drainage.

CONFIRMING OR DISCONFIRMING A HYPOTHESIS

Perhaps the two most important reasons to obtain an imaging study are to confirm or disconfirm a diagnostic hypothesis. Consider the cases of two patients who present to the emergency room with lower extremity swelling. Each may receive a lower extremity ultrasound examination to rule out the presence of deep venous thrombosis (DVT), a potentially life-threatening condition due to its association with pulmonary embolism, but the reasoning behind the test may be radically different. In the case of a chronically ill patient with a history of previous DVT who has recently stopped taking his or her anticoagulant medication, clinical suspicion of DVT may be very high. In this case, the study would likely be obtained primarily to confirm and localize recurrent thrombosis before an inferior vena caval filter is placed (Fig. 1–43). In another case, that of a previously healthy patient with clinical signs of cellulitis, clinical suspicion may be quite low. In this scenario, the study is obtained to verify that no life-threatening pathology is present before the patient is sent home on antibiotics. In the former case, the imaging study confirms a diagnostic impression before invasive therapy is instituted, while in the latter its purpose is to "rule out" an unlikely but life-

Figure 1–43. (A) The typical appearance of a bird's nest inferior vena cava filter, which has been deployed in a clear plastic tube. (B) Viewed on end, it is not difficult to appreciate how such a device could filter out emboli traveling cephalad from the deep veins of the pelvis and lower extremities. (C) When viewed in situ during an inferior vena cavagram, the wire mesh is often difficult to perceive. A number of different types of inferior vena cava filters are commercially available.

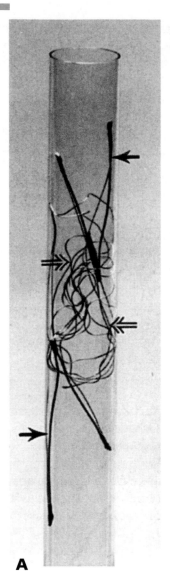

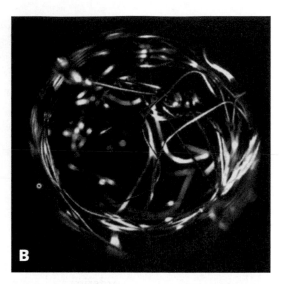

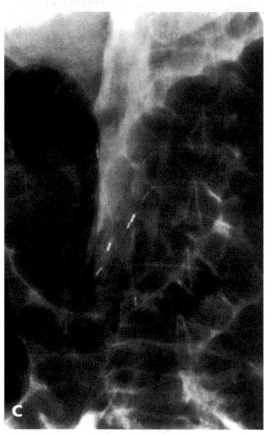

threatening pathology. In both cases, important clinical management decisions hang in the balance.

This raises an important issue in the specialty of medical imaging and in the broader arena of diagnostic reasoning. Except in the case of medical research or teaching, medical imaging studies should be performed only if they are likely to affect clinical management. Both clinicians and radiologists should always remember that: (1) no imaging study should be ordered unless it is likely to exert an important effect on clinical management; that is, if clinical management is the same whether the test is "positive" or "negative," then the test should not be performed; and (2) every imaging study should be performed and reported in such a way that its clinical utility is maximized. The radiologist's job is not to produce laundry lists of differential diagnostic possibilities, nor is it to recommend "clinical correlation" for every possible finding. Wherever possible, the radiologist's report should be clear and concise, and should answer as definitively as possible the clinical question at hand.

Outcomes

One of the effects of the advent of managed care in American medicine is to focus the attention of physicians on the outcomes of diagnostic testing, including their cost-effectiveness and the value of their contributions to the health of patients. The financial structure of medicine is changing in ways that discourage physicians from ordering unnecessary tests. In the days before utilization review and managed care, fee-for-service medicine meant that every physician in effect started the day with an empty pail, into which money was transferred for each test ordered or procedure performed. The more hysterectomies the surgeon performed, or the more chest X rays the radiologist read, the more money they found in their pails at the end of the day. In the environment of managed care, the referring physician begins every day with a pail of money, which grows lighter with each test ordered. Capitation means that physicians receive a certain amount of money in advance for each patient for whom they are responsible, which constitutes the pool of resources available for their care. A physician who orders too many tests will have no money left at day's end. In this environment, physicians are rewarded for limiting their use of diagnostic testing. One effect of this change in health care finance is to make referring physicians more circumspect about ordering medical imaging studies, and to increase the incentive for radiologists to perform studies only in cases where the result is likely to make a genuine difference in patient management.

The Radiologic Thought Process

The radiologic thought process can be divided into three components, each of which the student of diagnostic imaging must be familiar with. This familiarity is important for two reasons. First, nonradiologists are often faced with the task of analyzing imaging studies; for example, the emergency room physician who must make an immediate interpretation of a severely ill patient's chest radiograph. Second, optimal utilization of medical imaging studies requires some familiarity with how radiology is done, including the strengths and limitations of various studies, their role in various diagnostic algorithms, and the role of clinical information in radiologic diagnosis. Let us briefly review each of these three components. I have not labeled these components as stages, because they often take place simultaneously.

DETECTION

The first component of the radiologic thought process is the detection of lesions. This is the component on which novices usually focus their attention, although detection is only a small part of radiologic diagnosis. In order to detect lesions, knowledge of normal anatomy and the imaging characteristics of pathologic lesions is critical. Radiologists excel at lesion detection not because their eyes are any better in a physical sense than those of nonradiologists, but because of their deep understanding of normal anatomy and how it can be altered by various pathologic processes, which enables them to detect hundreds of pathologies. In fact, it is possible to train medical students and even nonmedical personnel to detect lesions such as pneumothorax just as well as radiologists in a very short period of time.

It should be emphasized that clinical information often plays a crucial role in the detection of lesions. For example, suppose a patient presents to the emergency room complaining of severe pain in a digit following a fall. It is vital that the referring physician furnish relevant information to the radiologist regarding the patient's clinical presentation. For one thing, the radiologist may suggest a different study based on this information. The clinician may reason that hand films would be the best examination, because they not only show the digit in question, but also help to rule out other unsuspected fractures, thus "killing two birds with one stone." However, hand films are less sensitive than finger films in detecting finger fractures. Moreover, additional views of the digit may be obtained in certain situations, in order to further increase sensitivity for the detection of fracture. The clinician's mission is not to "stump" the radiologist, because failure to detect a lesion reflects unfavorably on both the clinician and the radiologist. Rather, the radiologist and the clinician should seek to optimize each other's performance in the pursuit of optimal patient care. In the case of the possible finger fracture, examples of an inadequate clinical history would include, "Rule out fracture" or "Pain after fall." A good history would be, "Point tenderness in middle phalanx of fourth digit after fall."

DESCRIPTION

The second component of the radiologic thought process is the description of the finding. An accurate description is vital to good radiologic practice in part because it is often not possible to make a definitive diagnosis based solely on the radiologic findings. Moreover, an accurate description of the findings represents a vital step in reaching the correct diagnosis. Only when the finding is accurately described is it clear which differential diagnostic possibilities warrant strongest consideration. For example, determining whether pulmonary opacities seen on high-resolution CT are "ground glass," reticulonodular, or nodular in character powerfully influences the appropriate differential diagnosis. This is also true in the clinic, where an accurate description of a patient's chest pain may determine which of such diverse possibilities as myocardial ischemia or esophageal spasm is the more likely explanation.

Several key elements should be present in most descriptions of radiologic findings. These include the location of the lesion, its extent or size, and its general imaging characteristics. The latter includes general descriptors such as the clarity of its borders and its general morphology (round, stellate, cavitary), as well as more specific radiologic descriptors such as density (CT), echogenicity (ultrasound), signal intensity (MRI), and its behavior after the administration of contrast material.

One of the cardinal signs of a first-rate physician is the ability to accurately describe a patient's problem. This accuracy refers not only to technical precision, but to selecting out the most pertinent aspects of the case. Once an accurate description is in hand, it provides a benchmark against which to weigh each diagnostic hypothesis, to determine which provides the best fit.

DIFFERENTIAL DIAGNOSIS

The third and final component of the radiologic thought process is the production of a differential diagnosis. One factor in differential diagnosis that cannot be over-emphasized is the importance of adequate clinical history. Relatively few radiologic findings are pathognomonic (from the Greek roots meaning "disease" and "to know"). In most cases, the radiologist can at best generate an ordered list of likely explanations for a particular radiologic finding, which often will be powerfully influenced by clinical factors. For example, the differential diagnosis of many bone lesions is powerfully affected by whether or not the lesion is painful, with malignant lesions more likely when the patient is symptomatic. Yet there is no way the radiologist can discern if the patient experiences pain simply by inspecting the radiograph. In the case of an "infiltrate" on a chest radiograph, such clinical clues as whether the patient is febrile, whether the illness is acute or chronic, and whether the patient is immune compromised will exert a powerful effect on the differential diagnosis the radiologist constructs.

There is no single magic formula for producing an adequate differential diagnosis for the myriad radiologic findings that may arise in a dozen or more organ systems. However, it is possible to outline a general approach to differential diagnosis by which to order one's thoughts and ensure that the major categories of disease are at least considered. The mnemonic acronym is CITIMITV.

CONGENITAL

This category is especially important in pediatrics, but should be considered in adults as well. It includes heritable disorders, developmental anomalies, and anatomic variants. The remainder of the list consists of acquired disorders.

INFLAMMATION

In fact, some degree of inflammatory response is associated with all forms of cell and tissue injury. However, this category is meant to include noninfectious disorders that manifest themselves primarily as an inflammatory response, which may be either acute or chronic. An example of a noninfectious inflammatory disorder would be rheumatoid arthritis, which manifests as inflammation of the synovial membrane.

TUMOROUS

Cancer is the second leading killer in America, and results in approximately 575,000 deaths per year. From the Latin for "swelling," tumor simply implies an abnormal growth. From a differential point of view, two distinctions must be drawn. First, a tumor may be benign or malignant. In the case of a smooth, round lung nodule discovered on chest radiography, one would need to include in the differential diagnosis benign tumors such as a hamartoma, as well as malignant tumors such as an adenocarcinoma. The second distinction is between primary and metastatic lesions, which vary in relative frequency depending on the organ involved. In the case of the brain, primary malignancies are somewhat more common than metastases, while in the skeleton metastases outnumber primary malignancies by a factor of 50:1. In many cases, tissue biopsy is necessary to establish a definitive diagnosis.

INFECTIOUS

Major categories of infectious disease include viral, bacterial, and protozoal disorders. The immune status of the host is an important factor, because atypical or opportunistic infections become much more likely in the setting of impaired host response. Generally, clinical factors such as fever and an increased leukocyte count will favor an infectious etiology.

METABOLIC

Metabolic disorders relate to the endocrine system, nutritional disorders, and ion balance. Examples include Cushing's syndrome, hemochromatosis, and osteoporosis. In general, results of laboratory tests are crucial in establishing the diagnosis.

IATROGENIC

From the Greek *iatros* meaning the treatment of diseases (hence "pediatrics" for the medical specialty devoted to the treatment of children's diseases), iatrogenic disorders arise from medical interventions. Examples include drug reactions such as bleomycin-induced interstitial lung disease and venous thrombosis secondary to indwelling central venous catheters. Certain findings in hospitalized patients such as pneumothorax and small bowel obstruction are more often due to medical interventions than any other cause.

TRAUMATIC

Generally, the traumatic etiology of radiologic findings is obvious, as the patient is being evaluated explicitly to rule out traumatic injury. However, if the trauma is remote, the patient may not mention it. This history can be critical, for example, in the evaluation of many posttraumatic bone lesions, which can appear both radiologically and histologically like primary malignant bone tumors, due to the profuse osteoblastic activity they may provoke. The possibility of intentional trauma must always be borne in mind when evaluating pediatric images, because often the radiologist is the only physician who detects evidence of child abuse.

VASCULAR

Examples of vascular disorders include systemic lupus erythematosus and pulmonary embolism.

RADIOLOGIC ERROR

Error is a topic rarely addressed in medicine, perhaps in part because both physicians and patients have vested interests in the infallibility of medicine. Generally, radiology is probably even less forgiving of error than other specialties. If an internist fails to pick up a subtle breast nodule on physical examination, the existence of the finding is unlikely to be noted anywhere in the patient's medical record. A year later, when the nodule has grown into a mass, no one can be certain that the nodule was even present or large enough to be detectable when the physical examination was performed. By contrast, when a radiologist reading a mammogram misses subtle microcalcifications associated with a breast carcinoma, he or she has nowhere to hide. The microcalcifications will be on the film and available for detection by any physician (or malpractice attorney) by whom the study is subsequently reviewed.

Despite the antipathy toward error that exists in radiology, it has been estimated that even experienced radiologists may "miss" up to 25 to 30% of significant findings. Moreover, "overcalls," or false-positive results, may occur in as many as 1 to 2% of cases. Of the missed abnormalities, approximately 80% can be categorized as gross, meaning that they appear obvious when pointed out in retrospect. The other 20% of missed abnormalities are subtle or inconspicuous even on review. The significance of these research results is difficult to assess absent information on the clinical significance of the missed abnormalities. Failure to detect an incidental abnormality such as a cervical rib is of no clinical significance, whereas failure to detect a small primary lung carcinoma may deprive the patient of the opportunity for a curative resection.

The purpose of studying radiologic error is not to assign blame, but to improve performance. The three most common types of error are search errors, recognition errors, and decision-making errors. Search errors occur when the radiologist fails to fixate his or her central vision on the area of the film where the abnormality lies. These errors include so-called corner signs, in which the abnormality is at one of the corners of the film, at which the radiologist never looks. To avoid search errors, it is necessary to look at each portion of the film. This typically involves approximately 100 gaze fixations (each lasting a fraction of a second) for a single chest radiograph. A junior medical student will typically perform fewer fixations, centered on only a portion of the film—often the brightest areas (such as the heart on a chest radiograph) and the regions of highest contrast borders. An experienced radiologist, on the other hand, will distribute gaze fixations more evenly and will pay attention to darker and lower contrast regions of the film as well.

One of the most important steps to improving radiologic performance is taking care to search each image adequately. One of the most common errors in this regard has been called "satisfaction of search." This is defined as the decreased probability of finding additional abnormalities once an abnormality has been correctly identified. That is, once the radiologist has found something wrong, he or she immediately launches into a discussion of that abnormality, having prematurely terminated the search through the remainder of the film. This is an especially common error among neophytes, who often have difficulty finding any abnormality, and are so pleased with themselves when they do that they stop looking further. Another potential pitfall is the simple failure to devote adequate search time to each image. Doing so tends to increase the number of false-negatives. On the other hand, increasing search time can lead to an increase in the number of false-positives.

Recognition errors occur when an abnormality is scanned but not appreciated as an abnormality. To recognize an abnormality requires less visual acuity than a visual memory, which is composed of dozens or hundreds or thousands of similar visual experiences, against which the finding either does or does not stand out. Recognition differs between different people, depending on the depth and character of their previous experience. To perform well at recognition requires an understanding of normal radiologic anatomy and the myriad but characteristic ways in which various disease processes may manifest themselves.

Decision-making errors may account for slightly over one-half of all errors in radiologic diagnosis. In these errors, an abnormality is both scanned and recognized, but rejected as "noise" or a normal variant. Again, an experienced visual memory and an understanding of anatomy and pathophysiology may serve as the crucial factors in avoiding such errors. In addition, clinical information may play an important role in helping the radiologist to properly evaluate the significance of such findings.

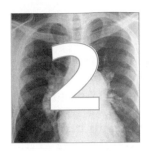

The Circulatory System: The Heart and Great Vessels

2

ANATOMY AND PHYSIOLOGY

IMAGING MODALITIES
- Radiography
- Angiography
- Computed Tomography
- Echocardiography
- Nuclear Cardiography
- Magnetic Resonance Imaging

PATHOLOGY
- Congenital
- Infectious
  - Rheumatic heart disease
  - Mitral stenosis
  - Mitral insufficiency
  - Aortic stenosis
  - Aortic insufficiency
- Inflammatory
  - Cardiomyopathy
- Vascular
  - Coronary artery disease

COMMON CLINICAL PROBLEMS
- Congestive Heart Failure
- Pulmonary Embolism

AORTA
- Anatomy and Physiology
- Pathology
  - Aneurysm
  - Dissection
  - Trauma

ANATOMY AND PHYSIOLOGY

Some of the greatest figures in the history of medicine and biology, including Aristotle, Galen, and Vesalius, never knew that the blood circulates through the body. William Harvey (1578–1657), perhaps the greatest English-speaking physician in history, was the first person to prove conclusively that the blood moves away from the heart through the arteries and back to the heart through the veins, and that the heart itself is the pump responsible for the blood's motion. However, despite his great triumph, even Harvey died having left a critical piece in the circulatory puzzle unfilled; namely, how the blood moves from the arteries to the veins. It was Malphigi, using the newly developed microscope, who demonstrated the existence of capillaries (from the Latin for "hair").

The circulatory (from the Latin *circulari,* "to form a circle") system transports gases, nutrients, waste products, cells, hormones, and a variety of other substances throughout the body. It may be divided into two components, the exchange portion and the conduction portion. At any moment, only about 5% of the blood is found in the portion of the circulatory system where exchange of materials between the blood and the extracellular fluid takes place, the capillaries. Nearly all of the 75 trillion living cells in the mature human body that are not bathed in blood are located within a few cell diameters of a capillary. The capillaries allow passive diffusion of metabolites to take place simultaneously over a very short distance and a very great surface area. The capillaries themselves are only 1 μm thick (an erythrocyte is 8 μm thick), thus enabling diffusion to take place across a very short distance, and hence more rapidly. The rate of diffusion is also critically augmented by the fact that the surface area of exchange is great. It is estimated that the total surface area available for metabolite exchange in the body's 40 billion capillaries is 600 m². With some notable exceptions, exchange of metabolites between the blood and the extracellular fluid occurs by passive diffusion, propelled by differences in metabolite concentration.

The other component of the circulatory system, the conduction portion, functions by active bulk flow, with the heart serving as the pump and the arteries, arterioles, venules, and veins serving as conduits. The conduits are not merely passive vessels, however, as the elastic recoil of the aorta is important is sustaining forward blood flow in diastole, and the relaxation and contraction of the arterioles is critical in distributing blood flow. The embryonic heart begins to beat around 3 weeks after conception, and over the course of a lifetime, contracts about 3 billion times. The right ventricle supplies the low-pressure, low-resistance pulmonary circulation, while the left ventricle supplies the high-pressure, high-resistance systemic circulation. Whereas the pulmonary circuit consists of a single pathway, the systemic circuit is actually comprised of a number of pathways (cerebral, coronary, mesenteric, etc.) arranged in parallel (Fig. 2–1). This difference is visible in the normal thickness of the two ventricles, with the left ventricle appearing much thicker than the right. The four valves permit blood to flow in only one direction through the heart (Fig. 2–2). Approximately 1% of cardiac muscle cells, including those in the sinoatrial (SA) and atrioventricular nodes, are autorhythmic, specialized for initiating and conducting the action potentials responsible for cardiac contraction.

Cardiac output is the product of stroke volume and heart rate. The normal cardiac output of 5 L/min may be increased during exercise by as much as eight times in highly trained athletes. Stroke volume, the amount of blood ejected from the ventricle with each contraction, is determined primarily by the end-diastolic volume. The Frank-Starling law of the heart states that the heart pumps all the blood returned to it; the more blood placed in the ventricle before it contracts, the greater its stroke volume. This both balances the output of the right and left sides of the heart, and also allows a rapid response to increased circulatory demands. During exercise, for example, increased skeletal muscle contractions and faster and deeper breathing increase venous return to the heart. Sympathetic stimulation can further increase stroke volume by increasing contractility, causing an increase in the ejection fraction (the ventricle squeezes out a greater proportion of the blood that fills it).

Heart rate is influenced primarily by autonomic input to the SA node. Parasympathetic stimulation decreases the rate of depolarization of the SA node, while sympa-

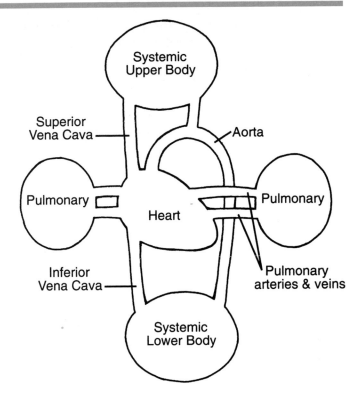

Figure 2–1. While the pulmonary circulation may be conceptualized as a single circuit, the systemic circulation consists of multiple circuits arranged in parallel.

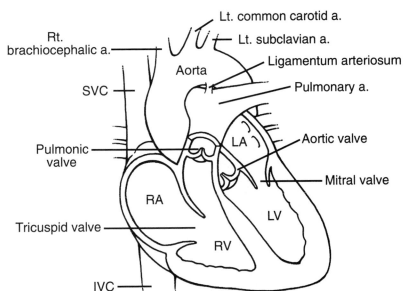

Figure 2–2. The four valves of the heart and their relationships to the great vessels.

thetic stimulation not only increases the SA node's rate of depolarization, but also increases the excitability of the arteriovenous node and conduction pathways. In addition, sympathetic stimulation increases contractility. As the heart rate begins to exceed 220 beats per minute, the time available for ventricular filling decreases to such a degree that cardiac output actually declines.

The heart's blood supply is the first to branch off from the aorta, with the coronary arteries (from the Latin *corona,* "crown") arising just above the aortic valve, and the

Figure 2–3. This diagram of the heart and great vessels also illustrates the principal branches of the coronary arteries arising from the aorta just above the aortic valve.

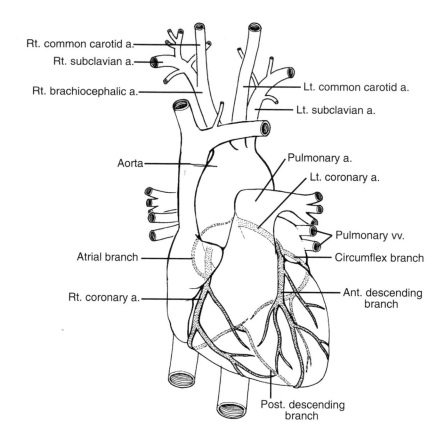

Rt. common carotid a.

Rt. subclavian a.

Rt. brachiocephalic a.

Lt. common carotid a.

Lt. subclavian a.

Aorta

Pulmonary a.

Lt. coronary a.

Pulmonary vv.

Atrial branch

Circumflex branch

Rt. coronary a.

Ant. descending branch

Post. descending branch

coronary veins returning blood to the right atrium (Fig. 2–3). Because of the high wall tension generated by the left ventricle during systole, approximately 70% of coronary blood flow occurs during diastole, propelled by the elastic recoil of the aorta (Fig. 2–4). This marks another reason that tachycardia ("fast heart") poses a threat to life, as the percentage of time the ventricle spends in diastole decreases with increasing heart rate. Normally, increased myocardial activity produces vasodilation of the coronary arteries and increased myocardial blood flow, but the balance between myocardial consumption and coronary supply may be tipped in favor of ischemia by occlusive atherosclerotic disease or vascular spasm.

The major resistance vessels are the arterioles, whose smooth muscle lining can be alternately tensed or relaxed to alter perfusion of a particular organ or tissue. An example of this mechanism is active hyperemia, in which increased carbon dioxide production in an area causes relaxation of arteriolar smooth muscle, with an increase in arteriolar radius, a decrease in arteriolar resistance, and increased perfusion of the area. Nonlocal modulators of blood pressure include both the nervous and endocrine systems, with the sympathetic nervous system playing a key role.

Most of the blood in the body, about 60% at rest, is found in the veins (Fig. 2–5). Veins serve as very low pressure conduits to return blood to the heart, and contain valves that permit flow in only one direction (cardiopetal). Negative thoracic pressure during inspiration, the squeezing of veins during skeletal muscle contraction, and the very low or even negative intraluminal pressure of the right atrium (due to reexpansion of the right ventricle during diastole) are all forces that favor blood return.

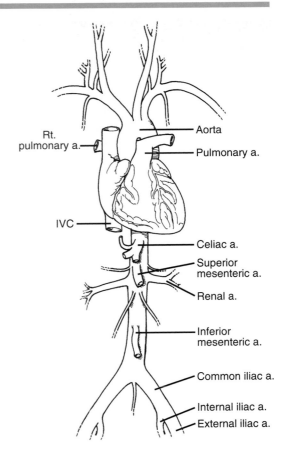

Figure 2–4. The aorta and its major branches. Note that a catheter inserted into one of the femoral arteries could be advanced upward through the aorta and into the mesenteric arteries, the brachiocephalic vessels, the coronary arteries, or the cardiac chambers themselves. This technique is employed in mesenteric angiography, cerebral angiography, coronary angiography, and cardiac angiography, respectively.

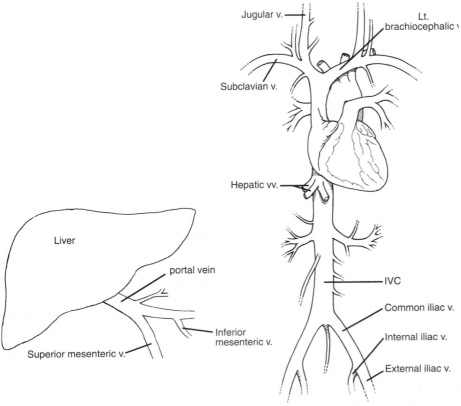

Figure 2–5. The major veins through which blood is returned to the heart. Note that a catheter inserted into the femoral vein could be advanced up through the right atrium, the right ventricle, and into the pulmonary arteries, as when a pulmonary arteriogram is performed. Of course, this could also be accomplished with a catheter inserted into a neck or arm vein, as well.

IMAGING MODALITIES

A variety of modalities are available for cardiac imaging, each with distinctive strengths and weaknesses. Determining which study is most appropriate to a particular clinical situation requires a knowledge of these strengths and weaknesses, as well as an understanding of the particular clinical question to be answered.

Radiography

The chest radiograph, often obtained for other reasons (e.g., "rule out congestive heart failure"), provides a wealth of information about the heart. While hypertrophy often produces little or no radiographic change, significant dilatation of cardiac chambers should be radiographically detectable on routine upright posteroanterior (PA) and lateral chest radiographs. When further information is required about specific chambers, oblique views may be helpful, although these are now only rarely obtained. On a PA view, the right heart border is made up by part of the right atrium, the upper left heart border is made up by part of the left atrium, and the mid and lower left heart border represents the left ventricle. The right ventricle, which is located anteriorly, is not seen. On the lateral view, the right ventricle makes up the anterior border of the heart, the left atrium makes up the posterosuperior border, and the left ventricle is the posteroinferior border.

Enlargement of each chamber produces a predictable change in appearance. Right ventricular enlargement causes filling in of the retrosternal clear space on lateral views. Right atrial enlargement is the most difficult to assess, but may cause bulging of the right heart border. Left ventricular enlargement increases the cardiothoracic ratio—the ratio of maximum width of the heart to the maximum width of the thorax, which is normally less than 0.50 (Fig. 2–6). It also causes the heart to bulge downward and to the left on the frontal view, and posteroinferiorly on the lateral view. Left atrial

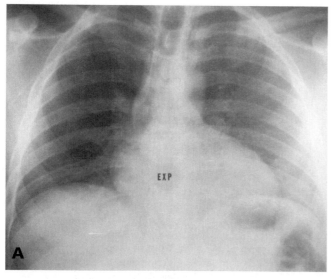
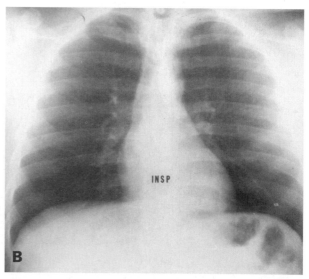

Figure 2–6. **(A)** This frontal chest radiograph demonstrates an increase in the cardiothoracic ratio, which measures approximately 0.55, and would seem to suggest cardiomegaly. However, in this case, the apparent cardiomegaly was technical rather than anatomical in nature, produced by marked underinflation of the lungs, which exaggerates the width of mediastinal structures, including the heart. EXP, expiration. **(B)** A follow-up film with adequate inspiration (INSP) demonstrates that the heart is normal in size and shape.

enlargement is manifest as a bulge below the pulmonary artery on the PA projection, as well as posterior displacement of the esophagus on the lateral view (best appreciated when the esophagus contains barium) (Fig. 2–7). When left atrial enlargement becomes pronounced, it may lift up the left mainstem bronchus.

The chest radiograph also provides information about pulmonary blood flow, with increased perfusion manifesting as increased diameter of the affected vessels. In the case of decreased flow, as in pulmonary embolism (PE), normal vasculature may be diminished or absent. Increased pulmonary vascular pressures manifest differently, depending on whether the veins or arteries are affected. Signs of pulmonary venous hypertension include enlargement of mediastinal veins such as the azygous vein; redistribution of pulmonary blood flow from the lower to the upper lung zones; perivascular edema, with associated loss of vessel definition and subsequent development of peribronchial cuffing (fluid around the bronchi); septal lines (Kerley's A-lines and B-lines); and frank airspace opacities, as fluid accumulates within the alveoli. Pulmonary artery hypertension produces central dilatation of the pulmonary arteries, which may be accompanied by peripheral pruning of vessels, especially when increased arteriolar resistance is the cause (Fig. 2–8).

Assessment of overall cardiac size and chamber contour is less reliable on portable radiographs, which are usually obtained with the patient in varying degrees of recumbency and in the anteroposterior (AP) projection (the film is placed under the supine patient's back and the X-ray beam enters from the front of the patient). As one would expect, the AP film tends to exaggerate the cardiac silhouette (the heart's shadow),

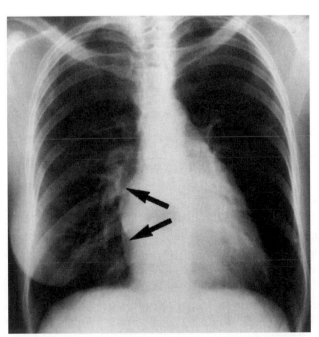

Figure 2–7. A chest radiograph demonstrates a classic plain radiographic appearance of left atrial enlargement due to rheumatic mitral valve disease. There is a prominent bulge of the left atrial contour, which actually becomes a border forming along the right side of the heart (arrows).

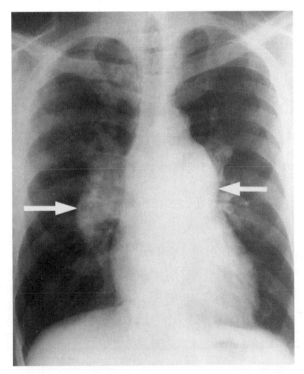

Figure 2–8. A frontal chest radiograph in a patient with a history of long-standing pulmonary artery hypertension demonstrates massive enlargement of the main pulmonary artery and the right and left pulmonary artery branches (arrows), with marked oligemia and "pruning" of the pulmonary vessels peripherally.

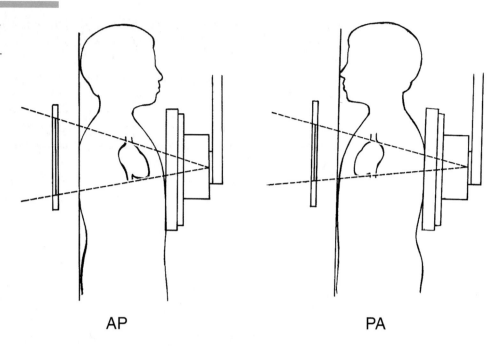

Figure 2–9. The effect of antero-posterior (AP) and posteroanterior (PA) chest radiographic technique on the size of the cardiac silhouette. The closer the heart is to the film, the less the degree of magnification, which makes the PA view the preferred technique for the assessment of cardiomegaly.

AP   PA

because the greater the distance between a shadow-casting object and the screen on which its shadow is cast, the larger its shadow appears (Fig. 2–9). Moreover, patients who require portable films are usually sicker (which is why they cannot come to the radiology department), and hence less able to take a deep breath; the resultant under-inflation is another common cause of apparent cardiomegaly, because the heart is not as stretched out along the craniocaudal axis. For these reasons, caution is warranted in assessing cardiomegaly on portable films. Furthermore, redistribution of pulmonary vascular flow from the lower lung zones to the upper lung zones cannot be diagnosed on a supine film, where it represents a normal finding (due to the loss of the gravitational gradient favoring flow to the lower lung zones).

Angiography

Cardiac angiography is most frequently performed to assess coronary artery disease. A catheter is usually placed into the femoral artery, advanced up through the aorta into the aortic root, and into the coronary arteries themselves (Fig. 2–10). Often, cannulating a particular artery requires the use of a specialized catheter, shaped to facilitate the particular maneuver being attempted. All catheter manipulation is performed under fluoroscopic monitoring, as is contrast injection. Cine films are obtained to allow the assessment of contrast flow patterns over time. It must be borne in mind that angiography visualizes only the contrast opacified lumen of the vessel, and does not provide direct visualization of the vascular wall itself. However, it is often possible to infer the nature of vascular pathology based on angiographic findings, such as the presence of a focal out-pouching within an area of luminal narrowing, indicating an ulcerating plaque.

Computed Tomography

Computed tomography (CT) may play an increasing role in cardiac imaging. Cardiomegaly, hypertrophic changes, pericardial disease, and coronary artery calcifica-

Figure 2–10. This coronary angiogram demonstrates a complete occlusion of the proximal left anterior descending coronary artery (arrow), with retrograde filling of this vessel via collaterals from a diagonal branch.

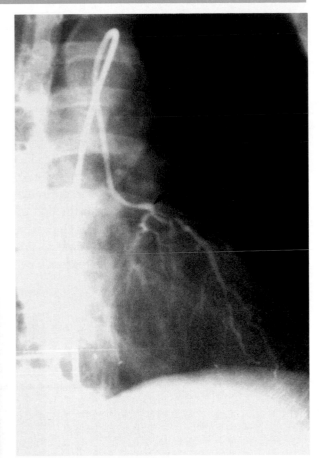

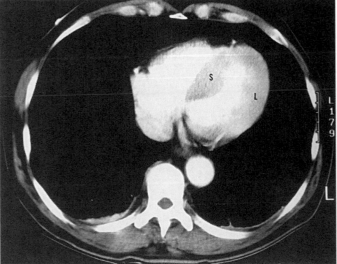

Figure 2–11. A 55-year-old hypertensive man underwent contrast-enhanced chest computed tomography to evaluate a known abdominal aortic aneurysm (not shown). An axial image through the level of the heart demonstrates marked thickening of the interventricular septum and lateral wall of the left ventricle, indicating the presence of a hypertrophic cardiomyopathy. L, lateral wall of left ventricle; S, interventricular septum.

tions are frequently diagnosed on routine thoracic CT examinations obtained for other reasons (Fig. 2–11). Ultrafast CT, which can complete data acquisition in 1/10 or 1/20 of a second, can eliminate the problem of cardiac motion and be used in cine format to observe the changes in morphology accompanying the cardiac cycle. Examples of uses for ultrafast CT include the assessment of morphologic and functional wall abnormalities associated with myocardial infarction, such as lack of wall thickening with systole and the presence of ventricular aneurysms, and in the determination of the patency of coronary artery bypass grafts. Ultrafast CT may also be helpful in assessing pericardial disease, such as restrictive pericarditis.

Echocardiography

Echocardiography is a major imaging examination in the United States, and recently has generated more revenue than any other diagnostic imaging study. The heart and great vessels are imaged using ultrasound, in three different modalities. M-mode, the first to be developed, produces a linear image of the changes in position of cardiac structures over time. As an example, M-mode enables the assessment of changes in the position of valve cusps over milliseconds, because thousands of pulses are sent and received by the transducer each second. Using gray-scale imaging, it is possible to produce two-dimensional "slice" images of the heart, which may be obtained via a transthoracic approach or from a transesophageal position, using a transducer mounted on the end of a flexible endoscope (Fig. 2–12). Finally, the Doppler technique enables the assessment of flow velocity and turbulence (Fig. 2–13). Using the Bernoulli equation (pressure in mm Hg = $4v^2$, where velocity is expressed in m/s), pressure changes can be estimated noninvasively.

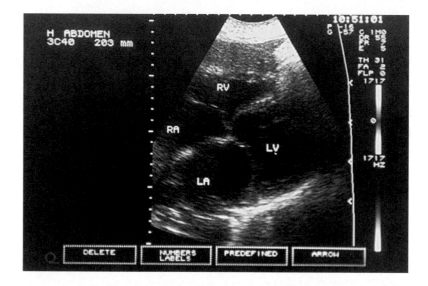

Figure 2–12. A "four chamber" ultrasonographic view of the heart obtained via a transthoracic approach reveals the four cardiac chambers, as well as the mitral and tricuspid atrioventricular valves. LA, left atrium; LV, left ventricle; RA, right atrium; RV, right ventricle.

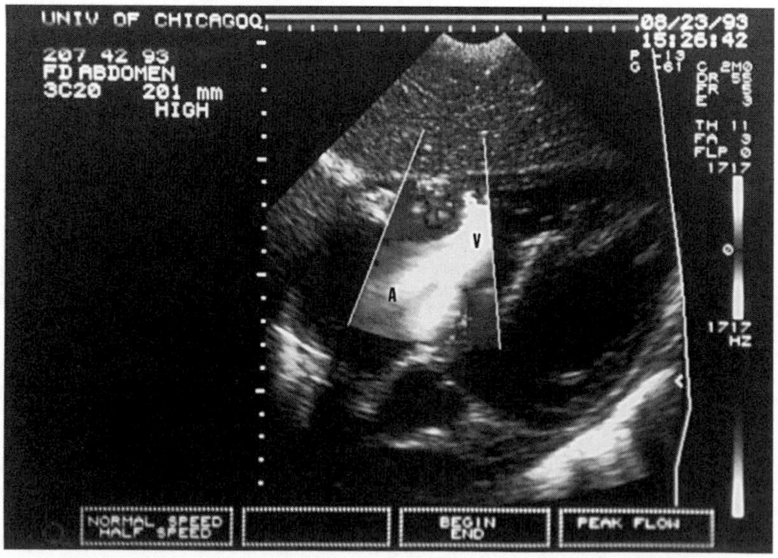

Figure 2–13. This gray-scale image of a duplex Doppler echocardiogram demonstrates blood flow across the tricuspid valve. By convention, blood flow toward the transducer (at the top of the image) is represented by red. Because this flow appeared red on the color image, we know that this represented flow in the expected direction, from the right atrium into the right ventricle. A, right atrium; V, right ventricle.

Figure 2–14. An axial sonogram of the heart reveals a rim of fluid outside the posterior wall of the left ventricle (black arrow), representing a pericardial effusion, as well as thickening of the left ventricular wall itself (white arrow).

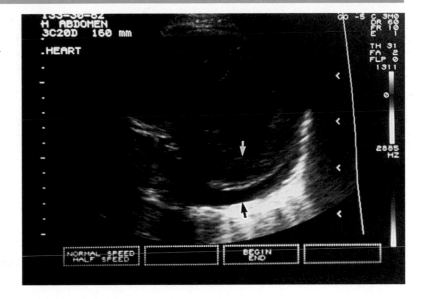

Echocardiography is the imaging modality of choice in the evaluation of valvular heart disease, where abnormalities of valve morphology, thickness, and motion can be readily detected. Stenosis manifests as abnormally high velocity across a valve, while regurgitant flow manifests as flow in the wrong direction (e.g., blue color flow when red is expected). Moreover, echocardiography permits assessment of the left ventricle, including chamber size, wall thickness, and function. It is useful in the diagnosis of the various types of cardiomyopathy (dilated, restricted, and hypertrophic). Pericardial effusions as small as 10 to 20 mL (Fig. 2–14) and cardiac masses, such as myxomas and rhabdomyosarcomas, are readily detected. Finally, the heart may also be stressed and visualized on echocardiography to assess exercise-related changes in wall contractility and ejection fraction.

Nuclear Cardiography

As will be discussed later, nuclear cardiography relies on the injection of radiotracer substances whose anatomic and physiologic localization provides information about cardiac structure and function. Acute myocardial infarctions can be diagnosed using labeled pyrophosphate compounds, which bind irreversibly to molecules in damaged myocardial cells and appear as "hot spots" on scintigraphy. Myocardial perfusion imaging relies on the fact that certain molecules, such as the potassium analogue thallium-201, are taken up by myocardial cells in proportion to regional blood flow. Ventriculography using labeled red blood cells provides assessment of cardiac size and function, with measurement of the cardiac ejection fraction. Positron emission tomography can be used to evaluate regional cardiac perfusion and metabolism.

Magnetic Resonance Imaging

Like echocardiography, magnetic resonance imaging (MRI) employs no ionizing radiation or contrast agents. Because data acquisition takes longer in MRI than in CT, cardiac and respiratory gating is essential. On conventional sequences, flowing blood appears as a signal void (black), although other "bright blood" sequences are also often employed. MRI is used to provide multiplanar imaging of cardiac anatomy and pathology, including aneurysms and thrombi, congenital heart disease, and aortic disease, such as dissecting aneurysms. MRI can be used to assess morphology throughout the cardiac cycle, averaging data acquisitions over hundreds of heart beats to produce views at each phase.

PATHOLOGY

Congenital

Congenital heart disease is discussed in Chapter 10.

Infectious

The pulmonary valve is rarely affected by noncongenital disease processes, leaving the mitral, tricuspid, and aortic valves as the principal sites of valvular heart disease. This discussion will focus on involvement of the mitral and aortic valves in rheumatic heart disease. The mitral valve consists of the annulus fibrosa, the valve cusps, the chordae tendineae, and the papillary muscles. In diastole, the valve opens as atrial pressure exceeds ventricular pressure, while in systole, when ventricular pressure exceeds atrial, the valve cusps close to prevent regurgitation. The aortic valve, which has no distinct fibrous annulus, opens when left ventricular pressure exceeds aortic pressure in systole, and closes in diastole as ventricular pressure falls. Blood is then trapped in the sinuses of Valsalva, from which it enters the coronary arteries and perfuses the heart, propelled by the elastic recoil of the aorta. The surface area of the mitral valve is approximately twice that of the aortic, 5 versus 2.5 cm^2 (Fig. 2–15).

RHEUMATIC HEART DISEASE

EPIDEMIOLOGY

By far the most common cause of acquired valvular heart disease is rheumatic fever, a systemic inflammatory process associated with infection by Group A β-hemolytic streptococcus and an ensuing autoimmune response. Perhaps as many as 3% of patients with epidemic streptococcal pharyngitis go on to develop rheumatic fever. Of patients who develop rheumatic fever, approximately one-third develop the sequela of rheumatic heart disease, with severe complications including death occurring decades later.

PATHOPHYSIOLOGY

When rheumatic fever involves the heart, all cardiac layers are affected, including the endocardium, myocardium, and pericardium. This contrasts with bacterial endocarditis, which involves the inner layer alone. The pathology of rheumatic heart disease stems primarily from fibrosis of the valve cusps and chordae, which may cause both stenosis (from fusion of the cusps) and regurgitation (from retraction of cusps and chordae). The valve most

Figure 2–15. A frontal chest radiograph in a patient with a history of prosthetic valve placement for rheumatic heart disease demonstrates the differences in size and position between the aortic and mitral valves. a, aortic valve; m, mitral valve.

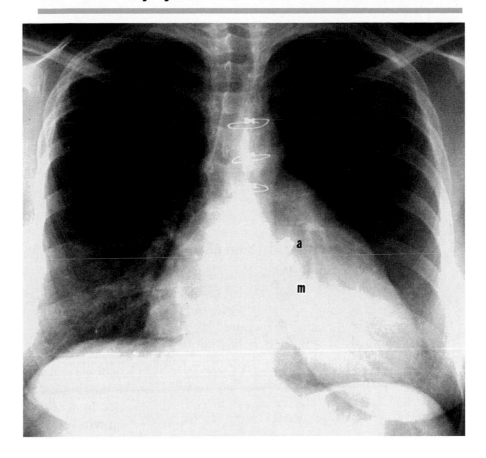

commonly affected is the mitral, which exhibits isolated involvement in 50% of cases. Another one-third of patients will exhibit a combination of mitral valve and aortic valve involvement. Isolated involvement of the aortic valve is uncommon.

CLINICAL PRESENTATION

More than 9 of 10 patients develop rheumatic heart disease between the ages of 5 and 15 years. Following the streptococcal pharyngitis, symptoms of rheumatic fever include fever, carditis, and polyarthritis.

IMAGING

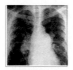 The hemodynamic consequences of stenosis and regurgitation and their imaging findings are predictable, based on physiologic principles. Stenosis of a valve produces proximal pressure overload. In the case of the aortic valve, the heart responds with left ventricular hypertrophy, which manifests as thickening of the wall without radiographically detectable evidence of cardiomegaly. Stenotic valves are often calcific, and these calcifications may be identifiable on chest radiographs. Insufficient or regurgitant valves, on the other hand, produce volume overload of cardiac chambers both proximal and distal to the lesion, with resultant radiographically detectable cardiomegaly. With progressive cardiomegaly, there is often progressive distortion of the supporting framework of the valve, which further aggravates regurgitation. In contrast to stenotic valves, insufficient valves rarely exhibit radiographically detectable calcifications. It should be noted that

diseased valves often exhibit a combination of stenosis and insufficiency; for example, nearly every stenotic valve will also leak to some degree.

MITRAL STENOSIS

EPIDEMIOLOGY

Mitral stenosis, the most common form of acquired valvular heart disease, afflicts women twice as often as men, and represents the most common cause of death in rheumatic heart disease.

PATHOPHYSIOLOGY

 As fibrosis progresses and the mitral valve orifice is reduced by 50%, an increased left atrial–left ventricular pressure gradient is required to propel blood into the left ventricle. Left atrial failure and dilation may ensue. Once the valve orifice reaches 1 cm², a 25 mm Hg gradient is required, and the increased left atrial pressure causes increased pulmonary venous and capillary pressures, reduced pulmonary compliance, and exertional dyspnea. It also causes pulmonary venous hypertension, with right-sided pressure overload and right ventricular hypertrophy and eventual failure.

CLINICAL PRESENTATION

Symptoms and signs usually develop in approximately two decades, and include exertional dyspnea, episodes of acute pulmonary edema, atrial fibrillation, and hemoptysis. On physical examination, the classic diastolic murmur includes accentuation of the first heart sound (due to snapping shut of the stenosed valve) and a mid-diastolic rumble (due to regurgitant flow across the valve). Once the patient becomes seriously symptomatic, death follows within 2 to 5 years unless the stenosis is relieved.

IMAGING

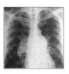 Radiographic findings include an initially normal-sized heart. The mitral valve itself is frequently calcified, and left atrial enlargement can often be detected, with elevation of the left main bronchus, a "double density" over the right atrium, and enlargement of the left atrial appendage. Another radiographic finding of left atrial enlargement is posterior displacement of the esophagus and left mainstem bronchus on barium swallow, as the left atrium forms the posterosuperior border of the heart. In advanced cases, the left atrium itself may calcify, although the high kilovoltage technique of contemporary chest radiography makes this difficult to detect (Fig. 2–16). Once right ventricular failure occurs, signs of right ventricular enlargement, such as filling in of the retrosternal clear space, begin to be detected. The condition is invariably accompanied by signs of pulmonary venous hypertension.

Radiographic findings vary depending on the severity of increased pulmonary venous pressure. At pressures up to 20 mm Hg, cephalization of pulmonary blood flow is seen, with increased caliber of upper versus lower lung zone pulmonary vessels. While the normal upper-to-lower vessel diameter ratio is approximately 1 to 3, in pulmonary venous hypertension it approaches 1 to 1, and may even reverse to some degree. This is thought to stem from predominately basilar perivascular edema (see the

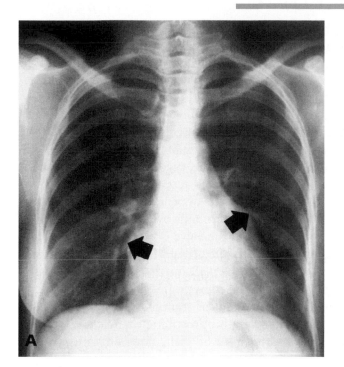

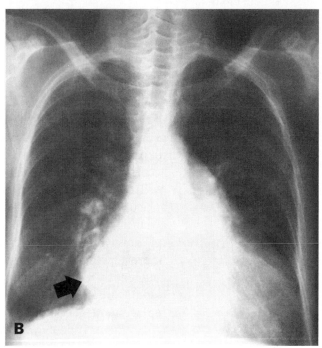

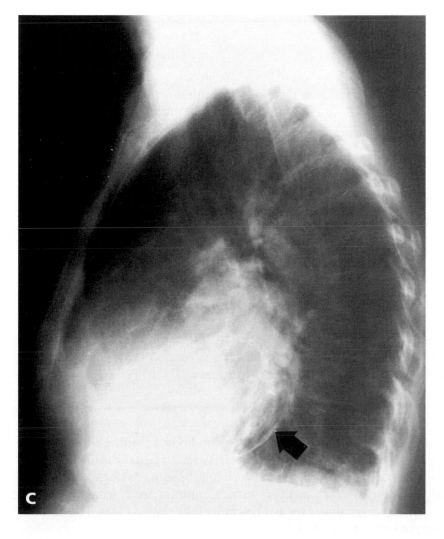

Figure 2–16. This woman had a history of rheumatic mitral valve disease. (**A**) Her frontal chest radiograph demonstrates left atrial enlargement, with a double density over the right heart border and bulging of the left atrial appendage (arrows). (**B,C**) Twenty years later, the left atrium creates a much more marked bulge (arrow) on the frontal view, and the lateral view (**C**) demonstrates calcification within the markedly enlarged left atrial wall (arrow).

discussion of Starling forces in the section on pulmonary edema), with reflex vasoconstriction and redistribution of blood flow to the upper lung zones. At pressures between 20 and 25 mm Hg, interstitial edema ensues, with plasma accumulating in the interstitium faster than pulmonary lymphatics can clear it. Once the pressure exceeds 25 mm Hg, alveolar edema results, with airspace infiltrates and pleural effusions.

Chronic pulmonary arterial hypertension manifests radiographically as enlargement of the arterial roots, with a paucity of peripheral lung vascular markings, the so-called pruned tree appearance. An uncommon but distinctive finding in mitral stenosis is pulmonary hemosiderosis, which follows hemorrhage from engorged capillaries, with the accumulation of hemosiderin, and a remarkable stippled appearance to the lungs.

Treatment of early mitral stenosis initially consists of penicillin prophylaxis, avoidance of physically strenuous activities, avoidance of volume overload, and treatment of atrial fibrillation. As the disease progresses and the valve orifice approaches 1 cm^2, mitral valvulotomy is generally indicated, which often results in striking symptomatic improvement and improved survival. This may be performed via cardiotomy, or percutaneously via a fluoroscopically guided balloon catheter. If valvulotomy is not sufficient, as in a patient with a significant component of regurgitation, prosthetic valve replacement may be necessary, using either a bioprosthetic or mechanical valve replacement. Patients with mechanical valves must be maintained on anticoagulants indefinitely, due to their increased thrombogenicity.

MITRAL INSUFFICIENCY

EPIDEMIOLOGY

Although rheumatic heart disease is the most common cause of mitral insufficiency, other causes include infectious endocarditis, papillary muscle rupture, and mitral valve prolapse.

PATHOPHYSIOLOGY

 Regardless of the cause, valvular insufficiency results in regurgitant flow of blood into the left atrium during left ventricular systole. As expected, the left atrium and left ventricle both dilate, as both must accommodate both normal and regurgitant volumes with every cycle. Typically, the left atrium dilates more than the left ventricle, and mitral insufficiency is associated with the so-called giant left atrium (Fig. 2–17). The giant left atrium is associated, in turn, with atrial fibrillation. Cardiac function is generally not severely affected because the condition develops gradually, and the left ventricle is able to accommodate the increased volume with little or no increase in end-diastolic pressure. Likewise, the left atrium simply expands, without an increase in pressure, and so the pulmonary edema and hemoptysis seen in mitral stenosis are relatively rare.

CLINICAL PRESENTATION

Chronic mitral regurgitation is a relatively benign condition, in which only a fraction of patients ever become symptomatic. Of all the left-sided lesions, it is the best tolerated. However, in acute mitral insufficiency, which may be seen in infective endocarditis or myocardial infarction with papillary muscle rupture, death from pulmonary edema and shock may result unless there is emergent valve replacement. The murmur of mitral regurgitation is, as expected, holosystolic.

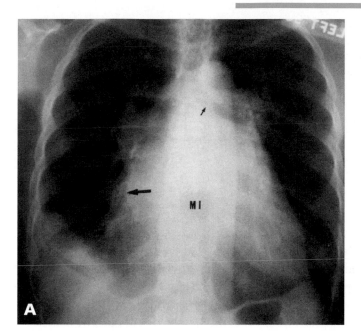

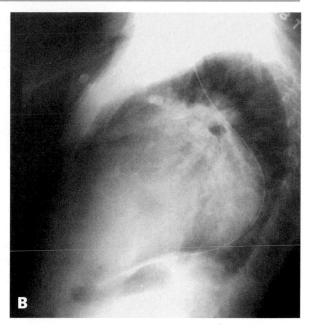

Figure 2–17. **(A)** This frontal chest radiograph from a patient with mitral insufficiency (MI) demonstrates massive left atrial enlargement, with a "double density sign" (arrow) and upward displacement of the left mainstem bronchus (small arrow). **(B)** A lateral chest radiograph in another patient with long-standing rheumatic mitral insufficiency demonstrates dramatic left atrial enlargement, which causes marked posterior displacement of the nasogastric tube within the esophagus.

IMAGING

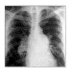 Radiologic findings eventually include left atrial enlargement in all cases, and left ventricular enlargement in some. It should be borne in mind that a chamber must double in size before enlargement is apparent on the chest radiograph. When chamber enlargement is not yet great enough to manifest on the radiograph, signs of mild to moderate pulmonary venous hypertension, such as equalization or cephalization of pulmonary blood flow, may nonetheless manifest. In contrast to mitral valve stenosis, the valve rarely calcifies in mitral insufficiency.

In the chronic form of mitral regurgitation, clinical monitoring focuses on the evaluation of left ventricular function, with treatment of congestive heart failure (CHF). Surgery may be required in some cases.

AORTIC STENOSIS

EPIDEMIOLOGY

The most common causes of aortic stenosis are rheumatic heart disease and congenital bicuspid aortic valve. In advanced age, even tricuspid aortic valves may undergo degeneration. Approximately one-half to three-quarters of patients who develop aortic stenosis from rheumatic heart disease are males. Likewise, approximately three-quarters of the 1% of persons with congenitally bicuspid aortic valves are males. By contrast, degenerative stenosis is seen with equal gender frequency, and is generally less severe.

PATHOPHYSIOLOGY

In the normal subject, the pressures in the left ventricle and aorta at systole are equal. In the patient with aortic stenosis, a pressure gradient develops across the aortic valve. Severe stenosis is usually defined as a valve orifice that measures 0.5 cm^2 or less (normal = 2.5 cm^2). When the pressure gradient reaches 50 mm Hg, the left ventricular demand for oxygen begins to increase precipitously, the chamber hypertrophies, and end-diastolic pressure rises due to the loss of compliance. Eventually, the pressure gradient may exceed 200 mm Hg.

CLINICAL PRESENTATION

Patients develop angina in mid-life without coronary artery disease, syncope (due to decreased systolic volume), and sudden death from ventricular fibrillation. The risk of sudden death is dramatically increased, and life expectancy is typically less than 5 years, when any of the following symptoms develop: angina pectoris, syncope, and dyspnea on exertion or orthopnea. The greater the degree of concurrent coronary artery disease, the earlier the patient with aortic stenosis is likely to present. The murmur of aortic stenosis peaks at mid-systole, and is associated with a *pulsus tardus et parvus* ("late and weak pulse"). If no murmur is heard, then it must be suspected that left ventricular output has declined to the point that flow across the valve is no longer sufficient to produce a murmur.

IMAGING

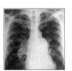

Radiologic findings include a normal heart size, but a more rounded appearance to the left ventricle. In adults, the aortic valve exhibits calcification. Echocardiography demonstrates a narrowed valve orifice and, by Doppler measurement, can be used to estimate the pressure gradient across the valve. In addition, both radiography and ultrasound may demonstrate poststenotic aortic dilatation.

Medical management of aortic stenosis consists of the use of digitalis and diuretics for CHF and the use of nitroglycerin for angina. Operative mortality is significantly reduced if valve replacement is undertaken prior to the development of heart failure, and significant improvement in long-term survival results. If the patient is a poor surgical candidate, transluminal balloon valvuloplasty may be warranted.

AORTIC INSUFFICIENCY

EPIDEMIOLOGY

Causes of aortic insufficiency include rheumatic heart disease, syphilis, connective tissue diseases (such as Marfan's syndrome and ankylosing spondylitis), myxomatous degeneration, and congenitally bicuspid aortic valve. Acute aortic regurgitation, as seen in trauma with aortic dissection or in endocarditis, represents a catastrophe, due to a rapidly progressive increase in end-diastolic pressure, pulmonary edema, and loss of cardiac output. Aortic insufficiency is the earliest of the rheumatic heart disease killers, and many patients become symptomatic before the age of 20 years.

PATHOPHYSIOLOGY

 Hemodynamically, chronic aortic insufficiency is associated with volume overload of the left ventricle, with resultant left ventricular dilatation and peripheral vasodilation. In addition, there is dilatation of the aortic root, which must accommodate an increased systolic volume. Left ventricular failure results from an unfavorable combination of increased cardiac output and oxygen consumption on the one hand (with every contraction, both the normal systolic volume and regurgitant volume must be pumped), and decreased coronary artery perfusion on the other (secondary to decreased aortic pressure during diastole, stemming from aortic dilatation and aortic valvular regurgitation).

CLINICAL PRESENTATION

Patients manifest the consequences of a reduction in peripheral arteriolar tone, in an effort to decrease the back pressure in the systemic arteries contributing to regurgitant flow. The most reliable of these is a very wide pulse pressure, on the order of 180/50. Patients also manifest a descrendo murmur after S_2.

IMAGING

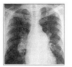 Radiographically, signs include left ventriculomegaly and hypertrophy, with a boot-shaped heart, and a widened ascending aorta. Left atrial enlargement may reflect both diminished left ventricular compliance and concurrent mitral valve disease. If the aorta is markedly widened, a primary aortic pathology such as syphilis or Marfan's syndrome should be suspected. Doppler echocardiography can very easily determine the presence of regurgitation (Fig. 2–18). Valve replacement must be undertaken before severe left ventricular failure occurs.

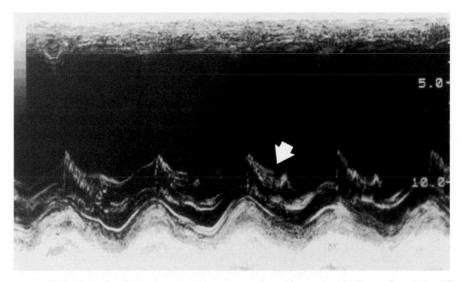

Figure 2–18. This M-mode echocardiogram demonstrates several interesting findings of aortic insufficiency. The thick black band across the middle of the image represents the left ventricular lumen, which is markedly enlarged due to the combination of normal left ventricular output and the large regurgitant volume. In addition, the mitral valve tracing is abnormal (arrow), due to the impact of the regurgitant aortic flow striking a mitral valve leaflet.

Inflammatory

CARDIOMYOPATHY

The term *cardiomyopathy* refers to processes that disrupt cardiac structure, cardiac electrical activity, and cardiac output. Several types of cardiomyopathy are recognized. Dilated cardiomyopathies account for 90% of cases in the United States, and most commonly result from coronary ischemia, toxins such as alcohol, or previous infection (most commonly viral). Patients present with CHF that may be right- or left-sided, and the most common radiographic finding is global cardiomegaly. The ventricles are hypokinetic and exhibit a decreased ejection fraction. Hypertrophic cardiomyopathy is most commonly familial or due to pressure overload. Because portions of the heart muscle thicken but the heart itself may not dilate, nearly 50% of patients may exhibit a normal chest radiograph. Cross-sectional imaging reveals abnormal thickness of the myocardium. Restrictive cardiomyopathy causes diastolic dysfunction (inability to dilate during diastole) and exhibits physiology similar to restrictive pericarditis. Causes include processes that infiltrate and stiffen the myocardium, such as amyloidosis and sarcoidosis. The chest radiograph often demonstrates normal cardiac size with pulmonary venous congestion.

Vascular

CORONARY ARTERY DISEASE

Even though the cardiac chambers are refilled with blood every second or so throughout life, the myocardium requires its own arterial supply, and the heart is in fact the first organ to receive freshly oxygenated blood from the left ventricle. The right and left coronary arteries originate in the right and left coronary sinuses of Valsalva. The right coronary artery (RCA) supplies the right ventricle and the atrioventricular node (in 90% of patients). The left coronary artery (LCA) divides into the anterior descending and circumflex arteries, the former supplying the ventricular septum and the anterior wall of the left ventricle, and the latter supplying the lateral wall of the left ventricle. Patients with the more common right-dominant systems have a posterior descending coronary artery that arises from the RCA, while in left-dominant systems it arises from the LCA. The posterior descending artery and posterolateral branches supply the inferior and inferolateral walls of the left ventricle.

EPIDEMIOLOGY

Coronary artery disease is by far the most common type of heart disease in the world, and constitutes the leading cause of death in the United States. One in every three deaths, a total of approximately 750,000 per year, results from coronary artery disease. By far the most common cause of coronary artery disease is progressive narrowing of the coronary lumen secondary to the formation of atherosclerotic plaques, which may be complicated in the acute setting by thromboembolism. Risk factors for atherosclerosis include cigarette smoking (nearly one out of three adult Americans), hypertension (one out of four adult Americans), and diabetes (16 million afflicted in the United States).

PATHOPHYSIOLOGY

 As the lumen of the coronary artery narrows, its resistance to flow increases, and the flow of blood distal to the diseased segment may be compromised. Fortunately, the coronary blood supply is relatively generous, and a severe degree of stenosis is necessary before lesions become hemodynamically significant. With distal arteriolar dilation and reduction in resistance, adequate flow can be maintained until the cross-sectional area of the lumen is reduced by more than 75%, at which point lesions become capable of causing physiologically significant ischemia. However, during exercise and increased myocardial demand, lesser degrees of attenuation may provoke symptoms and signs of myocardial ischemia.

The cellular pathophysiology of myocardial ischemia helps to explain its hemodynamic effects, as well as the use of the electrocardiogram (ECG) and cardiac enzyme levels in its diagnosis. When the flow of blood to the myocardium is reduced, regions of myocardium become hypokinetic due to the lack of cellular energy supplies. If a large enough area is affected, cardiac output may decline, and signs and symptoms of CHF may appear. In addition, cellular membrane pump function and ionic permeabilities are disrupted, changes reflected on the ECG as characteristic ST-segment and T-wave abnormalities, especially ST-segment depression and T-wave inversion. When ischemia progresses to the point of infarction, changes include the appearance of Q waves, ST-segment elevation, and peaked T waves. As myocardial cells die, they release their contents, including various myocardial enzymes, into the systemic circulation. Creatinine kinase peaks within hours, while serum glutamic oxaloacetic transaminase (SGOT) and lactate dehydrogenase (LDH) peak over the first 24 hours. Consequences may include sudden death from arrhythmia (secondary to ischemia in the conducting system), massive heart failure, or papillary muscle rupture.

CLINICAL PRESENTATION

Classic angina pectoris is a distinct type of chest pain that patients locate in the midchest and describe as a squeezing or tightening sensation, often employing a clenched fist to embellish their description. It often radiates into the arm(s) or up to the neck, and typically lasts for a period of seconds to minutes. Generally, chest pain can be described as anginal if it is substernal, is precipitated by exertion, and is promptly relieved with rest or nitroglycerin. When a patient's symptoms fulfill all three criteria, the pain is typical angina; if two of the three, it is called "atypical angina"; if one of the three, it is probably not anginal. While chest pain is an extremely common symptom, it indicates a significant medical problem in only a small percentage of cases. Other common sources of chest pain include anxiety with hyperventilation, esophageal pathology (reflux, spasm), chest wall problems such as costochondritis (Tietze's syndrome) and muscle strain, and pulmonary pathologies (asthma, pneumonia).

IMAGING

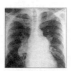 The imaging workup of myocardial ischemia is complex, and this discussion focuses on nuclear medicine imaging. The plain chest radiograph plays a limited role, due to the fact that its high specificity is matched by a relatively low sensitivity. Findings include calcification of the myocardial wall, which indicates previous infarction, and may be accompanied by left ventricular aneurysm (Fig. 2–19). Calcification of the coronary arteries, when seen, is highly specific for hemodynamically significant coronary artery disease, especially in patients under the

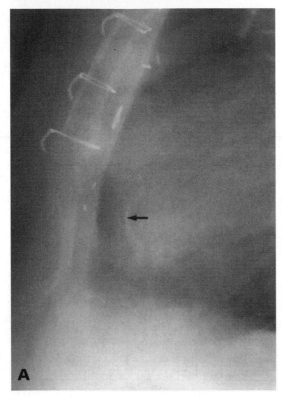

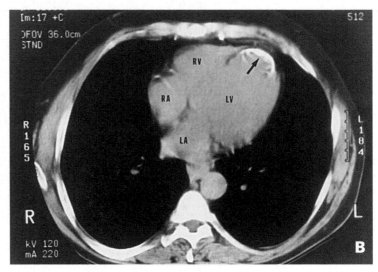

Figure 2–19. A 65-year-old man underwent plain chest radiography and a contrast-enhanced thoracic computed tomography examination to rule out a pulmonary malignancy. (A) A lateral view of the heart demonstrates a subtle rim of calcification along the anterior wall of the left ventricle (arrow). (B) An axial section through the heart with soft tissue windows demonstrates a calcified, rim-like bulge along the anterolateral cardiac border (arrow), which indicates that an old myocardial infarction has produced a true aneurysm of the left ventricle. Such aneurysms are visible on nuclear medicine or angiographic studies as akinetic segments, which represent calcified scar tissue. LA, left atrium; LV, left ventricle; RA, right atrium; RV, right ventricle.

age of 55 years. However, most chest radiographs are exposed at high kVp, meaning that calcifications tend to be "burned out." CT, especially fast CT, is much more sensitive in this regard.

Radioisotope perfusion imaging relies on the availability of tracers whose distribution corresponds to regional blood flow. Previously, thallium-201 chloride was the only commonly used tracer, although now technetium-99m (Tc-99m)-sestamibi is becoming more widely used. Both provide graphic demonstrations of the flow of blood to each portion of the myocardium, allowing the identification of regions of relatively decreased perfusion. This is not, however, equivalent to assessing the flow of blood within each coronary artery, as the development of collaterals may produce a relatively normal-appearing examination in patients with a severely occluded coronary artery branch.

Stress testing, using either exercise or pharmacologic stress, is employed in order to assess perfusion under conditions in which it is most likely to be abnormal. This increases the sensitivity of perfusion imaging for myocardial ischemia. The most common form of exercise testing is a treadmill test, with multiple, graded stages of increased workload according to a modified Bruce protocol. The patient who completes the protocol has exercised at least 9 minutes. The test may be aborted if the patient cannot continue due to fatigue, dyspnea, or severe angina, hypotension, or ECG changes. A common means of determining whether the myocardial workload was adequate is to calculate the "double product," which is the product of the heart rate and blood pressure. Another means is to determine whether the patient achieved 85%

of the maximum predicted heart rate (220–age in years). One would only expect to see a perfusion deficit in a resting patient when the stenosis was greater than 85%. During exercise, however, an artery with more than 50% stenosis cannot respond adequately to the myocardial demand for increased blood supply, and a defect is seen.

Thallium-201 exhibits biologic properties similar to potassium, meaning that, because of the action of the sodium-potassium adenosine triphosphatase (ATPase) pump, injected thallium tends to concentrate inside normally metabolizing cells. A scintigraphic image obtained soon after injection at peak exercise provides a useful "snapshot" of regional perfusion, with necrotic, fibrosed, or ischemic areas appearing as "cold spots" due to the lack of thallium uptake. To further determine whether the hypoperfused tissue is viable or not, a second set of images is acquired, at rest. Unless the stenosis is very severe, areas of viable tissue that are cold on exercise images will "fill in" on resting images. Hence a reversible defect (Fig. 2–20) indicates viable tissue, while an irreversible or fixed defect (Fig. 2–21) typically indicates dead tissue, most often scar.

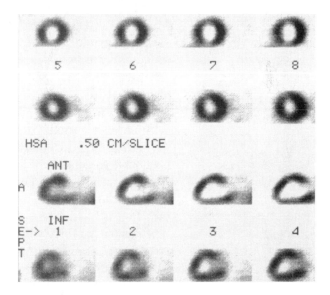

Figure 2–20. These single photon emission computed tomography (SPECT) images were obtained from a myocardial perfusion study using thallium-201 and technetium (Tc)-99m-sestamibi as radiotracers. The top two rows of images were obtained in the short axis, with sections obtained at 5 cm intervals from the heart apex through the base (recall that the apex of the heart is caudal to its base). On these short axis images, the left ventricular myocardium appears as a donut, with the anterior wall of the heart located superiorly, the left lateral wall of the heart on the viewer's right, the inferior wall inferiorly, and the interventricular septum on the viewer's left. The third and fourth rows represent vertical long-axis views, in which the anterior wall is located superiorly, the apex is on the viewer's left, and the inferior wall is inferiorly located. The first and third rows are stress images, which were obtained using Tc-99m-sestamibi. The second and fourth rows are rest images, in which thallium-201 was used. Compare the rest and stress images, to see if there are any perfusion defects on the stress images, and then examine the rest images to determine if they are reversible or irreversible. In this case, there is a defect in the inferior wall on the stress images that fills in completely on the rest images, indicating reversible ischemia. What coronary artery is likely compromised in this patient? Because the defect is in the inferior wall, the stenotic vessel is the right coronary artery. If the lateral wall were involved, we would say that the left circumflex artery was involved, while an anterior defect would indicate left anterior descending artery disease. The finding of a defect on the stress images establishes that coronary ischema is the source of a patient's chest pain. Moreover, reversible defects imply that viable myocardium is present, and that revascularization procedures such as angioplasty or coronary bypass may be of benefit. A fixed defect, on the other hand, may indicate infarcted myocardium, in which case the patient is unlikely to benefit from these procedures.

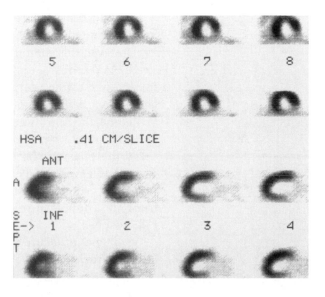

Figure 2–21. This myocardial perfusion study was performed and displayed as described in the previous figure. In this case, note the finding of an irreversible defect in the inferior wall, which most likely represents nonviable, scarred myocardium in the right coronary artery distribution.

COMMON CLINICAL PROBLEMS

Congestive Heart Failure

EPIDEMIOLOGY

CHF is a common clinical problem, and accounts for over 2 million hospital discharge diagnoses each year in the United States.

PATHOPHYSIOLOGY

Heart failure

Simply put, heart failure refers to the heart's inability to meet the body's demands for oxygen and nutrients and the removal of wastes. Failure of a ventricle produces increased back pressure in the vessels proximal to it, with resulting venous congestion—either systemic venous congestion from right heart failure or pulmonary venous congestion from left heart failure. Although there are myriad causes of heart failure, by far the two most common causes are ischemic damage to the myocardium and hypertensive heart disease, due to prolonged pumping against a chronically elevated systemic blood pressure.

When the heart fails, regardless of the cause, its contractility declines. As a result, it is unable to generate the same systolic pressures and stroke volumes it once did. The Frank-Starling curve describes the relationship between end-diastolic volume and stroke volume, and states that the ventricle pumps out the volume of blood with which it is filled. The greater the length to which cardiac muscle fibers are stretched, the greater the force with which they subsequently contract. Hence, filling either ventricle with more blood will cause it to contract more vigorously and eject more blood. The operation of this principle ensures that the outputs of the right and left sides of the heart are equalized, and that increased venous return (as in exercise) is accompanied by increased cardiac output. In heart failure, the Frank-Starling curve is shifted downward and to the right, meaning that the ventricle is able to eject less blood for a given end-diastolic volume (Fig. 2–22).

Early in heart failure, two compensatory mechanisms come in to play. First, the heart's sympathetic tone is reflexively increased, with a resultant increase in contractility. However, this gambit only works in the short term, as the heart becomes progressively less responsive to the increased sympathetic input. Second, the kidneys respond to decreased cardiac output with salt and water retention in an effort to expand circulating blood volume, and thereby increase end-diastolic volume and cardiac output. With time, the heart becomes progressively dilated, as it attempts to operate on a more favorable point on its Frank-Starling curve (longer cardiac muscle fiber length). Eventually, this dilatation becomes manifest on the chest radiograph as cardiomegaly, with such signs as widening of the cardiac silhouette and an increase in the cardiothoracic ratio. However, the chest radiograph is relatively insensitive to cardiomegaly, and the heart must double in volume before cardiomegaly can be reliably detected on routine radiographs.

Two types of failure occur: forward failure and backward failure. Forward failure of the left ventricle results in inadequate systemic perfusion. Backward failure of the left

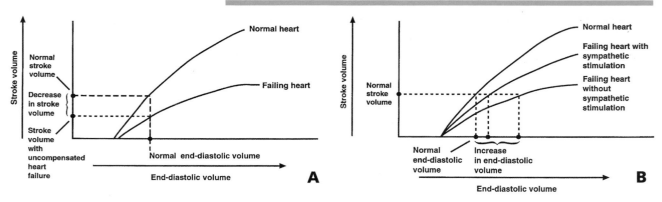

Figure 2–22. (A) The relationship between stroke volume and end-diastolic volume in the normal and failing heart. (B) The mechanisms of physiologic compensation, including sympathetic stimulation (which is only temporarily effective), and further dilatation when sympathetic stimulation ceases to be effective in maintaining cardiac output. These graphs help to explain the development of cardiomegaly in congestive heart failure.

ventricle results in increased pulmonary capillary pressures and an increased workload for the right ventricle; in fact, left heart failure is the most common cause of right heart failure. Accumulation of fluid in the lungs, pulmonary edema, results in decreased gas exchange, with decreased arterial oxygenation and increased carbon dioxide.

With further progression of heart failure, the heart reaches a point at which it is no longer able to pump a normal stroke volume, despite the operation of compensatory mechanisms. For a time, the patient is precariously balanced between adequate function and failure. Often, acute exacerbations of heart failure can be traced to relatively minor inciting events that tip the balance to failure, such as infections (with decreased cardiac function) and acute salt loads, as when a patient consumes a whole pizza containing more than a dozen grams of sodium. Normally, the short-term expansion of circulating volume would exert no deleterious consequences on myocardial function, but when the heart is already stretched to its limit, it cannot compensate for any further increase in end-diastolic volume. Treatment of CHF consists of the restriction of salt intake and the use of drugs such as digitalis, which increase cardiac contractility.

Pulmonary edema

As will be discussed in Chapter 3, the pulmonary capillaries and alveoli are so constructed as to take full advantage of Fick's law, which states that the rate of diffusion is increased as the distance across which it must take place is decreased. The alveolar walls are made up of a single layer of flattened type I pneumocytes, and the pulmonary capillaries surrounding each alveolus are also only one cell-layer thick. These structural characteristics mean that the air in the alveolar sac is separated from the red blood cells in the capillary by only 0.5 μm.

To understand the development of pulmonary edema, it is necessary to understand the Starling forces, which determine the net flow of fluid from the pulmonary capillaries into the pulmonary interstitium and alveolar spaces (Fig. 2–23). Essentially only two forces operate in each direction, the oncotic pressure (related to protein concentration) and the hydrostatic pressure. Like any other substance, water tends to flow from regions of higher concentration or pressure to regions of lower concentration or pressure. The concentration of water, so to speak, is highest in regions of low oncotic pressure (where the concentration of proteins is low).

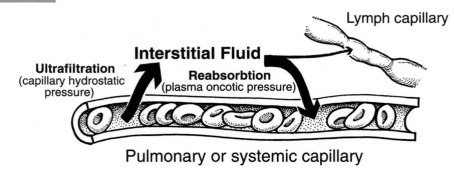

Figure 2–23. The movement of fluid between the pulmonary capillaries and the pulmonary interstitium. The most important force producing ultrafiltration of fluid from the blood into the interstitium is the pulmonary capillary hydrostatic pressure, which is higher at the arteriolar end than at the venular end of the capillary. The most important force returning fluid to the capillary is the plasma oncotic pressure, which remains constant at both ends of the capillary. The shifting balance between these two forces favors exit of fluid from the capillary at the arteriolar end, and reentry of fluid at the venular end. However, the net balance is not perfect, and a small amount of fluid remains in the interstitium, to be taken up and returned to the circulation by the lymphatics.

The plasma hydrostatic pressure is the force exerted on the inner walls of the capillaries by the pumping action of the heart, and amounts to approximately 35 mm Hg at the arterial end of the capillaries, and 15 mm Hg at the venous end. Hence this force tends to drive water from the capillary lumen into the interstitial tissues. The other force tending to move water into the interstitium is the interstitial oncotic pressure, which is normally close to zero, because high molecular weight plasma proteins cannot pass through the capillary membranes into the interstitium.

The other two Starling forces tend to move water in the opposite direction, from the interstitium into the capillary lumen. The plasma oncotic pressure is the result of the presence of high molecular weight plasma proteins, especially albumin, which cannot pass across the capillary membranes from the blood to the interstitial tissues. They keep the water concentration in the intravascular space lower than that in the extravascular space, thus tending to draw water from the interstitium into the blood vessels. The final force is the interstitial hydrostatic pressure, which is normally minimal.

The net Starling forces change as the blood moves from the arteriolar to venular ends of the capillaries, due to the change in the intraluminal hydrostatic pressure. At the arteriolar end, the net filtration pressure equals the sum of the hydrostatic pressure (35 mm Hg) and the osmotic force (–25 mm Hg), which is 10 mm Hg in favor of filtration, the net movement of fluid out of the capillary. By the time the blood reaches the venular end, it has lost 20 mm Hg of hydrostatic pressure, and the sum is –10 mm Hg, favoring absorption. Thus, under normal conditions, there is a nearly perfect balance between the filtration and absorption occurring along the capillary. In fact, however, a small amount of fluid is filtered every day.

Aside from the Starling forces, two other factors are important in determining the amount of fluid that collects in the lungs. The first is the lymphatic drainage of the lung. The lymphatics remove from the pulmonary interstitium the small amount of fluid that would otherwise accumulate there every day. The flow of lymphatic fluid is useful because it facilitates the clearance of minute particulate matter, including foreign material presented to immune cells in the lymph nodes into which lymphatics drain. These lymphatics course centrally within the alveolar and interlobular septae toward the hilum. The second additional factor that may contribute to pulmonary edema is the permeability of the capillary membrane itself. If the membrane becomes more permeable to the diffusion of plasma proteins, then the interstitial oncotic pressure will rise (reducing the concentration of water outside the capillaries), and fluid will tend to accumulate within the lung.

Based on these factors, pulmonary edema may result from any one of four different mechanisms. The first, and by far the most common, is an increase in pulmonary venous hydrostatic pressure, secondary to failure of the left ventricle and "damming up" of blood in the pulmonary capillaries. The second major mechanism is a reduction in the plasma oncotic pressure, with a resultant increase in the plasma concentration of water, and an increased gradient down which fluid tends to diffuse into the interstitium. Some investigators doubt that an isolated reduction in oncotic pressure can cause pulmonary edema by itself, but there is little doubt that it acts as an important cofactor in other conditions, such as left heart failure. Common causes of a reduction in plasma oncotic pressure would include the nephrotic syndrome, with loss of proteins in the urine; hepatic failure, which decreases synthesis of plasma proteins such as albumin; and severe burns, in which proteins are lost through the damaged or absent skin. The third common mechanism is an increase in capillary permeability, as occurs in the acute respiratory distress syndrome (ARDS). Conditions associated with ARDS include septicemia, shock, acute pancreatitis, inhalation injury, and direct chemical injury, as in aspiration or drowning. The fourth mechanism is an obstruction of venous drainage, as might result from the growth of a tumor.

It should be noted that the time course over which alterations in the Starling forces occur is critical in determining whether or not pulmonary edema is likely to result. Given enough time, the pulmonary lymphatics are able to increase their drainage of interstitial fluid several-fold. This explains the fact that patients in chronic CHF may exhibit quite elevated pulmonary venous pressures, yet relatively little or no evidence of pulmonary edema. Even though an increased amount of fluid is being transudated, the lymphatics have been able to increase their capacity over time. On the other hand, the previously healthy patient who suffers an acute myocardial infarction, with acutely increased left ventricular diastolic pressure and resultant increased pulmonary venous pressure, may develop radiographic evidence of pulmonary edema with only a relatively small increase in pulmonary venous pressure. Capillary leak due to release of a myocardial injury factor also plays a role in some of these cases. In the latter case, the pulmonary lymphatics have not been given sufficient time to respond to the increase in interstitial fluid.

CLINICAL PRESENTATION

The most common presenting symptom in CHF is dyspnea. Dyspnea refers to a subjective sensation of difficulty in breathing. It is usually accompanied by tachypnea, an increased respiratory rate, but need not be in every case. Dyspneic patients typically complain that they cannot catch their breath, or that their chest feels tight. A type of dyspnea commonly associated with CHF is orthopnea, dyspnea on assuming the supine posture, due to increased venous return to the failing left ventricle. The actual mechanisms underlying dyspnea have proven difficult to elucidate, but they probably involve abnormal activation of the neural centers of respiration in the brainstem, perhaps from stimulation of receptors in the upper and lower respiratory tracts.

The typical patient with cardiac dyspnea presents with a history of exertional dyspnea, which may eventually progress over years to dyspnea at rest. As we have seen, progressive failure of the left ventricle eventually produces left atrial hypertension. Left atrial hypertension causes pulmonary capillary hypertension, which in turn causes interstitial transudation of fluid, reduced pulmonary compliance, increased airways resistance, and increased work of breathing. The accumulation of fluid within the interstitium and airspaces also increases the distance across which oxygen and carbon dioxide must diffuse, decreasing the efficiency of alveolar gas exchange.

Shortness of breath (SOB) can usually be attributed to one of two fundamental categories of disease, cardiac or pulmonary. This dichotomy is reflected in the legion of requisitions seen in every busy radiology practice bearing the clinical history of "SOB. Pneumonia versus CHF." When a young, previously healthy adult patient presents to the emergency department acutely short of breath, the underlying pathology is almost certainly pulmonary in nature. On the other hand, when a patient with a history of CHF and multiple previous exacerbations presents with stereotypical symptoms, an exacerbation of CHF is the working diagnosis. The distinction between cardiogenic and noncardiogenic pulmonary edema is clinically important, because the usual therapies for CHF are unlikely to be of significant benefit in noncardiogenic pulmonary edema.

Many dyspneic patients prove less easy to categorize as cardiac or pulmonary on clinical grounds, and other clinical evidence must be sought to make this determination. One common difficulty is the fact that cardiac and pulmonary disease frequently coexist. Pulmonary function testing is often employed to determine whether the lungs are the likely culprit, and nuclear medicine and ultrasound are used to evaluate such cardiac parameters as ejection fraction. Blood gas analysis is also often employed. However, one of the most readily available and helpful means of distinguishing between cardiac and pulmonary dyspnea is plain chest radiography, and radiology plays a crucial role in the dyspneic patient.

IMAGING

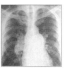 By far the most useful imaging study in suspected CHF is the PA and lateral chest radiograph, which demonstrates such characteristic findings as cardiac enlargement, pulmonary vascular redistribution (equalization or cephalization of pulmonary blood flow), unsharpness of the pulmonary vessels due to interstitial edema, pleural effusions, septal lines, and frank airspace opacities (Fig. 2–24).

Pulmonary edema begins within the interstitium, as the interstitial spaces immediately outside the capillaries become filled with fluid. Signs of edema at this point are subtle, and include loss of definition of the vascular markings (due to accumulation of fluid around the vessel walls), peribronchial cuffing (fluid around bronchi seen on end), and tram tracking (bronchi that appear thickened when seen from the side). Edema within the interstitium itself produces a ground-glass type of opacity, with airspaces surrounded by a very fine network of fluid-filled interstitium. As more fluid accumulates, septal lines begin to appear, which represent the fluid-distended interlobular septae in the periphery of the lung. Eventually, fluid begins to spill over into the alveoli, and fluffy airspace opacities begin to develop. These tend to be located in the mid- and lower lung zones (Fig. 2–25).

As noted in the discussion of valvular heart disease, the chest radiograph provides a reasonable measure of pulmonary venous pressure. At normal pressures less than 12 mm

Figure 2–24. This frontal chest radiograph demonstrates a classic appearance of congestive heart failure, with a marked increase in the cardiothoracic ratio due to multichamber cardiomegaly (arrows), distention of the azygous vein, bilateral pleural effusions with fluid in the minor fissure (white arrow), and bibasilar interstitial edema. A, azygous vein.

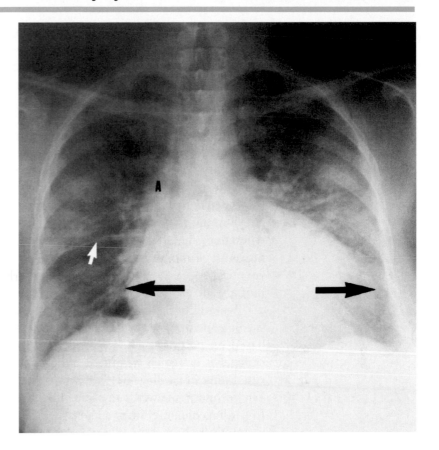

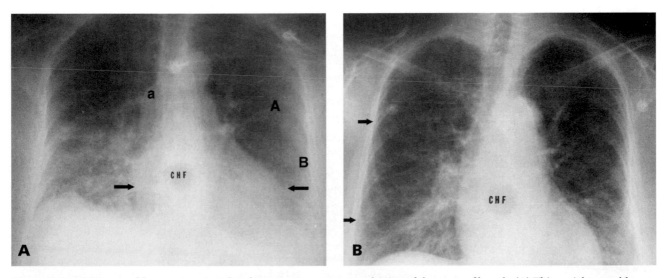

Figure 2–25. A 61-year-old woman presented to the emergency room complaining of shortness of breath. (**A**) This upright portable chest radiograph demonstrates a number of radiographic features of congestive heart failure (CHF), including cardiomegaly (small arrows), distention of the azygous vein (a), Kerley's A-lines (A) and B-lines (B), and diffuse bibasilar interstitial and airspace opacities, more severe on the right than on the left. (**B**) A film from another patient provides a clearer view of Kerley's B-lines (arrows). Kerley's A-lines are the several-centimeter long central linear opacities radiating outward from the central hilar regions. Kerley's B-lines, also known as septal lines, are the finer, shorter linear opacities extending perpendicularly from the peripheral pleura. The A-lines represent fluid accumulating in the central connective tissue septa, while B-lines represent fluid in the peripheral interlobular septa.

Hg, the radiograph is normal. At pressures of 12 to 18 mm Hg, redistribution of flow to the upper zones is the only finding. At pressures of 19 to 25 mm Hg, interstitial edema occurs, with loss of vascular definition, peribronchial cuffing, and septal lines. At pressures above 25 mm Hg, the alveoli begin to fill with fluid, and fluffy airspace opacities result. These findings may be associated with pleural effusion, which probably stems from the diffusion of fluid from congested visceral pleural lymphatics into the pleural space.

Noncardiogenic (nonhydrostatic) pulmonary edema will typically exhibit a quite different appearance from that seen in CHF. It is generally more peripheral, diffuse, and less gravity-dependent than cardiogenic edema (Fig. 2–26). For example, ARDS, which results from the leakage of protein-rich fluid across the pulmonary capillaries, is not associated with cardiomegaly and pulmonary vascular redistribution. Likewise, pleural effusions are not a typical part of ARDS, and the possibility of pneumonia should be entertained in ARDS patients who develop large effusions. Other examples of noncardiogenic pulmonary edema include the neurogenic, high-altitude, and reexpansion varieties (Fig. 2–27). Aside from myocardial ischemia, other causes of cardiogenic pulmonary edema include aortic stenosis, and mitral stenosis and insufficiency.

Two additional, nonradiologic maneuvers are helpful in distinguishing between cardiogenic and noncardiogenic pulmonary edema, both of which are predictable based on pathophysiologic grounds. First, the placement of a pulmonary artery catheter is extremely helpful, as the pulmonary capillary wedge pressure will be elevated only in cardiogenic pulmonary edema (due to increased left atrial pressures). The second maneuver is the transbronchial sampling of edema fluid from the lungs. In cardiogenic pulmonary edema, the fluid is low in protein, while in ARDS, the fluid is protein-rich. It should be noted, however, that the two types of pulmonary edema may coexist in the same patient. For example, a burn patient with ARDS is likely to be aggressively hydrated in an effort to maintain circulating volume, which may produce the distention of mediastinal veins often seen in CHF.

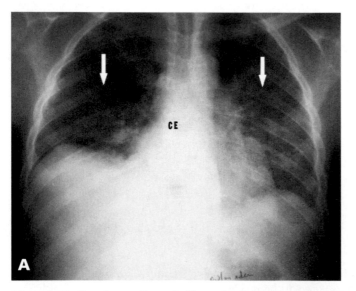
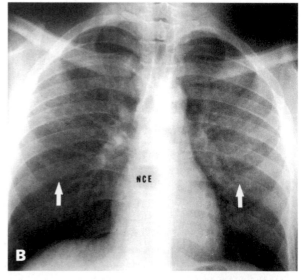

Figure 2–26. Two chest radiographs illustrating the distinction between the hydrostatic and capillary leak forms of pulmonary edema. (A) The first film is from a patient with a history of renal failure and acutely increased left ventricular pressure due to a myocardial infarction, and demonstrates an enlarged cardiac silhouette, enlargement of the azygous vein, and a predominately central and basilar pattern of edema (arrows). CE, cardiogenic edema. (B) The second film is from a patient with a drug-related capillary leak edema, and demonstrates a normal heart size, no azygous distention, and a diffuse, more peripheral and upper edema pattern (arrows). NCE, noncardiogenic edema.

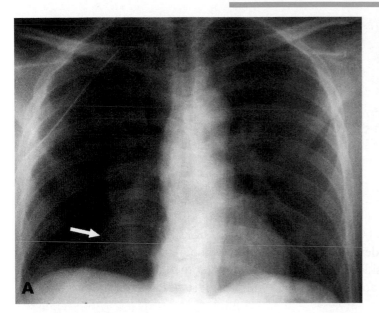
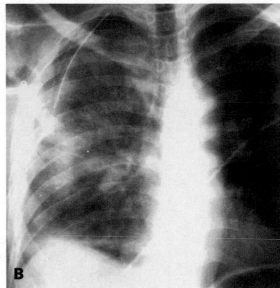

Figure 2–27. This patient suffered complete collapse of the right lung. (A) A frontal chest radiograph demonstrates the collapsed lung around the right hilum (arrow), as well as a chest tube that had not adequately evacuated the pneumothorax and required repositioning. (B) A follow-up film demonstrates reexpansion of the right lung, which is now diffusely edematous—a dramatic example of reexpansion pulmonary edema secondary to a sudden shift in the Starling forces favoring transudation of fluid into the lung.

Pulmonary Embolism

EPIDEMIOLOGY

Thrombosis (from the Latin for "clot") within the deep veins of the leg with embolism (from the Greek for "wedge") of clot to the pulmonary arteries probably occurs more than 600,000 times per year in the United States, and results in nearly 200,000 deaths annually. Many of these patients suffer massive embolism and die before therapy is possible, with 11% of patients dying within 1 hour of the onset of symptoms. However, many more do not die suddenly. In those in whom the diagnosis is made and correct therapy instituted, over 90% survive, while only 70% of undiagnosed patients survive. The accurate diagnosis of PE is therefore extremely important clinically speaking, as tens of thousands of lives may be saved each year across the nation.

Risk factors for PE include immobilization, recent surgery, hypercoagulable state, malignancy, a history of previous deep venous thrombosis (DVT) or PE, and perhaps estrogen therapy. Of note is the fact that these risk factors contribute to the probability of PE by predisposing to DVT. This explains why many high-risk patients (such as older patients undergoing hip or knee prosthetic joint placement) are placed in compression hose and/or given heparin prophylaxis.

PATHOPHYSIOLOGY

The pathophysiology of PE is complex. The vast majority of emboli originate in the deep veins of the legs between the knees and hips (DVT). Emboli originating in right atrial thrombi are rare. Once thrombi have formed, embolized up the vena cava, passed through the

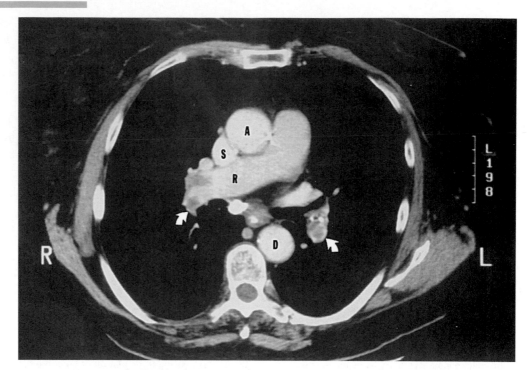

Figure 2–28. This axial image from a contrast-enhanced thoracic computed tomography (CT) scan demonstrates multiple bilateral filling defects within the pulmonary artery branches (arrows), indicating pulmonary embolism (PE). Using helical scanning and bolus contrast infusion, CT is establishing itself as an excellent means of diagnosing PE. A, ascending aorta; D, descending aorta; R, right main pulmonary artery; S, superior vena cava.

right heart, and lodged in the pulmonary arteries, several outcomes are possible (Fig. 2–28). The first, massive embolus (with death in half of cases), results from severe impairment of right ventricular output, with cor pulmonale, distention of neck veins, and hypotension. Another outcome may be pulmonary infarction (in about 10% of cases), in which the bronchial artery component of the lung's dual blood supply is not sufficient to compensate for pulmonary artery obstruction. Most cases of PE result in neither of these outcomes, however, and while the patient may not die during the initial episode, failure to diagnose the condition often results in recurrent and fatal embolism.

PE causes some degree of mismatch between pulmonary ventilation and perfusion (V/Q mismatch), in which portions of the lung are ventilated but not perfused. This produces an immediate widening of the arterial-alveolar PO_2 gradient, with inability to achieve the expected degree of arterial oxygenation on oxygen supplementation, based on blood gas measurement.

CLINICAL PRESENTATION

Patients who do not die suddenly from massive pulmonary emboli typically present with sudden onset of dyspnea. Many patients complain of chest pain. Physical examination often reveals tachypnea and tachycardia. The ECG may demonstrate right ventricular strain or right axis deviation, although nonspecific ST- and T-wave changes are more common. However, the clinical diagnosis of PE is notoriously unreliable, and the first and most crucial step is simply to suspect PE.

IMAGING

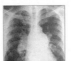

Plain radiography

A not infrequent chest radiographic finding is a normal examination, although a number of nonspecific findings, including atelectasis (due to impaired surfactant production secondary to decreased perfusion), may be seen. A more specific but rare finding is that of the so-called Hampton's hump, a pleural-based opacity pointing toward the heart (corresponding to the "wedge-shaped defect" discussed later) (Fig. 2–29). An even rarer but more specific sign is called "Westermark's sign," and consists of absent or markedly diminished pulmonary vascularity in the affected region.

Lower extremity ultrasound

When the diagnosis is suspected and there is no other obvious etiology, such as a pneumonia on chest X ray, one of two diagnostic courses of action should be consid-

Figure 2–29. A 68-year-old man complained of the abrupt onset of acute right-sided pleuritic chest pain. (A) A chest radiograph demonstrates bilateral, pleural-based, wedge-shaped opacities (arrows) suspicious for "Hampton's humps." (B) An axial computed tomography image of the thorax at the level of the left atrium demonstrates multiple Hampton's humps (arrows) in this patient with angiographically proven pulmonary emboli. Because infarction is present in less than 10% of cases of pulmonary embolism (PE) (only a fraction of which exhibit this sign on plain radiographs), the Hampton's hump is an insensitive but relatively specific sign of PE.

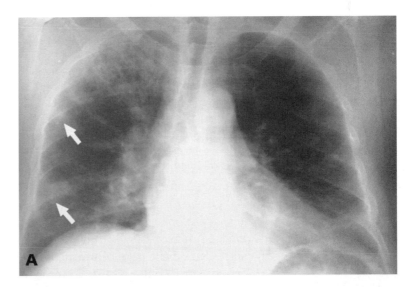

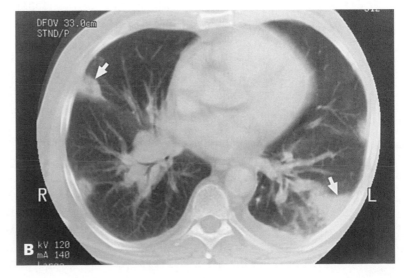

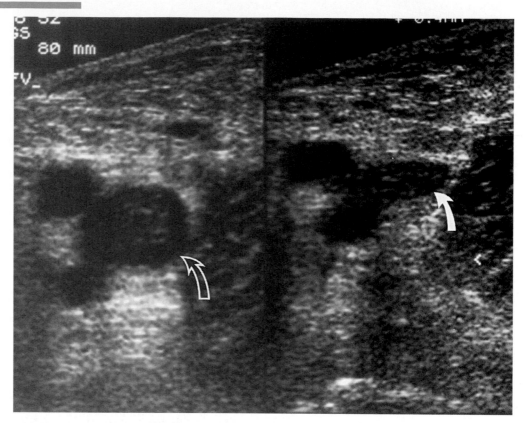

Figure 2–30. This split-screen transverse image of the proximal femoral vessels demonstrates the classic sonographic findings of deep venous thrombosis (DVT). The image on the left was obtained without compression and shows the superficial and deep femoral arteries, with the common femoral vein (CFV) (open arrow) in between. Note the presence of echogenic material, representing thrombus, within the CFV. The image on the right, obtained with transducer-applied compression of the vessels, shows that the CFV is incompletely compressible (arrow), indicating DVT.

ered. In many patients, pulmonary symptoms are mild or nonexistent, and DVT is suspected on the basis of unilateral lower extremity swelling, erythema, or a palpable venous cord. In these cases, lower extremity duplex Doppler imaging is the study of choice, focusing on the superficial femoral vein between the inguinal ligament and the knee. A normal vein is thin walled, completely compressible (pressure applied with the transducer causes complete apposition of the far and near walls), and the vessel lumen is anechoic on gray-scale images and fills completely with color flow. However, when a clot is present, the vessel wall may be thickened or irregular, the lumen may demonstrate internal echoes, and most importantly, the vessel is incompletely compressible and does not fill from wall to wall with color flow (because of the presence of internal thrombus) (Fig. 2–30). When lack of compressibility or incomplete color flow is demonstrated, DVT therapy is warranted.

Ventilation/perfusion scan

If the patient exhibits more than minimal pulmonary symptoms and signs, the study of choice is a nuclear medicine ventilation/perfusion lung scan (V/Q scan).

The rationale behind the V/Q scan is straightforward. If there is a clinically significant PE, a segmental region of diminished or absent perfusion should be detectable (segmental because the pulmonary parenchyma is supplied by segmental arteries; this is not to say, however, that the perfusion deficit could not be lobar or even involve an entire lung in the case of a "saddle" embolus obstructing the left or right main pulmonary artery). If there is no segmental perfusion defect, the patient does not have PE. If there is a perfusion defect, a diagnosis of PE is possible, but must be confirmed by an assessment of the ventilation of that portion of the lung. If the perfusion defect is due to underlying lung disease (with outright destruction of capillaries as in emphysema of necrotizing pneumonia, or with airspace disease and decreased perfusion due to a hypoxia-stimulated autoregulatory response), then the ventilation will be abnormal in that region as well. A "classic" PE, then, is an "unmatched" perfusion defect; that is, a perfusion defect without associated ventilation defect (Fig. 2–31).

However, it must be noted that PE with infarction (producing hemorrhage and/or atelectasis) will demonstrate a matched defect, as will processes such as pneumonia or focal edema. In these cases, however, the chest radiograph will demonstrate nonspecific consolidation. Hence, whenever the chest radiograph shows a region of consoli-

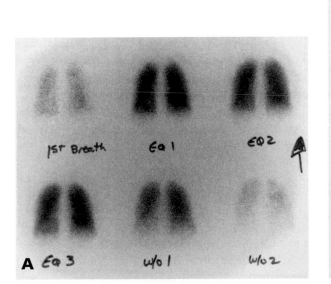
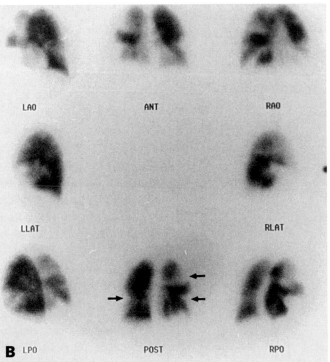

Figure 2–31. A 59-year-old human immunodeficiency virus-positive man presented to the emergency department severely short of breath and tachypneic. The chest radiograph provided no explanation for the patient's symptoms, and a ventilation/perfusion lung scan was requested to rule out pulmonary embolism (PE). **(A)** Ventilation images demonstrate normal radiotracer distribution on the single breath, equilibrium, and washout images. **(B)** However, perfusion images obtained in the standard projections demonstrate multiple bilateral wedge-shaped perfusion defects (arrows), indicating a high probability of acute PE. No further imaging is required in such situations, and the patient was placed immediately on anticoagulant therapy.

dation, the V/Q scan cannot be expected to provide definitive information about that region. This is why a V/Q scan should never be ordered or interpreted in the absence of a current chest radiograph.

Pulmonary perfusion is assessed by means of the injection of Tc-99m-labeled macroaggregated albumin into a peripheral vein. Approximately 500,000 particles are injected, and these travel through the heart, out the pulmonary outflow tract, and into the pulmonary arterioles, where they become lodged. In other words, the most commonly employed diagnostic test in the evaluation of PE involves the intentional production of PE! However, this apparently large number of particles actually embolizes only approximately 1 of every 1000 pulmonary capillaries, and thus the hemodynamic effect, even in the most critically ill patients, is negligible. In rare cases in which a right-to-left shunt exists (raising the possibility of cerebral embolization), or when the patient suffers severe pulmonary hypertension, the number of particles may be reduced. Images are obtained in multiple projections by placing the patient in front of a scintillation detector and recording the number and location of the radioisotope emissions from the thorax.

Ventilation scanning is most often performed using xenon-133 gas, although Tc-99m-DTPA aerosol is used instead in many centers. Imaging consists of inhalation, rebreathing, and "washout" phases obtained over several minutes, usually in a single posterior projection. While ideally the perfusion images would be performed first to determine if there is a perfusion deficit (if not, the diagnosis of PE is already excluded), the ventilation portion is usually performed first because the higher-energy emissions from the Tc-99m used in the perfusion study would interfere with detection of the xenon-133 emissions.

Broadly speaking, the results of V/Q scans are reported according to four classifications. A normal scan means that no suspicious perfusion defects were detected, and effectively rules out PE. A low probability scan consists of perfusion defects unlikely to represent emboli, such as small defects, nonsegmental abnormalities, or larger, matched defects of the sort expected in chronic obstructive pulmonary disease (COPD) (with delayed washout of tracer on ventilation images), and is traditionally believed to be associated with a 10 to 15% incidence of PE. A high probability scan consists of multiple unmatched, segmental perfusion defects, with no other likely etiology than PE, and is associated with at least an 85% incidence of PE. Intermediate (or indeterminate) probability scans include those in which there is extensive pulmonary consolidation or COPD, both of which compromise the specificity of the scan, as well as cases in which there is only a single defect.

Pulmonary angiography

The "gold standard" for diagnosing PE is the pulmonary angiogram. This study involves passing a catheter from a peripheral vein (typically the common femoral vein) through the right side of the heart and into the pulmonary outflow tract under fluoroscopic guidance, with selective catheterization of either the right or left pulmonary artery. Iodinated contrast material is then injected, and multiple rapid-sequence X-ray images are obtained. Relative contraindications to pulmonary angiography include severe pulmonary hypertension, left bundle branch block (because conduction through the right branch may be temporarily disturbed as the catheter passes through the right ventricle, producing complete heart block), and a history of

Figure 2–32. This "black bone" digital image from a pulmonary angiogram demonstrates intraluminal filling defects (arrows) within the proximal branches of the right pulmonary artery, yielding a diagnosis of pulmonary thromboembolism.

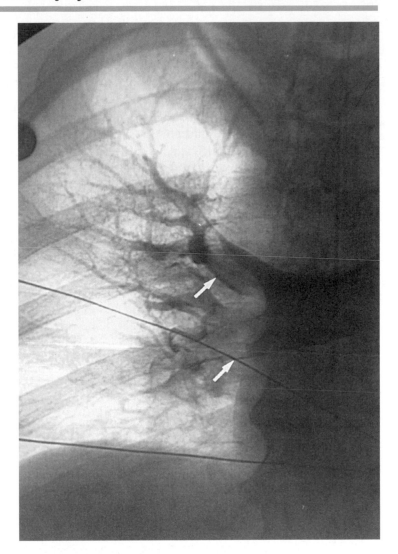

severe contrast reaction. The conclusive sign of PE is the demonstration of an intraluminal filling defect within one of the pulmonary arteries (Fig. 2–32).

Therapy of PE

Treatment of PE may consist of surgical thrombectomy or intravascular thrombolytic therapy, but these are rarely utilized in most centers. The strategy of therapy in most cases is the use of anticoagulants to prevent clot propagation and recurrence. Effective prophylaxis can be achieved in high-risk patients without symptoms or signs through low-dose subcutaneous heparin. Once DVT or PE has occurred, immediate treatment consists of higher doses of heparin, aimed at keeping the partial thromboplastin time 1.5 to 2.0 times control. After the acute stage, patients generally receive at least 3 months of oral coumadin therapy. As previously noted, these steps significantly decrease the risk of death from PE.

In view of the great benefits of anticoagulant therapy, why not simply place all patients with suspected DVT or PE on anticoagulants, without going to the additional effort and expense of lower extremity ultrasound, V/Q scan, or pulmonary angiography? The answer, of course, is that anticoagulation carries a 10 to 20% risk of complications. Patients on heparin therapy may experience bleeding at intravascular insertion sites, in the gastrointestinal (GI) tract or retroperitoneum, or from wounds. Coumadin poses similar risks, and also interacts adversely with a number of other drugs, which may affect its degradation (barbiturates), absorption (cholestyramine), or metabolism (disulfuram), or simply increase the risk of hemorrhage through other mechanisms of anticoagulant function (aspirin). The principal contraindications to anticoagulant therapy are a history of significant hemorrhage, as from a central nervous system (CNS) or GI source, and recent major surgery. Inability to obtain adequate anticoagulation, as in a noncompliant patient, is another not uncommon problem.

What can be done in the patient with documented DVT or PE, in whom anticoagulation is contraindicated or cannot be achieved? In these cases, percutaneous placement of an inferior vena cava (IVC) filter in the angiography suite may be warranted, which can be performed through the same puncture site immediately after pulmonary angiography. The collapsed, net-like filter is placed into the infrarenal IVC, where it is allowed to expand and engage the walls of the vein. Thus positioned, it traps emboli originating in the legs and pelvis, preventing them from reaching the heart and lungs. Once trapped, the emboli are usually lysed by intrinsic thrombolytic mechanisms.

AORTA

Anatomy and Physiology

The thoracic aorta may be divided anatomically into three sections. The most proximal is the ascending aorta, which extends from the aortic root to a point immediately proximal to the (right) brachiocephalic artery, and includes the sinuses of Valsalva and the right and left coronary arteries. The next portion is the arch, which gives rise to the brachiocephalic artery (giving rise to the right subclavian and common carotid arteries), the left common carotid and subclavian arteries, and terminates at the ligamentum arteriosum. The third portion is the descending aorta, which extends down to the diaphragm.

The thoracic aorta serves two important physiologic functions. First, it serves as the conduit for the entire output of the left ventricle. Second, its elastic recoil enables it to serve as a pressure reservoir, storing the kinetic energy of systolic ejection, then releasing it during diastole, thereby ensuring that the blood pressure never drops to zero, and maintaining forward flow of blood throughout the cardiac cycle. This is especially important with respect to the heart's own blood supply; the tension within the myocardium during systole prevents significant coronary artery blood flow during that phase of the cardiac cycle, and the energy stored in the aorta's elastic walls propels blood to the left ventricle during diastole.

Pathology

While numerous disease processes may affect the aorta, three merit attention here: aneurysm, dissection, and trauma.

ANEURYSM

EPIDEMIOLOGY

The vast majority of aortic aneurysms in the United States are atherosclerotic, related to the high prevalence of tobacco use, hypertension, diabetes, and atherogenic diet. Other types of aneurysms include traumatic (secondary to penetrating trauma or deceleration injury), mycotic, and syphilitic.

PATHOPHYSIOLOGY

 Pathologically, there are two types of aneurysms. A true aneurysm involves all three layers of the vessel wall (intima, media, and adventitia), while a false aneurysm consists of a rupture of the vessel wall, with the hemorrhage contained by the adventitia (Fig. 2–33). Morphologically, aneurysms may be described as fusiform (circumferential dilation) or saccular (eccentric outpouching).

The treatment of thoracic aortic aneurysms consists primarily of antihypertensive medications. If the patient is symptomatic, there has been a rapid increase in size, or the aorta is greater than 6 cm in diameter, surgical resection and vascular grafting are often performed. Why are large aneurysms more worrisome? The answer hinges on the law of Laplace, which states that the tension in the wall of a vessel is proportional to the transmural pressure multiplied by the radius. Assuming the mean arterial pressure remains constant, the tension in the wall, which is the force that will cause rupture, increases in direct relation to the radius. Hence, the larger the diameter of an aneurysm, the more likely it is to rupture. A 6-cm aneurysmal segment of aorta has twice the wall tension of a healthy 3-cm segment.

CLINICAL PRESENTATION

Most patients with thoracic aortic aneurysms are asymptomatic, but a small minority will present with symptoms such as deep, diffuse chest pain, hoarseness, and even

True aneurysm   False aneurysm

Figure 2–33. The morphologic distinction between a true aneurysm (left) and a false aneurysm (right). Note that the true aneurysm involves an outward bulge in all three layers of the vessel wall, while the false aneurysm consists of a rupture of the vessel wall, with the hemorrhage contained by the adventitia.

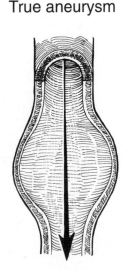

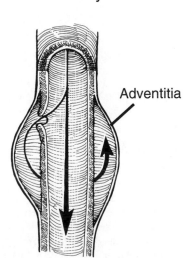

Adventitia

hemoptysis or hematemesis (secondary to communication with the tracheobronchial tree or esophagus).

IMAGING

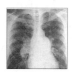

A number of radiologic modalities are useful in assessing for the presence of an aortic aneurysm. Patients with atherosclerotic aneurysms typically demonstrate plain radiographic signs of advanced atherosclerosis, including enlargement of the aortic silhouette, and tortuosity and calcification of the aorta and other arteries, including the coronary arteries (Fig. 2–34). Enlargement of the aorta or a change in its contour can be assessed by comparison to previous films (Fig. 2–35). Angiography is the traditional mainstay of aneurysm assessment, although the contrast column will trace out only the patent portion of the lumen, thus underestimating the diameter of a thrombus-containing vessel. CT provides a better estimate of vessel diameter, as well as the character of any thrombus. A nontraumatic aneurysm rarely ruptures if its diameter is less than 5 cm. Signs of rupture by CT include a sudden increase in the size of the aorta, the appearance of a pleural effusion (hemothorax), or the presence of a high-attenuation hematoma around the aorta. MRI provides a similar assessment to that of CT, but requires no intravascular contrast (Fig. 2–36).

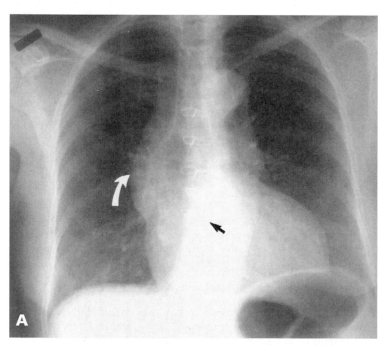

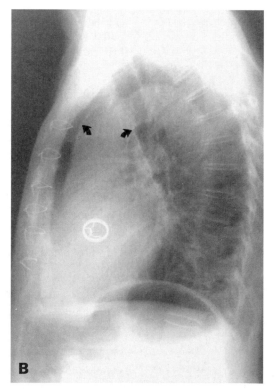

Figure 2–34. A 69-year-old woman presented for routine chest radiography. (A) The posteroanterior chest radiograph demonstrates probable enlargement of the ascending aorta (white arrow) and a prosthetic aortic valve (black arrow). (B) The lateral view confirms a fusiform aneurysm of the ascending aorta with calcified walls (arrows), measuring approximately 5 cm in diameter. The prosthetic aortic valve is reidentified, positioned at the junction of the left ventricular outflow tract and the aneurysmal ascending aorta. Likely etiologies of an ascending aortic aneurysm include atherosclerosis, syphilis, and connective tissue diseases such as Marfan's syndrome.

Figure 2–35. A 70-year-old woman who presented with back pain underwent a lumbar spine series. While mild degenerative changes are visible at multiple levels, the most remarkable finding is a calcified abdominal aortic aneurysm, which measures 5.5 cm in maximal diameter (arrow). The possibility of processes such as dissection and rupture cannot be ruled out on the basis of this film, and further evaluation with computed tomography (CT) or ultrasound generally warrants consideration. In this case, no additional pathology was detected on CT (not shown), and the patient declined surgical repair. She is being followed for complications with annual ultrasound examinations.

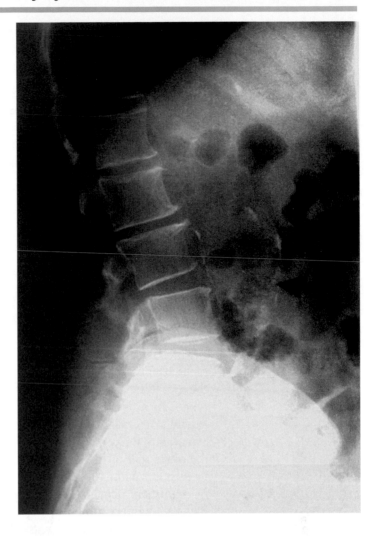

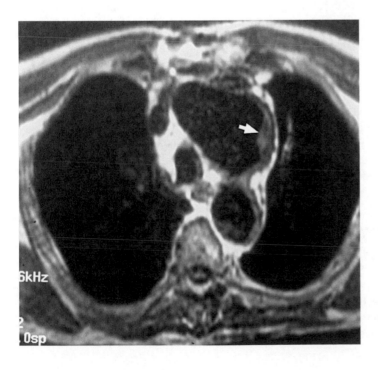

Figure 2–36. A 73-year-old man presented with dysphagia and underwent a barium esophagram (not shown), which demonstrated extrinsic pressure on the esophagus from a thoracic aneurysm. A contrast-enhanced computed tomography examination was requested, but was not performed because of the patient's elevated creatinine and the risk of contrast-induced renal failure. Instead, magnetic resonance imaging was performed. An axial spin echo ("black blood") image at the level of the aortic arch demonstrates a 5 cm saccular aneurysm of the aortic arch, which contains a small amount of mural thrombus (arrow). Aneurysms of more than 5 cm in diameter are at increased risk of rupture, which may extend into the pericardial sac and produce pericardial tamponade.

DISSECTION

EPIDEMIOLOGY

Aortic dissection is most common in hypertensive men in the sixth and seventh decades of life. Other risk factors include connective tissue disorders such as Marfan's syndrome, coarctation of the aorta, and bicuspid aortic valve. Marfan's syndrome is related to an autosomal-dominant defect in connective tissue protein synthesis, resulting in an abnormal arterial media, and is associated with such physical examination findings as large height, asthenic build, scoliosis, and ectopia lentis. Untreated, patients are at very high risk of premature death from valvular insufficiency and aortic dissection, typically involving the ascending aorta.

PATHOPHYSIOLOGY

 Aortic dissection involves disruption of the aortic intima and dissection of blood into the media, where it often tracks longitudinally within the vessel wall. This creates two "lumens": a true lumen through which blood continues to flow, and a false lumen within the vessel wall, which expands to some degree and tends to occlude flow. Dissections are classified into two types according to the Stanford system: A and B. A type A dissection involves at least the ascending aorta, and a type B involves only the descending aorta (Fig. 2–37). The type A form is the most dangerous, because of three potential complications: it may extend proximally to involve the aortic root, causing acute aortic insufficiency; it may extend into the coronary arteries, compromising cardiac perfusion; and it may rupture the outer wall of the false lumen, causing hemopericardium and cardiac tamponade or even exsanguination.

Treatment depends on the type of dissection. The type B form is usually treated medically, with control of hypertension utilizing a combination of nitroprusside and a beta-blocker, aiming to decrease the shear stress on the vessel. Type A dissections are typically treated surgically, which may be performed emergently if the patient cannot be stabilized medically. Signs of stabilization include resolution of pain and lack of radiographic evidence of dissection propagation.

CLINICAL PRESENTATION

Acute aortic dissection is typically heralded by the onset of severe, "tearing" chest pain, and may be accompanied by symptoms of the various complications, such as myocardial infarction, stroke (if the dissection compromises the carotid or vertebral arteries), and dyspnea (from acute aortic regurgitation).

IMAGING

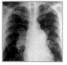 The radiologic evaluation begins with the plain film, which again may show aortomegaly, a disparity in the sizes of the ascending and descending portions of the aorta, a new left pleural effusion, and a change in the position of preexisting intimal calcifications due to the accumulation of blood within the vessel wall. CT is a relatively quick and noninvasive examination that will often demonstrate the intimal flap, the extent of the tear in the vessel wall, and the presence or absence of extravasation (Fig. 2–38). MRI provides multiplanar imaging

Figure 2–37. A 67-year-old hypertensive man presented to the emergency room with severe tearing chest pain. He was hemodynamically stable, and a contrast-enhanced thoracic computed tomography examination was ordered to rule out an aortic dissection. (A) An axial image from that study at the level of the ascending aorta reveals an intimal flap in both the ascending and descending portions of the aorta (arrows), indicating a type A dissection. (B) A subsequent gradient refocused magnetic resonance image ("bright blood") at a higher level reveals extension of the dissection into the great vessels, with intimal flaps visible in the right brachiocephalic artery, and the left common carotid and subclavian arteries. The patient immediately underwent surgical placement of a prosthetic aortic valve and aortic root. b, right brachiocephalic artery; c, left common carotid artery; s, left subclavian artery.

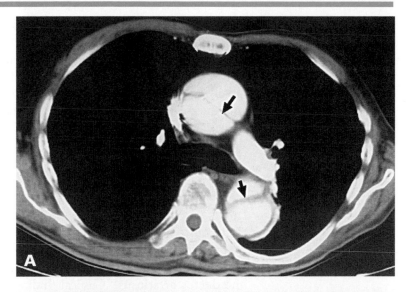

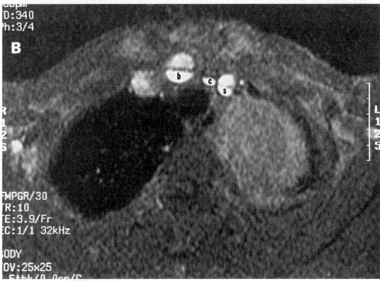

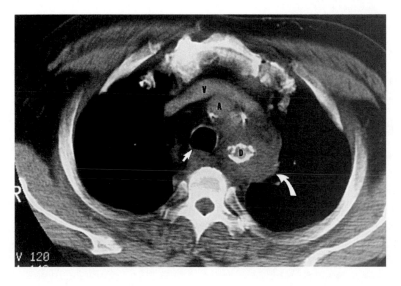

Figure 2–38. A middle-aged man with a long history of diabetic vasculopathy presented with severe chest pain. A contrast-enhanced thoracic computed tomography exam was obtained to evaluate a possible aortic dissection. An axial image just below the level of the aortic arch demonstrates the markedly calcified intima of the descending aorta, which is surrounded by abnormal soft tissue density (curved arrow). While in other clinical settings this finding might represent a tumor or adenopathy, in this case it indicated the presence of aortic extravasation. The straight arrow indicates the air-containing trachea. A, ascending aorta; D, descending aorta; V, left brachiocephalic vein.

capability, but is less appropriate in most acute situations. Transesophageal echocardiography can be performed at the bedside, and constitutes the most commonly employed technique at many institutions. Angiography remains the gold standard, because the precise entry site and extent of the false lumen can be identified, the involvement of the aortic branches, including the coronary arteries, can be assessed, and the aortic valve itself can be evaluated.

TRAUMA

The sequelae of thoracic trauma include both aortic aneurysm and dissection, which have been discussed. Other aortic sequelae include transection and laceration, which are fatal in more than 90% of cases. Except in cases of penetrating trauma, where the mechanism of injury is obvious, it is thought that most injuries result from "pinching" of the aorta between the anterior chest wall and the vertebral column, which explains the relatively high percentage of injuries at the ligamentum arteriosum (remnant of the ductus arteriosus). Clinical findings in aortic injury include asymmetric upper extremity pulses, a disparity between upper and lower extremity blood pressures, chest pain, and dyspnea.

Radiologic findings include those previously mentioned for aneurysm and dissection. Caution is warranted in the interpretation of the chest radiograph, as even severe aortic injury may demonstrate no plain radiographic abnormalities. In addition, abnormalities such as widening of the mediastinum may reflect not traumatic rupture of the aorta, but other less serious mediastinal injuries, or may even be iatrogenic, related to central line insertion. However, a high clinical suspicion is warranted in every case, and aortography is the examination of choice. The key findings to be excluded are intimal tear, aneurysm, dissection, and extravasation.

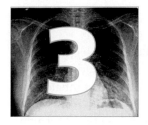

3 The Respiratory System

ANATOMY AND PHYSIOLOGY

The primary function of the respiratory system is to permit gas exchange—the diffusion of oxygen from the atmosphere into the bloodstream, from which it is extracted to support cellular metabolism, and the diffusion of metabolically produced carbon dioxide from the blood into the atmosphere. The respiratory system also performs a number of secondary functions, including moistening inhaled air to prevent alveolar linings from drying out, enhancing venous return to the heart during inspiration, helping to maintain acid-base balance, enabling speech, defending against inhaled foreign matter, and activating a variety of blood-borne materials that pass through it, as in the conversion of angiotensin I to angiotensin II by angiotensin-converting enzyme (ACE) in the pulmonary capillaries.

The upper respiratory tract includes many of the pharyngeal structures discussed in Chapter 4, and functions primarily to conduct air to and from the sites of actual gas exchange. The trachea (from the Latin *trachia,* "windpipe") begins at the larynx in the neck and extends approximately 12 cm to the tracheal bifurcation in the chest (Fig. 3–1). It is surrounded anteriorly and laterally by U-shaped cartilages, which often calcify with age, particularly in elderly women. By far the most common malignancy of the larynx and trachea is squamous cell carcinoma, which is strongly associated with cigarette smoking. Lining the upper respiratory tract are ciliated cells that project into a sticky luminal layer of mucus, which constitute the mucociliary elevator (Fig. 3–2). Particulate matter of a certain size is trapped in this mucus layer and then propelled by ciliary motion upward toward the throat, where it can be expectorated or swallowed.

The mainstem bronchi of each lung arborize into lobar and segmental bronchi, which correspond to pulmonary divisions (Fig. 3–3). The right lung has upper, middle, and lower lobes, while the left lung has an upper lobe (including the lingula) and lower lobe. Each lung is invested by a double-layered serosal membrane, the pleura (Greek, "rib"), made up of inner visceral (Latin, *viscus,* an inner part of the body) and outer parietal (Latin, "wall") layers. The lobes are divided from one another by invaginations of the visceral pleura, called fissures. The right lung contains two fissures: the major fissure, which separates the upper and middle lobes anteriorly from the lower lobe posteriorly, and the minor fissure, which separates the upper lobe from the middle lobe. The left lung contains one fissure, the major fissure, which separates the upper and lower

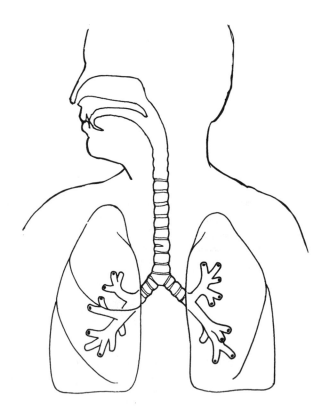

Figure 3–1. Trachea, mainstem bronchi, and segmental bronchial branches.

Figure 3–2. This scanning electron micrograph displays the extensively ciliated surface of the normal bronchiolar mucosa, which is integral to the function of the mucociliary elevator.

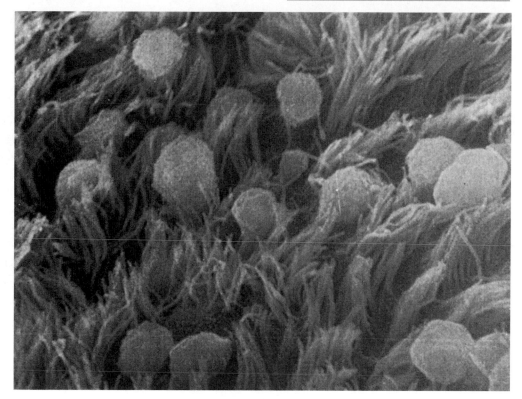

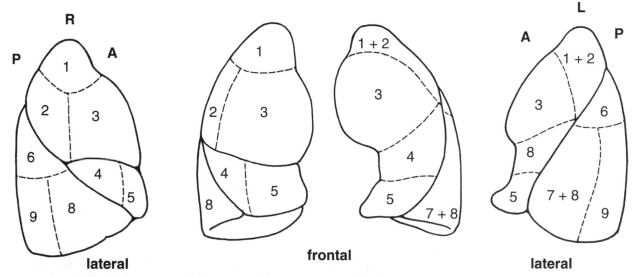

Figure 3–3. The lobar and segmental anatomy of the lung. Upper lobe: 1, apical segment; 2, posterior; 3, anterior. Middle lobe (R) or lingula (L): 4, lateral; 5, medial. Lower lobe: 6, superior; 7, medial basal; 8, anterior basal; 9, lateral basal; 10, posterior basal. Note that the left upper lobe includes the lingula, and in the left lower lobe the anterior and medial basal segments are combined. The posteromedully located posterior basal segment of the lower lobes (10), is not seen on these drawings.

lobes. The fissures are best visualized on lateral radiographs. The lobes are then divided into segments, each of which is supplied by segmental bronchi and vessels.

Clusters of tiny alveolar air sacs are found at the end of each terminal bronchiole, the last purely air-conducting structure of the airways (Fig. 3–4). The acinus (from the Latin, "grape") is a grape cluster-like structure distal to the terminal bronchiole. Each acinus measures approximately 7 mm in diameter and contains approximately 400

Figure 3–4. An alveolus, including type I and type II pneumocytes and the pulmonary capillaries.

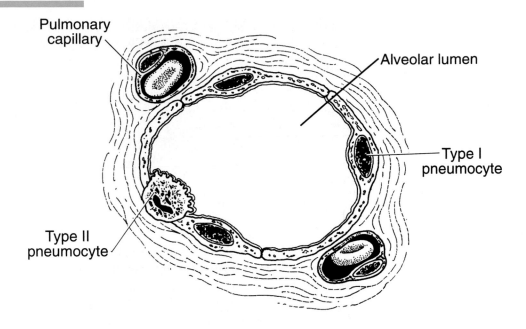

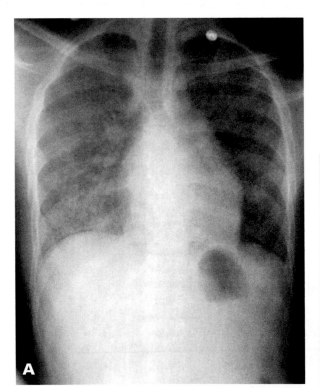

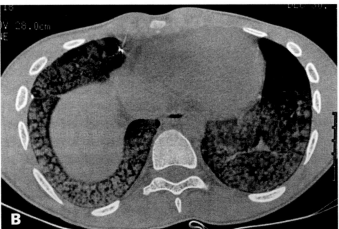

Figure 3–5. A 15-year-old male with a history of idiopathic pulmonary hemorrhage presented to the emergency room with acute hemoptysis and shortness of breath. (A) A portable anteroposterior chest radiograph demonstrates diffuse bilateral alveolar opacities, slightly worse on the right. (B) An axial image from a high-resolution thoracic computed tomography beautifully demonstrates the acinar character of these opacities. Comparing the 1 cm hash marks on the right side of the image, innumerable 7 mm acinar opacities are visible, representing blood-filled acini. Each acinus contains approximately 400 alveoli. The relative sparing of the left upper lobe is perplexing. The two bright foci at the borders of the right middle lobe represent surgical staples from a previous open lung biopsy.

alveoli (Fig. 3–5). Before high-resolution computed tomography (CT), the acini could only be seen on autopsy. With the advent of high-resolution CT, it has become possible to inspect pulmonary subsegmental anatomy during life. High-resolution CT is performed by examining very narrow slices of the lung, approximately 1 to 1.5 mm in width, and utilizing a high spatial frequency reconstruction algorithm. The secondary pulmonary lobule is the elemental pulmonary component visible by high-resolution CT and appears as a polygonal structure measuring 1.5 to 2 cm in diameter. Pulmonary arteries and bronchioles are centrally located within the secondary lobule, while the veins and lymphatics are peripherally located. Each secondary pulmonary lobule contains three to five acini.

There are approximately 300 million alveoli (from the Latin for "hollow cavity") in the lungs (Fig. 3–6). They are adapted to two key physical parameters of diffusion: distance and surface area. The first is Fick's law, which states that the shorter the distance across which diffusion must take place, the more rapidly it occurs. Atmospheric air in the alveolar lumen is separated from erythrocytes in the pulmonary capillaries only by the walls of the alveoli, which consist of a single layer of flattened alveolar cells, and the one cell-thick capillary endothelium, with a total width of only 0.2 μm (a red blood cell is approximately 7 μm in diameter). The alveoli also exploit the principle that the greater the surface area along which diffusion takes place, the more rapid its rate. The total respiratory surface area available for gas exchange in the lungs is approximately 75 m^2 (about the size of a doubles tennis court), but would be only about 0.01 m^2 if the lungs consisted of a single hollow chamber of the same dimensions (Fig. 3–7).

The epithelial cells of the alveoli are of two types, each called pneumocytes, from the Greek, *pneuma-*, "to breathe," and *kytos*, "hollow," from which the combining form *-cyte*, "cell," is derived. Type I pneumocytes are the flattened squamous cells that cover approximately 95% of the alveolar surface area. Type II pneumocytes are cuboidal cells that secrete pulmonary surfactant, the phospholipoprotein complex that reduces the surface tension between water molecules lining the alveoli and thereby prevents alveolar collapse at low lung volumes, as well as reducing the work of breathing by

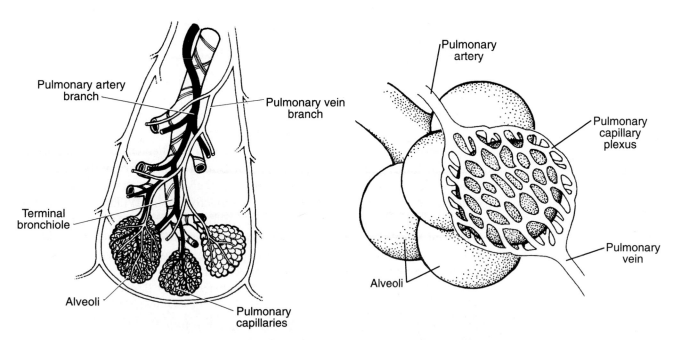

Figure 3–6. The relationship between an alveolus and its capillaries.

Figure 3–7. This light micrograph of the alveolar wall demonstrates the presence of numerous pulmonary capillaries and pneumocyte cell membranes across which gas exchange takes place in the alveoli. Note the erythrocytes within the capillaries. The lumen of the alveolus represents the airspace, and the walls of the alveolus represent the interstitial space.

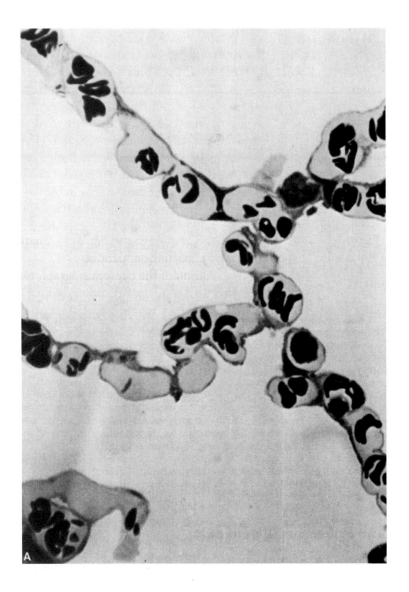

increasing lung compliance. Fortunately, lung compliance is so high that only approximately 3% of energy expenditure is devoted to respiration during quiet breathing. Type II pneumocytes are capable of mitosis and represent the source of type I pneumocytes. Also present within the lumen of the alveoli are alveolar macrophages, which play a defensive role against microbes and particulate matter.

The airspaces are not completely isolated from one another, either functionally or anatomically. Functionally, the condition of one alveolus affects its neighbors through the phenomenon of interdependence. Each alveolus is surrounded by other alveoli, to which it is connected by strands of connective tissue. When any one alveolus starts to collapse, its neighbors are stretched, and their recoil in turn helps to keep the collapsing alveolus inflated. Moreover, there are anatomic channels of collateral air drift between the airways, including the pores of Kohn (interalveolar passages) and canals of Lambert (communications between preterminal bronchioles and alveoli). These communications may prove both beneficial and harmful—beneficial in that they allow collateral air drift behind an area of airway obstruction, but harmful in that they also provide a route of intersegmental dissemination in processes such as lobar pneumonia.

IMAGING MODALITIES

The Chest X Ray

Chest radiography is the most frequently performed radiologic study in the United States, representing approximately 35% of examinations in many hospitals. In certain acute situations, a basic understanding of the chest radiograph may save a patient's life. In the nonacute setting, even basic radiographic findings may profoundly alter patient management. The chest radiograph's ubiquity and clinical value provide both the student and physician who understand it well an opportunity to shine among colleagues and teachers (Fig. 3–8). Figures depicting normal chest radiographic anatomy are found in the appendix.

Although the chest radiograph is routine, it also presents one of the most complex interpretive tasks faced by radiologists and nonradiologists alike; hence, a systematic approach is crucial. The following presents one reasonable algorithm for evaluating the chest radiograph. This preliminary discussion is supplemented in the remainder of the chapter with more detailed discussions of specific pathophysiologic processes and additional imaging modalities.

TECHNICAL FACTORS

The basic chest examination consists of two films, one taken in frontal projection and the other in lateral projection. Frontal chest radiographs come in two principal

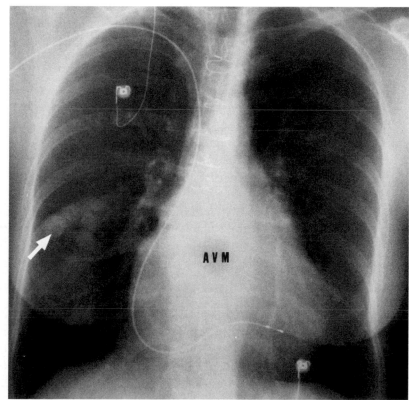

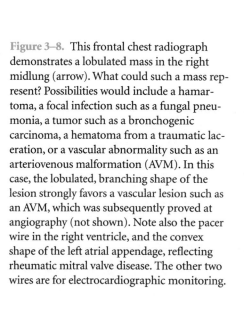

Figure 3–8. This frontal chest radiograph demonstrates a lobulated mass in the right midlung (arrow). What could such a mass represent? Possibilities would include a hamartoma, a focal infection such as a fungal pneumonia, a tumor such as a bronchogenic carcinoma, a hematoma from a traumatic laceration, or a vascular abnormality such as an arteriovenous malformation (AVM). In this case, the lobulated, branching shape of the lesion strongly favors a vascular lesion such as an AVM, which was subsequently proved at angiography (not shown). Note also the pacer wire in the right ventricle, and the convex shape of the left atrial appendage, reflecting rheumatic mitral valve disease. The other two wires are for electrocardiographic monitoring.

varieties, posteroanterior (PA) and anteroposterior (AP). These designations refer to the path taken by the X-ray beam through the patient, with the X-ray film cassette touching the patient's chest in the PA radiograph, and touching the patient's back in the AP radiograph. The PA radiograph is exposed with the patient standing, hands on hips with palms facing backward to rotate the scapulae out of the lung fields, and at maximal inspiration to "spread out" the pulmonary parenchyma as much as possible. If possible, PA and lateral films should be obtained in every patient, because they provide optimal plain radiographic evaluation of the thorax (Fig. 3–9). However, many hospitalized patients are too ill to come to the radiology department and stand for a PA film, and for this reason they must be examined by portable radiography. In this case, a single frontal film is generally obtained in the AP projection, because only the film cassette and not the X-ray tube can be placed under the bed-bound patient. In some hospitals, 50% of chest radiographs are portable examinations.

Four technical factors should be evaluated on every chest radiograph: penetration, rotation, inspiration, and motion. The portable AP radiograph is generally inferior to a standard PA radiograph in each of these respects. Penetration refers to the degree of under- or overexposure of the film. On a properly penetrated film, the intervertebral disk spaces and branching pulmonary vessels should be faintly visible behind the heart. Because the portable film is obtained under less controlled conditions, proper penetration is more difficult to achieve, although new digital techniques available at some institutions may allow correction for under- or overexposure.

When a patient is said to be rotated on a chest radiograph, it means that the patient was facing slightly to the right or to the left when the film was exposed. Rotation is detected as an asymmetry in the distance between the medial margins of the right and left clavicles and the midline, represented by the spinous processes of the vertebral bodies.

Inspiration is assessed by counting the number of posterior ribs visible above the hemidiaphragm, which should number 10 on each side. Bed-bound patients are generally not able to inspire as deeply as ambulatory patients. An underinflated radiograph exaggerates heart size and obscures visualization of the pulmonary parenchyma.

Motion is assessed by noting the sharpness of the hemidiaphragms and pulmonary vessels, which appear blurred if the patient was breathing at the time the film was exposed. Because portable radiography units are generally not as powerful as fixed units, longer exposure times are necessary to adequately expose the film, resulting in greater potential for motion artifact.

Several additional differences between PA and AP chest radiographs deserve mention. One is the magnification of heart size present on AP films, which may be as great as 20%, and may be further exacerbated by underinflation. On a standard PA film, the cardiac silhouette should not comprise more than 50% of the width of the thorax. The heart appears larger on an AP film because, being an anterior thoracic structure, it is farther away from the film, causing it to cast a larger shadow. Many patients with apparent cardiomegaly on portable radiographs will turn out to have normal-size hearts when a PA examination is obtained. Cardiac magnification may also result from anatomic anomalies such as a pectus excavatum deformity (Fig. 3–10).

Another difference is the apparent pulmonary vascular redistribution present on AP films, due to the patient's supine position. On a normal upright film, the lower lung zone pulmonary vessels are approximately three times the diameter of the upper zone vessels, due to gravity-dependent distribution of flow. On supine films, there appears to be pulmonary vascular redistribution, with upper zone vessels equal in size

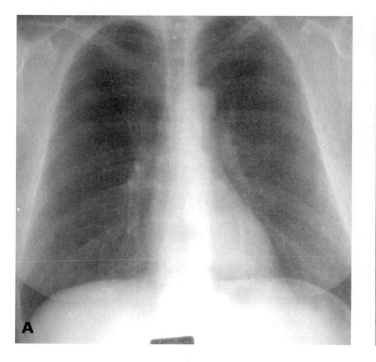

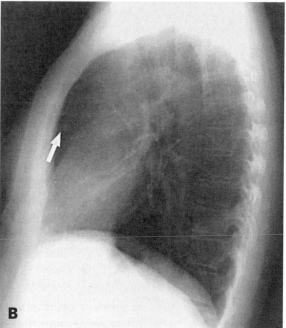

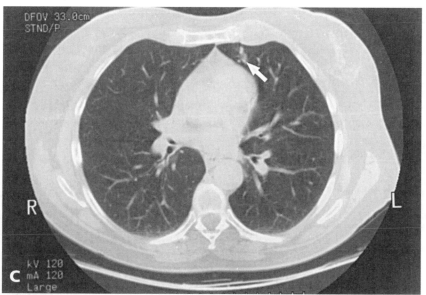

Figure 3–9. A 52-year-old woman presented with a history of persistent cough. (**A**) The posteroanterior chest radiograph reveals no detectable abnormality. (**B**) On the lateral view, however, a 1.5 cm nodule is seen in the retrosternal clear space (arrow), which was shown on computed tomography (**C**) to be located in the medial aspect of the left upper lobe (arrow). Biopsy revealed small cell lung carcinoma. The nodule was not seen on the frontal view because its medial location caused it to be superimposed over the aorta. This case dramatizes the importance of obtaining and carefully inspecting the lateral view. R, right; L, left.

to the lower zone vessels. This erroneously suggests pulmonary venous hypertension, as in congestive heart failure (CHF).

Another difference between upright PA and supine AP films is the relative insensitivity of the latter to pleural effusions and pneumothoraxes. Pleural effusions can be detected in even small amounts as blunting of the costophrenic angles on upright

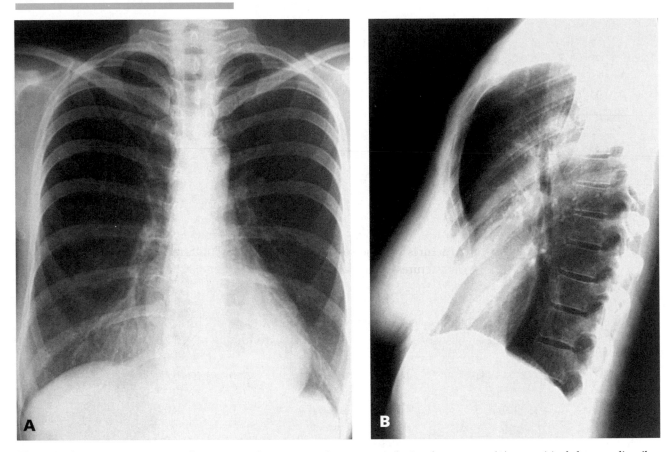

Figure 3–10. This young woman with symptoms of an upper respiratory tract infection demonstrates (**A**) a surprisingly large cardiac silhouette, with a cardiothoracic ratio that measures nearly 0.50, despite the fact that her lungs are well inflated. Note also that the right heart border is somewhat indistinct. (**B**) The lateral view explains why, revealing a prominent pectus excavatum deformity, which flattens the heart.

Figure 3–11. A 68-year-old woman with colon carcinoma complained of abdominal pain and was found to have a tense abdomen. A portable chest radiograph reveals a critical finding—the presence of tiny crescents of gas under each hemidiaphragm, indicating pneumoperitoneum. The patient's colon carcinoma had perforated the bowel wall, and she was taken emergently to surgery. Note also the presence of ill-defined consolidation in the base of the left lung, likely secondary to aspiration.

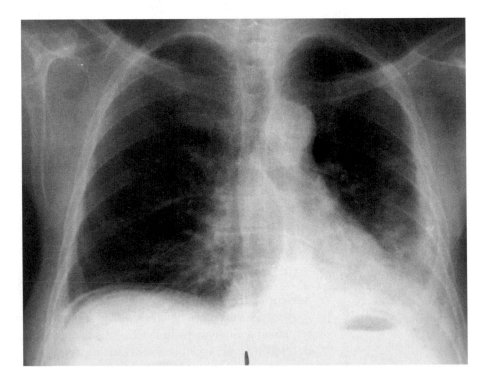

films, but layer out behind the lung on supine films. A small pneumothorax is readily detected on an upright film as an apical separation between the lung and the thoracic wall, but on supine films air within the pleural space tends to spread out along the anterior thoracic wall and is not seen in tangent.

SEARCH PATTERN

A commonly employed approach to the chest radiograph utilizes an "A-B-C" (*a*bdomen-*b*ones-*c*hest) approach. The value of this approach, which puts the chest itself last, is the fact that it ensures that other easily overlooked areas outside the chest are inspected on each film. Key abdominal findings that should be sought out on chest radiographs include pneumoperitoneum, gastrointestinal (GI) dilatation (obstruction), and masses (Fig. 3–11). Inspection of the bones should include not only the osseous structures but the soft tissues as well. Key findings in the osseous structures include rib fractures, vertebral compression fractures, blastic or lytic bone lesions, and evidence of metabolic bone disease, such as hyperparathyroidism. Important findings in the soft tissues would include evidence of a previous mastectomy (missing breast shadow) and calcifications within soft tissue tumors. In children, the portion of the skeleton visualized on the chest radiograph should always be inspected for evidence of child abuse, such as posterior rib fractures.

In order to ensure that easily overlooked structures within the chest are attended to, it is again helpful to save the lungs for last. A good place to begin is the airway. This includes inspection of the trachea and major bronchi for evidence of foreign bodies, displacement, or luminal attenuation (Fig. 3–12). Next the pleural space should be inspected, looking for processes such as pleural effusions, pleural plaques, pleural-based masses, and pneumothorax. The mediastinum should then be carefully evaluated, looking for widening of the paratracheal stripe (which should measure less than 3 to 4 mm), fullness in the AP window and azygoesophageal recess, and bulging of the paraspinal lines. The hila should be then inspected for evidence of fullness and for

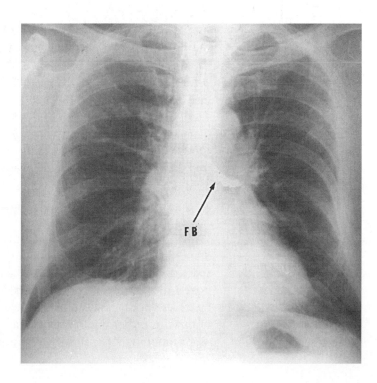

Figure 3–12. This elderly woman presented to the emergency room acutely short of breath. Although the patient had no history of dyspnea, initial clinical suspicion focused on asthma. However, a frontal chest radiograph clearly reveals the cause of the patient's symptoms. In the left mainstem bronchus is a serrated, gently curved foreign body (FB) measuring 1 cm in width and several centimeters in length (arrow). This represented the patient's denture, which she had unknowingly aspirated while eating.

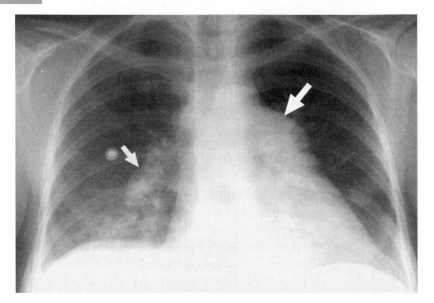

Figure 3–13. A 33-year-old woman who complained of dyspnea on exertion demonstrates striking evidence of pulmonary hypertension, with massive dilatation of the main (large arrow) and right (small arrow) pulmonary arteries and pruning of pulmonary vessels peripherally. The perfectly round opacity in the right midlung is a metallic button on the patient's gown. According to Ohm's law (flow = pressure difference/resistance [I = P/R]), elevated pulmonary arterial pressure may result from an increase in pulmonary blood flow, an increase in pulmonary vascular resistance, or increased left atrial pressure. An example of increased pulmonary blood flow would be a left-to-right shunt, such as a ventricular septal defect. An example of increased pulmonary vascular resistance would be pulmonary embolism. An example of pulmonary venous hypertension would be mitral stenosis. In this case, the patient suffered from mixed connective tissue disease, which had produced increased pulmonary vascular resistance, chronic pulmonary hypertension, and cor pulmonale (right ventricular hypertrophy).

dilatation of the pulmonary arteries (Fig. 3–13). Abnormalities in the mediastinum and hila often indicate the presence of masses or adenopathy. The general shape and size of the heart, as well as the symmetry and distribution of pulmonary perfusion, should always be evaluated (discussed at length in Chapter 2) (Fig. 3–14).

Finally, the lungs themselves should be examined. Key parameters include lung volumes, unilateral differences in density, and the presence of focal or diffuse opacities. Some key findings to exclude on every chest radiograph include pneumothorax, subtle nodules that may represent early lung carcinomas, and small pleural effusions that may provide the only radiographic evidence of pathology such as tuberculosis (TB). Subtle nodules that may be missed are often found in the upper lung zones, in the paramediastinal regions, and "behind" the ribs and clavicles.

PULMONARY PARENCHYMAL PATTERNS

While numerous patterns of pulmonary parenchymal abnormality may be seen, a fundamental distinction to be drawn is that between airspace and interstitial disease. Airspace disease represents filling of the pulmonary acini, the 8 mm respiratory units composed of respiratory bronchioles, alveolar ducts, and alveoli (Fig. 3–15). Airspace opacities appear fluffy and ill-defined and often become confluent to form larger regions of opacity. Other findings in airspace disease include air bronchograms (lucent tubular and branching structures representing aerated bronchi surrounded by opaque acini),

Figure 3–14. A frontal chest radiograph of a 5-year-old girl demonstrates subtle but definite asymmetry in pulmonary perfusion, with far more pulmonary vascular markings on the right than on the left. The differential diagnosis of this finding would include congenital hypogenetic lung syndrome, pulmonary artery occlusion from stenosis or pulmonary embolism, and airway obstruction. In this case, the diagnosis was a pulmonary sling, an aberrant origin of the left pulmonary artery from the right pulmonary artery, with decreased left pulmonary blood flow. Note that the patient is rotated somewhat to the right on this view.

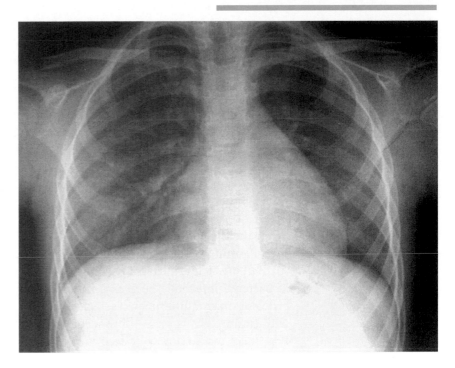

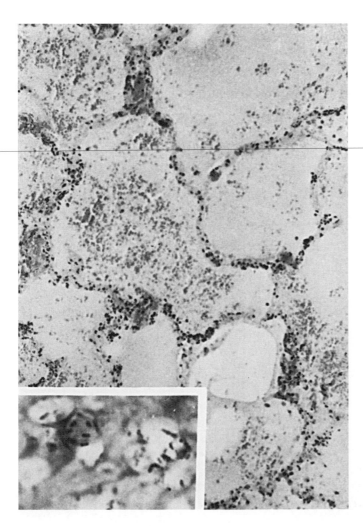

Figure 3–15. This light micrograph (× 300) of the lung demonstrates filling of the airspaces with a combination of edema and hemorrhage in a patient with pneumococcal pneumonia. The inset (× 2000) proves that the edema fluid teems with bacteria.

absence of volume loss (the acini remain filled, with replacement of air by fluid or tissue), and a nonsegmental distribution (pores of Kohn and channels of Lambert allow intersegmental communication). Interstitial disease, on the other hand, tends to produce opacities that can be characterized as reticular (delicate lines of opacity), nodular, reticulonodular, or ground glass (hazy increase in density). It represents the accumulation of fluid or tissue within the pulmonary interstitium, which includes not only the potential space between alveoli but the lymphatics and veins as well. Commonly a parenchymal abnormality is difficult to characterize as distinctly airspace or interstitial, and often some combination of airspace and interstitial opacities is present (Fig. 3–16).

AIRSPACE DISEASE

While the complete differential diagnosis of an airspace pattern of pulmonary opacification is quite lengthy, only five fundamental substances can be responsible for the airspace filling. These include pus, tumor, protein, water, and blood. Pus is seen primarily in bacterial infections, such as pneumococcal pneumonia, although other infectious processes may fill the airspaces, including TB and fungal pneumonias. Alveolar filling with tumor cells is seen in bronchoalveolar carcinoma and lymphoma (Fig. 3–17). Proteinaceous fluid may be seen in the acute respiratory distress syndrome (ARDS), secondary to the leakage of plasma across damaged pulmonary capillary endothelium, or in alveolar proteinosis. Water indicates pulmonary edema, including cardiogenic pulmonary edema (often accompanied by an enlarged cardiac silhouette and other signs of CHF, such as bilateral effusions and pulmonary venous hypertension) and noncardiogenic pulmonary edema, such as volume overload or renal failure (Fig. 3–18). Blood may be due to trauma, bleeding diathesis, infarct, or vasculitis (as in Goodpasture's syndrome) and is a common postmortem finding, presumably due to ischemic hemorrhage.

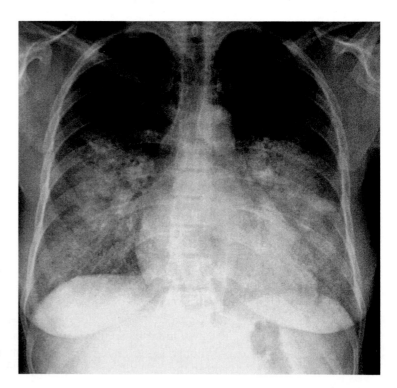

Figure 3–16. A 46-year-old substance-abusing woman presented to the emergency room with a cough productive of blood-tinged sputum. Her chest radiograph reveals diffuse bilateral mixed interstitial and airspace opacities in both mid- and lower lung zones. Such a pattern is not typical for community-acquired pneumonia or edema, and this process was presumed to represent "crack lung," a disorder associated with the use of crack cocaine.

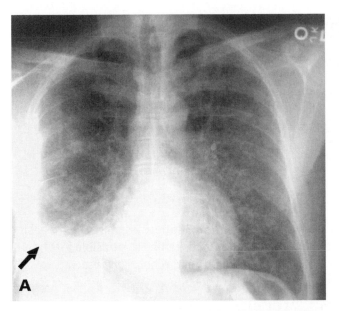

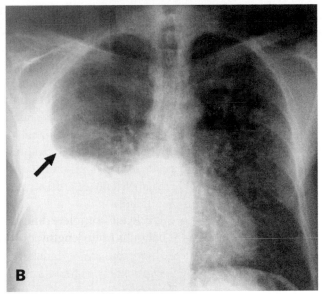

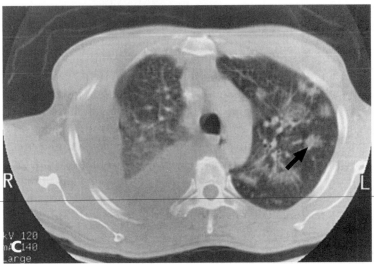

Figure 3–17. (A) A posteroanterior chest radiograph in a 55-year-old man with known bronchoalveolar carcinoma demonstrates multiple bilateral nodular airspace opacities and a right pleural effusion (arrow). (B) A follow-up film several months later demonstrates worsening of the right effusion, which now occupies the caudal half of the right hemithorax (arrow). (C) An axial computed tomography image at the level of the aortic arch displays the multiple focal, ill-defined airspace opacities to better advantage (arrow). Note again the large right pleural effusion. Bronchoalveolar carcinoma is a subtype of adenocarcinoma, which tends to grow slowly and often demonstrates no adenopathy.

INTERSTITIAL DISEASE

While the differential diagnosis of interstitial disease extends to encompass over 100 distinct pathologic processes, most cases can be traced to one of several major categories of disease (Fig. 3–19). Infectious causes of interstitial disease include viruses, mycoplasma, TB, and *Pneumocystis carinii*. Tumor cells may fill the interstitium, as in lymphangitic spread of breast carcinoma. Inflammatory causes include collagen vascular diseases such as rheumatoid arthritis, drugs, and the pneumoconioses. Water within the interstitium generally reflects a less severe degree of pulmonary edema than

Figure 3–18. An anteroposterior chest radiograph of a 30-year-old woman with acute glomerulonephritis demonstrates a classic picture of noncardiogenic pulmonary edema (NCE), with a cardiac silhouette that is not enlarged (given the portable technique), and the presence of bilateral, predominately perihilar ill-defined airspace opacities.

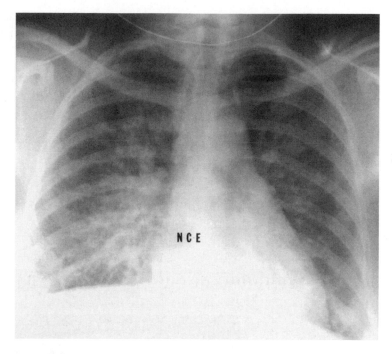

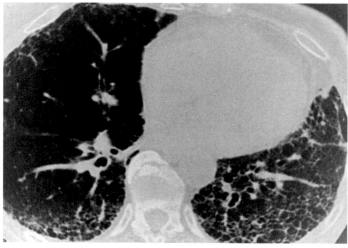

Figure 3–19. This axial image through the lung bases from high-resolution thoracic chest computed tomography demonstrates typical changes of idiopathic pulmonary fibrosis, the result of progressive inflammation and fibrosis of the lung parenchyma of unknown etiology. A number of processes, including collagen vascular diseases, drug toxicities, and inhalational lung diseases can also produce this end-stage appearance of chronic interstitial lung disease. Once the process reaches this stage of "honeycombing" and traction bronchiectasis (from fibrosis), the prognosis tends to be poor, on the order of several years.

that seen in airspace disease, most commonly due to CHF. Some cases of interstitial lung disease are idiopathic, as in idiopathic pulmonary fibrosis.

ATELECTASIS

Atelectasis refers to unaerated lung, which may range in extent from a subsegmental portion of parenchyma to an entire lung, in which case it is more commonly referred to as collapse. Patients with atelectasis will become dyspneic if the degree of underaeration is sufficient to compromise total pulmonary gas exchange. Reasoning pathophysiologically, it is possible to predict all of the types of ateletasis that are seen in clinical practice.

Resorptive atelectasis refers to the collapse of airspaces distal to a bronchial obstruction. Important causes of obstruction in adults include mucus plugs and tumors, especially bronchogenic carcinomas (Fig. 3–20). Mucus plugs are commonly seen in patients with obstructive airways disorders (asthma, chronic bronchitis) and

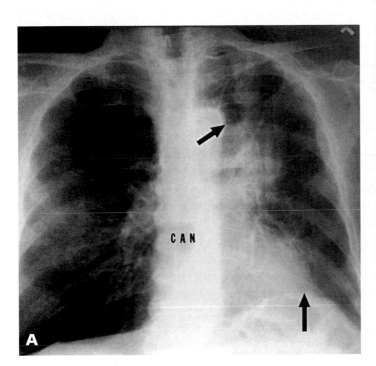

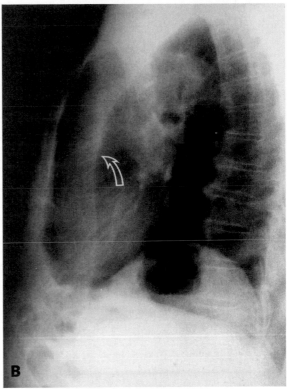

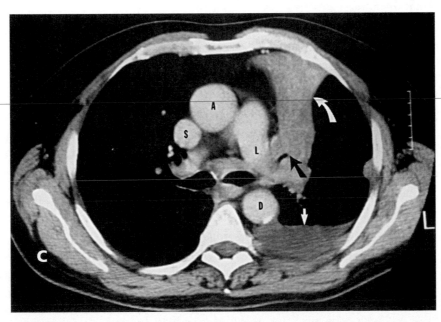

Figure 3–20. A 60-year-old man with a 100 pack-year smoking history complained of a persistent cough. **(A)** An anteroposterior chest radiograph demonstrates multiple indirect signs of left-sided atelectasis, including a relatively small left hemithorax, shift of the heart and mediastinal structures to the left, and elevation of the left hemidiaphragm (large arrow). In addition, there is an ill-defined opacity in the left suprahilar region that is highly suspicious for a mass, likely a bronchogenic carcinoma producing left upper lobe collapse. Note the medial lucency produced by upward migration of the superior segment of the left lower lobe (small arrow). **(B)** The lateral view is confirmatory, demonstrating anterior displacement of the left major fissure (open arrow), a direct sign of lobar collapse. **(C)** An axial image from a thoracic computed tomography scan demonstrates the mass obstructing the left upper lobe bronchus (black arrow), as well as the anteriorly collapsed left upper lobe (curved white arrow), a characteristic pattern. Also note the malignant left pleural effusion (white arrow), as well as the pleural-based metastasis along the lateral aspect of the left thorax. A, ascending aorta; D, descending aorta; L, left pulmonary artery; S, superior vena cava.

patients whose ventilatory function is compromised, rendering them unable to cough (such as patients on mechanical ventilation). How does resorptive atelectasis occur? Regardless of the type of obstructing lesion, once an airway becomes completely occluded, the airspaces distal to it cannot be ventilated (except perhaps by the pores of Kohn and canals of Lambert). Over a period of minutes to hours, the gas in the involved airspaces is taken up by the blood in the pulmonary capillaries. Oxygen is rapidly absorbed, due to the high oxygen affinity of hemoglobin, while nitrogen, which is poorly soluble in plasma, is slowly absorbed. As the gas exits the airspaces, they become progressively smaller and eventually collapse completely. Complete atelectasis of a lobe may occur within minutes in a patient breathing 100% oxygen. In intubated patients, another common cause of resorptive atelectasis is endotracheal tube malposition. For example, if the tip of the tube is located in the right mainstem bronchus, the left lung may receive no ventilation, causing it to collapse.

Passive or relaxation atelectasis occurs as a result of a space-occupying process in the (extrapulmonary) pleural space. The two most common processes are pleural effusion and pneumothorax. Another cause is tumor within the pleural space. One such tumor is malignant mesothelioma, a neoplasm related to asbestos exposure, which often completely encases the lung (Fig. 3–21). In each of these conditions, inward displacement of the visceral pleura away from the chest wall results in decreased lung volume, with a resultant decrease in airspace ventilation. The intrapulmonary counterpart of passive atelectasis is compressive atelectasis, which occurs when lung tissue is compressed by an adjacent intraparenchymal space-occupying lesion. One of the most common etiologies is a large space-occupying bulla in bullous emphysema. Transthoracic bullectomy and lung reduction surgery have become important means of restoring ventilatory function to such patients. Naturally, another cause of compressive atelectasis is a large lung tumor.

Adhesive atelectasis occurs due to loss of pulmonary surfactant, which is produced by type II pneumocytes. The water molecules lining the alveoli tend to exert an attractive effect on one another (surface tension). The effect of these attractive forces would be to increase dramatically the work of inflating the airspaces, were it not for the surfactant's ability to diminish surface tension. Respiratory distress syndrome of the newborn, also called hyaline membrane disease, is perhaps the best known manifestation, caused when an immature lung that has not yet begun producing sufficient quantities of surfactant is forced to take on the task of respiration. Atelectasis in pulmonary embolism (PE) also results in part from a local surfactant deficiency in infarcted lung. One of the most common manifestations of adhesive atelectasis is a "plate-like" linear opacity, representing underinflation or collapse of a subsegmental portion of lung (Fig. 3–22).

Cicatricial atelectasis is exactly what its name implies—the loss of volume in lung tissue produced by pulmonary parenchymal scarring. The most common cause of cicatricial atelectasis is postinfectious, with TB and necrotizing pneumonia being the most prevalent. Another common cause of cicatricial atelectasis is radiation therapy, which actually causes at least two forms of atelectasis. High pulmonary parenchymal doses are commonly seen in the treatment of Hodgkin's disease of the mediastinum and in the treatment of lung carcinomas, particularly small cell carcinoma. In the case of mediastinal irradiation, a characteristic paramediastinal pattern of atelectasis and scarring, paralleling the radiation port, is often seen. In the acute phase of radiation injury, damage to type II pneumocytes causes passive atelectasis. Over the course of the succeeding months, pulmonary scarring and cicatricial atelectasis ensue, probably due to capillary endothelial damage.

The most reliable of the radiographic findings in atelectasis is displacement of one

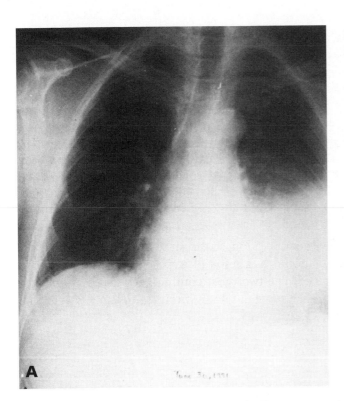
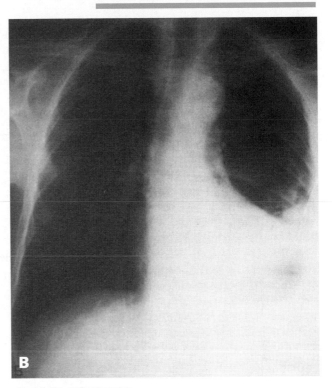

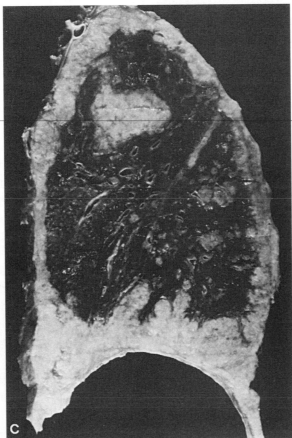

Figure 3–21. (A) The chest X ray of a 49-year-old man with a history of asbestos exposure demonstrates a left pleural effusion. (B) After the effusion was drained, underlying pleural tumor masses were revealed. (C) An autopsy specimen of the same patient demonstrates malignant mesotheolioma completely encasing the lung.

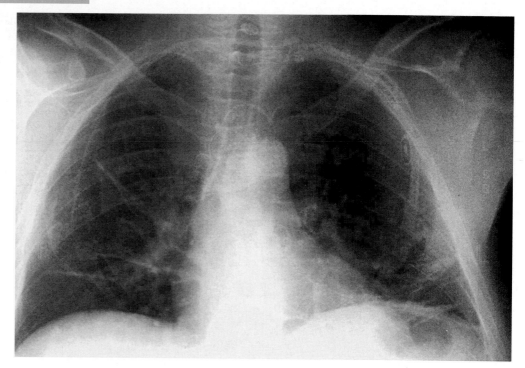

Figure 3–22. A 30-year-old man underwent a transsphenoidal hypophysectomy for a adrenocorticotropic hormone (ACTH)-secreting tumor of the anterior pituitary gland (Cushing's disease). His postoperative chest radiograph 2 days later demonstrates bilateral linear opacities representing subsegmental atelectasis. What caused this striking pattern of atelectasis? One hypothesis relates to the sudden withdrawal of his abnormally high serum levels of glucocorticoids. In premature infants, pulmonary surfactant production can be stimulated by the administration of steroids. Could it be that this patient's type II pneumocytes had become accustomed to high levels of glucocorticoids, and that their production of surfactant declined in response to the abrupt drop-off in steroid levels after the ACTH-secreting tumor was removed, thus resulting in adhesive atelectasis?

or more of the interlobar fissures, which is pulled toward the collapsed lobe. Another is displacement of pulmonary vessels, such as downward and medial displacement of the interlobar pulmonary artery in lower lobe collapse. Other signs include ipsilateral elevation of the hemidiaphragm and shift of mediastinal structures such as the heart or trachea toward the involved side. Often the collapsed portion of lung will be evident as a region of increased opacity, while the unaffected portion may appear more lucent, due to compensatory hyperexpansion. A common finding is the presence of linear, plate-like opacities in one or both lungs, which may represent either atelectasis or scarring. As always, comparison with previous radiographs can prove extremely helpful, as can follow-up examination. When the finding is new, or if it resolves subsequently, the diagnosis of atelectasis is quite likely, while if the finding was present years before or does not change on follow-up, it represents scarring.

CLINICAL HISTORY

The importance of the clinical history in interpreting chest radiographs cannot be overemphasized. Absent such a history, the radiologist often can do little more than describe the findings and provide a long list of possible etiologies, which presents relatively little help to the clinician. On the other hand, even a brief clinical history can often enable the radiologist to narrow down considerably the differential diagnosis. Critical parameters to be included on every chest radiograph requisition include the following: age, gender, acute or chronic presentation, febrile or afebrile, significant medical and surgical history (such as immune compromise, collagen vascular disease, malignancy, etc.), pertinent occupational history (such as exposure to silica or grain silos), drug therapy (such as penicillin or adriamycin), results of pertinent tests (such as TB, human immunodeficiency virus [HIV], blood coagulation profile, etc.), and, where possible, a clinical question that the test is obtained to answer.

Examples of a good clinical history would include "55-year-old retired shipyard worker with 80 pack-year smoking history who presents with 20-lb weight loss over 3 months and new onset of right pleuritic chest pain," or "35-year-old HIV-positive woman with acute onset of cough and chills." The former points toward a malignancy such as lung carcinoma or mesothelioma, while the latter suggests an infectious etiology, including the possibility of an opportunistic organism. An example of a suboptimal clinical history in either of these settings would be "Rule out infiltrate."

Other Imaging Modalities

Digital radiography has provided several benefits over conventional techniques, including more consistent quality and reduced repeat rates, particularly in portable radiography. Digitization enables postprocessing of image data to provide edge enhancement, improved contrast resolution, and manipulation of window and level settings to enhance visualization of the different regions of the chest, such as the lungs and the mediastinum. Dual energy subtraction techniques, now available on some dedicated upright (not portable) chest units, make it possible to "subtract out" the bones from a chest radiograph, permitting improved visualization of the pulmonary parenchyma. Alternatively, it is possible to "subtract out" the lungs, to determine whether a suspected pulmonary nodule may in fact represent a lesion within a bone.

CT and high-resolution CT have dramatically enhanced thoracic imaging because of their vastly superior contrast resolution and ability to distinguish between anatomic and pathologic structures based on cross-sectional projections, eliminating the superimposition of structures that characterizes PA and lateral chest radiographs. Iodinated contrast material is used to evaluate vascular disease, to characterize the enhancement characteristics of lesions, and to distinguish hilar nodes from vascular structures. CT is commonly employed to better evaluate lesions detected on plain radiography, such as pulmonary nodules and hilar or mediastinal masses, to stage lung cancers, to rule out occult thoracic metastases in malignancies with a propensity to metastasize to the lung, and to evaluate vascular pathology such as suspected aortic dissection. Three-dimensional reconstructions in the sagittal and coronal planes occasionally prove helpful; for example, in evaluating hilar lesions and suspected diaphragmatic injury. Recently, contrast-infused CT has emerged as a sensitive and highly specific means of evaluating suspected PE. High-resolution CT provides more precise characterization of calcifications within pulmonary nodules and more precisely characterizes parenchymal lung diseases and bronchiectasis. It represents the most sensitive method of in vivo detection of emphysema.

Magnetic resonance imaging (MRI) enjoys several advantages over CT which can prove helpful in select situations. Its ability to image directly in multiple planes provides superior assessment of many apical, hilar, and subcarinal lesions. Its superior contrast resolution can often clearly distinguish between tumor and normal adjacent tissue such as muscle and fat. Its ability to distinguish between various tissue types and between flowing blood and stationary tissue without exogenous contrast can prove quite helpful in patients with a contraindication to iodinated contrast material (Fig. 3–23).

Disadvantages of MRI include decreased spatial resolution, insensitivity to calcification, and profound motion artifacts if good electrocardiographic and respiratory gating of image acquisition are not achieved. MRI is also more time-consuming and expensive than CT. CT is generally the preferred modality in noncardiovascular situations.

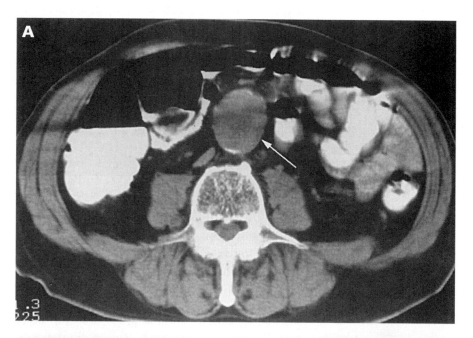

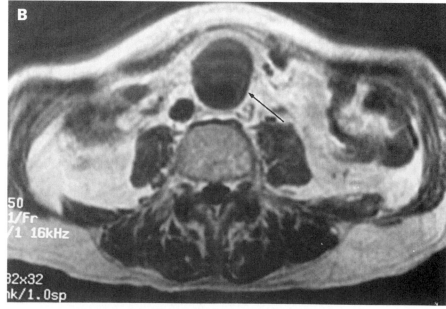

Figure 3–23. (**A**) A nonenhanced axial abdominal computed tomography (CT) image and (**B**) a nonenhanced axial spin echo magnetic resonance image at the same level demonstrate magnetic resonance imaging (MRI)'s ability to evaluate vascular structures—in this case, the abdominal aorta (arrow)—without the use of intravascular contrast material. In this case, the patient's creatinine was abnormally high, and the risk of renal failure precluded the use of iodinated contrast material. The nonenhanced CT demonstrates only a fusiform distal abdominal aortic aneurysm, but does not distinguish between flowing blood and thrombus. The MRI demonstrates that most of the aneurysm is filled with intermediate signal intensity clot, while the posterior portion contains signal void, indicating flowing blood.

Ultrasound is used primarily in the adult in the evaluation of pleural effusions and masses, anterior mediastinal masses, and chest-wall processes.

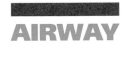

AIRWAY

Asthma

EPIDEMIOLOGY

Asthma is the most important cause of acute airway obstruction, which represents one of the most common presenting complaints in U.S. emergency rooms. Asthma is characterized as acute and reversible airway obstruction and afflicts approximately 1 in every 50 adult Americans. Precipitants of acute attacks vary from patient to patient, but include airway irritants such as dust and noxious chemicals, inflammatory mediators such as histamine, and a variety of antigens associated with allergy, such as ragweed pollen. Additional stimuli include exercise, cold, and, in some patients, nonsteroidal anti-inflammatory agents. Many patients will give a family history of the disorder or report a history of allergic symptoms.

PATHOPHYSIOLOGY

The airways obstruction has two components. The first is bronchospasm, mediated by hyperreactivity of smooth muscle surrounding both the small and large airways. The second component of obstruction is chronic inflammation, which includes excessive mucus production and thickening of airway membranes. A number of different factors contribute to the clinical picture, including increased airways resistance (which increases in inverse proportion to the fourth power of the radius), decreased airflow rates and forced expiratory volumes, hyperinflation of the lungs (which may remain inflated at autopsy even when the pleural cavity is opened), increased work of breathing, and ventilation/perfusion (V/Q) mismatches.

CLINICAL PRESENTATION

The asthmatic suffering from an acute exacerbation presents with dyspnea, wheezing, and cough. Clinical signs of more severe airway obstruction include the recruitment of accessory muscles of respiration, such as the sternocleidomastoids, and the development of a pulsus paradoxus (a greater than 10 mm Hg drop in systolic blood pressure with inspiration). Only approximately 3% of metabolic energy expenditure is normally devoted to respiration in quiet breathing, but this may increase to 30% or more in patients with obstructive disease (or poorly compliant lungs), with the result that breathing itself becomes exhausting. In severe cases, blood gases typically reveal hypoxemia and hypercarbia, and a rise in the $PaCO_2$ is an indication that the patient is decompensating and may require transfer to the intensive care unit. If the attack progresses to the point that the airways are plugged with mucus, the patient becomes refractory to bronchodilators and the state of status asthmaticus ensues. At this point, intubation is often required.

IMAGING

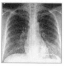

Radiologic evaluation consists almost exclusively of chest radiography. The radiographic signs of an acute asthma exacerbation are predictable, based on the pathophysiology. Air trapping and hyperinflation are produced by the tendency of narrowed airways to collapse under the increased positive intrathoracic pressures necessary to exhale against increased airways resistance (which explains why wheezes are most prominent in the expiratory phase of respiration). Signs of hyperinflation include flattening of the diaphragms, attenuation of vascular markings, and an increase in both lung height and AP diameter, with expansion of the retrosternal clear space.

Atelectasis is a frequent finding, and is related to the resorption of oxygen from respiratory bronchioles and alveoli distal to a plugged airway. Bronchial wall thickening may be visualized as peribronchial cuffing and tram tracking, which refer to thickened bronchi seen on end and lengthwise, respectively. In rare cases, mucus plugs with a branchlike structure may be visualized within the bronchial tree.

It should be noted, however, that chest radiography is not performed in order to diagnose an asthma exacerbation, which can usually be based on strictly clinical grounds. The clinician does not need a chest X ray to determine if a patient is suffering an asthma attack, and the study is often normal in any case, even when the attack is severe. Chest radiography is performed to rule out other possible etiologies of dyspnea and to assess for the complications of asthma, such as pneumothorax and pneumomediastinum, which may result from high expiratory pressures or positive pressure ventilation, with resultant alveolar rupture (Fig. 3–24). When such complications arise, the plan of therapy may require expansion to include such maneuvers as the insertion of a chest tube. A chest radiograph is also useful in excluding other lesions

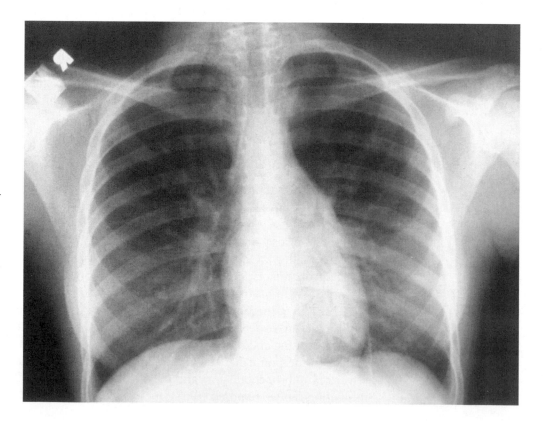

Figure 3–24. A 10-year-old girl presented to the emergency room with dyspnea. The posteroanterior view of the chest demonstrates hyperexpanded lungs, as well as a more significant finding—linear lucencies extending from the mediastinum up into the neck, indicating pneumomediastinum and cervical emphysema. Although not necessarily life-threatening in itself, such a finding warrants close clinical monitoring.

that may masquerade as asthma, such as pneumonia or tracheobronchial obstruction. Such mimics require therapies different from the standard asthmatic regimen, such as antibiotics or surgery.

Chronic Bronchitis and Emphysema

EPIDEMIOLOGY

Common causes of chronic and unremitting airways obstruction include chronic bronchitis and emphysema, which usually coexist in varying proportions in any particular patient. Chronic bronchitis is a clinical diagnosis, defined as cough and sputum production during at least 3 months for 2 consecutive years. Emphysema is a pathologic diagnosis, defined as destruction of lung tissue with enlargement of airspaces (Fig. 3–25).

PATHOPHYSIOLOGY

 Both diseases are characterized by chronic alveolar hypoventilation, which results in a tendency to hypercarbia and hypoxemia. In chronic bronchitis, blood is shunted past unventilated alveoli, while in emphysema, the alveoli themselves are destroyed. Early in the course of the disease, the V/Q mismatch is less severe in emphysema than in chronic bronchitis,

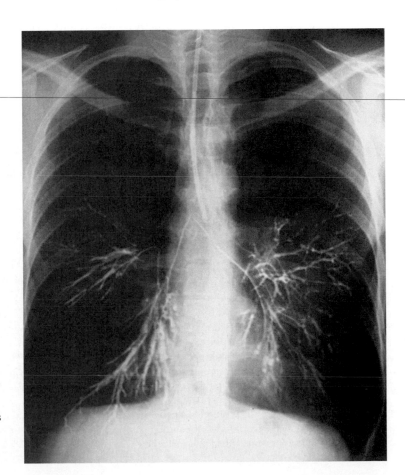

Figure 3–25. Bronchograms are rarely performed since the advent of computed tomography, but this bronchogram provides a dramatic demonstration of the destruction of airspaces and airways seen in severe emphysema. Although all lung zones are involved, the disease is most severe in the upper lung zones, which is characteristic of the centrilobular emphysema associated with cigarette smoking. Note also that the lungs are large, a characteristic finding in this process.

because both airspaces and capillaries are destroyed. The single most important causative agent is cigarette smoke, although another important cause of emphysema is α-1-antitrypsin deficiency (Fig. 3–26). α-1-Antitrypsin is an endogenous protease inhibitor which, in effect, prevents pulmonary autodigestion.

CLINICAL PRESENTATION

Although both disorders are chronic and unremitting, patients tend to present during exacerbations, generally precipitated by upper respiratory infections (with increased sputum production and bronchospasm), episodes of CHF, or even PE. Patients with chronic bronchitis are especially likely to be chronically colonized by bacteria, probably due to a combination of defective mucociliary clearance and impaired immune response. Pulmonary function testing reveals a prominent deficit in forced expiratory volume in chronic bronchitis, and a loss of diffusing capacity (measured with carbon monoxide) in emphysema.

IMAGING

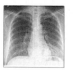 The chest radiograph is insensitive in the diagnosis of chronic bronchitis and emphysema, and approximately 50% of patients with clinically diagnosed chronic obstructive pulmonary disease (COPD) will have normal chest radiographs. Radiography is employed primarily to assess complications of these disorders, such as pneumonia, pneumothorax (thin-walled bullae may rupture into the pleural space), and lung cancer (both emphysema and bronchogenic carcinoma are, of course, tobacco-related). However, the chest radiograph can suggest the diagnosis.

Radiographic signs suggestive of chronic bronchitis include indications of bronchial thickening, such as peribronchial cuffing and tram tracking, and there is

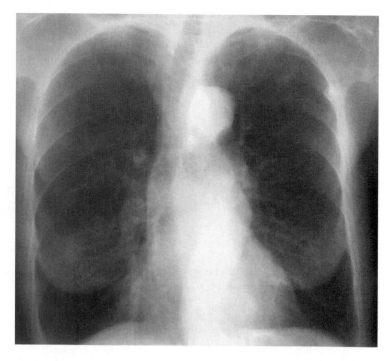

Figure 3–26. A 70-year-old woman's chest radiograph reveals the ravages of a lifetime of cigarette smoking. Note that her lungs are large and that pulmonary vessels appear markedly sparse in some areas; for example, the right base. These findings are suggestive of emphysema. In addition, the cardiothoracic ratio is at the upper limits of normal, and the aorta is unfolded, bulging to the left at the level of the pulmonary artery. When one finds evidence of emphysema, the probability of other smoking-related disorders is increased, as this patient demonstrates. Note the spiculated nodule in the left upper lobe, which was found at biopsy to represent an adenocarcinoma. Note also the position of a pseudonodule in the right lung base relative to the contour of the right breast; this represents a shadow cast by the nipple of the right breast.

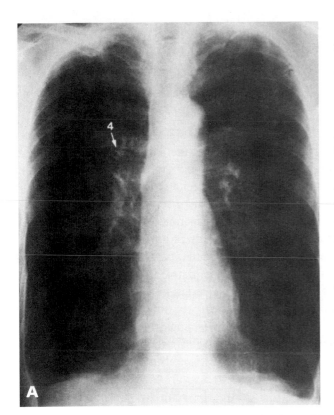

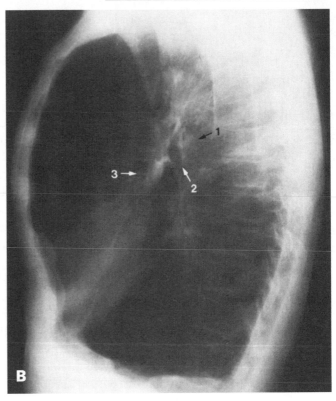

Figure 3–27. This 65-year-old man exhibits several radiographic signs of emphysema. (A) On the frontal view, the lungs are large, and the hemidiaphragms are flattened. (B) On the lateral view, a "barrel chest" becomes apparent, with anterior convexity of the sternum and mild diaphragmatic inversion. 1, left descending pulmonary artery; 2, left mainstem bronchus; 3, anterior segmental artery; 4, upper lobe bronchus.

often a diffuse but nonspecific increase in lung markings. Plain radiographic findings in emphysema include hyperinflation with flattening of the diaphragms and expansion of the retrosternal airspace, diffuse lucency from destruction of lung tissue, and bullae (thin-walled cysts left in the wake of lung destruction) (Fig. 3–27).

Because pulmonary artery hypertension is often a feature of COPD, prominent central pulmonary arteries may be noted in both chronic bronchitis and emphysema. High-resolution CT is the most sensitive in vivo technique available in detecting and characterizing the morphologic changes of emphysema.

PLEURA

Pleural Effusion

EPIDEMIOLOGY

Pleural effusion is the abnormal accumulation of fluid between the visceral and parietal pleura. Strictly speaking, a pleural effusion is not a disease, but a sign of disease that usually requires further diagnostic evaluation. Statistically, the most common causes of pleural effusions are, in descending order of frequency, CHF, bacterial pneumonia, malignancy (especially lung and breast cancer), PE, viral pneumonia, and cirrhosis of the liver.

PATHOPHYSIOLOGY

The normal amount of fluid in the pleural space of each lung is several milliliters. Its accumulation is governed by the Starling forces (discussed in Chapter 2), with flow of fluid from the parietal pleura and resorption of fluid at the visceral pleura. When thoracentesis is performed, the aspirated fluid may be classified as bloody, chylous, purulent, or serous.

Another important distinction is that between transudative and exudative effusions. Transudates are characterized by low protein (effusion/serum protein < 0.5), and are most commonly produced by elevated pulmonary venous pressures in CHF. Another means of determining if an effusion is transudative is by measuring its lactate dehydrogenase, which will be less than 200 IU. Exudates are produced by inflammatory or infiltrative processes, and have a higher protein concentration due to increased capillary permeability. When an exudative effusion is found in an adult, carcinoma is the single most likely cause. The finding of malignant cells within the fluid generally signifies diffuse involvement. Infections that frequently produce pleural effusions include TB, *Klebsiella, Staphylococcus aureus,* and anaerobes. Such infections within the pleural space may produce the sequela of calcified pleural plaques (Fig. 3–28).

CLINICAL PRESENTATION

Large effusions often present with dyspnea, because the fluid beneath or around the lung prevents its normal inspiratory expansion and tends to produce passive atelecta-

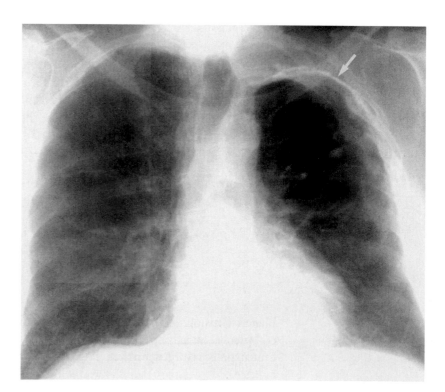

Figure 3–28. This posteroanterior chest radiograph in an adult with a history of childhood tuberculosis (TB) demonstrates multiple sequelae of TB, including parenchymal scarring and calcified granulomata, as well as a prominent calcified pleural plaque in the left apex (arrow).

sis of adjacent lung. Other common presenting complaints in patients with pleural effusions include cough and chest discomfort or pain, which is often pleuritic in nature. Signs raising suspicion for pleural effusion on physical examination include diminished breath sounds, and dullness to percussion, with adjacent increased breath sounds due to overlying atelectatic lung.

IMAGING

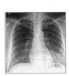 Radiography is useful in the detection and quantitation of pleural effusions. Upright positioning is preferred, because it will cause fluid to collect at one end of the lung (the lower). The lateral radiograph is more sensitive than the frontal, because the posterior aspect of the costophrenic sulcus, the most dependent portion of the pleural space in the upright position, is much better visualized. A small amount of pleural fluid, less than 75 cc, will tend to collect in a subpulmonic location, between the lung and the diaphragm, and may be undetectable, although its presence is suggested when the hemidiaphragm appears to be elevated, especially laterally, or when the gastric bubble appears unusually distant from the base of the left lung. However, as the amount of fluid approaches 100 cc, it tends to spill into the costophrenic sulcus, and becomes visible as a blunting of the usually sharp posterior angles on the lateral radiograph, with a meniscus-like appearance. As more fluid accumulates (> 200 cc), the costophrenic angles will become blunted on the frontal projection as well.

If an effusion is suspected but cannot be demonstrated on routine upright views, a decubitus film, with the patient lying on the side, may show a small amount of fluid layering out along the lateral chest wall. This technique is sensitive for effusions as small as 10 cc. In large effusions, fluid may be seen tracking into the fissures, especially on the lateral view.

On portable radiography, with the patient in a supine position, sensitivity for the detection of pleural effusion is markedly decreased, and if clinical concern is high, upright radiographs should be obtained, if at all possible. If not, ultrasound may warrant consideration. Plain radiographic findings in the supine position include diffuse opacification of the hemithorax, because the effusion layers out behind the lung, and blunting of the costophrenic angle. On occasion, the fluid will accumulate at the lung apex, in which case it produces a white "apical cap."

A common clinical problem is an effusion that has become loculated due to adhesions between the visceral and parietal pleura, which is commonly seen in infectious and neoplastic effusions. Loculated fluid may simulate a pleural mass. The presence of loculations can make diagnostic thoracentesis more difficult and may also render therapeutic taps (aimed to relieve dyspnea by withdrawing a large amount of fluid) unsuccessful, due to the presence of multiple noncommunicating loculations. In this case, a decubitus film will demonstrate whether the fluid is loculated, because trapped fluid will not layer out along the lateral chest wall.

Ultrasound and CT may prove helpful in guiding thoracentesis in cases of loculation, because they can help to select out the largest pocket. They may also be necessary to determine whether an area of presumed pleural fluid may in fact consist, at least in part, of collapsed lung. Imaging guidance increases the probability of obtaining fluid and decreases the rate of complications, such as hepatic or splenic laceration, pulmonary hemorrhage, and pneumothorax. In the case of a diagnostic tap, what should be done with the fluid? Because the range of possible etiologies for effusions is fairly broad, pleural fluid should be routinely sent for chemistry, cell count and differential, culture and sensitivity, gram stain, acid-fast bacilli, and cytology.

Pneumothorax

EPIDEMIOLOGY

Pneumothorax, the presence of air within the pleural space, may result from trauma or occur spontaneously.

PATHOPHYSIOLOGY

In the setting of penetrating trauma, pneumothorax may result from the introduction of air through the chest wall. If the wound does not seal itself, there is a leakage of air through the chest wall and into the pleural space, creating a so-called sucking chest wound. In this situation, the negative intrathoracic pressure created with each inspiration causes additional air to enter the pleural space, which may rapidly eventuate in a tension pneumothorax. In tension pneumothorax, the continued accumulation of air in the pleural space causes complete collapse of the affected lung, with a shift of the mediastinum toward the contralateral side. Death may rapidly ensue, largely due to the compromise of venous return to the heart produced by the distortion of normal mediastinal anatomy, as well as V/Q mismatching and hypoxemia. Blunt trauma may cause pneumothorax when a rib punctures the pleura or when tracheobronchial rupture results (Fig. 3–29). The latter condition is associated with pneumomediastinum and persistence of pneumothorax even after functional chest tube placement.

Spontaneous pneumothorax may be idiopathic or related to preexisting lung disease. Idiopathic pneumothorax typically occurs in men in the third or fourth decades, especially in tall and asthenic individuals. Such patients are sometimes found to have bullae or blebs in the lung apices. A bulla is defined as a thin-walled gas collection that is greater than 1 cm in diameter, while a bleb is a collection of gas less than 1 cm wide

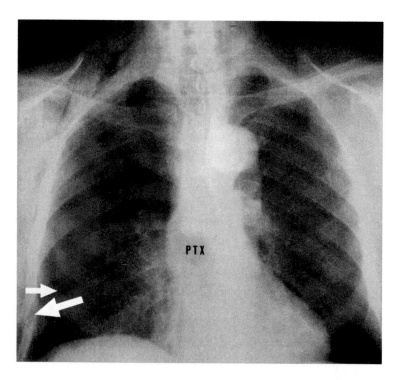

Figure 3–29. This patient suffered blunt trauma to the right chest wall. Note the displaced fracture of one of the right lateral ribs (small arrow), which has resulted in a right pneumothorax (PTX) (large arrow) and air tracking in the subcutaneous tissues up into the base of the neck. This appearance is typical of a pneumothorax, with a visceral pleural line bounded on one side by the collapsed lung and on the other by lucent air within the pleural space.

within the layers of the visceral pleura. COPD is the most common predisposing condition in spontaneous pneumothorax, and there is an association with Marfan's syndrome.

Regardless of the patient's underlying condition, positive pressure ventilation is a risk factor, and intubation should generally be avoided in patients with pneumothorax if a chest tube is not in place. The most common cause of pneumothorax in hospitalized patients is iatrogenic, secondary to central venous catheter placement. An upright chest radiograph should be obtained in every patient who has undergone placement of a central line, in part to confirm line position, but also to rule out the presence of a pneumothorax.

CLINICAL PRESENTATION

The usual presentation of pneumothorax is the sudden onset of dyspnea and chest pain. Patients with more serious tension pneumothorax are tachypneic, tachycardic, hypotensive, and cyanotic.

IMAGING

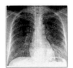 Whenever possible, upright radiographs should be obtained in suspected pneumothorax, because up to one-third of pneumothoraxes may be inapparent on supine films. An upright chest radiograph demonstrates a small pneumothorax as an apical visceral pleural line displaced away from the chest wall, with an absence of lung markings peripheral to it. Larger pneumothoraxes are also suggested by asymmetrical lucency of the involved hemithorax (Fig. 3–30). Potential mimics include skin folds, which often extend peripherally beyond the chest wall, and bullae. If a patient cannot sit or stand upright, a lateral decubitus film should be obtained with the affected side up, which will cause intrapleural air to collect just below the chest wall. CT is more sensitive than plain radiography, but should be reserved only for difficult cases due to its increased cost.

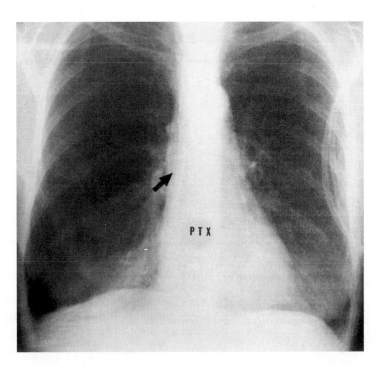

Figure 3–30. This posteroanterior chest radiograph in a patient who underwent insertion of a right subclavian central venous catheter (arrow) demonstrates increased lucency of the right hemithorax as compared to the left. This was due to a large right pneumothorax (PTX), which resulted from puncture of the pleura during insertion of the catheter. Note a nodular opacity in the right lower lung, just above the diaphragm. We can be confident that this does not represent a lung cancer for two reasons. First, the lung has collapsed medially beyond this point, and therefore the nodule cannot be within the lung. Second, this represents a typical location for a breast nipple, and this opacity did in fact represent a nipple shadow.

MEDIASTINUM

Anatomy and Imaging

The mediastinum is the narrow, vertically oriented, "white" mid-portion of the chest located between the two lungs on a frontal chest radiograph. Its contents include the heart and great vessels, the trachea and main bronchi, the esophagus, and numerous lymph nodes. Understanding the anatomy of the mediastinum on the frontal and lateral chest radiographs is critical to detecting and evaluating abnormalities. The mediastinum is usually divided into anterior, middle, and posterior compartments (Fig. 3–31). The middle mediastinum contains the pericardium and its contents, as well as the great vessels and trachea and mainstem bronchi. Structures anterior to it are in the anterior mediastium, and posteriorly located structures are in the posterior mediastinum.

The compartmental location of a mass is often suggested on the frontal radiograph; for example, a left-sided anterior mediastinal mass will not efface the border of the descending aorta, whereas a posterior mediastinal mass often will (Fig. 3–32). This stems from the fact that, because the descending aorta is located in the posterior mediastinum, only a posterior mediastinal mass will be contiguous with it. However, the key radiographic projection for determining the location of a mediastinal mass is the lateral, which eliminates the superimposition of the mediastinal compartments characteristic of the frontal view.

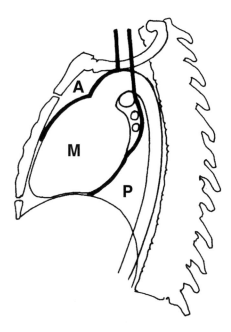

Figure 3–31. The three compartments of the mediastinum, as revealed on the lateral chest radiograph. While these divisions do not correspond to any intrinsic anatomic divisions, they are extremely useful in formulating appropriate differential diagnoses for masses in the different compartments. A, anterior; M, middle; P, posterior.

A = anterior to heart & great vessels

M = heart, aorta & branches,
pulmonary arteries, trachea

P = behind heart

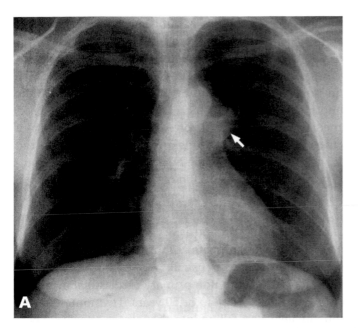 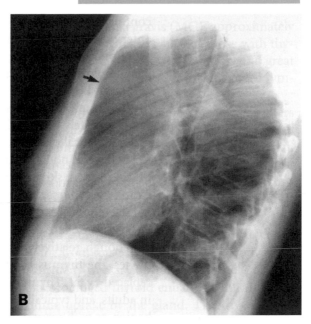

Figure 3–32. A 37-year-old woman complained of chest and arm pain. (A) Her posteroanterior chest radiograph demonstrates a prominent mediastinal bulge (arrow) in the region of the aorticopulmonary window (the space between the aortic arch and the main pulmonary artery). Where is this mass likely located within the mediastinum? Note that the left lateral borders of both the aortic arch and the descending aorta are clearly seen. This suggests that the mass is likely in the anterior mediastinum, where it would not be in contiguity with the aorta. (B) The lateral radiograph confirms the anterior location of the mass, which fills in the normally vacant retrosternal clear space (arrow). The differential diagnosis of an anterior mediastinal mass in this patient would include thymic lesions such as thymoma, germ cell tumor, and lymphatic masses such as sarcoidosis or lymphoma. In this case, biopsy yielded a large cell lymphoma.

Examples of relatively common mediastinal abnormalities include mass, infection, and hemorrhage, any one of which may manifest as diffuse mediastinal widening or a more focal contour abnormality. CT is generally the examination of choice in further evaluating an abnormality seen on chest radiography. MRI is superior in the evaluation of suspected vascular pathology, such as aortic dissection, as well as in the evaluation of masses in the posterior mediastinum, and in patients for whom iodinated contrast poses special risk. This discussion focuses on the differential diagnosis of mediastinal masses, based on the compartments of the mediastinum—a classic radiologic differential.

Mediastinal Mass

ANTERIOR MEDIASTINUM

The anterior mediastinum, often referred to as the prevascular compartment, is bounded by the sternum anteriorly and the heart and great vessels posteriorly. The normal anterior mediastinum is a relatively "empty" compartment, containing only the internal mammary vessels and lymph nodes and the thymus. Aside from the lymph nodes and thymus, two additional types of tissue may be present within the anterior mediastinum and give rise to masses: thyroid tissue and germ cells. Thyroid tissue may be present due to the extension of a goiter or carcinoma from the relatively

Teratomas and other germ cell neoplasms such as seminomas and choriocarcinomas are typically found in patients under the age of 40 years. Malignant germ cell tumors are seen almost exclusively in men. Teratomas contain ectodermal, mesodermal, and endodermal tissues, and often contain calcifications, fat, and even teeth. Choriocarcinoma is usually associated with elevated levels of human chorionic gonadotropin, which may produce gynecomastia.

MIDDLE MEDIASTINUM

The middle or vascular compartment of the mediastinum contains the heart and pericardium, the aorta and its great branches, the central pulmonary artery and veins, the trachea and mainstem bronchi, and numerous lymph nodes. Due to the presence of the aorta and its great branches, the differential diagnosis of middle mediastinal masses includes vascular lesions (Fig. 3–35). Among the most common vascular lesions is generalized aortomegaly, often seen in patients who are advanced in years or who have suffered long-term hypertension. As the aorta enlarges, it often becomes tortuous, swinging out farther laterally than normal on the frontal projection and farther posteriorly on the lateral view. Such tortuosity is particularly worthy of comment in patients less than 50 years of age, where such changes cannot be ascribed to normal aging, and likely stems from hypertension, increased cardiac output (as in chronic anemia), or accelerated atherosclerosis. The presence of a focal aneurysm merits concern largely due to the danger of rupture, which increases in proportion to the size of the aneurysm. Aortic aneurysms are further discussed Chapter 2.

Congenital malformations of the foregut may also produce middle mediastinal masses. Bronchogenic cysts result from aberrant budding of the tracheobronchial tree, producing a cystic structure lined by respiratory epithelium (with a pseudostratified columnar epithelium containing mucus glands) and containing cartilage within its

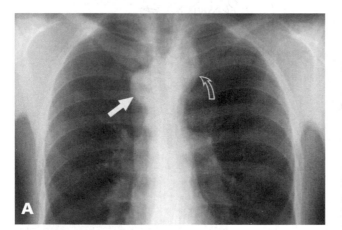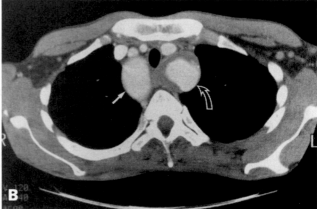

Figure 3–35. (A) The chest radiograph of this 30-year-old man demonstrates a markedly abnormal mediastinal contour, with bilateral paratracheal mass-like opacities producing mass effect on the trachea and a mild to moderate degree of luminal attenuation. The fact that no normal aortic arch contour is seen along the left mediastinal border is a strong hint that the right-sided mass (arrow) represents a right aortic arch. This suggests a possible explanation for the left-sided mass (curved arrow); namely, that it represents an aberrant left subclavian artery. (B) An axial image from a contrast-infused thoracic computed tomography scan demonstrates both the right aortic arch (small arrow) and the aneurysmal aberrant left subclavian artery (curved arrow). The presence of aneurysmal dilatation explains the prominent left mediastinal contour abnormality. Note the presence of nonenhancing mural thrombus surrounding much of the contrast-containing patent lumen.

walls. They do not communicate with the tracheobronchial tree unless infected. The lesions are usually subcarinal in location, contain water-density fluid, and do not enhance with contrast administration. Neurenteric cysts are lined by enteric epithelium, usually do not communicate with the GI tract, and are associated with vertebral body abnormalities such as anterior spina bifida or hemivertebrae.

Adenopathy is by far the most common middle mediastinal mass, the differential for which includes bronchogenic carcinoma, lymphoma and leukemia, metastases, sarcoidosis, and infection. The finding of middle mediastinal adenopathy in patients with lung carcinoma will generally be accompanied by detection of the primary tumor. However, in some cases of small cell carcinoma, the adenopathy may be the more striking of the two. Bilateral involvement is associated with a poorer prognosis than unilateral involvement, which is generally on the same side as the tumor. Occasionally, the nodes may calcify, which can be seen in treated malignancies, granulomatous diseases, and the pneumoconiosis silicosis (Fig. 3–36).

Sarcoidosis is a granulomatous disease of unknown etiology that is more common in blacks than whites and is commonly seen in the age range of 20 to 40 years. TB may exhibit an appearance similar to that of sarcoidosis, although the granulomas in sarcoidosis are noncaseating. Patients commonly present with malaise, fever, and ery-

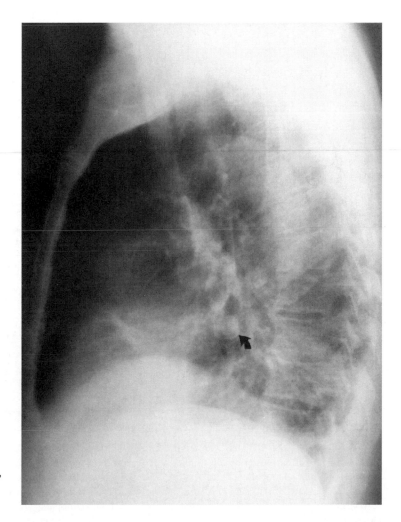

Figure 3–36. This lateral chest radiograph demonstrates multiple calcified mediastinal lymph nodes (arrow) in a patient with silicosis. This pattern of calcification is sometimes described as "eggshell" in appearance. Silicosis is associated with inhalation of silica dust, which can occur in occupations such as mining and sandblasting.

thema nodosum, although many patients with early disease are asymptomatic. Approximately one-quarter of patients will also have pulmonary symptoms such as dyspnea and cough. In 80% of patients, radiographic findings include enlargement of the mediastinal and hilar nodes, the so-called 1-2-3 sign of right paratracheal and right and left hilar adenopathy (Fig. 3–37). Involvement of the lung is less frequently seen, manifesting as an interstitial abnormality that tends to spare the lower lung zones, and progresses to fibrosis in 20% of cases of long-standing involvement (Fig. 3–38). The staging of sarcoidosis correlates with the probability of resolution. Stage I disease, with bilateral hilar nodal enlargement, resolves in 75% of cases. Stage II disease, with both

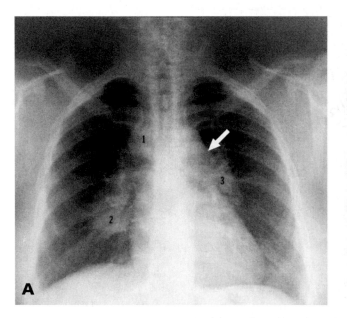
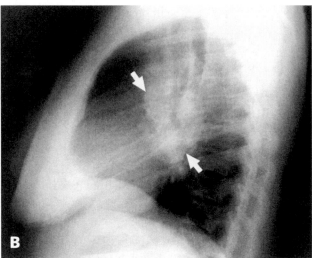
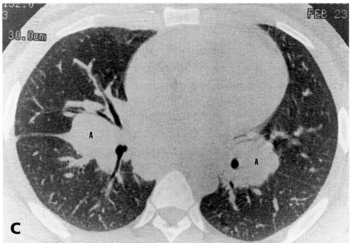

Figure 3–37. A 30-year-old black woman presented with persistent cough, and was found on physical examination to have bibasilar crackles. (A) An anteroposterior chest radiograph demonstrates prominent right paratracheal (1), aortopulmonary window (arrow), and bilateral hilar adenopathy (2 and 3), the "1-2-3" sign. No pulmonary parenchymal abnormalities are seen. (B) The lateral view shows a prominent "donut" sign of hilar adenopathy (arrows). (C) An axial image from a high-resolution chest computed tomography scan with "lung window" settings demonstrates bilateral hilar adenopathy (A), as well as a diffuse fine nodularity throughout the lung parenchyma, as well as thickening of subpleural lines, indicating pulmonary parenchymal involvement.

Figure 3–38. This posteroanterior chest radiograph in a patient with a history of long-standing sarcoidosis (SAR) demonstrates characteristic changes of end-stage disease, with severe upper lobe fibrosis that has produced bullae in both apexes. In addition, there is a round, mass-like opacity within a cavity in the left upper lobe (arrow), which represents a mycetoma, the infestation of one of the cavities with aspergillus.

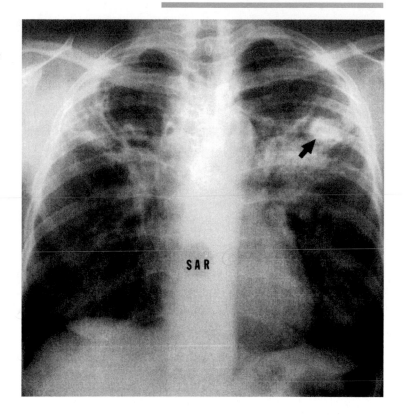

hilar and pulmonary parenchymal disease, resolves in 30%. In stage III, when strictly parenchymal disease is seen, only 10% of patients resolve.

Among the infectious causes of middle mediastinal adenopathy are TB, histoplasmosis, and coccidiodomycosis. Primary TB manifests as homogenous lobar opacification with ipsilateral mediastinal or hilar adenopathy, both of which may eventuate in calcified granulomata, producing the so-called Ranke complex. Reactivation TB is seen most commonly in the upper lung zones and often cavitates. Histoplasmosis is endemic in the Ohio, Mississippi, and St. Lawrence river valleys in the United States, and typically produces a flu-like syndrome that resolves with no sequelae save for the presence of calcified granulomata within the lungs, mediastinal lymph nodes, or the spleen and liver (Fig. 3–39). Coccidioidomycosis is endemic to the southwestern United States, and may produce "valley fever" when associated with arthralgias and erythema nodosum. Adenopathy is seen in approximately 20% of infected individuals.

POSTERIOR MEDIASTINUM

The posterior mediastinum lies behind the heart and great vessels and includes the esophagus, descending aorta, azygous and hemiazygous veins, and the intercostal and paraspinal nerves.

The most common posterior mediastinal masses are neurogenic tumors (Fig. 3–40). Tumors arising from peripheral nerves are neurofibromas or schwannomas, while those arising from the sympathetic ganglia are usually gangliomas. The former are usually seen in the 20 to 40 year age range, while the latter are usually seen before age 20 years. Both neurofibromas and schwannomas are more common in patients with type I neurofibromatosis (NF-I), the most common of the phakomatoses. The phakomatoses include NF-I, an autosomal dominant disorder including café au lait

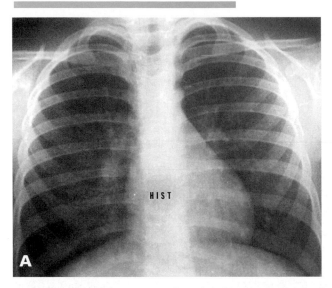

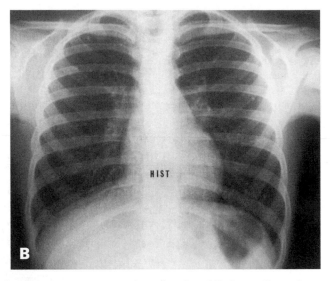

Figure 3–39. This young patient from the Ohio River valley developed respiratory symptoms, and was found on (**A**) chest radiography to have a diffuse bilateral pattern of pulmonary nodules, due to histoplasmosis (HIST). (**B**) A follow-up film several years later shows multiple bilateral calcified nodules.

spots, neurofibromas, optic gliomas, and spinal lesions; NF-II, the so-called central NF, which includes bilateral VIIIth cranial nerve masses; tuberous sclerosis, which manifests with seizures, mental retardation, and adenoma sebaceum; Sturge-Weber disease, which consists of a facial angioma and ipsilateral cerebral atrophy and calcification; and von Hippel-Lindau disease, which is associated with central nervous system (CNS)

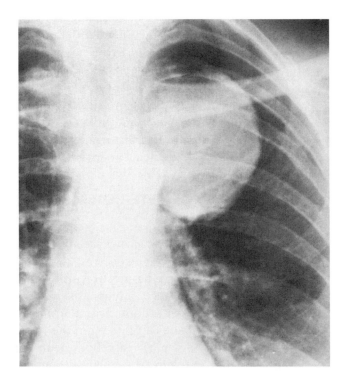

Figure 3–40. This coned-down view of a chest radiograph demonstrates a left-sided mediastinal mass. We know that it cannot be located in the anterior mediastinum, because it extends above the clavicle. Moreover, the fact that it does not obscure the lateral border of the aortic arch (a middle mediastinal structure) suggests that it does not lie within the middle mediastinum either. Hence, it is likely a posterior mediastinal mass, and therefore a neurogenic tumor. At surgery, a schwannoma was removed.

and retinal hemangioblastomas and renal cell carcinoma. Both neurofibromas and schwannomas appear as round paraspinal soft tissue masses. Biopsy of these lesions may prove quite painful, secondary to their neural origin.

Other paravertebral abnormalities include infection, enlargement of the azygous vein, and extramedullary hematopoiesis. Paravertebral abscesses are often related to spinal infection, with staphylococcus the most common organism. Salmonella is often seen in sickle-cell disease. Both present with rapid onset of fever and leukocytosis. TB presents more indolently, with Pott's disease manifesting as slow collapse of one or more vertebral bodies, often with acute kyphosis or "gibbus" deformity, and a paraspinal mass. Enlargement of the azygous vein may reflect increased venous pressure or flow (such as volume overload in a renal failure patient who has missed a dialysis appointment), as well as either inferior or superior vena caval obstruction. In inferior vena cava (IVC) obstruction, the azygous provides venous drainage into the superior vena cava (SVC) for structures below the level of the obstruction. The azygous may also drain supradiaphragmatic structures, when the SVC is obstructed between its junction with the azygous vein and the heart. Extramedullary hematopoiesis is seen with ineffective production or excessive destruction of erythrocytes, such as thalassemia and sickle-cell disease. The paraspinal mass represents hyperplastic marrow that has extruded from the vertebrae or ribs.

LUNG

Congenital

Congenital diseases of the lung are also discussed Chapter 10. Congenital pathologies that may present in the adult include bronchogenic cyst and Kartagener's syndrome. Bronchogenic cysts arise from an abnormal branching of the tracheobronchial tree, producing cysts that are lined with respiratory epithelium. Most are found in the mediastinum, but 10 to 20% are located in the lung. They are initially seen as well-defined, thin-walled cysts that demonstrate water attenuation by CT, but may develop a communication with the bronchial tree and become air filled. They are commonly seen in the subcarinal or parahilar regions. Kartagener's syndrome results from a deficiency in the dynein arms of cilia, resulting in immotile cilia. Patients present with recurrent respiratory infections and hearing difficulties. Radiographic findings include complete thoracic and abdominal situs inversus (on chest radiograph, cardiac apex and gastric bubble on the right), bronchiectasis, and sinusitis (Fig. 3–41).

Infectious

PNEUMONIA

EPIDEMIOLOGY

It is estimated that approximately 2.5 million cases of pneumonia are diagnosed each year in the United States, and it is the sixth most common proximate cause of death.

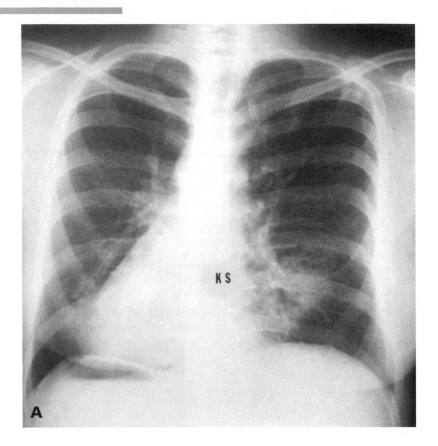

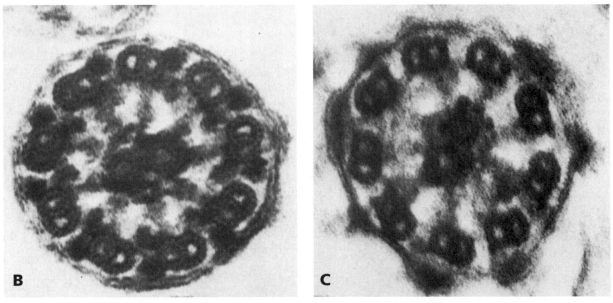

Figure 3–41. A 15-year-old boy presented with symptoms of a respiratory tract infection. (A) A focal interstitial opacity in the lower left lung represented an acute pneumonia, which was responsible for the patient's presentation. The other findings can prove difficult for a neophyte to detect. What are they and what do they imply about the health of this patient's future offspring? The critical findings are a right-sided cardiac apex, a right-sided gastric bubble, and bronchiectatic changes in both lower lobes. The patient's paranasal sinus films (not shown) demonstrated mucosal thickening, indicating chronic sinusitis. These findings are diagnostic of Kartagener's syndrome (KS), which can be traced to a deficiency in the dynein arms of cilia. The patient's ability to father children is in doubt, as associated amotility of the sperm produces infertility. (B,C) These electron micrographs (× 250,000) illustrate (B) a normal cilium with two dynein arms projecting in a clockwise rotation from each of the nine peripheral doublet microtubules, and (C) a patient whose cilia lack both inner and outer dynein arms, which render them immobile.

PATHOPHYSIOLOGY

Pneumonias can be divided into community-acquired and nosocomial infections. Most pneumonias result from inoculation with inhaled or aspirated microorganisms. Although pneumonia may occur in otherwise perfectly healthy patients of any age, certain factors predispose to its development, including impairment of specific immune responses of the sort seen in HIV disease or organ transplantation with immunosuppression, disruption of non-specific airway defenses such as mucociliary clearance due to cigarette smoke or tracheal intubation, and chronic lung diseases such as chronic bronchitis or cystic fibrosis, which interfere with local pulmonary defense mechanisms and render the lung a more microbially hospitable environment. The very young and very old are at particular risk, as are patients suffering from chronic debilitating diseases. Another important risk factor for pneumonia is impaired oropharyngeal function, as seen, for example, in alcohol intoxication, stroke, and head and neck cancer, all of which predispose to aspiration (Fig. 3–42). An important risk factor for pneumococcal pneumonia is splenectomy, which occurs spontaneously during the natural history of sickle-cell disease.

CLINICAL PRESENTATION

The patient who contracts bacterial pneumonia usually presents with sudden onset and rapid progression of symptoms, with little or no prodrome. A patient who feels well in the morning may appear toxic by evening, with high fever and complete prostration. Pneumococcal pneumonia in particular often manifests initially by one or several bouts

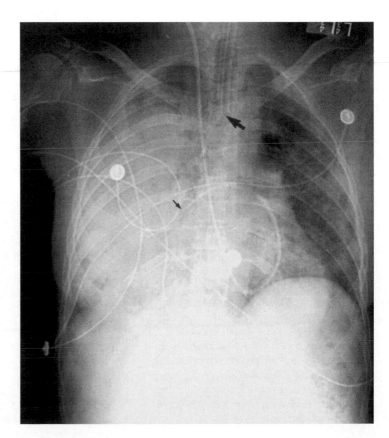

Figure 3–42. A 56-year-old substance-abusing woman suffered an episode of massive aspiration. On which side was she lying when the aspiration occurred? She was lying on her right side, as revealed by the much greater severity of the airspace opacities on that side, due to the gravity-dependent delivery of a greater volume of gastric contents to the right lung. Soon after the aspiration episode, she began to develop severe shortness of breath, impaired gas exchange, and stiff lungs, requiring mechanical ventilation. This clinical picture resulted from gastric acid-induced damage to the pulmonary capillaries, which causes an acute capillary-leak edema: acute respiratory distress syndrome. Note the good position of the endotracheal tube tip approximately 4 cm above the carina (large arrow) and the pulmonary artery catheter entering the right interlobar pulmonary artery (small arrow).

of rigors, presumably reflecting bacteremia. The pneumococcus represents the most common cause of community-acquired pneumonia in virtually all age groups. Staphylococcal and gram-negative pneumonias are common in hospitalized or debilitated patients, and *Klebsiella* is often seen in alcoholics (Fig. 3–43). Anaerobic bacterial pneumonias usually arise from aspiration, and patients with poor dental hygiene are at increased risk. The so-called atypical pneumonias include viral and mycoplasmal infections, which present with a more insidious onset, usually over several days.

IMAGING

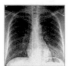

Upper respiratory tract infections are usually diagnosed and treated on clinical grounds, without the aid of medical imaging. A chest radiograph is obtained in suspected acute bronchitis only to rule out the presence of a coexisting pneumonia. Prior to the discovery of the X ray, lower respiratory tract infections were diagnosed based on history and physical examination findings, including constitutional symptoms such as malaise and fever, respiratory

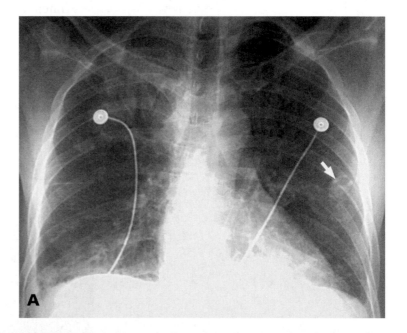

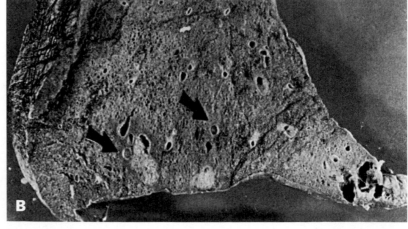

Figure 3–43. **(A)** This frontal chest radiograph of a 35-year-old intravenous drug abuser demonstrates multiple patchy airspace opacities and nodules throughout both lungs, several of which demonstrate cavitation (arrow). These lesions were found to represent staphylococcal septic emboli. **(B)** This photograph of a gross lung specimen from another patient demonstrates the typical appearance of such cavitated septic emboli (arrows).

symptoms such as productive cough and pleuritic chest pain, and auscultatory findings such as tubular breath sounds. An old radiologic adage, "one look is worth a thousand listens," conveys the central role now played by the chest radiograph in the diagnosis of pneumonia.

The chest radiograph is helpful not only in determining whether a patient has a pneumonia, but also in suggesting what pathogens are likely to be involved, based on the radiographic pattern. Three classic patterns of pulmonary opacification are recognized: bronchopneumonia, lobar pneumonia, and interstitial pneumonia. While other diagnostic modalities such as blood and sputum cultures may play an important role in guiding therapy in difficult cases (although both are often nondiagnostic), the chest radiograph alone often proves adequate to select an effective antibiotic regimen.

Bronchopneumonia

Bronchopneumonia is initially centered in the lobular bronchi, and thus presents with a patchy, inhomogeneous airspace opacification, which may eventually spread out to involve the whole lobule. The opacities themselves are airspace in appearance, meaning that they exhibit an ill-defined, fluffy appearance, secondary to the fact that they represent pus-filled alveoli (Fig. 3–44). Lobules within multiple lobes are typically involved, giving the process a patchy appearance, although over several days they may coalesce and become more homogeneous. Because the airways themselves are filled with pus, air bronchograms (see below) are not seen, and loss of volume in affected areas may occur, due to airway obstruction and atelectasis. Other common sequelae include cavitation and abscess formation secondary to necrosis, as well as the development of parapneumonic effusions and empyemas (Fig. 3–45). The classic organism responsible for such patchy airspace infiltrates is *Staphylococcus aureus,* although Gram negatives such as *Escherichia coli* and *Pseudomonas* are also seen. Staphylococcal

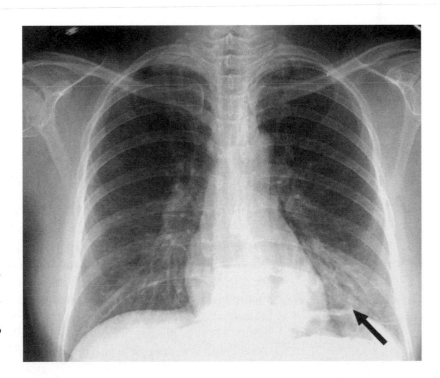

Figure 3–44. This posteroanterior chest radiograph in a 38-year-old woman demonstrates a typical appearance of a left lower lobe bronchopneumonia (arrow), with ill-defined, nodular, confluent opacities that represent a patchy distribution of pus-filled acinar units. Note also the presence of biapical scarring, reflecting previous radiation therapy.

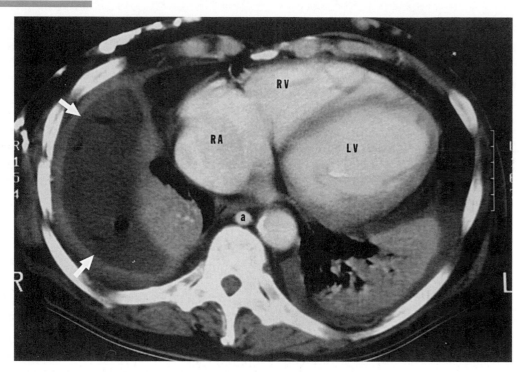

Figure 3–45. A 60-year-old man with a history of pneumonia exhibited persistent fevers and no radiographic improvement despite antibiotic therapy. An axial image from a contrast-enhanced computed tomography scan of the thorax demonstrates a classic appearance of an empyema, pus within the pleural space. Findings include a lenticular (lens-shaped), smooth-walled fluid collection (arrows) surrounded by the enhancing, thick rinds of the parietal and visceral pleura. In this case, multiple tiny gas collections are visible within the fluid, raising suspicion for bronchopleural fistula formation, the development of a communication between a bronchus and the pleura space. In contrast to parapneumonic pleural effusions, empyemas generally require chest tube drainage. Note the consolidation and small effusion at the left lung base. a, azygous vein; LV, left ventricle; RA, right atrium; RV, right ventricle.

pneumonia generally responds slowly to appropriate antibiotic therapy, and many patients are left with permanent lung damage.

Lobar pneumonia

Lobar pneumonia begins not within the lobular bronchi, but within the distal airspaces, and spreads via the pores of Kohn and the canals of Lambert to produce nonsegmental lobar opacification. With time, the infection may spread to involve the entire lobe, producing a classic lobar pattern that is strongly associated with pneumococcal pneumonia (Fig. 3–46). Fortunately, rapid deployment of antibiotics has rendered such classic presentations relatively less common, as the infection is often arrested before it has time to involve an entire lobe. Because only the terminal airspaces are usually involved, with sparing of the bronchi, so-called air bronchograms are often seen, which represent air-filled bronchi surrounded by pus-filled airspaces, and appear as tubular and branching lucencies within the consolidation (Fig. 3–47). Likewise, the lack of airway involvement renders postobstructive atelectasis uncommon, and lung volumes are usually preserved. Pneumococcal pneumonia is generally treated with low-dose penicillin and manifests a dramatic response within 1 or 2 days.

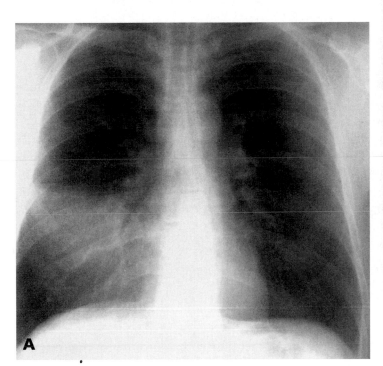
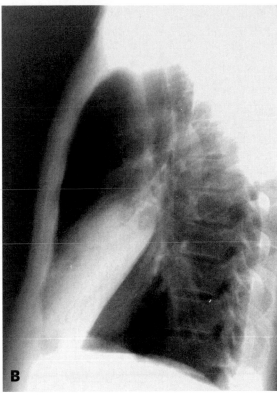

Figure 3–46. A 49-year-old man presented with the acute onset of fever, prostration, and a cough productive of rusty-brown sputum. (A) The posteroanterior chest radiograph demonstrates airspace consolidation in the right middle lobe, with obscuration of the right heart border due to the contiguity of the pus-filled airspaces and the heart (the so-called silhouette sign). (B) The lateral view confirms the airspace infiltrate and volume loss in the right middle lobe, which is bounded by the minor fissure superiorly, and the major fissure posteroinferiorly. The patient was successfully treated for a presumed pneumococcal pneumonia.

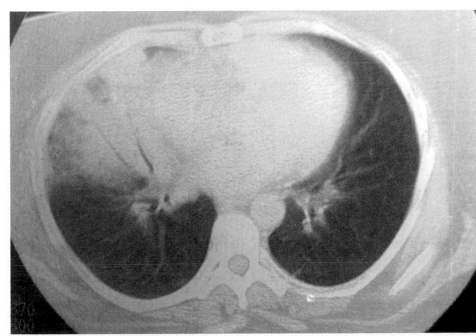

Figure 3–47. A 45-year-old man complained of cough and chest pain. An axial image from a thoracic computed tomography scan (obtained for other reasons) demonstrates dense airspace consolidation in the right middle lobe, which contains several air bronchograms. The fluffy, ill-defined margins of the opacities and the presence of air bronchograms are classic for an airspace process, in this case a community-acquired pneumococcal pneumonia.

The chest radiograph normally lags far behind the clinical response, and residual radiographic abnormalities may be seen for weeks, particularly in older patients.

Interstitial pneumonia

Interstitial pneumonia involves not the alveoli or airways, but the pulmonary interstitium along the bronchi and bronchoalveolar walls. The opacities of an interstitial process are not fluffy and ill-defined, but reticular (linear) and nodular in appearance, appearing like a white chicken wire fence superimposed on a black background. Air bronchograms are not seen because the alveoli remain aerated, although atelectasis may be seen secondary to thickening and eventual obstruction of small airways. The most common pathogens are mycoplasma and viruses. Mycoplasma is commonly seen in young adults and decreases dramatically in incidence during the fourth decade (Fig. 3–48). Most viral pneumonias are due to influenza, and hence tend to occur in epidemics, as distinct from the community-acquired bacterial pneumonias.

TUBERCULOSIS

EPIDEMIOLOGY

At the turn of the century, TB was one of the most common causes of death in the United States, often striking children and young adults. Fortunately, until the mid-1980s, the incidence of TB in the United States decreased at a rate of approximately 3% per year, most likely due to a combination of improved nutrition and increasingly effective antimicrobial therapy. However, with the advent of HIV disease and the rising number of immunocompromised patients, the incidence of TB is now increasing.

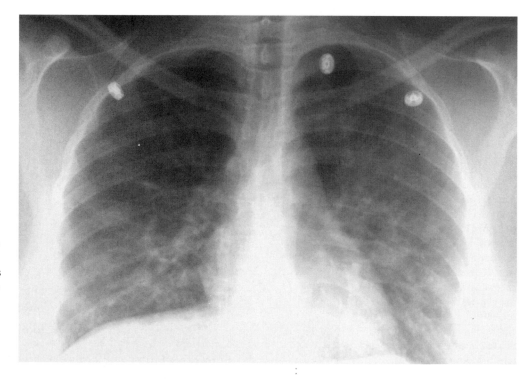

Figure 3–48. This posteroanterior chest radiograph in a young woman who presented with chest pain and cough demonstrates a typical bilateral interstitial pneumonia due to mycoplasma, with infiltration of the alveolar walls and interlobular septa producing linear opacities. Note three metallic snaps on the patient's gown superimposed over the upper thorax.

Individuals at increased risk include not only HIV-positive and immunosuppressed patients, but alcoholics, intravenous drug abusers, and immigrants from areas with a high incidence of tuberculous infection. Recently, strains of multidrug-resistant TB have begun to appear. If present trends continue, TB will constitute one of the most important public health problems in the United States within the first few decades of the next century.

PATHOPHYSIOLOGY

 Approximately 10 to 20% of cases of active disease in the United States are primary TB, which occurs by person-to-person pulmonary transmission. Infected droplets measuring approximately 5 μ in diameter (roughly the size of an erythrocyte) are inhaled into the mid- and lower lung zones (where aeration is greatest). The host response leads to macrophage and lymphocyte infiltration, with the release of lysosomal enzymes and subsequent caseation necrosis and calcification. A vigorous immune response by a healthy host often terminates the infection within several months. The only sequelae may be parenchymal and nodal calcifications and an enhanced response to tuberculous antigens, manifested as greater than 10 mm of induration after purified protein derivative skin testing. Reactivation TB results when the initial infection is merely walled off but not completely irradicated. Months or even decades later, immune impairment associated with aging, disease, or immunosuppression may allow reactivation of the infection.

CLINICAL PRESENTATION

Primary TB, which classically afflicts children, is often asymptomatic, or produces relatively slight clinical symptoms. Some patients may present with an acute pneumonic process. The patient with postprimary TB usually presents with chronic cough, weight loss, night sweats, and fever.

IMAGING

 In primary TB, the radiographic presentation may include focal airspace opacity, or an isolated pleural effusion. The parenchymal lesion is often located in the (better aerated) lower lobes. Lymphatic spread to regional lymph nodes may produce adenopathy (Fig. 3–49). The combination of a calcified parenchymal opacity (the Ghon lesion) and ipsilateral hilar adenopathy is referred to as the Ranke complex.

The reactivation phase of the infection is associated with upper lobe consolidation, a distribution that is usually attributed to the higher oxygen tensions found in the higher lung zones. The upper lobe pneumonia is often necrotizing, producing cavities that range in size up to 10 cm. These may exhibit thin or thick walls and may contain air-fluid levels. From a clinical point of view, cavitation—particularly with air-fluid levels—indicates that the infection is likely to be at a highly infectious stage, when coughing can spread infected particles throughout both the patient's own airways (transbronchial spread) and room air, infecting others. Diffuse hematogenous dissemination may produce a "miliary" pattern on chest radiograph, consisting of innumerable tiny opacities throughout all lung fields (Fig. 3–50). The term *miliary* derives from the fact that the innumerable tiny nodules were thought to resemble a host of

Figure 3–52. This left bronchogram was performed by introducing a catheter through the trachea and into the left mainstem bronchus, after which contrast was injected. Note the reduced number of bronchial divisions and airspaces in the upper lung as compared to the mid- and lower lung zones. These findings reflect destruction of lung tissue from a previous tuberculous lung infection.

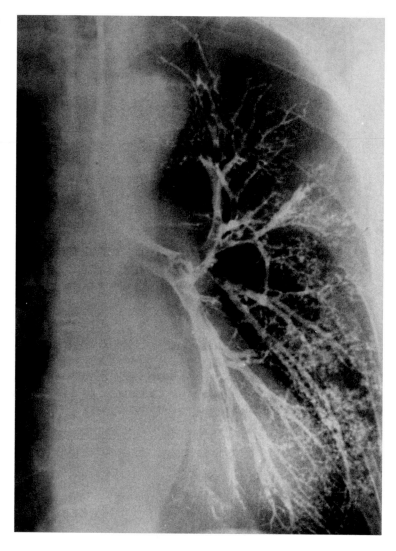

mother–fetus/infant route. Worldwide, approximately 70% of cases are thought to involve a heterosexual route.

AIDS, which represents a late stage in the natural history of HIV infection, is seen at any one time in only a small percentage of the HIV-infected population. HIV especially targets the CD4-positive helper T cells of the immune system, whose numbers are progressively depleted over the natural history of the infection. Because the helper T cell acts as a kind of field marshall of both the humoral and cellular immune responses, this depletion results in increased susceptibility to a host of opportunistic infections and malignancies. Clinical findings supportive of a diagnosis of AIDS include a CD4 count below 200/mm^3 and opportunistic infections such as *Pneumocystis carinii* pneumonia (PCP).

Pneumocystis carinii pneumonia

The most typical pulmonary disease seen in HIV-positive patients is PCP, which represents the initial manifestation of AIDS in up to 60% of patients, generally those with a CD4 count below 300/mm^3. It is estimated that between 50 and 80% of AIDS patients develop at least one episode of PCP, which proves fatal in between 10 and 20% of patients. Pneumocystis is classified as a protozoan, and clinical infection represents reactivation of latent disease. Patients present with dyspnea, fever, and a nonproductive cough. Radiographic findings include a normal chest radiograph in 10%, but up to 80% of patients demonstrate a diffuse, bilateral pattern of reticular interstitial infiltrates, which may progress to diffuse airspace consolidation over a period of days (Fig. 3–53). In febrile immunocompromised patients with a normal chest radiograph, nuclear medicine gallium-67 scanning demonstrates diffuse bilateral pulmonary activity that may antedate chest radiographic findings by as much as 2 weeks (Fig. 3–54). On plain chest films, pleural effusions are rare, and their presence should prompt suspicion of another process. High-resolution CT is more sensitive and spe-

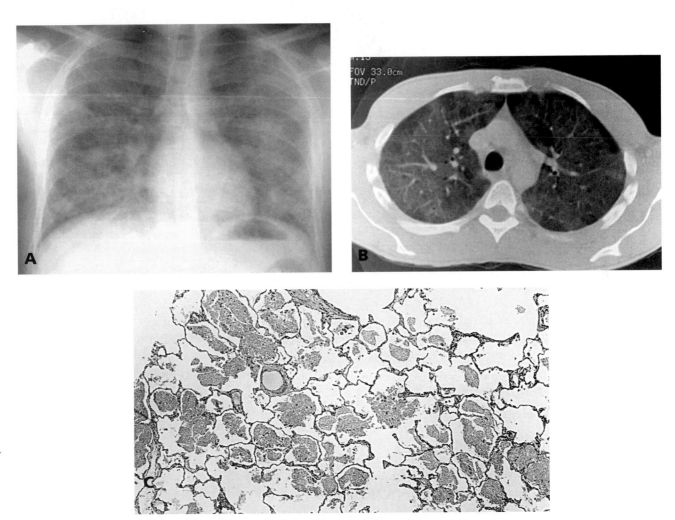

Figure 3–53. A 38-year-old human immunodeficiency virus-positive man presented with a several day history of sore throat and myalgia progressing to respiratory distress. (**A**) A frontal chest radiograph demonstrates diffuse, bilateral airspace consolidation. (**B**) An axial image from a chest computed tomography scan obtained at the same time demonstrates the typical "ground-glass" appearance of *Pneumocystis carinii* pneumonia (PCP), which consists pathologically of a combination of organisms and proteinaceous exudate lining the airspaces. Note the relative sparing of the "cortex" or periphery of the lungs, often seen in PCP. The patient responded well to appropriate antibiotics. (**C**) This light micrograph of a lung specimen demonstrates a classic reaction pattern to *Pneumocystis,* with intraalveolar foamy material and relatively scant interstitial infiltrates.

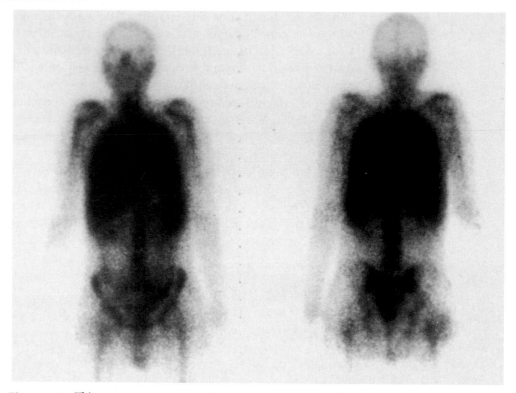

Figure 3–54. This young man receiving radiation and chemotherapy for Hodgkin's lymphoma complained of tightness in the chest but was otherwise well. A chest radiograph was negative for pneumonia. He underwent a routine gallium-67 citrate scan to assess his response to therapy. While the scan demonstrates no evidence of abnormal radiotracer activity in the lymphatic system, indicating a good tumor response, it does reveal striking diffuse bilateral pulmonary activity (the anterior image is on the left, and posterior on the right). The patient was found to be suffering from *Pneumocystis carinii* pneumonia (PCP). This case illustrates the excellent sensitivity of the gallium scan for the detection of PCP, which approaches 100%.

cific than plain radiography, and typically demonstrates diffuse ground-glass opacities, with thin-walled cysts in some cases. Subpleural cysts can result in spontaneous pneumothorax.

Other fungal infections

Other fungal infections also occur by reactivation of latent infection. Cryptococcus is the second most common fungal pneumonia seen in AIDS and often presents with an interstitial infiltrate or isolated pleural effusion. The vast majority of patients have disseminated disease at the time of presentation, with severe headache and other signs of meningitis in most patients. Histoplasmosis most often exhibits a nodular pattern. Coccidioidomycosis most often exhibits a diffuse interstitial pattern with thin-walled cavities.

Mycobacteria

Reactivation TB can occur at any point in HIV disease. In a majority of patients who eventually develop TB, TB will be the initial manifestation of HIV infection. Early in the course of HIV infection, pulmonary TB is radiographically indistinguishable from reactivation TB in the non-HIV-infected patient, with a tendency to upper lobe predominance, cavitation in up to one-half of cases, and pleural effusions in one-quarter. Late in HIV infection, with CD4 counts below 50/mm^3 and a virtual absence of cellular immunity, the usual host response to the organism is lacking, and atypical findings predominate. These include adenopathy and pleural effusions in over one-half of patients, with no cavitation, and a miliary pattern of pulmonary opacities. Mycobacterium avium complex rarely presents as a pulmonary disease.

Bacteria

It must not be forgotten that run-of-the-mill bacterial pneumonias are common in HIV disease, with an incidence approximately six times that in the general population. Bacterial pneumonia is most commonly seen early in the course of HIV infection. In fact, the occurrence of more than one bacterial pneumonia in a year in a previously healthy patient may be an indication for HIV testing, and multiple bacterial pneumonias constitute an AIDS-defining illness. The most common organisms are the usual organisms seen in non-HIV-infected patients, including *Staphylococcus pneumoniae* and *Haemophilus influenza*.

Kaposi's sarcoma

Although its incidence is declining, Kaposi's sarcoma (KS) remains the most common malignancy in HIV disease and constitutes an AIDS-defining illness. Most patients are homosexual men, and a herpes virus has been implicated as the causative agent. Only about 5% of patients demonstrate pulmonary involvement, which is almost always preceded by visceral manifestations. Radiographic findings include nodules and/or coarse interstitial opacities radiating outward from the hila (Fig. 3–55). Pleural effusions and adenopathy are relatively common. If the diagnosis is uncertain, nuclear medicine studies can be helpful; KS is thallium-avid but gallium-negative.

Lymphoma

AIDS-related lymphoma is an aggressive non-Hodgkin's B-cell disorder with extranodal involvement in nearly all patients. Approximately 10% of patients demonstrate thoracic involvement, including single or multiple masses, interstitial or alveolar opacities, and effusions, with adenopathy in 20%. Lymphoma is both thallium- and gallium-avid, which distinguishes it from KS. The prognosis is poor, with a median survival of approximately 6 months.

Lymphocytic interstitial pneumonitis

Lymphocytic interstitial pneumonitis (LIP) is an AIDS-defining illness in children, in whom it is most common. Pathologically, it consists of a mixed infiltrate of lymphocytes, plasma cells, and histiocytes in the pulmonary interstitium. The disorder is also seen in non-AIDS conditions such as Sjogren's syndrome (immune-mediated destruction of exocrine glands resulting in mucosal and conjunctival dryness), in which it can be associated with malignant transformation. This is not the case in AIDS-associated LIP. LIP is an indolent process that persists for months, without response to antibiotics. Radiographic findings consist of nonspecific persistent reticulonodular opacities. The diagnosis is established by biopsy.

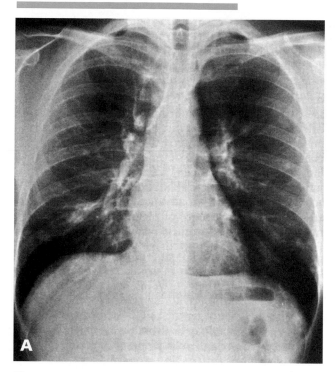
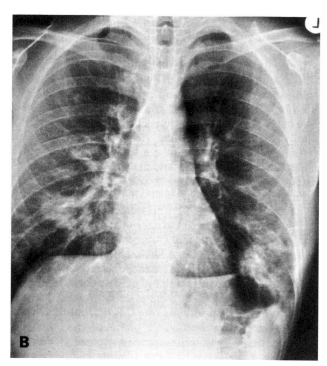

Figure 3–55. (A) A frontal chest radiograph in this acquired immunodeficiency syndrome patient demonstrates bilateral scattered nodular opacities and interstitial opacities radiating outward from the hila. (B) A follow-up film 3 months later demonstrates progression of disease, Kaposi's sarcoma.

Tumorous

METASTATIC DISEASE

Pulmonary malignancy arising from another primary is more common than primary lung carcinoma. In fact, the lung is the single most frequent site of metastatic disease in the human body. Why? The answer lies in the fact that the lung constitutes the first capillary bed distal to the circulation of most organs and tissues. The most important exception to this statement is the liver, which, because of the hepatic portal system, represents the first capillary bed distal to most of the GI tract, including the stomach, pancreas, and colon. Because the liver "sees" the venous blood from the pancreas first, it would be unusual to find pulmonary metastases in a pancreatic carcinoma patient whose liver was free of disease. Neoplasms that commonly metastasize to lung include GI tract malignancies, melanoma, sarcomas, and carcinomas of the breast, kidney, and lung. Plain chest radiography, and in some cases CT, is mandatory in any patient diagnosed with such a tumor, because the presence of pulmonary metastases dramatically alters prognosis and therapy.

Hematogenous dissemination is the most common route of metastatic spread to the lung. Additional paths of metastasis include direct extension, pleural spread (typically producing a malignant pleural effusion), transbronchial spread (a frequent route for bronchoalveolar carcinoma), and lymphogenous dissemination. At least three-quarters of patients with lung metastases will have implants elsewhere in the body as well. Hematogenous spread occurs when a tumor invades venules or lymphatics, and cells break off and travel in the blood, become trapped in a distal capillary bed, take root, and spread beyond the capillary into surrounding tissue. It is estimated that only 1 in 100,000 cells released into the bloodstream is able to complete this course.

Where are metastases most frequently found within the lungs? Predictably, in the regions that enjoy the greatest perfusion: the bases. Most metastases will be multiple and bilateral as well, although up to 10% of metastases may be solitary (Fig. 3–56). Cavitation is a common feature of squamous cell carcinomas, while calcification may be seen in osteogenic sarcoma and mucin-producing tumors such as certain gastric, colorectal, and ovarian carcinomas.

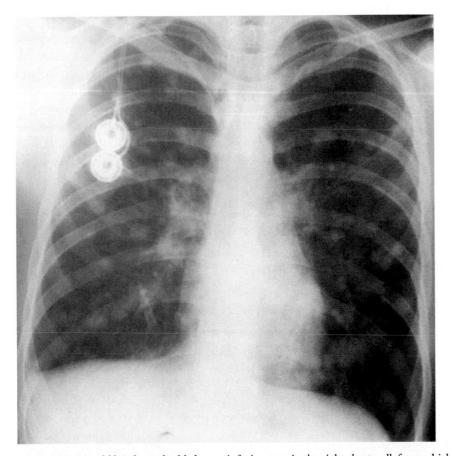

Figure 3–56. A 16-year-old boy has a double lumen infusion port in the right chest wall, from which a catheter extends through the right subclavian vein and down into the superior vena cava. Whenever one sees such a device, suspicion for a malignancy requiring cytotoxic chemotherapy should be increased. In this case, both lungs contain multiple bilateral nodules, ranging in size up to approximately 1 cm. The multiplicity of these lesions and their distribution throughout both lung fields strongly favors hematogenous metastases. What is the likely primary? Note that even though these nodules are relatively small, they appear quite dense, at least as dense as the adjacent ribs. This suggests that they may be calcified. What tumor in a 16-year-old could produce multiple calcified pulmonary nodules? The most likely culprit is a bone-forming tumor, such as an osteogenic sarcoma, which was the diagnosis in this case. Occasionally, nonosteogenic metastatic lesions may also calcify in response to therapy.

PRIMARY LUNG CANCER

EPIDEMIOLOGY

Often called bronchogenic carcinoma because these malignant neoplasms can be traced to exposure to inhaled carcinogens, the lung cancers have dramatically risen in incidence during the twentieth century. While only several hundred cases were reported annually in the United States at the turn of the century, approximately 200,000 lung cancers are now diagnosed each year, and lung cancer is the leading cause of cancer mortality, resulting in 95,000 deaths per year among men, and 60,000 deaths per year among women. In the 1980s, it surpassed breast cancer as the number one cancer killer of American women, a distinction it has held for decades in men (Fig. 3–57).

PATHOPHYSIOLOGY

The trends in lung cancer incidence are traceable to cigarette smoking. Approximately 90% of lung cancer deaths are directly attributable to tobacco, with a strong correlation between the level of risk and the number of pack-years smoked, and a decline in risk with smoking cessation (although it takes 10 to 20 years for risk to return to normal). Tobacco use in American men and women has dramatically declined since 1965, when more than 60% of men and 30% of women smoked, but cigarette use has dramatically risen in other nations, such as the Philippines, Korea, and Poland, which must brace their health care systems for epidemics of lung cancer.

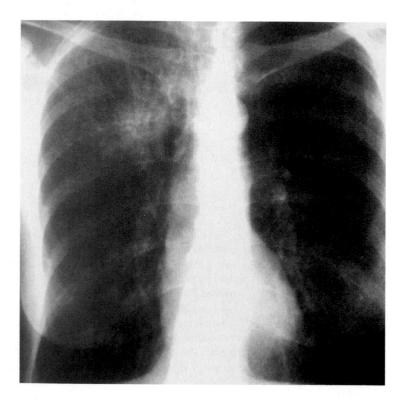

Figure 3–57. This posteroanterior chest radiograph demonstrates a classic appearance of a primary lung carcinoma, with a large spiculated mass in the right upper lobe. Note the linear soft-tissue radiations extending outward from the tumor, particularly superolaterally, sometimes referred to as a "corona radiata" (from the Latin for "crown" and "spoke"). The corona radiata is not specific for malignancy, however, and may be seen in any process that provokes a desmoplastic response. The radiographic margins of a tumor provide a "visual biopsy" of its biological behavior. In this case, the infiltrative appearance of the lesion, with intricate interdigitation of tumor and normal lung tissue, constitutes a strong indicator of invasive behavior.

Other risk factors for the development of lung cancer include exposure to environmental agents such as radon, various occupational exposures including asbestos and uranium, and a number of preexisting diseases, such as pulmonary fibrosis and scleroderma. In many situations, the risks are additive. For example, while the average smoker has a relative risk of contracting lung cancer 10 times that of a nonsmoker, that risk rises to 50 times normal when the smoker has a history of occupational asbestos exposure (Fig. 3–58).

Despite recent developments in medical and surgical therapies, the outlook remains bleak. The only hope for cure lies in complete resection of all tumor cells, yet three-quarters of tumors are deemed inoperable at preoperative staging, to which another 10% are added based on operative findings. Five-year survival is approximately 10%.

CLINICAL PRESENTATION

Lung cancer presents with a variety of symptoms. Tumors involving central bronchi present with respiratory symptoms, such as cough, hemoptysis, and postobstructive pneumonia. Pleural involvement may produce pleuritic chest pain or local chest-wall pain, as well as dyspnea from effusions. Well-known syndromes associated with lung cancer include paraneoplastic syndromes (such as Cushing's syndrome in a patient with corticotropin-producing oat cell carcinoma), Pancoast's syndrome (pain, hand weakness, and Horner's syndrome secondary to a superior sulcus tumor impinging on the brachial plexus and sympathetic ganglia), and SVC syndrome (distention of head, neck, and upper limb veins due to compression or invasion of the SVC).

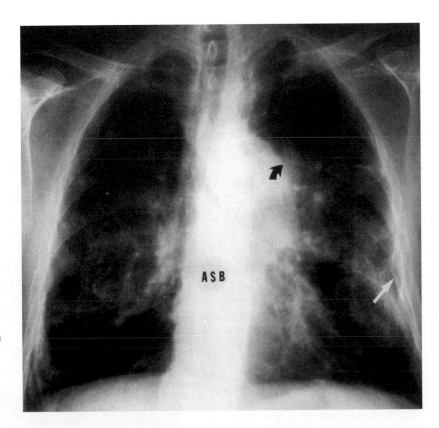

Figure 3–58. This elderly male smoker demonstrates multiple important sequelae of his occupational asbestos exposure. The first is the presence of asbestosis (ASB), as manifested by pulmonary fibrosis in the mid- and lower lung zones, as well as fibrosis involving the mediastinal pleura and paracardiac lung, which produces the so-called shaggy heart sign. A second is the presence of calcified pleural plaques (white arrow). The third is a left suprahilar mass (black arrow), which represented a bronchogenic carcinoma.

IMAGING

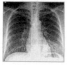 It is often said that all pneumonias in patients over 35 years of age should be followed to the point of radiographic resolution. Why? Because the pneumonia may be trying to tell us something; namely, that one of the patient's bronchi harbors an obstructing lesion. Hence, recurrent pneumonias in the same site should prompt a search for an endobronchial lesion, which will likely be either a squamous cell carcinoma, a carcinoid tumor, or a foreign body.

There are four histologic types of bronchogenic carcinoma, each with its own characteristic biologic behavior and imaging characteristics.

Histologic types

The most common primary pulmonary malignancy, adenocarcinoma, is increasing most rapidly in incidence, and now accounts for 50% of lung cancers. On light microscopy, this tumor forms glandular or papillary structures. It is the most common type in women and has the weakest association with cigarette smoking. While the primary lesion exhibits relatively slow growth, it tends to metastasize early. Radiologically, three-quarters of these lesions present peripherally in the lung, most often as a solitary nodule or mass, and often in the upper lobes (Fig. 3–59). A variant of adenocarcinoma, bronchoalveolar carcinoma, disseminates along the tracheobronchial tree. It characteristically presents as a small peripheral nodule or as persistent airspace opacities (a "pneumonia" that fails to respond radiographically to antibiosis). It has a much better prognosis if removed before it reaches 3 cm in size.

The second most frequent form, accounting for approximately one-third of cases, is squamous cell carcinoma, so named because it exhibits the keratinization and intercellular bridges one expects in squamous epithelium. Squamous cell carcinoma typically arises centrally within a bronchus, spreading by endobronchial growth. On radiographs, it often appears as a hilar or perihilar mass, and produces segmental or lobar atelectasis and/or consolidation secondary to bronchial obstruction (Fig. 3–60). However, up to one-third of lesions may present peripherally. It is the most common type to cavitate and also constitutes the most common etiology of Pancoast's syndrome. It has

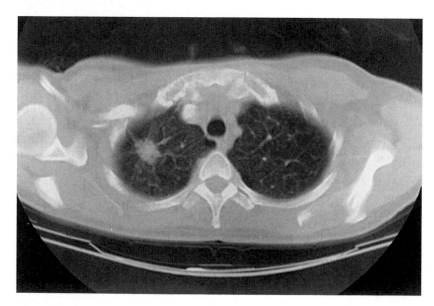

Figure 3–59. A 42-year-old woman had smoked two packs of cigarettes per day for 25 years. A chest radiograph (not shown) suggested a possible lesion in the right upper lobe, and a thoracic computed tomography scan was obtained for further characterization. It demonstrates a 3 cm spiculated mass in the right apex, which proved on biopsy to be a primary adenocarcinoma. The term *spiculation* refers to the strands of tumor cells or reactive fibrosis seen radiating centrifugally from the central tumor.

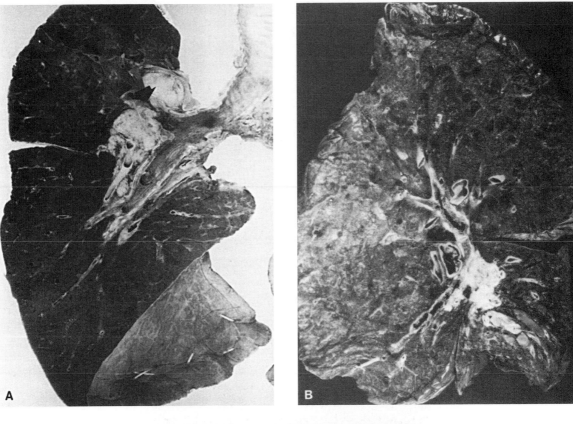

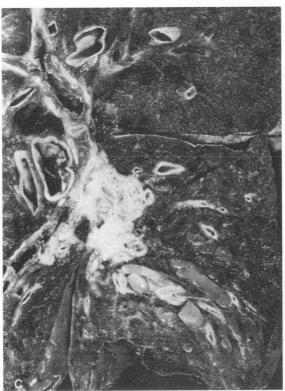

Figure 3–60. (A) This gross specimen photograph of a squamous cell lung carcinoma demonstrates a classic appearance, with tumor arising centrally in the upper lobe bronchus (arrow). (B) Another specimen demonstrates a squamous cell carcinoma arising in a lower lobe bronchus. (C) A close-up view of the tumor shows that the lower lobe has undergone obstructive atelectasis, with the development of purulent bronchiectasis.

the best overall prognosis, with significant potential for cure if tumors are removed prior to metastatic spread.

The third most common cell type is small cell carcinoma, including the so-called oat cell variety, so named because its cells are small, round, and possess hyperchromatic nuclei. It is the most strongly associated with cigarette smoking. Small cell carcinoma most often presents as a large, central mass and is very likely to be metastatic at the time of detection, with 80% of patients demonstrating extrathoracic metastatic disease (Fig. 3–61). It is associated with significant degrees of mediastinal and hilar adenopathy in most cases. Paradoxically, while small cell carcinoma exhibits the best response to radiation and chemotherapy, it also has the shortest median survival, approximately 1 to 2 years.

Large cell lung carcinoma most often presents as a large, peripheral mass. Unfortunately, it exhibits the worst combination of biological behaviors, growing rapidly and metastasizing early. However, its prognosis remains more favorable than that of small cell carcinoma.

Solitary pulmonary nodule

One of the classic differential diagnoses in radiology is that of the solitary pulmonary nodule (SPN). SPNs are defined as single pulmonary lesions measuring less

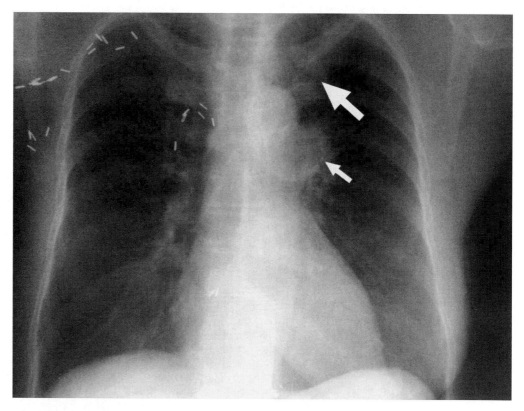

Figure 3–61. This posteroanterior chest radiograph in a 71-year-old woman reveals evidence of a previous mastectomy and axillary lymph node dissection, with absence of the right breast shadow and multiple surgical clips in the right axilla. In addition, there is a several centimeter mass in the medial aspect of the left upper lobe (large arrow), which is associated with a mass in the left aorticopulmonary window (small arrow). These findings represent a primary small cell carcinoma with mediastinal lymphadenopathy.

than 3 cm in diameter, and at least 150,000 of these lesions are biopsied or excised each year. In descending order of frequency, the most likely etiologies for a solitary nodule are granuloma (TB, histoplasmosis, etc.), bronchogenic carcinoma, carcinoid tumor, and metastasis. The best morphologic predictor of benignity is central calcification (Fig. 3–62). Other radiologic characteristics that favor benignity include small size (although every 6 cm lung cancer was once a 1 cm tumor, and this criterion should not influence diagnostic workup), well-defined borders (although many lung cancers are well-defined), and patterns of calcification, such as complete, laminated, or "popcorn" calcification (the latter indicating a hamartoma). The fact that carcinomas may arise in preexisting granulomas means that this criterion must be applied with caution. An additional criterion is the patient's age. Nodules in patients younger than 35 years of age rarely represent carcinomas. On the other hand, a nodule in a 60-year-old heavy smoker is very likely to represent a lung cancer.

Where possible, the single most important determination to be made in the evaluation of a SPN is whether the nodule is a new or changing finding. If it has been stable for more than 2 years, it is almost certainly benign. The key to determining change is the acquisition of previous chest radiographs. A time-consuming, worrisome, and expensive diagnostic workup can often be completely avoided if a nodule is found to

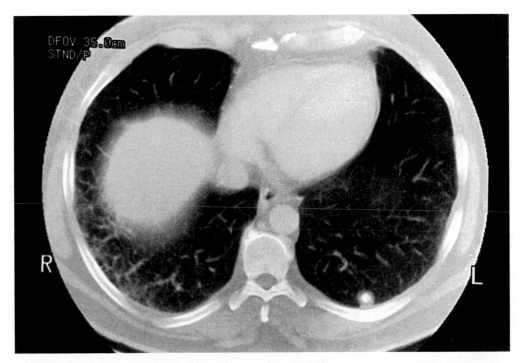

Figure 3–62. This asymptomatic 64-year-old man was found to have a pulmonary nodule near the left lung base on routine chest radiographs (not shown). No previous chest radiographs were available, and lung cancer figured prominently in the differential diagnosis. In an effort to better characterize the nodule, a thoracic computed tomography examination was performed, which would not only better characterize the nodule but also provide staging information if the lesion turned out to be malignant. This axial image demonstrates that the lesion is densely calcified centrally, indicating that it represents a benign granuloma. A malignant tumor, which tends to grow in an irregular and even destructive fashion, would not exhibit such a symmetrical, perfectly round, central calcification. Note that the lesion is contiguous with the pleura posteriorly.

have been present for years. Generally, a lesion that has been stable in size for 2 years can be diagnosed as benign, because the typical doubling time of a primary lung malignancy is approximately 120 days. However, changes in size may be subtle; a lesion that doubles in volume increases in diameter by only approximately 25%, indicating that accurate measurements are critical in assessing for change.

Tissue diagnosis

The radiologist's role in the diagnosis of lung cancer extends beyond the radiographic detection of tumors to include the acquisition of tissue for diagnosis. Using fluoroscopic or CT guidance, it is possible to obtain both fine needle aspirates and core needle biopsies of nodules, masses, and adenopathy, as well as suspected metastatic lesions. Such procedures enable tissue typing of most tumors, with a better than 90% rate of success, at lower cost, and with a lower rate of complication than surgical procedures such as thoracotomy. The principal complication of transthoracic needle biopsy is pneumothorax, which occurs in approximately 20% of cases. However, in 90% of pneumothoraxes, the degree of respiratory compromise is clinically insignificant, and the placement of a pleural vent is not required. Additional complications of transthoracic needle biopsy include bleeding and hemoptysis. Other means of obtaining tissue include bronchoscopy for central endobronchial lesions, and thoracoscopy and even thoracotomy in patients for whom the risk of pneumothorax is unacceptable (e.g., a patient with severe bullous emphysema).

Staging

Whether lung cancer is primary or metastatic, staging is another routine function of the radiologist. It is important for several reasons. First, in the case of metastatic disease, a small percentage of patients may benefit from resection of their pulmonary metastases, such as patients with melanoma or osteogenic sarcoma. In addition, patients with metastatic disease elsewhere in the body, such as the liver or CNS, generally should be spared thoracotomy. Similar reasoning applies in the staging of primary lung carcinoma, where surgery with curative intent should be undertaken only in the minority of patients in whom cure is possible; that is, patients whose tumors have not already spread to other organs. Staging is also important in the evaluation of treatment protocols.

The staging of lung cancer employs the familiar TNM (*tumor-node-metastasis*) system. T refers to the size, location, and extent of the primary tumor; N to local nodal involvement; and M to the presence or absence of distant metastatic disease, including lymphatic involvement. Among the most common examinations used in staging are CT scans of the chest and upper abdomen, and radionuclide bone scans to assess skeletal involvement.

Unfortunately, none of the cross-sectional imaging techniques (CT, MRI, or ultrasound) can demonstrate abnormal internal nodal architecture, and the criteria for metastatic nodal involvement are based on size, which has limitations. For example, if the radiologist reports every node larger than 1 cm in short axis as probably involved, which is standard practice for most nodal groups, nearly one-third of the nodes called abnormal will be free of metastatic disease, while nearly one-tenth of smaller nodes will show evidence of micrometastasis. Nuclear medicine studies using tumor-specific radiopharmaceuticals may provide a more sensitive and specific means of tumor staging in the future.

Inflammatory

ASPIRATION

EPIDEMIOLOGY

Clinical risk factors for aspiration can be divided into two principal categories: CNS disorders and swallowing disorders. Common CNS conditions include recent general anesthesia, alcoholism, and seizure disorders. Important predisposing conditions in children are mental retardation and cerebral palsy. Common swallowing disorders include head and neck cancers, previous head and neck surgery or irradiation, and esophageal motility disorders, including gastroesophageal reflux. In hospitalized patients, the presence of endotracheal tubes and nasogastric tubes, which interfere with normal oropharyngeal function, are also risk factors.

PATHOPHYSIOLOGY

 Aspiration of oropharyngeal contents into the tracheobronchial tree and airspaces poses a threat for two principal reasons. First, the normal oropharyngeal flora consists of dozens of species of bacteria, both aerobic and anaerobic, that are capable of causing pneumonia if they reach the lungs in sufficient quantities. The virulence of oropharyngeal contents is increased in patients with poor oral hygiene, in whom mixed anaerobic infections are especially common. Because halitosis serves as an indicator of bacterial overgrowth, many of these patients will have noticeably bad breath.

The second reason that aspiration poses a threat to the lungs relates to the irritative properties of gastric contents. The low pH of gastric secretions, with a hydrogen ion concentration approximately 10,000 times that found in the pulmonary interstitium, means that even a small quantity of aspirate can produce a profuse chemical pneumonitis in exposed regions of lung. Moreover, aspirated food particles can both induce a foreign-body granulomatous response and serve as a culture medium for bacterial growth.

CLINICAL PRESENTATION

A history of coughing or choking when eating and repeated unexplained pneumonias are the most important clinical indicators that an ambulatory patient may have aspirated. Patients with aspiration pneumonitis often exhibit a low-grade fever and productive cough.

IMAGING

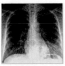 Lung zones affected by aspiration will vary depending on the amount of aspirate and the patient's position at the time the episode occurred. Generally, the aspirated material will travel to the most gravity-dependent portions of the lung. In the upright position, this most commonly includes the posterior basal segments of the lower lobes (Fig. 3–63). In supine patients, the left lower and superior segmental lobes are most commonly involved. The usual radiographic pattern of acute aspiration consists of airspace opacities in the

Figure 3–63. A 74-year-old woman underwent a barium esophagogram to evaluate dysphagia. A single swallow produced substantial aspiration of the contrast bolus. Note barium outlining the distal trachea and mainstem bronchi (long arrow). As expected in this upright patient, most of the contrast bolus has found its way to the most gravity-dependent portion of the lung, the posterior basal segment of the lower lobe (thick arrow).

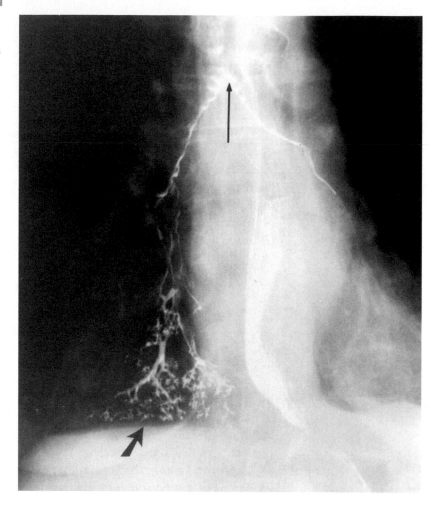

affected portions of lung. Atelectasis may also be seen, presumably secondary to pneumonitic damage to type II pneumocytes or obstruction of airways by food particles. The picture usually begins to improve within several days, unless complicated by infection or ARDS. Repeated bouts may lead to a chronic aspiration pattern, characterized by interstitial opacities and scarring.

INHALATIONAL LUNG DISEASE

A variety of inhaled inorganic dust particles may overwhelm the lung's intrinsic clearance mechanisms and produce a pneumoconiosis. The pneumoconioses include silicosis, coal worker's pneumoconiosis, and asbestos-related disease. All produce tiny nodules that may progress through inflammation to fibrosis to end-stage lung disease. Macrophages ingest the dust particles but are unable to digest them, with the release of phagolysosomal enzymes and the formation of granulomas.

Asbestos exposure may cause not only interstitial lung disease, but pleural diseases as well. These include pleural plaques (which may calcify), pleural effusions, and malignancies. The most common malignancy in asbestos exposure is lung cancer, although malignant mesothelioma has a more specific correlation with asbestos exposure, with a 5000 to 10,000 times increased incidence. The risk of bronchogenic carcinoma and carcinomas of GI tract is also increased. Radiographically, mesothelioma manifests as pleural thickening and/or effusion, diffuse encasement of the lung with volume loss, or pulmonary metastases.

Metabolic

Cystic fibrosis is often called the most common fatal genetic disease in Caucasians, with an incidence of 1 in 2000 persons in the United States. It is caused by a defect in a membrane ion transport protein of mucous-secreting cells, which results in the production of thick, tenacious mucus by exocrine glands and resultant impaired mucociliary transport. Pulmonary manifestations are universal and include mucous plugging, recurrent infections, especially with pseudomonas, and progressive respiratory failure. Other clinical manifestations include pancreatic insufficiency, sinusitis, and infertility in males. Radiographic findings include bronchiectasis, disordered aeration (secondary to mucous plugging), pneumonia, and predominantly upper lobe involvement (Fig. 3–64). Complications include pneumothorax, hemoptysis, aspergillus superinfection, and pulmonary hypertension and cor pulmonale.

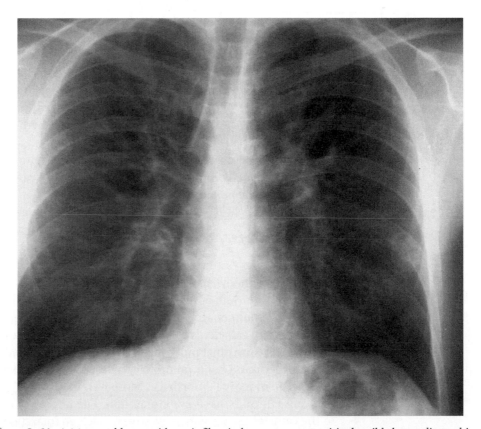

Figure 3–64. A 26-year-old man with cystic fibrosis demonstrates surprisingly mild chest radiographic abnormalities, which testify to the effectiveness of recent improvements in the clinical management of this disease. Note the diffuse bilateral interstitial abnormality, which is most severe in the lung apexes, where it is also accompanied by bronchiectasis (which is well seen in the medial aspect of the right upper lobe). A more focal opacity in the periphery of the left midlung represents an acute infectious process.

Iatrogenic

MEDICAL DEVICES

One of the most common reasons for obtaining a chest radiograph in hospitalized patients is to assess the results of medical interventions, such as the placement of central venous catheters and intravascular monitoring devices. The first order of business in reading the chest radiograph of any intensive care unit patient is to verify the correct position of medical devices and ensure the absence of placement complications.

Central venous catheters

The most frequent use of central venous catheters is the administration of medications, such as antibiotics and cytotoxic chemotherapeutic agents, although other uses such as parenteral feeding and central venous pressure monitoring are also common. Both intravenous medications and feeding solutions are often too irritating to smaller peripheral vessels and must be administered centrally, where they are immediately diluted in larger volumes of blood. By far the most common routes of catheter insertion are the jugular and subclavian venous approaches. The latter is generally more comfortable for the patient, who may have a catheter in place for weeks or months. Recently, the insertion of smaller caliber central venous catheters via a peripheral route has also become popular.

Regardless of the route of insertion of a central venous catheter (assuming it is above the heart), the optimal position of its tip is within the SVC, between the brachiocephalic veins and the right atrium. The normal SVC overlies the right mediastinum running craniocaudally, and the distal portion of the catheter should follow this route. Types of malposition include location outside the SVC, such as in smaller vessels or in the heart (which can precipitate arrhythmias), or outside the vascular space altogether, in which case hematoma formation is likely (Fig. 3–65). An extravascular location is often associated with poor blood return following catheter insertion. Another important complication of central venous catheter insertion is pneumothorax, produced by puncture of the pleura.

Pulmonary artery catheters

Pulmonary artery catheters are routinely employed in critically ill patients to monitor pulmonary hemodynamics and cardiac output. The catheter is usually placed into the right subclavian vein and allowed to follow the flow of blood through the right heart and into the pulmonary outflow tract. The key consideration in placement of a pulmonary artery catheter is to ensure that the tip is not located more peripherally in the lung than the proximal pulmonary arteries. If it is located more peripherally, inflation of the balloon to obtain pulmonary artery "wedge" pressures may rupture the vessel, causing pulmonary hemorrhage. Moreover, the tip itself may occlude a smaller vessel and cause thrombosis or even infarction. The finding of a wedge-shaped opacity distal to the catheter tip is highly suggestive of such an infarction.

Balloon pumps

In patients with cardiogenic shock, an intra-aortic counterpulsation balloon pump may be inserted to augment cardiac output. The balloon is pneumatically inflated

Figure 3–65. This patient complained of a sensation of tightness in the right side of her chest and shortness of breath 1 day after the insertion of a right subclavian central venous catheter. Because blood could be withdrawn through the catheter, no postprocedure chest radiograph was obtained, and the patient received several liters of fluid through the catheter before eventually becoming symptomatic. A portable chest radiograph was then obtained, which revealed that the central line is more medial than expected in position within the central upper mediastinum (arrow). Unfortunately, the entire volume of intravenous fluid entered the right hemithorax, resulting in a near-complete right hydrothorax and shift of mediastinal structures to the left. This illustrates the importance of obtaining a chest radiograph after insertion of a central line, even if no complication is suspected.

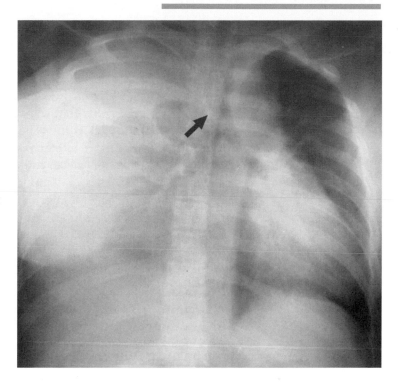

during diastole, which increases intra-aortic pressure and augments coronary perfusion. During systole, it deflates, thereby reducing afterload and left ventricular work. The catheter is generally placed from a femoral approach and should be positioned so that its radiopaque tip is distal to the left subclavian artery, the last of the great vessels branching off from the aortic arch. If the tip is placed proximal to the left subclavian artery, it may cause dissection or occlusion of the carotid and subclavian arteries.

Pacemakers

Cardiac pacemakers are commonly employed to treat arrhythmias, and are generally implanted under the skin of the chest or abdomen, with leads tunneled subcutaneously up to the subclavian vein site where they enter the central veins and descend to the heart. A similar device is the implantable automatic defibrillation device, which can cardiovert the patient automatically in the field. Pacemakers may be unipolar or bipolar. Unipolar pacer lead tips should be located near the apex of the right ventricle, while bipolar leads are generally located in the right atrial appendage and the right ventricular apex. Aside from the usual complications of central line placement, complications with the placement of pacer wires include puncture of the myocardium and the development of hemopericardium. In addition, the pacemaker device and leads should be inspected to ensure that there is no disruption in the wiring that could render the device nonfunctional.

Endotracheal tubes

Patients on mechanically assisted ventilation generally require endotracheal intubation to ensure that only the respiratory tract, and not the digestive tract, is ventilated.

The radiopaque walls of the endotracheal tube are generally visible on portable chest radiographs descending through the pharynx into the trachea. The tip of the tube should be located approximately 5 cm above the carina in most adult patients. It must be borne in mind that the tip of the tube will change in position with changes in head position. With the chin tilted down toward the chest, the tip will move closer to the carina, while elevating the chin will cause the tip to move away from the carina. A tip located too high may allow the balloon cuff to impinge upon the vocal cords. A tip located too low may move into one of the mainstem bronchi, almost always the right, causing underventilation of the contralateral lung. Another concern is the degree of inflation of the cuff. An overinflated cuff can press on the tracheal mucosa with sufficient force that it overcomes capillary perfusion pressure and causes necrosis, with resultant tracheomalacia. At a minimum, the cuff should not cause the walls of the trachea to bow laterally.

Chest tubes

Chest tubes are inserted primarily to drain gas or fluid from the pleural space. Thus, the tube can only perform its intended function if it is located within the pleural space, in communication with the collection it is intended to drain. One sign that the tube is improperly positioned is persistence of the pneumothorax or hydrothorax. An even more worrisome sign is an increase in gas, which may indicate more serious complications, such as an air leak from the tracheobronchial tree.

Nasogastric tubes

Nasogastric tubes are commonly inserted to decompress the stomach, as in bowel obstruction, or for aspiration or lavage of gastric contents, as in upper GI bleeding. The tip of the tube is routinely visualized on portable chest radiographs and should be located in the gastric body or antrum (Fig. 3–66). If the tip is located within or below the pyloric channel, the tube may not achieve its intended purpose. Similarly, a tube located too high, within the esophagus, may not communicate with the gastric lumen at all. Strictly speaking, the tip of the tube is less important in this regard than its side port, which is generally located 5 to 7 cm above the tip. It is the side port, and not the tip, that is used for injection or aspiration. Enteric feeding tubes, such as Dobhoff tubes, are positioned in the distal duodenum or proximal jejunum.

Traumatic

Trauma may injure the lung by a variety of mechanisms, including direct impact by a penetrating object and shear injuries due to torsion at interfaces between fixed and mobile structures. Aside from bone fractures and pneumothorax, one of the most common manifestations of chest trauma is pulmonary contusion (Fig. 3–67). Contusion occurs when vessels rupture, with filling of adjacent interstitium and alveoli with blood and associated edema. Interstitial and airspace opacities usually appear approximately 6 hours after the injury, and require approximately 1 week to resolve. When abnormalities persist beyond that point, consideration should be given to the possibility of superinfection and ARDS.

Figure 3–66. The frontal chest radiograph in an 18-year-old woman demonstrates an endotracheal tube well positioned in the esophagus and striking gaseous distention of the stomach in the left upper quadrant, as well as a nasogastric tube. Why is the stomach so distended, in spite of the fact that a nasogastric tube has been placed? The answer, of course, is that the naso-gastric tube is strikingly malpositioned. Its tip does not reach the gastric lumen, and therefore cannot decompress it. Instead of passing down through the mediastinum and into the left upper quadrant, the tube deviates leftward at the level of the tracheal bifurcation and is superimposed over the left lower lung. Why? The tube was inadvertently inserted into the tra-chea instead of the esophagus and extends down into a left lower lobe bronchus. Immediately after this radiograph was seen, the tube was repositioned.

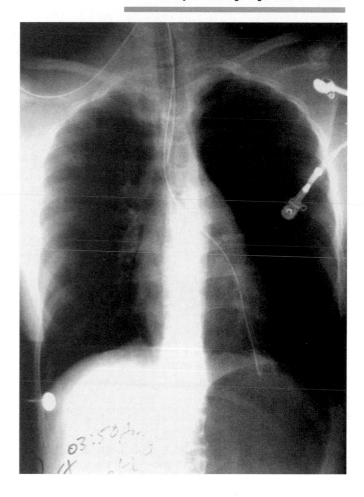

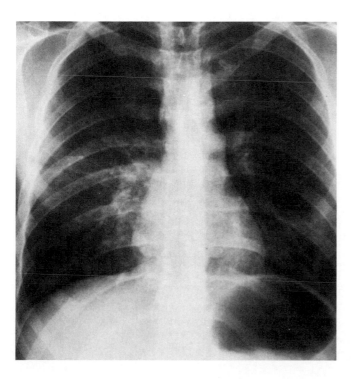

Figure 3–67. This 18-year-old suffered blunt chest trauma after a motorcycle accident. The frontal chest radiograph demon-strates an ill-defined opacity in the right lower lung, which rep-resented a pulmonary contusion.

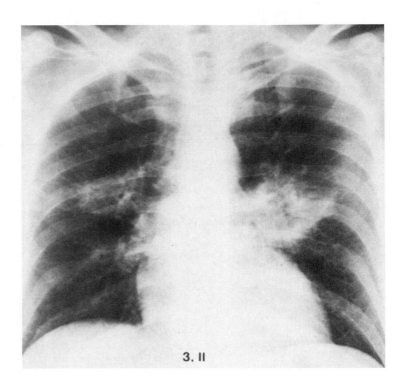

Figure 3–68. A 37-year-old man with maxillary sinusitis and proteinuria demonstrates chest radiographic findings of multiple areas of pulmonary consolidation with cavitation, which in light of the clinical history are strongly suggestive of Wegener's granulomatosis.

Vascular

The lung is prey to injury in collagen vascular diseases and vasculitides. The most common collagen vascular disease to involve the lung is rheumatoid arthritis. Common findings include rheumatoid lung nodules and fibrosing alveolitis, in addition to pleuritis and pleural effusions. Like other collagen vascular diseases such as ankylosing spondylitis and systemic lupus erythematosus, rheumatoid arthritis tends to involve the lower lung zones, where blood flow is greatest. An important vasculitis affecting the lung is Wegener's granulomatosis, which is a systemic disease that involves the upper respiratory tract and kidneys as well. Vascular destruction manifests in the lungs as multiple cavitating nodules and interstitial lung disease (Fig. 3–68).

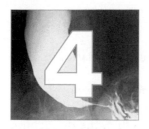

4 The Digestive System

The abdomen extends inferiorly from the diaphragm through the pelvis, and includes tissues from most of the major organ systems. This chapter focuses on the imaging of the digestive system, including both the alimentary canal and the solid organs that participate in digestion.

THE DIGESTIVE TRACT

Anatomy, Physiology, and Imaging

The digestive tract begins at the lips and ends at the anus. From a strict anatomic point of view, the luminal contents of the digestive tract are not inside but outside the body and do not become truly internalized until they enter into capillaries or lymphatics by passing through the mucosal cells lining the gut.

The major divisions of the digestive tract include the mouth, the oropharynx (from the Latin for "mouth" and "throat"), the esophagus (from the Greek *oisophagos,* "passage for food"), the stomach (from the Greek *stoma,* "mouth"), the duodenum (from the Latin *duo,* "two" + *den,* "ten," because it is 12 fingers' breadth long), the jejunum (from the Latin *jejunus,* "empty," because it was thought to be empty at death), the ileum (from the Latin *ileus,* "flank"), the colon, the rectum (from the Latin for "straight," as in rectitude), and the anus (from the Latin for "ring," as in annular) (Fig. 4–1). Let us briefly consider each of these divisions in turn.

OROPHARYNX

STRUCTURE AND FUNCTION

The pharynx is usually divided by anatomists into three segments, the nasopharynx (from the skull base to the soft palate), the oropharynx (from the soft palate to the hyoid bone), and the hypopharynx (from the hyoid bone to the cricopharyngeus muscle). The oropharynx functions in the mechanical breakdown of food through chewing, in the chemical breakdown of food through salivary amylase, in speech, and in swallowing. Because the digestive and respiratory systems share a common pathway in

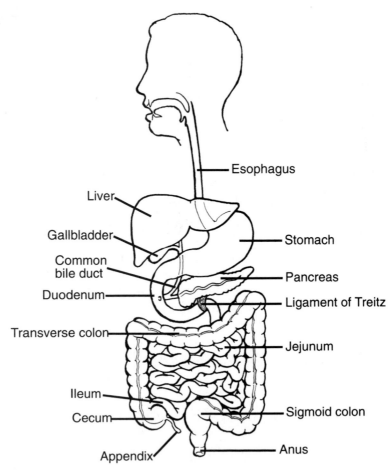

Figure 4–1. Parts of the gastrointestinal tract.

the oropharynx, swallowing represents a critical function, ensuring that ingested material does not reach the lungs. Aspiration refers to the passage of liquid or solid oral contents into the trachea.

IMAGING

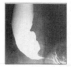 Though not a standard phase of a barium swallow examination, double-contrast pharyngography is performed in cases where dysphagic symptoms are suspicious for a pharyngeal, as opposed to esophageal, abnormality, such as choking. Pharyngography involves double-contrast views of the oropharynx and hypopharynx in both anteroposterior (AP) and lateral projections, with and without phonation and the Valsalva maneuver (Fig. 4–2). Structures to be evaluated include the valleculae (the symmetric pouches in the recess between the base of the tongue and the epiglottis) and the pyriform sinuses (the lateral pouches between the larynx and hypopharynx). Asymmetry in these structures suggests neuromuscular impairment or a space-occupying lesion such as a carcinoma (Fig. 4–3).

An important type of imaging in this area is the oropharyngeal motility (OPM)

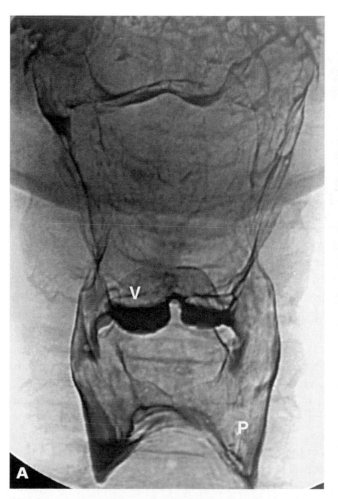 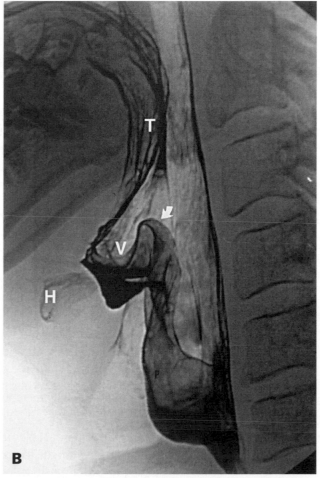

Figure 4–2. These (A) frontal and (B) lateral projection digital radiographs from a double-contrast pharyngogram exquisitely demonstrate the normal structures of the pharynx. The epiglottis is designated by the white arrow. The hyoid bone (H) separates the oropharynx from the hypopharynx. P, pyriform sinus; T, base of tongue; V, vallecula.

Figure 4–3. This frontal view of a double-contrast pharyngogram demonstrates a lobulated mass arising from the lateral aspect of the left pyriform sinus (open arrows), outlined by barium coating its surface. Squamous cell carcinoma is the most common lesion to produce such an appearance. Note the median glossoepiglottic fold (arrow), which separates the right vallecula (V) from the left. P, right pyriform sinus.

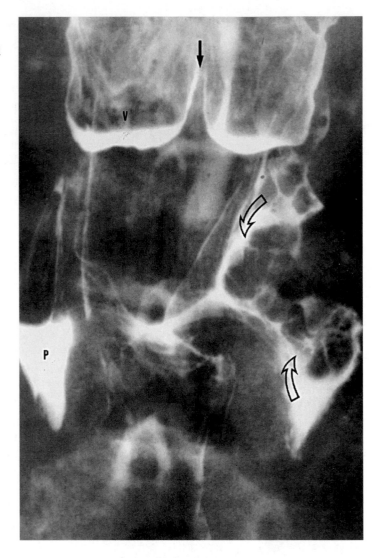

study, which is frequently employed to evaluate patients with known or suspected swallowing disorders secondary to tumor (such as head and neck cancer) or neuromuscular dysfunction (such as the postcerebrovascular accident patient). The patient is monitored fluoroscopically in the lateral projection while boluses of barium or food mixed with barium are transferred from the lips to the upper esophagus. The OPM study can be used to determine whether patients can be fed orally, and to counsel patients regarding appropriate types of food to eat, as well as compensatory chewing and swallowing maneuvers. Patients who exhibit significant aspiration should not be fed orally, due to the risk of aspiration pneumonitis and pneumonia (see the discussion of pneumonia in Chapter 3).

If swallowing is to occur normally, food must be prevented from reentering the mouth, from entering the nasal passages, and most importantly, from entering the trachea. Normal swallowing involves: (1) suppression of respiration by the medullary swallowing center; (2) elevation of the uvula to prevent nasal reflux; (3) positioning of the back of the tongue to prevent oral reentry; and (4) posteroinferior reflection of the epiglottis and apposition of the vocal cords to prevent penetration into the glottic region, which would result in aspiration.

ESOPHAGUS

STRUCTURE AND FUNCTION

The esophagus extends from the pharyngoesophageal sphincter at the level of C5–6 to the gastroesophageal (GE) junction. Its proximal one-third is predominately striated muscle, while the distal two-thirds are smooth muscle. The fact that it lacks an outer serosal layer is often invoked to explain the tendency for neoplasms to spread quickly from the esophagus to other mediastinal structures. The most important function of the esophagus, of course, is to transport swallowed material from the pharynx to the stomach, through the coordinated muscular contractions known as peristalsis (from the Greek *peri-*, "around," and *stallein,* "to place").

In a normal individual, esophageal peristalsis is so efficient that it is possible to drink liquids while suspended upside down. The primary wave requires 5 to 9 seconds to move the bolus into the stomach. If the bolus becomes lodged for some reason, or if an esophageal motility disorder is present, a secondary wave arises, which is more forceful than the primary wave. The secondary wave is initiated not via the central nervous system swallowing center through the vagus nerve (as is the primary wave), but by the intrinsic nerve plexuses of the esophagus. Tertiary contractions are nonproductive fasciculations seen exclusively in motility disorders.

IMAGING

 Radiologic evaluation of the esophagus is performed in both single- and double-contrast fashion, with the patient in both upright and prone positions. Upright views are obtained in double-contrast (Fig. 4–4). With adequate air distention and luminal coating, double contrast visualization of mucosal detail and the detection of subtle mucosal lesions is excellent. Single-contrast views with the patient prone are performed to assess motility and to aid in the demonstration of mass lesions and filling defects, which are often best evaluated with a greater degree of luminal distention than double-contrast views provide. In addition, the presence and degree of GE reflux, the major cause of heartburn, is best assessed at this stage. The esophagus, stomach, and duodenum are often imaged together in a so-called upper gastrointestinal (GI) examination (Fig. 4–5). Computed tomography (CT) and magnetic resonance imaging (MRI) are used primarily to evaluate the extent of disease, usually in the setting of an esophageal carcinoma. Endoluminal ultrasonography also provides visualization of local tumor extent.

STOMACH

STRUCTURE AND FUNCTION

The stomach, which stores and liquifies food and initiates protein digestion, is divided arbitrarily into the fundus, the body, and the antrum (Fig. 4–6). The fundus is that portion of the stomach that lies above the GE junction. The body comprises the central two-thirds, extending from the fundus to the incisura angularis. The body and the fundus contain the chief cells, which secrete pepsinogen, and the parietal cells, which secrete hydrochloric acid and intrinsic factor. Normal gastric pH is approximately 2,

Figure 4–4. This spot film from a double-contrast esophagogram demonstrates two prominent indentations along the left side of the proximal esophagus. They are quite smooth and form obtuse angles with the esophageal lumen, suggesting that they reflect pressure from structures extrinsic to the esophagus. What is the differential diagnosis of these contour abnormalities? In this case, there is no differential, because these represent normal impressions on the esophagus by the aortic arch (solid arrow) and the left mainstem bronchus (open arrow). As this case illustrates, a thorough knowledge of normal anatomy, including so-called normal variants, is critical in interpreting imaging studies.

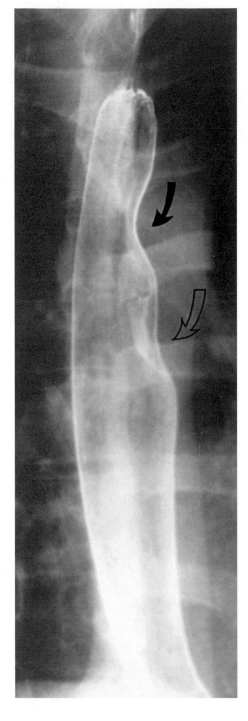

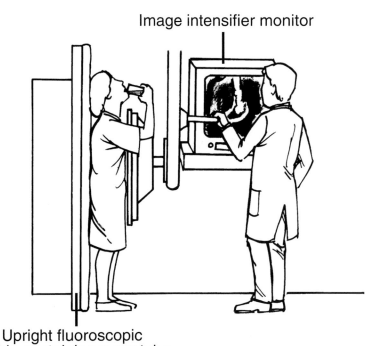

Image intensifier monitor

Upright fluoroscopic
table containing x-ray tube

Figure 4–5. This diagram illustrates an upper gastrointestinal examination, in which a patient drinks barium and fluoroscopic monitoring is used to obtain images of the esophagus, stomach, and duodenum.

A

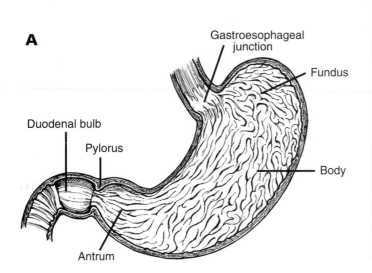

Gastroesophageal junction

Fundus

Duodenal bulb

Pylorus

Body

Antrum

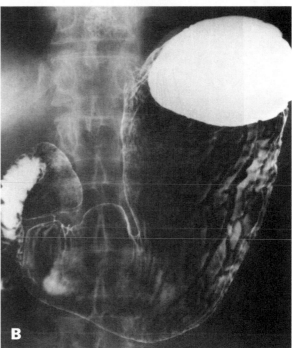

B

C

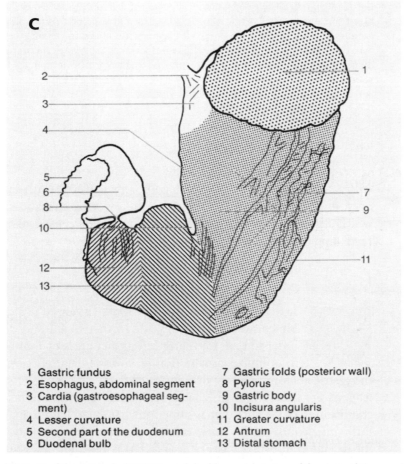

1 Gastric fundus
2 Esophagus, abdominal segment
3 Cardia (gastroesophageal segment)
4 Lesser curvature
5 Second part of the duodenum
6 Duodenal bulb
7 Gastric folds (posterior wall)
8 Pylorus
9 Gastric body
10 Incisura angularis
11 Greater curvature
12 Antrum
13 Distal stomach

Figure 4–6. (A) Parts of the stomach. (B,C) Normal double-contrast view of the stomach in a supine patient.

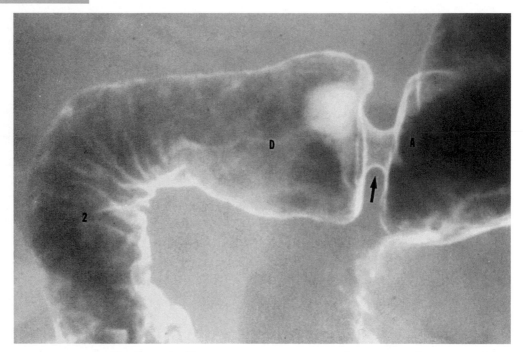

Figure 4–7. A spot film from a double contrast upper gastrointestinal examination demonstrates the distal gastric antrum (A), pylorus (arrow), duodenal bulb (D), and upper half of the second portion of the duodenum (2). The pylorus is critical in normal digestion because it enables the small bowel to digest and absorb over a period of hours a large quantity of food that may have been consumed in only minutes, by releasing food at a slow controlled rate from the stomach into the duodenum. Patients who have undergone pyloroplasty or partial gastrectomy may experience a "dumping syndrome" due to the dumping of large quantities of gastric contents into the small bowel at once. These patients experience nausea, weakness, and palpitations, followed by reactive hypoglycemia, due to the large osmotic load and premature unregulated absorption of glucose.

with a hydrogen ion concentration approximately 10,000 times that of the blood. The antrum, extending from the body to the pylorus, contains gastrin-secreting cells, which stimulate secretion by the parietal and chief cells. The pylorus is important in regulating the rate of gastric emptying (Fig. 4–7).

IMAGING

 Like the esophagus, the stomach is visualized using both single- and double-contrast techniques, the former to fill and distend the stomach in order to look for filling defects and areas of mural rigidity, and the latter to optimize visualization of mucosal detail. Because different portions of the gastric anatomy are best demonstrated from different points of view, multiple projections are necessary, with changes in patient positioning between each. Moreover, compression of the abdomen is sometimes helpful to flatten out the stomach, especially during the course of the single-contrast phase of an examination. CT is less useful for the detection of primary gastric lesions but is good for assessing the extent of disease, such as whether a lesion extends through the wall of the stomach or whether metastatic lesions are present in the liver.

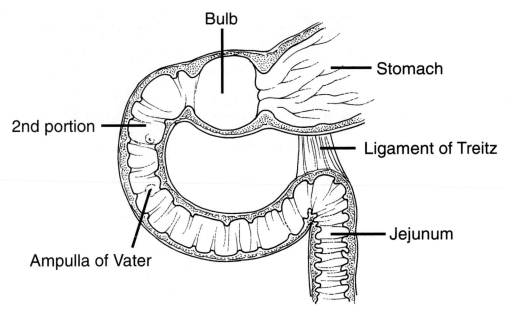

Figure 4–8. This diagram illustrates the appearance of the portions of the duodenum on both single- and double-contrast studies.

DUODENUM

STRUCTURE AND FUNCTION

The duodenum functions principally in digestion, the breakdown of food molecules (Fig. 4–8). It extends from the pyloric canal to the ligament of Treitz, the traditional boundary between the upper and lower GI tracts. The duodenum is divided into four parts. The first part, referred to as the bulb, is surrounded by visceral peritoneum on all sides, and it represents the only portion of the duodenum that is intraperitoneal. More than 90% of peptic ulcers occur in the duodenal bulb.

The remainder of the duodenum is retroperitoneal. The second, or descending, portion of the duodenum contains along its medial aspect the ampulla of Vater, through which the biliary system and exocrine pancreas secrete their alkaline digestive juices into the small bowel. The third portion of the duodenum extends horizontally to the left to a point between the aorta and inferior vena cava (Fig. 4–9). At that point, the fourth portion of the duodenum begins to ascend upward and to the left, terminating at the ligament of Treitz, which marks the boundary between the duodenum and the jejunum. The ligament of Treitz is commonly located immediately to the left of the L2 vertebral body.

The distinction between the different portions of the duodenum is important, for example, when a tumor is found. A tumor arising in the first portion of the duodenum is quite unlikely to be malignant, whereas a tumor in the fourth portion carries a very high risk of malignancy.

IMAGING

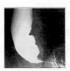

Contrast examination of the duodenum is also performed with both single- and double-contrast techniques. Mass lesions, which appear as filling defects, are well imaged in single-contrast fashion, as is the degree of luminal distensibility. The double-contrast technique is generally supe-

Figure 4–9. A 63-year-old man presented with a history of recurrent vomiting after meals. An upper gastrointestinal examination was performed, with injection of contrast medium through the patient's indwelling nasogastric tube. (**A**) A frontal spot film demonstrates a prominent narrowing of the third and fourth portions of the duodenum, producing a string-like appearance (small arrows). In addition, the body and antrum of the stomach are narrowed as well (large arrows). The fact that the stomach is involved discounts intrinsic duodenal lesions such as Crohn's disease and lymphoma and increases the probability of extrinsic processes such as a pancreatic mass. (**B**) An axial image from a noncontrast abdominal computed tomography scan discloses the etiology, a large abdomonal aortic aneurysm (A), over which the duodenum is draped and narrowed (arrow). A knowledge of regional anatomy is critical in arriving at a rational differential diagnosis.

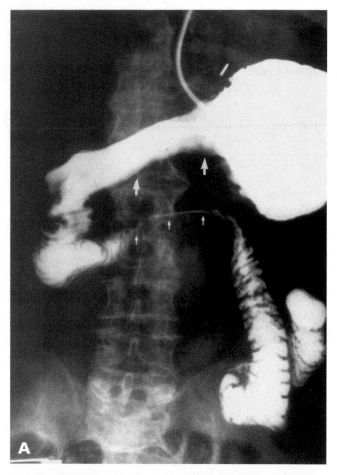

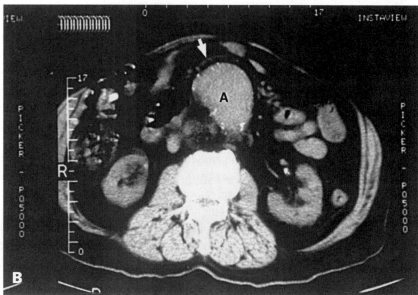

rior for the evaluation of the fold pattern and smaller mucosal lesions (Fig. 4–10). As in the esophagus and stomach, the primary role of CT is to determine the extent of disease, including transmural involvement and local or distant metastases. If CT is to accurately characterize the primary lesion, adequate distention of the lumen is critical, as redundant folds in a collapsed viscus can easily simulate a neoplasm.

Figure 4–10. Spot film of the duodenal sweep from a double-contrast upper gastrointestinal examination reveals nodular duodenal fold thickening (arrows) in the "C" loop, indicating severe duodenitis, which in this case was secondary to peptic disease.

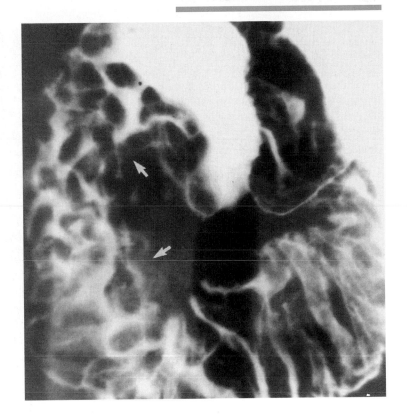

MESENTERIC SMALL BOWEL

STRUCTURE AND FUNCTION

The mesenteric small bowel functions primarily in the absorption of nutrients. It extends from the ligament of Treitz to the ileocecal valve. It is so named because it is suspended from the small bowel mesentery, which extends obliquely from the left upper quadrant into the right lower quadrant. While the mesenteric small bowel itself measures approximately 7 m in length, its mesentery is only a little more than 1 ft (i.e., 30 cm) in length, indicating that the small bowel mesentery is a highly folded structure. The mesentery not only suspends the small bowel mesentery from the posterior abdominal wall, but also contains blood vessels, lymphatics, and nerves.

The mesenteric small bowel is divided into the jejunum and the ileum, with the ileum constituting the distal 60% of its length. On intraluminal contrast studies, the jejunum has a wider lumen, a thicker wall, and more folds per centimeter than the ileum. The surface area of the small bowel is remarkably increased by the presence of mucosal folds (valvulae conniventes), villi, and microvilli. Though only about 7 m in length if fully extended, these structures create a surface area of 300 m^2, about the size of a doubles tennis court.

IMAGING

Common indications for imaging the small bowel include abdominal pain, malabsorption, diarrhea, and blood in the stools. Techniques for imaging the small bowel include the so-called small bowel follow-through, a dedicated small bowel series, and enteroclysis. The small bowel follow-through represents a continuation of an upper GI series, in which the patient

Figure 4–11. An overhead film from an enteroclysis (small bowel enema) demonstrates the exquisite small bowel mucosal detail revealed by this technique. Note that the jejunum, which contains more folds per centimeter than the ileum, is located primarily in the left upper quadrant, while the ileum, with its more rarefied fold pattern, is located primarily in the right lower quadrant.

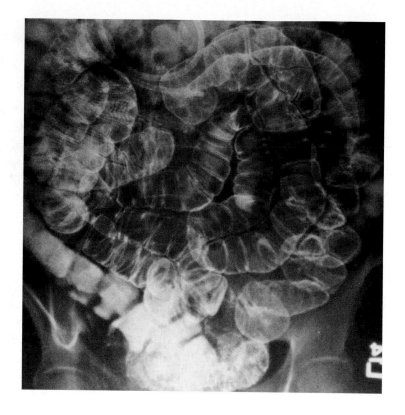

drinks a barium preparation under fluoroscopic monitoring and spot films are taken of the esophagus, stomach, and duodenum. In the follow-through, the same contrast is followed beyond the duodenum into the mesenteric small bowel, with overhead films taken at 15- to 30-minute intervals until contrast is seen in the colon. Additional spot films with compression are taken of the terminal ileum and of any findings of interest. The follow-through is somewhat less sensitive than the dedicated small bowel series, in which a barium preparation optimized for the small bowel is employed. Another means of visualizing the terminal ileum is by refluxing contrast introduced for a barium enema through an incompetent ileocecal valve, which can be followed where indicated by per rectal air insufflation to provide double-contrast visualization.

The gold standard of small bowel imaging is the enteroclysis, which is performed by oral intubation of the jejunum, followed by injection of barium, which is followed in turn by a continuous infusion of methylcellulose solution. As the barium shot is pushed along the lumen by the methylcellulose chaser, the mural surfaces become outlined, the lumen becomes mildly distended, and the mucosal fold pattern and areas of stenosis or dilatation are optimally visualized (Fig. 4–11). Disadvantages of enteroclysis include the need for more specialized equipment, patient discomfort associated with intubation, and higher cost.

LARGE INTESTINE

STRUCTURE AND FUNCTION

The functions of the large intestine include absorption, storage, and elimination (Fig. 4–12). It measures approximately 1.5 m in length, and includes the cecum; appendix; ascending, transverse, and descending portions of the colon; sigmoid colon; rectum;

Figure 4–12. Topography of the colon in relation to other abdominal organs.

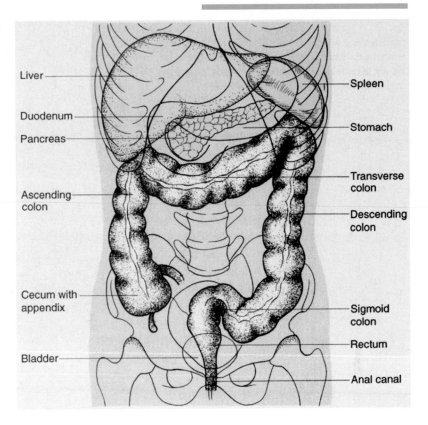

Liver
Duodenum
Pancreas
Ascending colon
Cecum with appendix
Bladder

Spleen
Stomach
Transverse colon
Descending colon
Sigmoid colon
Rectum
Anal canal

and anal canal. The blood supply of the intestine from the ligament of Treitz through the splenic flexure of the colon is from the superior mesenteric artery, with the inferior mesenteric artery supplying the more distal large intestine. Both the ascending and descending portions of the colon are extraperitoneal in location, which is important in understanding the spread of intraperitoneal inflammatory and neoplastic processes. Some patients have unusually long segments of colon, most commonly the sigmoid or transverse colon, referred to as a "redundant" colon, which may require extra maneuvers on endoscopic or endoluminal contrast examinations in order to visualize the entire colon.

IMAGING

Common indications for imaging the colon include rectal bleeding, abdominal pain, anemia, and weight loss. Because a complete evaluation of the colon requires patient mobility (to direct flow of contrast and/or air through the colon), some elderly and debilitated patients may be poor candidates for a barium enema. Before any contrast study is undertaken, a plain radiograph of the abdomen should be obtained to ensure that the colon is properly cleansed and that no residual contrast material from another examination is present. Fecal debris can easily masquerade as a polypoid lesion (Fig. 4–13). The standard preparation protocol employed in colonoscopy will interfere with a double-contrast barium enema, because the colonic mucosa is typically too wet to permit proper barium coating. The examination is performed using a barium-containing bag connected by a tube to the rectal tip. In double-contrast examinations, an insufflator is employed to introduce air into the colon via the rectum (Fig. 4–14).

Figure 4–13. This spot film from a double-contrast barium enema seems to demonstrate a large, polypoid lesion filling much of the rectum. In fact, however, this "lesion" merely represents stool in the rectum. This image dramatizes the importance of adequate bowel preparation.

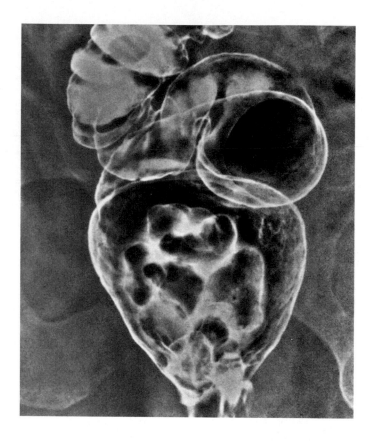

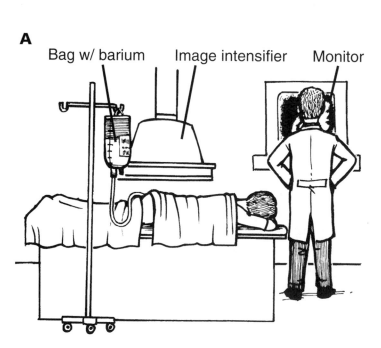

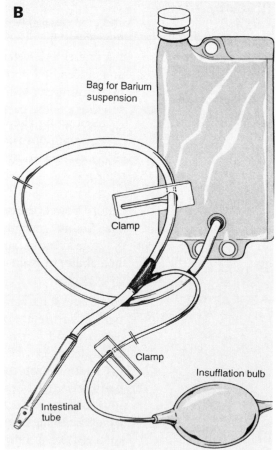

Figure 4–14. (**A**) A patient undergoing barium enema. (**B**) Intestinal tube and insufflator attached to barium reservoir.

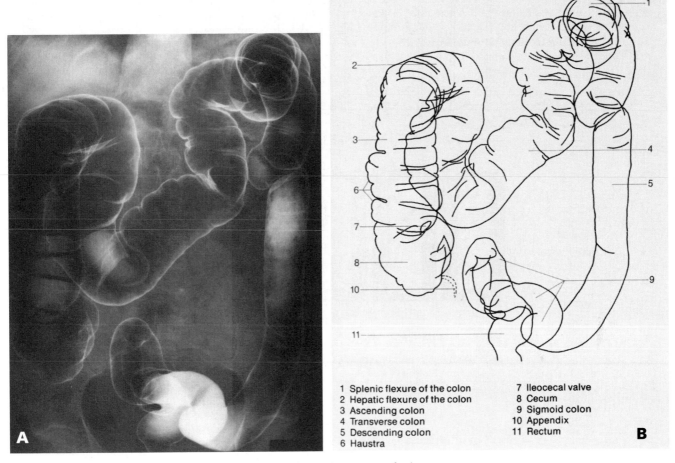

1 Splenic flexure of the colon
2 Hepatic flexure of the colon
3 Ascending colon
4 Transverse colon
5 Descending colon
6 Haustra

7 Ileocecal valve
8 Cecum
9 Sigmoid colon
10 Appendix
11 Rectum

A   B

Figure 4–15. Normal double-contrast colonic anatomy.

In imaging the colon, a single-contrast examination is preferred to evaluate patients with obstructing lesions and fistulas, as well as those who do not exhibit the mobility required for a double-contrast examination (Fig. 4–15). The double-contrast technique is especially useful for demonstrating small polypoid lesions and evaluating mucosal detail, which is particularly important in such situations as suspected inflammatory bowel disease. CT and MRI are best for evaluating the distant spread of primary colonic malignancies and determining the nature of extrinsic processes affecting the large intestine, such as pelvic malignancies. Both CT and MRI are more limited in their ability to evaluate the local extent of tumor.

Basic Patterns of Gastrointestinal Tract Abnormalities

Nearly all radiologically detectable GI tract lesions can be categorized according to a relatively small number of radiographic patterns. These patterns may be further grouped into three basic categories: lesions projecting into the gut lumen, lesions affecting the structure of the gut wall itself, and lesions projecting away from the lumen of the gut. Additional processes include distention and narrowing of the gut.

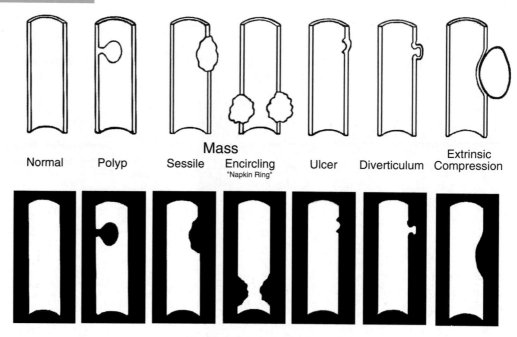

Mass

Normal   Polyp   Sessile   Encircling   Ulcer   Diverticulum   Extrinsic
                              "Napkin Ring"   Compression

Single contrast appearance

Figure 4–16. Paradigmatic abnormalities visible on barium studies: filling defects (polyps and masses), and extramural projections (ulcers, diverticula, and fistulae).

In interpreting a contrast study of the GI tract, one effective strategy for ensuring a thorough evaluation is to train the eye to follow the natural course of the contrast agent from proximal to distal. A good grasp of normal anatomic patterns is crucial. Generally, if the observer can bear in mind each of the five fundamental patterns of GI abnormalities—filling defects, intrinsic mural abnormalities, extraluminal projections, distention, and narrowing—few radiologically detectable pathologies will be missed (Fig. 4–16).

FILLING DEFECTS

The principle types of lesions that project into the gut lumen are polyps and masses. They are referred to as filling defects because they represent areas that should normally fill with barium but instead are occupied by tissue and thus remain unfilled. The contour of the displaced barium provides a silhouette of the abnormal tissue.

POLYPS

Polyps (from the Greek *polypous*, meaning "many-footed") are produced by excessive growth of the mucosa of the bowel wall, which may be up to several centimeters in diameter. They may be benign or malignant, and their morphology may be described as sessile or pedunculated (Fig. 4–17). A sessile polyp (from the Latin *sedere*, "to sit") refers to a broad-based lesion that is not attached to the mucosa by a peduncle. In contrast, a pedunculated polyp (from the Latin *pes*, meaning "foot") is attached by a

Figure 4–17. This overhead film from a double-contrast barium enema reveals multiple polyps, both sessile and pedunculated (arrows), scattered throughout the colon. In practice, spot films of involved regions should be obtained during the examination to better characterize the size, form, and margins of these lesions and assess the probability of malignancy.

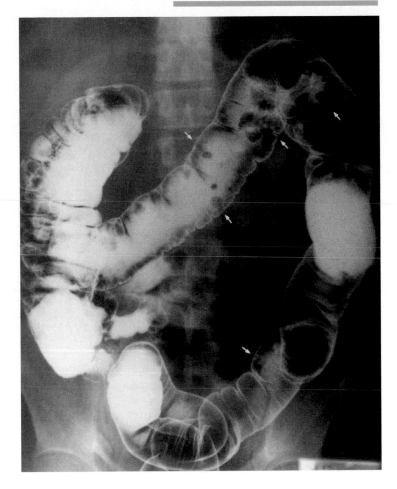

stalk to the mucosa. Unless they are large, polyps are usually identified on single-contrast studies as filling defects in the contrast column, or on double-contrast studies outlined by a thin rim of contrast.

Polyps come in multiple histologic types. Nonneoplastic polyps include hyperplastic polyps (overgrowth of otherwise normal cells), inflammatory polyps, and hamartomatous polyps, which represent an abnormal proliferation of tissues that are otherwise normally present.

Neoplastic polyps include adenomas and carcinomas. Adenomas are composed of benign-appearing glandular epithelium. As the polyp extends outward from the mucosal surface, its lack of attachment to deeper layers of the bowel wall enables it to be pulled farther out into the lumen and eventually to be pulled downstream by peristalsis, which is why so many polyps have a pedunculated appearance (Fig. 4–18). Histologic characteristics of a polyp indicative of benignity include lack of cellular atypia, few mitotic figures (suggesting low growth rate), low nucleus/cytoplasm ratio, and lack of spread beyond the mucosa. Dysplastic polyps are those that demonstrate a greater degree of atypia. The term *carcinoma* is reserved for malignant epithelial growths. Unequivocally carcinomatous polyps will demonstrate evidence of local and/or discontinuous (metastatic) tumor spread. A carcinoma in situ is a growth of cancerous-appearing cells that appears well-contained, without evidence of local, lymphatic, or vascular invasion.

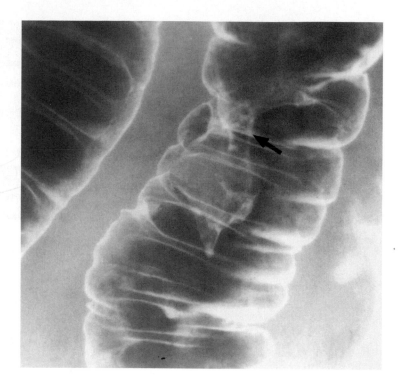

Figure 4–18. This spot film from a double-contrast barium enema reveals a classic appearance of a pedunculated adenomatous polyp, which is called pedunculated because it is connected to the bowel by a stalk (arrow). When one polyp is discovered, there is a 50% chance that additional polyps will be found elsewhere in the colon. Moreover, the fact that this polyp measures more than 2 cm in diameter implies an approximately 40% probability of malignancy.

MASSES

Masses are lesions measuring more than a few centimeters in size and may grow primarily in an exophytic fashion into the lumen or intramurally. The term *polyp* is sometimes used as a modifier to describe masses, a polypoid mass being one with multiple excrescences or outgrowths extending from its surface.

A mass that grows exophytically out into the lumen is more likely to cause early obstruction, bleed more easily, and grow down into the wall later, and therefore tends to be discovered at an earlier, more resectable stage. Other tumors tend to spread intramurally, producing either an annular constricting lesion, the so-called napkin-ring lesion seen in many colorectal carcinomas, or a diffusely infiltrating lesion, as in the so-called *linitis plastica*, or "leather bottle," lesion of scirrhous gastric carcinoma.

Lesions originating from below the mucosa, typically the submucosa, produce a different margin with the luminal surface from that of mucosal tumors. A submucosal tumor pushes a segment of the mucosa outward from beneath, tending to produce smoothly tapered, obtuse angles with the bowel wall. A mucosal tumor, on the other hand, grows out from the surface of the mucosa and tends to have a more abrupt zone of transition with the luminal surface and acute angles.

INTRINSIC WALL ABNORMALITIES

Changes within the bowel wall itself that may affect the radiographic appearance of the gut include a number of processes. One of the most important is a change in the fold pattern, which may occur anywhere from the esophagus to the rectum. Increased prominence or thickening of the folds typically reflects either an inflammatory process (such as gastritis), edema, or infiltration by cells or cellular products (Fig. 4–19). Edema is by far the most common cause and may result from any of the usual physiologic forces that cause interstitial fluid accumulation, including

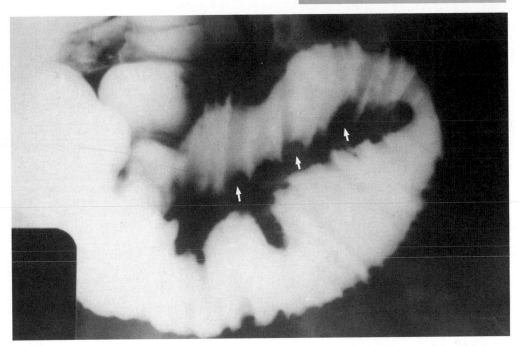

Figure 4–19. This spot film from a small bowel series demonstrates marked thickening of the folds in this segment of small bowel (arrows). The differential diagnosis of fold thickening includes causes of submucosal edema such as ischemia and enteritis, submucosal tumor such as lymphoma, and submucosal hemorrhage from such causes as coagulopathy. However, in this patient with a clinical history of malabsorption, etiologies such as Whipple's disease and celiac sprue are more likely. In this case, active sprue was the culprit. Sprue reflects an intolerance to the gluten found, for example, in wheat.

ischemia, congestive heart failure, and hypoproteinemia. Causes of infiltration of the gut wall, which typically results in both thickening and rigidity, include lymphoma and amyloidosis.

EXTRALUMINAL PROJECTIONS

ULCERS

Common lesions extending away from the lumen of the gut are ulcers, which appear as extraluminal collections of barium. A variety of ulcer types exist, including the peptic ulcerations in peptic ulcer disease; aphthous ulcers, most commonly associated with Crohn's disease; the collar-button ulcers of ulcerative colitis; and malignant patterns of ulceration. In the case of peptic ulcers, a benign ulcer usually exhibits intact epithelium extending right up to its edge, because it is produced by the erosion of the gut wall by intraluminal forces. A malignant ulcer, on the other hand, demonstrates a heaped-up mound of irregular tissue around its edges, because it results from necrosis of the central portion of the tumor (Fig. 4–20). Other criteria of benignity are considered in the discussion of peptic ulcers in Chapter 6.

DIVERTICULA

Another type of lesion extending away from the lumen are diverticula, from the Latin *devertere*, meaning "to turn aside" (as in "divert"). In the presence of these

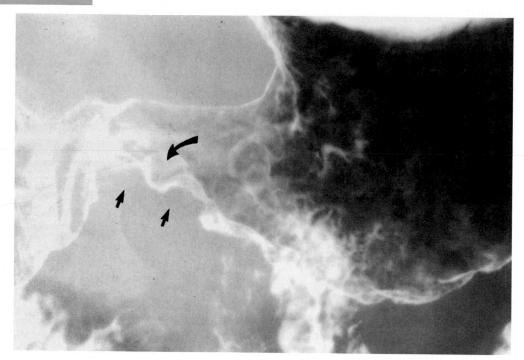

Figure 4–20. This spot film of the gastric antrum from an upper gastrointestinal examination demonstrates an irregular mucosal filling defect along the inferior margin of the antrum, which contains a central ulceration (curved arrow). Imaging features favoring a malignant etiology include the mass-like appearance of the heaped-up folds, the fact that the ulcer crater does not project beyond the expected margin of the gastric wall (arrows), and the lack of normal distensibility and peristalsis observed in this area during fluoroscopy. Endoscopic biopsy revealed gastric adenocarcinoma.

lesions, the barium in the gut lumen literally turns to one side when it reaches the diverticulum, which it fills in an orientation perpendicular to the gut lumen (Fig. 4–21). So-called false diverticula represent outpouchings that do not contain all layers of the bowel wall. The most important diverticula are the colonic variety, which can become obstructed by inspissated luminal material, resulting in inflammation and infection. Colonic diverticula are further discussed in the diverticulitis section of Chapter 6.

DISTENTION

One of the most commonly sought findings on plain films of the abdomen is distention, or dilatation of the bowel (Fig. 4–22). This usually reflects the presence of an obstruction distal to the dilated segment. If the only dilated viscus is the stomach and the remainder of the bowel is airless, one might suspect a gastric outlet obstruction. On the other hand, if the entire small and large bowel were distended down to the sigmoid region, one would expect an obstructing process in that location.

Obstructions are often divided into mechanical and nonmechanical classes. The most common mechanical obstructions in adults include postsurgical adhesions, hernia, and masses. The most common nonmechanical obstruction is ileus, which is always seen in the postoperative setting, and may also result from pain (such as an obstructive ureteral stone), inflammation (such as appendicitis), ischemia, and

Figure 4–21. A frontal spot film from an upper gastrointestinal examination demonstrates an incidental finding of a giant duodenal diverticulum, arising from the superior aspect of the fourth portion of the duodenum (arrow).

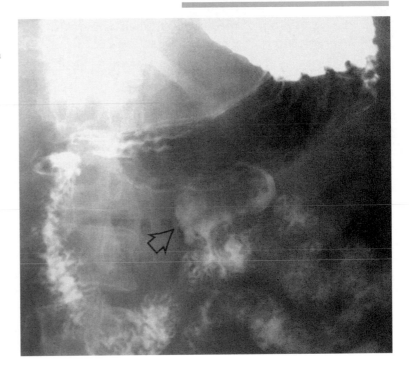

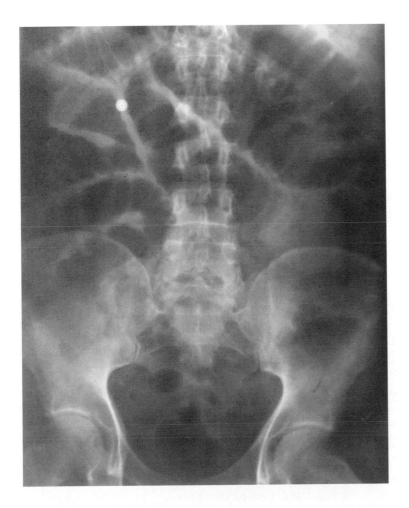

Figure 4–22. This supine abdominal radiograph of the abdomen reveals multiple gas-filled, dilated segments of small bowel in the mid- and upper abdomen, which resulted from a sigmoid diverticular abscess (not seen), producing a focal ileus of the distal small bowel adjacent to it and distention of the more proximal small bowel.

medications (such as narcotic analgesics). Obstruction is further discussed in Chapter 6.

NARROWING

Focal or diffuse narrowings of the bowel most often reflect either normal anatomic structures or muscular spasm. However, they may also reflect a number of pathologic processes, in which case the narrowing will persist. Long segment narrowing is a common sequela of Crohn's disease, in which transmural inflammation results in fibrosis and stricture (Fig. 4–23). A similar appearance may occur from almost any process that results in scarring, although the narrowing is often more focal. Carcinomas may cause irregular strictures, as in the well-known "apple core" annular constricting lesion of colon carcinoma.

Processes outside the bowel may also cause narrowing due to extrinsic compression. While a postoperative adhesion produces proximal bowel dilatation, the site of the adhesion itself will appear as a tight stenosis, often with angulation and fixation of the adhesed bowel segment. Extra-GI tumors and fluid collections, as well as inflammatory masses, may likewise compress the bowel, producing what is often referred to as "mass effect."

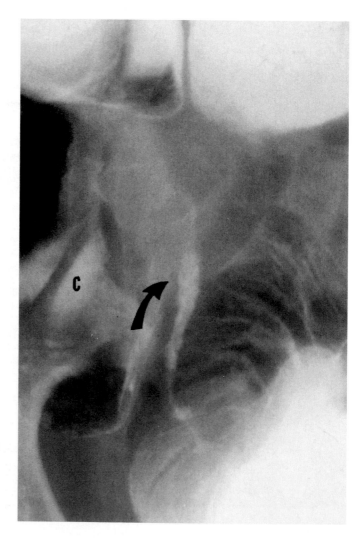

Figure 4–23. A spot film of the ileocecal region from a small bowel series demonstrates the classic "string sign" of the terminal ileum in Crohn's disease (arrow), which in this case consists of a combination of chronic scarring and an acute exacerbation of inflammation and edema. The terminal ileum is by far the most likely segment of small bowel to be involved by Crohn's disease, and after resection, disease frequently recurs in the "neoterminal" ileum. C, cecum.

Select Pathologies

ESOPHAGUS

CONGENITAL

The most important congenital abnormalities of the esophagus are esophageal atresia and tracheoesophageal fistula, which are discussed in Chapter 7 and in Chapter 10.

INFLAMMATORY

The most common cause of inflammation of the esophagus is reflux esophagitis, in which an incompetent lower esophageal sphincter allows acidic gastric contents access to the esophageal mucosa, often associated with symptoms of heartburn. While most patients with reflux do not have hiatal hernias, there is an increased incidence of reflux in this condition, which involves herniation of a portion of the stomach up through the diaphragm into the thorax (Fig. 4–24). Radiologic findings of reflux include actual visualization of retrograde flow of contrast from the stomach into the esophagus, thickening of esophageal folds, granularity of the mucosa, and strictures. Another common cause of esophagitis, which is associated with postinflammatory stricture formation, is chemical ingestion, especially corrosives such as lye. The strictures asso-

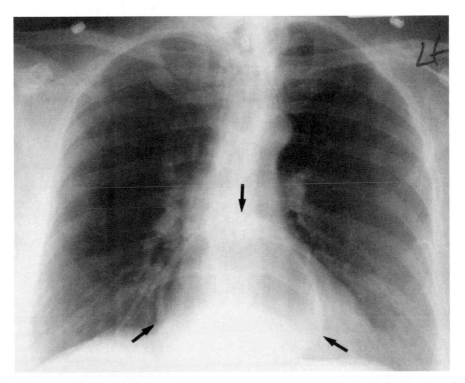

Figure 4–24. A posteroanterior chest radiograph in a 58-year-old woman admitted with an acute asthma exacerbation demonstrates a large lower mediastinal mass containing an air-fluid level, representing a large hiatal hernia (arrows). Ninety-five percent of hiatal hernias are of the sliding variety, in which the gastroesophageal (GE) junction is above the diaphragm. In the other type, paraesophageal hernias, the GE junction is in its normal location, below the diaphragm, but part of the gastric fundus herniates up through the diaphragmatic hiatus.

ciated with lye ingestion are typically fusiform and long, often involving the whole esophagus (Fig. 4–25).

Achalasia is an acquired esophageal motor disorder, characterized by failure of the lower esophageal sphincter to relax, secondary to degeneration of Auerbach's plexus. Most cases occur idiopathically in young patients and present with dysphagia and weight loss. Radiologic findings include absence of normal peristalsis, dilatation, and a persistent beak-like tapering of the distal esophagus, often associated with an obstructive air-fluid level (Fig. 4–26). Complications include aspiration (manifesting acutely as aspiration pneumonitis and/or pneumonia, and chronically as interstitial lung disease) and carcinoma.

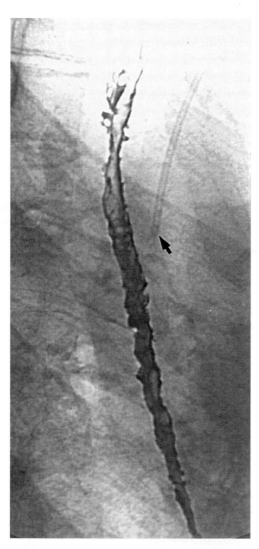

Figure 4–25. This 16-year-old boy attempted suicide by ingesting lye. An oblique film from a barium esophagogram performed in the upright position demonstrates a long, nodular stricture of the mid- and distal esophagus, with areas of ulceration. Note also a central venous catheter extending into the superior vena cava (arrow), which was inserted to provide nutritional support while the esophagus healed.

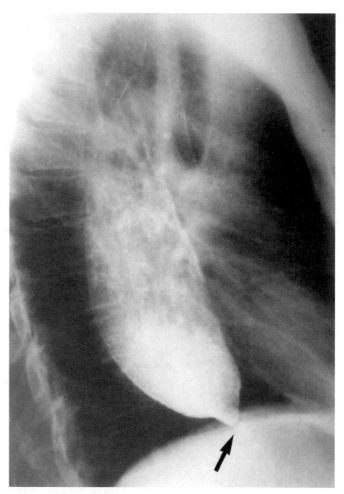

Figure 4–26. This upright lateral view of the thorax from a barium swallow examination demonstrates a markedly dilated mid- and distal esophagus; a prominent air-fluid level containing a mixture of swallowed secretions, debris, and contrast; and a "bird-beak"-like tapering of the distal esophagus (arrow). These findings result from a combination of esophageal aperistalsis and failure of the lower esophageal sphincter to relax. Emptying occurs only when the pressure due to the height of the fluid column is sufficient to overcome the tonic contraction of the lower esophageal sphincter, meaning that emptying is facilitated in the upright position. Other causes of megaesophagus include scleroderma, diabetic neuropathy, and dilatation due to obstructing tumor or postinflammatory stricture.

TUMOROUS

Both benign and malignant tumors are seen in the esophagus. By far the most common benign tumor is the leiomyoma, a smooth muscle tumor that is usually asymptomatic and typically presents as a smooth intramural mass.

The most common malignant tumor of the esophagus is squamous cell carcinoma, which arises in a mucosal lining that is normally composed of stratified squamous epithelium. Nearly two-thirds of primary esophageal malignancies are squamous cell carcinomas, and they are more common in men (M:F = 4:1) and blacks. Risk factors include alcohol and tobacco abuse, as well as medical conditions such as lye stricture and achalasia. The radiologic appearance is a polypoid, ulcerative, or stenotic mass in the mid- or distal esophagus. The tumor is typically advanced at diagnosis, with local spread to the trachea, aorta, or pericardium; lymphatic metastases to the mediastinal and celiac nodes; and hematogenous dissemination, especially to the liver. The primary lesion is best imaged by barium swallow, while CT and MRI are used primarily in staging (Fig. 4–27).

An esophageal tumor of rapidly increasing incidence is adenocarcinoma, which

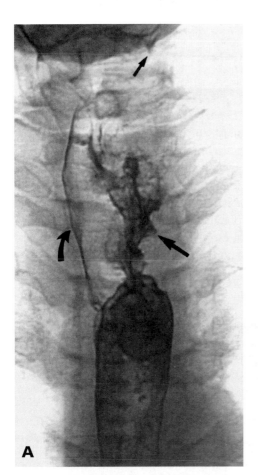

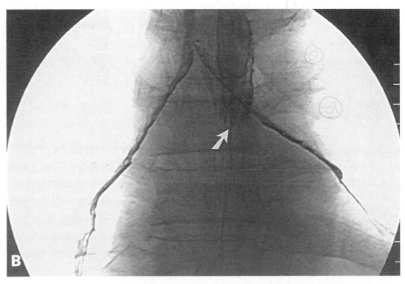

Figure 4–27. A 64-year-old man presented with a 2-month history of odynophagia and dysphagia, as well as a 22 Kg weight loss. A barium swallow was requested. (**A**) A spot film obtained after a single test swallow of barium reveals a 4 cm circumferential narrowing of the proximal esophagus, with proximal and distal shouldering. [We know we are in the proximal esophagus because the inferior margins of the pyriform sinuses are visible at the top of the image (small arrow)]. Note the ulceration along the left side of the irregularly narrowed segment (large arrow). What accounts for the smooth rim of barium projected to the right of the esophageal lesion (curved arrow)? (**B**) A second spot film at the level of the carina reveals some contrast in the mid-esophagus below the lesion (arrow), as well as contrast outlining the distal trachea and mainstem bronchi. Although only a single swallow of contrast medium was taken, the degree of esophageal obstruction was great enough to cause aspiration of a significant portion of the bolus. As is typically the case, this patient reported a long history of cigarette smoking and alcohol use.

Figure 4–28. This double-contrast esophagogram reveals a nodular mucosal pattern, suggestive of reflux esophagitis, as well as a mid-esophageal stricture. These findings are suggestive of Barrett esophagus.

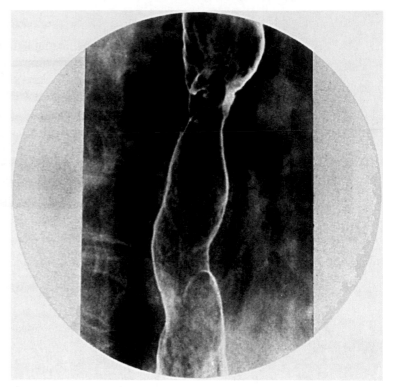

now constitutes approximately one-third of primary esophageal malignancies. It is associated with Barrett esophagus, which consists of columnar metaplasia of the esophageal mucosa, presumably secondary to chronic reflux. Barrett esophagus is most common among white males and may develop in as many as 10% of patients with chronic reflux. The most important radiologic indicator of Barrett esophagus in a patient with mucosal changes of reflux esophagitis is a mid-esophageal stricture (Fig. 4–28). Up to 10% of patients with Barrett esophagus eventually develop adenocarcinoma. The tumor is usually found in the distal esophagus, and typically has a polypoid or ulcerative appearance, not unlike that of squamous cell carcinoma.

INFECTIOUS

Infectious lesions of the esophagus are most commonly seen in immunocompromised patients. Causative organisms include herpes simplex, which produces small, discrete ulcerations; *Candida,* which produces raised, plaque-like lesions; and cytomegalovirus (CMV), which produces large ulcerations (Fig. 4–29).

IATROGENIC

There are several iatrogenic lesions of the esophagus. Medications such as tetracycline, aspirin, and potassium supplement tablets may produce esophagitis if they become lodged in the esophagus. For this reason, patients should be encouraged to drink a full glass of water and to remain upright when taking such pills. Another important iatrogenic lesion is perforation, which is seen in a small percentage of patients who have undergone endoscopy or following dilatation for achalasia. The risk of perforation is increased in patients with esophageal diverticula, such as Zenker's diverticulum. This

Figure 4–29. A 35-year-old human immunodeficiency virus-positive man with a CD4 count of 24 presented with dysphagia. A spot film from an upper gastrointestinal examination demonstrates a subtle, plaque-like filling defect in the distal esophagus (arrow). A subsequent endoscopic study confirmed the characteristic whitish plaques of candidiasis.

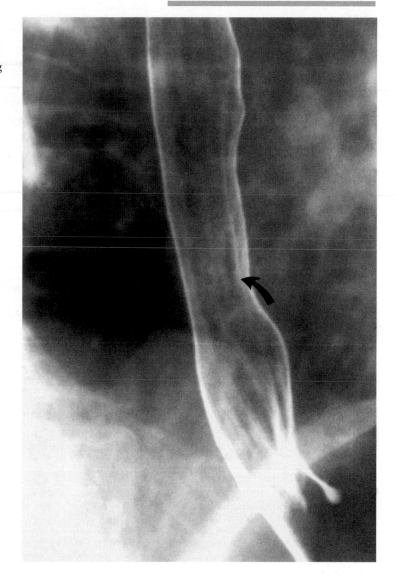

increased risk stems from the fact that these luminal projections may be inadvertently intubated during insertion of a nasogastric tube or endoscope.

TRAUMATIC

There are two important traumatic lesions of the esophagus. Mallory-Weiss tear is most commonly seen in alcoholics who have experienced prolonged episodes of vomiting. It involves a tear of the esophageal mucosa, which is frequently associated with hematemesis and hematochezia. The radiographic finding is mucosal disruption at the tear. Boerhaave's syndrome involves a transmural rent in the esophagus, usually due to a sudden increase in intraluminal pressure secondary to vomiting or trauma. The perforation is usually on the left side, just above the diaphragm. The patient presents with sudden onset of severe epigastric pain, which can progress rapidly to shock. Plain film findings include pneumomediastinum and a left-sided pleural effusion. Oral contrast administration demonstrates left-sided extravasation into the mediastinum and pleural space. Due to a mortality rate of 25–50%, emergent thoracotomy is often indicated (Fig. 4–30).

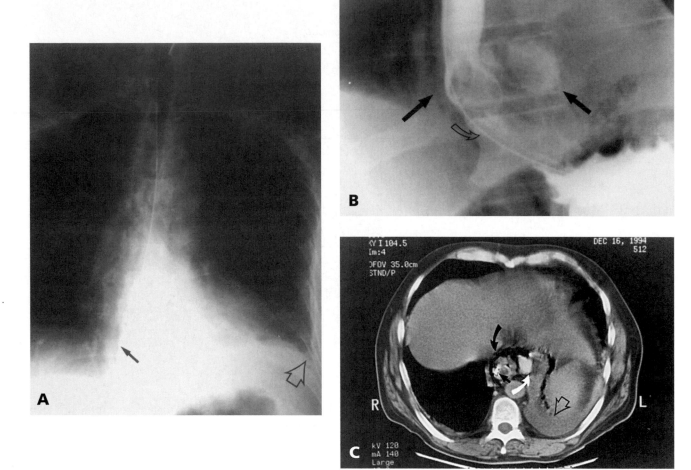

Figure 4–30. A 59-year-old man presented to the emergency room with a history of prolonged retching and the sudden onset of hematemesis and severe epigastric pain. (A) A portable frontal chest radiograph demonstrates a dense opacity in the retrocardiac region of the left base, a left pleural effusion (open arrow), and vertical linear lucencies suggestive of pneumomediastinum (arrow). Under fluoroscopic monitoring, a limited esophagogram was performed with water-soluble contrast medium. (B) A spot film at the level of the gastroesophageal junction (GEJ) demonstrates extravasation of contrast from the left side of the esophagus (arrow) and also better demonstrates the paraesophageal air (long arrow). Note also nasogastric tube (open arrow). (C) An axial section from a thoracic computed tomography scan just above the GEJ clearly demonstrates the pneumomediastinum (curved arrow), extravasated contrast material adjacent to the esophagus, and a left pleural effusion (open arrow). It is estimated that 90% of cases of Boerhaave's syndrome involve tears of the left posterolateral aspect of the esophagus. In contrast to Mallory-Weiss tears, which involve only the esophageal mucosa, Boerhaave's syndrome implies a transmural disruption.

VASCULAR

The most important vascular lesion of the esophagus is esophageal varices (Fig. 4–31). In patients with severe hepatic cirrhosis and portal hypertension, the portal vein is often decompressed via the coronary and azygous veins (which connect to the superior vena cava [SVC]), producing thin-walled, dilated veins in the lower esophagus. These are called "uphill varices," because the flow of blood is from the abdomen into the thorax. "Downhill varices" occur in obstruction of the SVC caudal to its anastamosis with the azygous vein, with flow of blood from the thorax into the abdomen

Figure 4–31. "Uphill" and "downhill" esophageal varices typically result from portal hypertension and superior vena cava obstruction, respectively. In uphill esophageal varices with portal hypertension, increased portal venous pressure is decompressed through the coronary vein and into the esophageal/azygous system, while downhill varices result from obstruction of the superior vena cava below the level of the insertion of the azygous vein, which allows decompression in the opposite direction.

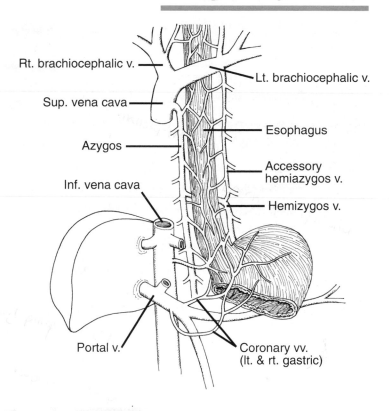

(Fig. 4–32). One of the greatest dangers with esophageal varices is erosion of the vein walls from GE reflux, which can produce massive and often fatal GI bleeding. A relatively new treatment for varices is transjugular intrahepatic portosystemic shunt (TIPS), which is discussed in the interventional section of Chapter 1.

STOMACH

INFLAMMATORY

Gastritis is a relatively common condition, with an increased incidence in patients using nonsteroidal anti-inflammatory drugs, alcoholics, and seriously ill patients. It consists of erosions of the gastric mucosa, which are usually rapidly reversible. Radiologic findings include small erosions and fold thickening.

A complete discussion of peptic ulcer disease is found in Chapter 6. Gastric ulcers are seen radiographically as persistent collections of barium that project beyond the gastric lumen, often with a raised rim of surrounding edema. Ulcers may be benign or malignant. Signs of a benign gastric ulcer include mucosal folds extending up to the crater, penetration beyond the expected luminal margin, and normal peristaltic activity (Fig. 4–33). Malignant ulcers occur in the midst of a neoplasm manifesting aberrant behavior and typically do not exhibit these signs. Definitely benign ulcers can be followed up with repeat upper GI examination at 6 weeks to ensure complete healing, whereas malignant-appearing or indeterminate ulcers should undergo biopsy (Fig. 4–34).

Both gastritis and peptic ulcer disease are associated with the presence of *Helicobacter pylori,* a urease-producing organism whose metabolic byproducts include

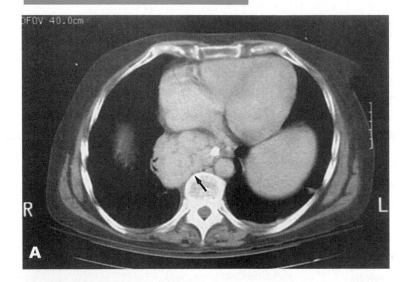

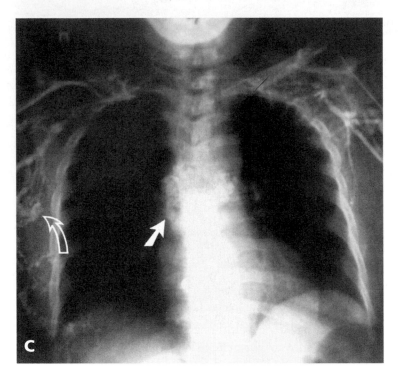

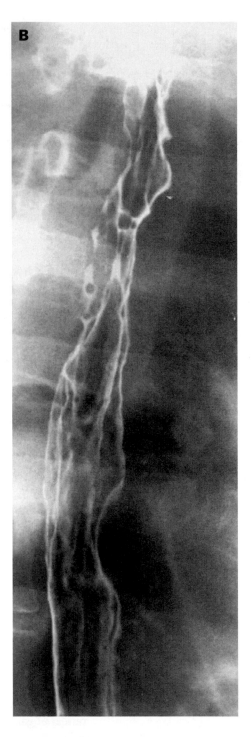

Figure 4–32. A middle-aged woman presented with acute upper gastrointestinal hemorrhage. Upper endoscopy (not shown) revealed esophageal varices, etiology unknown. A contrast-enhanced computed tomography scan of the thorax and abdomen was subsequently obtained for other reasons. (**A**) An axial image at the level of the heart reveals a polylobulated enhancing mass (arrow) arising from the right side of the nasogastric tube-containing esophagus. These represent the tangled mass of uphill esophageal varices. (**B**) A spot film from an esophagogram in another patient shows serpentine filling defects in the upper esophagus, representing "downhill" varices. (**C**) A frontal view of the thorax from an upper extremity venogram, performed by injection of iodinated contrast medium into an upper extremity vein, demonstrates the etiology of these downhill esophageal varices—multiple calcified lymph nodes in the mediastinum (arrow), associated with previous radiation therapy of a mediastinal lymphoma, which has produced distal superior vena cava (SVC) obstruction. Note also the recruitment of prominent chest-wall collateral vessels, especially on the right (curved arrow).

(continued)

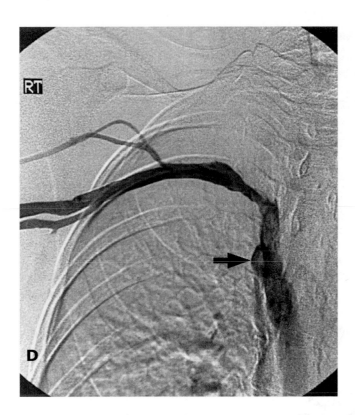

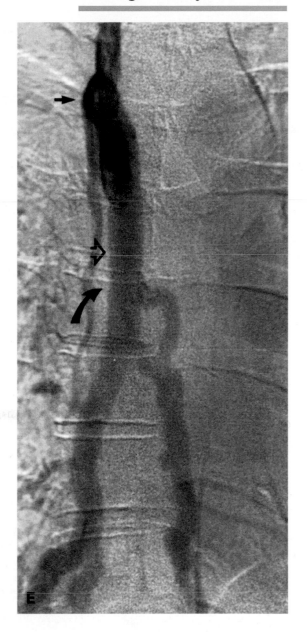

Figure 4–32. *(continued)* (**D**) Digital subtraction films from another patient with SVC obstruction due to previous radiation therapy demonstrate the mediastinal venous anatomy. Injection of an antecubital vein produces filling of the axillary and subclavian veins, as well as the SVC. However, there is essentially no flow in the SVC below the point of its junction with the azygous vein (arrow), and the axygous vein itself is unusually dilated. (**E**) Another image centered over the mediastinum shows the junction of the azygous vein and SVC (arrow), the large azygous vein draining inferiorly (open arrow), and the points of junction with the dilated hemiazygous veins (curved arrow).

ammonia and other alkaline substances. The association in the case of duodenal ulcers is felt to be as high as 99%, but perhaps only as high as 80% in cases of gastritis. Radiologic findings are nonspecific, and the diagnosis requires endoscopic biopsy or aspiration of gastric contents and urease assay.

TUMOROUS

The most common primary malignancy of the stomach is adenocarcinoma. At one time the most common malignancy in the United States, its incidence has markedly decreased, and now only 25,000 cases per year are diagnosed. Gastric adenocarcinoma is much more common in Japan. Men are more commonly affected than women, with a peak age of incidence in the sixth decade. Predisposing conditions are all associated

Figure 4–33. This spot film of the stomach from a double contrast upper gastrointestinal examination reveals a focal collection of barium protruding beyond the expected margin of the lesser curve of the stomach (arrow), with multiple thin mucosal folds radiating outward from its center. These are typical findings of a benign gastric ulcer. At least 95% of all gastric ulcers are benign, and approximately 90% are due to peptic ulcer disease. Other causes include medications such as corticosteroids and aspirin.

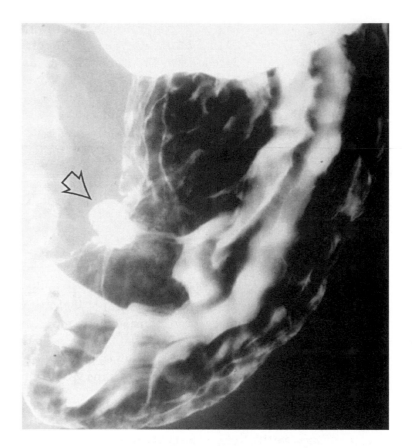

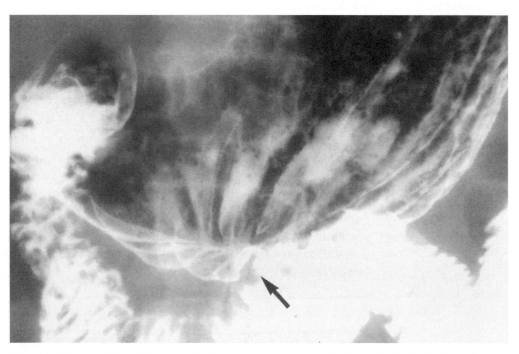

Figure 4–34. A spot film of the stomach from an upper gastrointestinal examination in the frontal projection demonstrates a "spoke wheel" pattern of mucosal folds radiating outward from a point along the greater gastric curvature (arrow). This is a typical appearance of a benign gastric ulcer that has healed with residual scarring. Such an appearance effectively rules out the presence of malignancy, and no further imaging or biopsy is required.

with gastritis and include achlorhydria and previous gastrojejunostomy (with reflux of alkaline bile). Two types are recognized, polypoid and infiltrating. The latter may produce a *linitis plastica,* or "leather bottle" stomach, characterized by thickened, stiff walls (Fig. 4–35). Many gastric adenocarcinomas present as malignant-appearing ulcers, likely because the tumor lacks the usual mucosal defenses against gastric acid. Because the disease has usually penetrated the submucosa or spread to the lymph nodes at the time of diagnosis, 5-year survival is only about 10%.

The most common metastatic neoplasms to involve the stomach are breast carcinoma, melanoma, and lung carcinoma. In a patient with acquired immunodeficiency syndrome (AIDS), Kaposi's sarcoma and lymphoma must be considered. Often gastric metastases will be multiple in number and exhibit a "bull's-eye" appearance, consisting of a mucosal filling defect with a central ulceration.

METABOLIC

One "metabolic" disorder seen in the stomach is Menetrier's disease, which involves a combination of protein-losing enteropathy, achlorhydria, and an increased incidence of adenocarcinoma. Men are more commonly affected than women, and the usual age of diagnosis is in the sixth or seventh decade of life. The loss of protein, which produces edema and an increased incidence of infection, can be traced to proliferation of the superficial layer of the gastric mucosa, which becomes "leaky." This proliferation

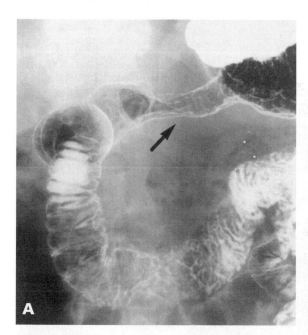
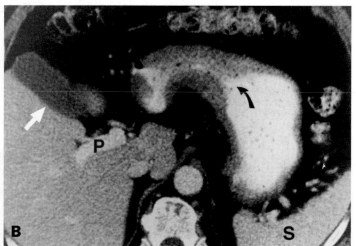

Figure 4–35. A 55-year-old man with a history of progressively severe epigastric pain and weight loss underwent esophagogastroduodenoscopy (EGD), which was negative. However, an upper gastrointestinal barium examination was markedly abnormal. **(A)** A frontal spot film reveals marked narrowing and rigidity of the gastric antrum (arrow), with complete absence of peristaltic waves under fluoroscopic monitoring. This finding indicates the presence of a *linitis plastica* gastric malignancy, most likely a scirrhous adenocarcinoma. Endoscopy was repeated with instructions to take deep biopsies of the superficially normal-appearing gastric antrum. These confirmed the diagnosis. **(B)** An axial image from a staging computed tomography examination clearly demonstrates the diffuse concentric wall thickening of the gastric antrum (arrow, which also indicates the direction of barium flow from the gastric body into the antrum). P, portal vein; S, spleen; white arrow indicates the gallbladder.

produces characteristic giant rugal folds on barium examination. The achlorhydria is secondary to atrophy of the deeper glandular layer of the mucosa.

A second metabolic disorder of the stomach is Zollinger-Ellison syndrome, which consists of recurrent treatment-resistant peptic ulcers, diarrhea, and abdominal pain. In 90% of cases, a gastrin-secreting tumor is present, often in the pancreas or duodenum. Approximately one-half of these prove to be malignant.

IATROGENIC

Numerous iatrogenic conditions are seen in the postoperative stomach. Commonly performed gastric procedures include the Nissan fundoplication, in which a portion of the stomach is wrapped around the distal esophagus to reduce GE reflux; the Billroth I, in which the distal stomach is resected, and the remainder of the stomach is anastamosed to the duodenum; and a Billroth II, in which the distal stomach is resected and a gastrojejunostomy is performed (Fig. 4–36). Early complications for which contrast studies (not barium) are often requested include suspected anastomotic leak and obstruction (often secondary to edema). Later complications include gastritis (often secondary to bile reflux), recurrent ulcers, and gastric carcinoma, which occurs in approximately 1 in 20 patients at two decades.

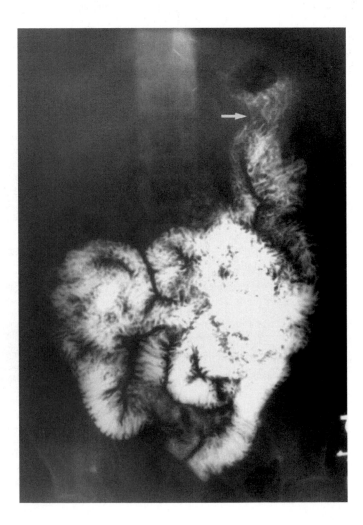

Figure 4–36. This overhead film from a dedicated small bowel series demonstrates typical post-Billroth II anatomy, with failure to visualize the normal duodenal C-loop and visualization of an anastomosis between the gastric remnant and jejunum (arrow).

SMALL BOWEL

CONGENITAL

The most common congenital anomaly of the small bowel is a Meckel's diverticulum. Resulting from failure of closure of the omphalomesenteric duct, which connects the primitive yolk sac to the bowel lumen through the umbilicus, Meckel's diverticulum is characterized by the rule of 2s: It occurs in 2% of the population, it is usually located within 2 ft of the ileocecal valve, it usually measures approximately 2 inches in length, it usually presents with complications before 2 years of age, and approximately 20% of patients suffer complications. Complications stem from the presence of gastric mucosa within the diverticulum, the acidic secretions of which can produce inflammation, ulceration, and bleeding. The lesion is difficult to detect radiographically, because the diverticulum usually does not fill with barium. The imaging study of choice is a nuclear medicine technetium (Tc)-99m-pertechnetate scan, which will show accumulation of radiotracer in the ectopic gastric mucosa (Fig. 4–37). Another congenital abnormality is the enteric duplication cyst, which usually presents as a mass displacing adjacent bowel.

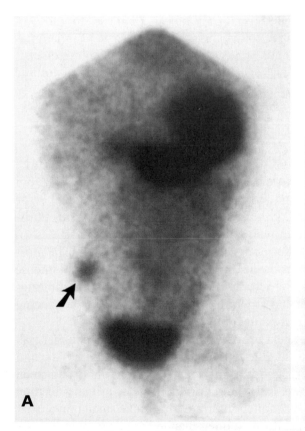
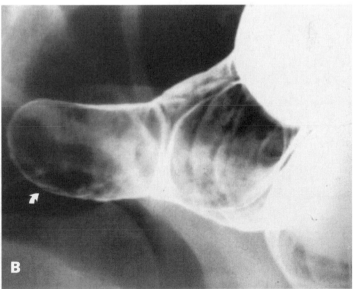

Figure 4–37. (A) This frontal image of the abdomen from a nuclear medicine Meckel scan demonstrates expected radiotracer activity in the stomach and bladder. However, there is an additional area of activity in the right lower quadrant, representing a Meckel's diverticulum (arrow). Approximately 50% of Meckel's diverticula contain sufficient gastric mucosa to secrete technetium-99m-pertechnetate. The sensitivity of the study may be further increased by the administration of pentagastrin, which promotes acid secretion from gastric mucosa. (B) A spot film from a barium examination demonstrates the actual "diverticulum" extending outward from the lumen of the ileum (arrow).

INFLAMMATORY

The most important inflammatory disease of the small bowel is Crohn's disease. It is characterized pathologically by transmural inflammation of the bowel. Because the entire wall is involved, there is a corresponding predilection in this disorder to extraluminal manifestations, such as abscess and fistula formation. Crohn's disease most often affects young adults, who present with diarrhea, abdominal pain, lassitude, and weight loss—nonspecific symptoms that often lead to a long delay in diagnosis. Although Crohn's disease can involve the GI tract anywhere from the mouth to anus, it involves the small bowel alone in 30% of cases, the large bowel alone in 30% of cases, and both in the remaining 40% of cases.

Imaging

 Radiographic findings in Crohn's disease include aphthous ulcers (tiny craters up to several millimeters in diameter), cobblestoning (linear ulcerations with intact intervening mucosa), stricturing and rigidity (the "string sign" when severe), and fistula formation (Fig. 4–38). A fistula (from the Latin for "pipe") is an abnormal communication between two hollow viscuses or a viscus and the skin. Another characteristic finding is discontinuous involvement, or so-called skip lesions separated by normal bowel. Fistulization and skip lesions are not characteristic of ulcerative colitis, the other major type of inflammatory bowel disease. Unlike ulcerative colitis, surgery is not curative in Crohn's disease, and recurrences are typically located just distal to the site of anastamosis. Multiple bowel resections can result in malabsorption syndromes.

TUMOROUS

The small bowel is the segment of the GI tract least often involved by neoplasms. The most common primary small bowel neoplasm is carcinoid tumor, which arises from endocrine cells deep in the mucosa and secretes vasoactive substances such as serotonin. This may produce the carcinoid syndrome, which consists of cutaneous flushing, cramps, and diarrhea, and is seen mainly in patients with liver metastases. In patients without liver metastases, the hormones are inactivated by the liver. The most common location of carcinoid tumor is the ileum, where serotonin induces an intense desmoplastic reaction that can cause strictures and fibrosis. Radiographic findings include small filling defects, kinking and stricture of bowel, and strongly enhancing liver metastases, due to the very vascular nature of the tumor (Fig. 4–39).

Adenocarcinoma is the most prevalent primary malignancy of the proximal small bowel. It has a relatively poor prognosis, due to the high incidence of lymphatic and hematogenous spread at the time of diagnosis. Lymphoma is another important small bowel malignancy, and the small bowel is the most common site of primary GI tract lymphoma. Because it arises in and most often infiltrates the ample small bowel lymphoid tissues, especially in the terminal ileum, it often manifests radiographically with wall thickening, effacement of folds, and luminal widening.

Metastases occur either by intraperitoneal seeding from ovarian, gastric, or colon carcinoma, or by hematogenous spread, with implants of melanoma, breast, or lung carcinoma along the antimesenteric border (Fig. 4–40). Many patients with Kaposi's sarcoma will exhibit umbilicated nodules (a nodule with a small central cavity) in their small bowel mucosa.

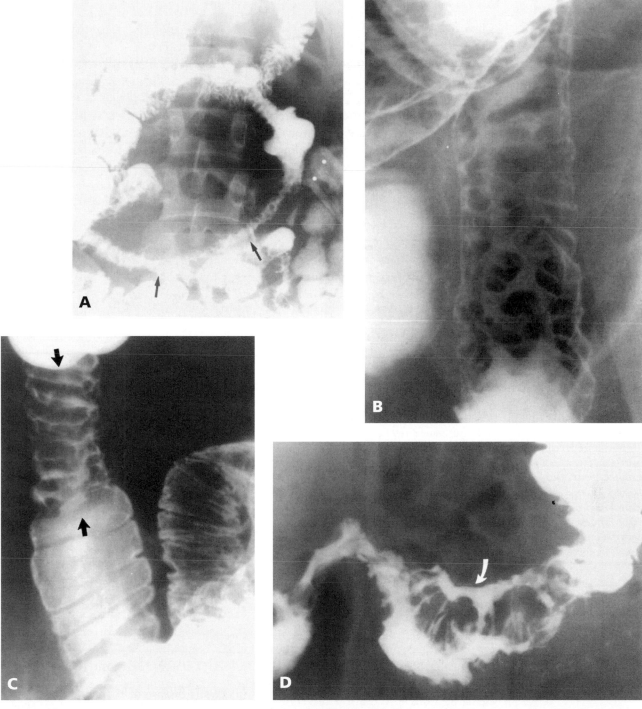

Figure 4–38. A 30-year-old man presented with a history of fever, abdominal cramping, weight loss, and bloody diarrhea. (A) A spot film from his small bowel series demonstrates a long segment of luminal narrowing, a "cobblestone" pattern of nodular inflammation and edema (arrows), and linear ulcerations that may eventuate in fistulae. Mural thickening of this segment can be inferred from the distance separating it from other segments of the bowel. Note the slightly radiopaque compression paddle used to move overlapping segments of the bowel out of the field of view, which contains two tiny round radiopaque markers (on the right side of the film). (B) A spot film of the ileum in another Crohn's disease patient demonstrates the classic appearance of "cobblestoning," with interlacing linear ulcers surrounding nodular mounds of edematous mucosa. Contrast material fills the gutters of the linear ulcerations, while the focal areas of edematous muscosa appear as filling defects. (C) Another film shows the discontinuous character of Crohn's disease, with a markedly abnormal segment of small bowel interposed between two normal segments (arrows). (D) A spot view from a small bowel series in another patient demonstrates prolific intramural fistula formation within the wall of a segment of the small bowel, indicating the transmural nature of the inflammatory process (arrow).

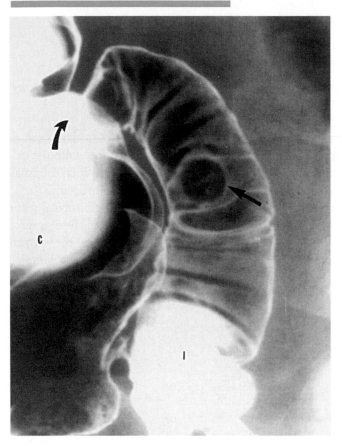

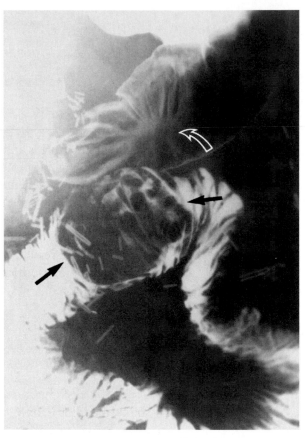

Figure 4–39. This spot film from a small bowel series in which air has been introduced via the rectum to distend the distal small bowel demonstrates a round, well-demarcated filling defect in the terminal ileum (arrow), which was proven at surgery to represent a carcinoid tumor. Most carcinoid tumors arise from the gastrointestinal tract, although the bronchial tree is another common site of origin. The appendix is the most common site, followed by the terminal ileum. Note the location of the ileocecal valve (curved arrow). C, cecum; I, terminal ileum.

Figure 4–40. This patient with a history of metastatic melanoma had previously undergone a resection of a small bowel metastasis (note surgical clips) and presented with new symptoms of a proximal small bowel obstruction. A spot film from a small bowel series demonstrates a large filling defect expanding and partially obstructing this segment of jejunum (arrows), representing another deposit of melanoma. Also note the radiant fold pattern in the gastric antrum, indicating an unrelated healed peptic ulcer (open white arrow).

INFECTIOUS

Acute gastroenteritis is the most common infectious disease of the small bowel, secondary to such pathogens as *Campylobacter jejuni* and *Staphylococcus aureus,* for which imaging is rarely employed. Patients with AIDS are predisposed to a number of enteritides, including cryptosporidium, CMV, and mycobacterium-avium-intracellulare. These manifest radiographically with nonspecific fold thickening.

An uncommon systemic infectious disease that usually involves the GI tract is Whipple's disease, which is caused by a Gram-positive actinomycete and is usually seen in middle-aged Caucasian males. It also involves the joints and the central nervous system in many patients. Radiographic findings include coarse, thickened bowel folds, predominately in the proximal small bowel.

METABOLIC

Common metabolic diseases of the small bowel include lactase deficiency, amyloidosis, and sprue. Disaccharides such as lactose are not properly digested by the jejunum if sufficient quantities of lactase are not produced, a condition seen more commonly in blacks, Orientals, and Arabs. Radiographic findings include bowel dilatation without fold abnormalities.

Amyloidosis, a systemic condition, complicates inflammatory disorders such as rheumatoid arthritis and may also occur in primary form. It is associated with deposition of eosinophilic proteinaceous material that stains with Congo red. When the small bowel is involved, it demonstrates impaired motility and diffusely thickened folds.

Sprue comes in several forms, only one of which is discussed here. Nontropical sprue presents with steatorrhea and weight loss and is due to the toxic effect of gluten, a protein found in wheat and other grains, on the small bowel mucosa of susceptible individuals. While the remainder of the bowel wall is normal, the mucosa becomes denuded and flattened. The radiographic picture is a dilated jejunum with a sparse fold pattern.

VASCULAR

The most important vascular pathology of the small bowel is arterial ischemia, which is usually secondary to thrombosis or embolism of the superior mesenteric artery (SMA). The SMA supplies the bowel between the duodeno-jejunal junction at the ligament of Treitz and the splenic flexure of the colon. Venous thrombosis is also a possibility, most commonly due to low flow states such as congestive heart failure and portal hypertension or hypercoagulable states. Plain films show an ileus pattern with evidence of bowel wall thickening (separation of loops). On CT, a filling defect can be often visualized within the SMA or vein.

COLON AND RECTUM

INFLAMMATION

Ulcerative colitis is the most important inflammatory disorder of the colon. Symptoms include bloody diarrhea, abdominal pain, and blood in the stools. When severe, systemic symptoms such as weight loss and anorexia may appear. Associated conditions include sclerosing cholangitis, arthritis, and ocular and dermatologic disorders. In contrast to Crohn's disease, ulcerative colitis is restricted to the mucosa, involves only the colon, virtually always begins in the rectum, does not involve the anus, does not produce skip lesions (i.e., involves the colon diffusely instead of in a discontinuous fashion), carries a 10- to 30-fold increased risk of malignancy, and can be cured with colectomy (Fig. 4–41).

Imaging

 Radiographic findings include a granular-appearing mucosa, collar-button ulcers (due to undermining of the mucosa), foreshortening of the colon, and a lack of normal haustrations (Fig. 4–42). Pseudopolyps represent small areas of relatively normal mucosa surrounded by erosions. An acute life-threatening complication is toxic megacolon, which is caused by transmural colitis, loss of motor tone, and rapid dilatation of the colonic lumen. Signs of

Figure 4–41. A 32-year-old woman with a long history of ulcerative colitis presented for barium enema with complaints of a right upper quadrant abdominal mass. (**A**) A single overhead radiograph from the barium enema demonstrates a relatively featureless, ahaustral appearance to the colon, indicative of chronic inflammation. In addition, there is an area of annular (from the Latin for "ring") narrowing of the colon in the hepatic flexure (arrow), suspicious for a carcinoma. (**B**) An axial image from a follow-up computed tomography scan obtained to stage the presumed carcinoma demonstrated a 9 cm mass in the hepatic flexure (arrow), associated with infiltration of the surrounding fat and numerous pathologic mesenteric lymph nodes in the center of the abdomen, which could be enlarged due to the chronic inflammation or tumor. No evidence of distant metastases was found. At surgery, an infiltrative adenocarcinoma was resected. White arrows indicate the ureters.

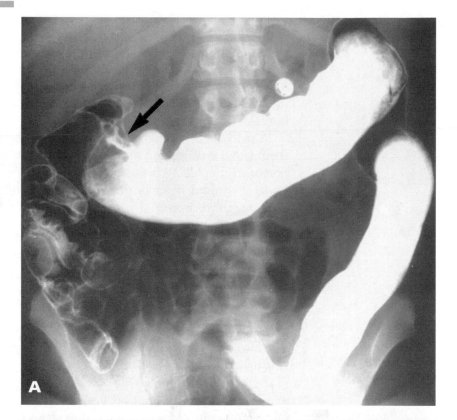

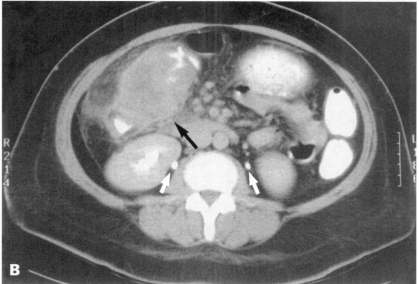

toxic megacolon in a patient with ulcerative colitis include systemic toxicity and profuse bloody diarrhea associated with mucosal sloughing. Plain film findings include marked dilatation of the colon, which, because the transverse colon is the most anterior segment, normally manifests as a dilated (> 6 cm), gas-filled transverse colon on supine radiographs (Fig. 4–43). Performance of a barium enema is strictly contraindi-

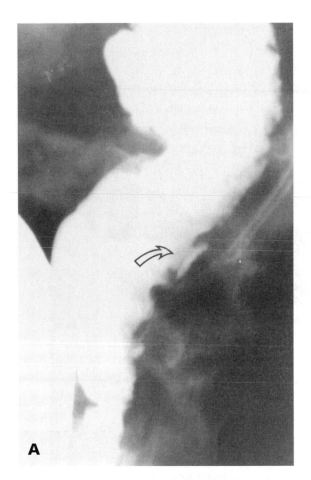

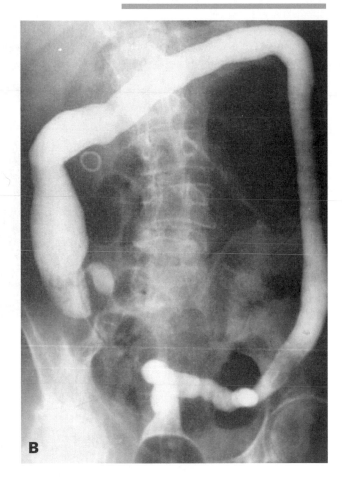

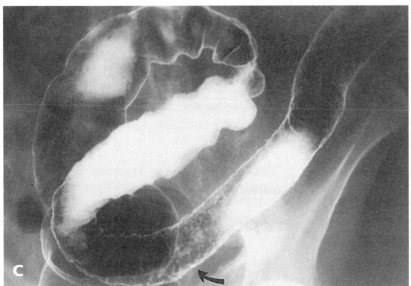

Figure 4–42. (A) This spot film from a single-contrast barium enema reveals a shallow mucosal ulceration that has spread out laterally to undermine the mucosa, producing the classic appearance of a "collar-button" ulcer in ulcerative colitis (arrow). (B) This overhead film from a single-contrast barium enema in another patient reveals a foreshortened, featureless-appearing large bowel, sometimes referred to as a "lead pipe colon," indicating a long-standing disease. (C) A spot film from a double-contrast barium enema in a third patient reveals a granular-appearing mucosa in an otherwise ahaustral colon (arrow), indicating a reactivation of inflammation in a patient with chronic ulcerative colitis.

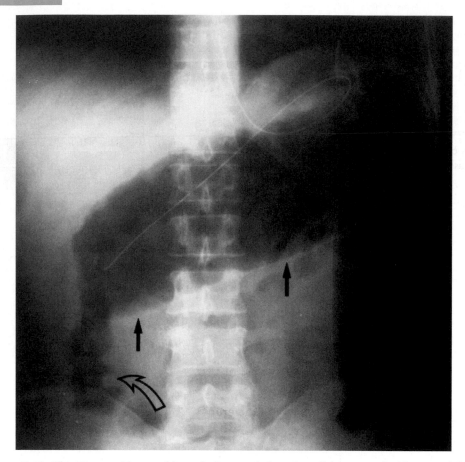

Figure 4–43. This 40-year-old man with newly diagnosed ulcerative colitis presented with severe abdominal pain and rebound tenderness. A supine radiograph of the abdomen demonstrates a nasogastric tube coiled in the gastric fundus, with its tip extending to the expected location of the first portion of the duodenum. There is dilation of the transverse colon (arrows), which measures 6 cm in maximal diameter, as well as a somewhat ahaustral appearance of the colon. The ascending and transverse colon demonstrate thumb-sized luminal indentations (open arrow), called "thumbprinting," and are indicative of bowel wall edema. In a patient with ulcerative colitis, this is highly suggestive of toxic megacolon, which was subsequently confirmed at surgery. Toxic megacolon occurs when mucosal inflammation becomes transmural, with bowel wall edema and ischemia, and a substantial risk of perforation and mortality. Barium enema is contraindicated, due to the risk of perforation.

cated in toxic megacolon, due to the danger of perforation. Overall mortality is as high as 20%.

TUMOROUS

Epidemiology

Colorectal cancer is the second most common cause of cancer death in the United States, with about 60,000 deaths annually. Approximately 150,000 new cases are diagnosed each year. A person's lifetime risk of developing colon cancer is 6%, and once the diagnosis is made, the 5-year survival rate is approximately 40%. Early, small, and hence local disease enjoys the best prognosis. Surgical resection constitutes the only opportunity for cure, although surgery may also be performed for palliation (e.g., to relieve an obstruction) (Fig. 4–44).

Figure 4–44. This spot film from a single-contrast barium enema demonstrates a classic "apple core" annular constricting carcinoma of the colon, with only a thread-like residual lumen within the lesion (arrows). It is called "apple core" because the barium within the attenuated lumen resembles the remainder of an apple after large bites have been taken out circumferentially around its equator. This degree of luminal attenuation is invariably associated with obstructive symptoms, and even though a lesion of this magnitude typically carries a poor prognosis, surgery is necessary to relieve the associated obstruction.

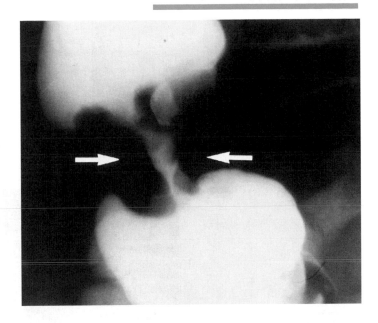

Pathophysiology

A variety of observations support the theory that carcinomas originate in adenomas, including the similar distribution of the two types of lesions in the colon, the parallel incidence rates of adenomas and carcinomas in different countries, the fact that endoscopic removal of adenomas reduces the incidence of carcinoma, and the finding of adenomas, carcinomas in situ, and invasive carcinomas together in some pathologic specimens. It probably takes at least 10 years for an adenoma to develop into a carcinoma, and the majority of adenomas appear never to realize their malignant potential.

While numerous types of polyps, or mucosal elevations, may develop in the colon, including the most common hyperplastic variety (which has no malignant potential), the two types of adenomatous polyps of concern with regard to colorectal carcinoma are tubular adenomas and villous adenomas. Tubular polyps appear pedunculated (on a stalk), while villous polyps are often sessile (appearing to "bulge out" from the mucosa). When an adenoma is discovered, size is crucial in determining its probability of harboring a cancer. Those less than 1 cm in size have a less than 1% chance of malignancy, which increases to 10% for those between 1 and 2 cm and may be as high as 40% for those over 2 cm (Fig. 4–45).

When one adenoma is discovered, there is a 30% probability that the colon harbors another adenoma, and there is a 40% probability that another will develop in the future. The corresponding figures for synchronous ("same time") carcinomas are 5% and for metachronous ("later time") carcinomas, 10%. Hence, once an adenoma or carcinoma is discovered, it is vital that the remainder of the colon be examined, with regular follow-up in the future.

Imaging

The radiologist plays several roles in colorectal cancer. The barium enema, either single or double contrast, is the radiologic mainstay in the screening and detection of new disease, as well as in the detection of recurrent disease. CT provides the primary modality for the staging of disease, in which MRI and endorectal ultrasound may also play a role.

THE SOLID ORGANS OF DIGESTION

Generally, solid organs will be better evaluated by cross-sectional imaging studies than by fluoroscopic contrast studies, in which masses and other pathologic processes in these organs can only be inferred by their effect on gut morphology. In interpreting cross-sectional imaging studies of the abdomen, in which the sheer amount of anatomy can at first appear overwhelming, it is important to adopt an ordered approach to consistently exclude common or important abnormalities.

Search Pattern

When faced with a CT or MRI study of the abdomen, the following represents a reasonable approach. First, examine each organ for size, shape, homogeneity, and abnormal areas of enhancement. Crucial parameters include the presence of masses or mass effects (such as displacement of blood vessels or adjacent organs), fluid collections, regions of altered brightness on nonenhanced or enhanced images, and adenopathy. The organs and areas to be systematically inspected include the liver, gallbladder, spleen, pancreas, adrenal glands, kidneys, GI tract, mesentery, retroperitoneum, and vessels (aorta and iliac branches, celiac axis, SMA, and the inferior vena cava and its iliac and femoral branches, as well as the portal vein and superior mesenteric veins). In addition, the bones and soft tissues should be examined.

Select Pathologies

LIVER

CONGENITAL

Hemochromatosis is one of the most common genetic diseases, which often presents due to its manifestations in the liver. The disease is inherited as an autosomal recessive trait and is found in heterozygous form in up to 10% of the white population. Although congenital, it rarely manifests before the third or fourth decade. It is characterized by a defect in intestinal iron absorption, which is normally downregulated when systemic iron stores are sufficient. Secondary hemochromatosis occurs in individuals who require multiple blood transfusions.

Both primary and secondary forms result in iron deposition in such organs as the liver, the pancreas, and the skin, producing the classic triad of hepatic cirrhosis, diabetes, and bronze pigmentation ("bronze diabetes"). The definitive diagnosis is established by hepatic biopsy, but can be suggested by elevated serum ferritin levels. Often, the diagnosis is not suspected, but can be suggested in the appropriate clinical setting by such imaging findings as hyperechoic liver on ultrasound, a markedly increased density of the liver on noninfused CT images (> 75 HU, and significantly denser than the spleen), and marked hypointensity of the liver on T2-weighted images. Therapy usually consists of phlebotomy.

INFLAMMATORY

A common "inflammatory" lesion of the liver is cirrhosis, which involves destruction of hepatocytes and hepatic lobular architecture, with replacement by scarring and regenerating hepatic nodules. Cirrhosis was so named by Laennec based on the yellowish appearance of the diseased liver, after the Greek *kirrhos,* meaning "tawny." The most common cause in the United States is alcoholism, although patients with hepatitis B are also at considerably increased risk. Patients present with failure to thrive, jaundice (due to disordered bilirubin metabolism), ascites, signs of portal hypertension, and abnormal liver function tests.

Imaging

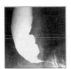

Liver biopsy is the definitive test, but the presence of cirrhosis can be suggested by multiple imaging studies. Ultrasound signs include hepatomegaly and irregularity of the hepatic surface, ascites, and evidence of portal hypertension, including varices and splenomegaly. CT findings include heterogeneity of the hepatic parenchyma, nodularity of the liver surface, ascites, and signs of portal hypertension. In sclerosing cholangitis, which is characterized by progressive fibrotic inflammation of the biliary tree leading to biliary obstruction and cirrhosis, percutaneous cholangiography demonstrates multiple focal strictures of the bile ducts.

TUMOROUS

The liver, along with the lung, is one of the two organs most often involved by metastatic malignancy, and hepatic metastases are 20 times more prevalent than primary hepatic malignancies. Approximately one-third of patients who die of malignancy demonstrate at least pathologic evidence of hepatic metastases. The liver is the most common site of metastatic disease in colorectal carcinoma, and other common sources of hepatic metastases include digestive system sites such as the stomach and pancreas, as well as the breast and lung (Fig. 4–48). As many as 15 to 20% of patients actually die of hepatic disease, rather than their primary tumor.

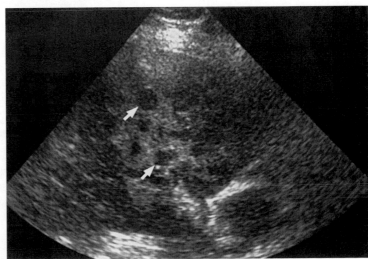

Figure 4–48. A 70-year-old woman with a history of breast cancer presented with elevated liver function tests. A sagittal (longitudinal) sonogram through the inferior aspect of the right lobe of the liver demonstrates multiple hypoechoic lesions (arrows), which is the most common appearance of hepatic metastases. Characteristically hyperechoic metastases include gastrointestinal malignancies and hepatocellular carcinoma.

While the liver is subject to a number of primary malignancies, hepatocellular carcinoma is the most important, and constitutes the most common visceral malignancy worldwide. Risk factors include chronic hepatitis B and C, cirrhosis, and metabolic disorders such as glycogen storage diseases. Of the 5000 cases diagnosed each year in the United States, approximately 4000 occur in men. Patients present with a right upper quadrant mass and evidence of liver failure, including jaundice and ascites. α-Fetoprotein levels are often elevated, and can be used to help distinguish hepatocellular carcinoma from metastatic carcinoma.

On imaging of hepatocellular carcinoma, CT demonstrates a hypodense, enhancing lesion that often invades vascular structures such as the portal vein (Fig. 4–49). Ultrasound usually demonstrates a hypodense mass that may invade vessels and is associated with high velocity flow on Doppler imaging. Both CT and ultrasound provide excellent guidance for biopsy.

Cavernous hemangioma is the most prevalent nonmalignant tumor, and is found in approximately 5% of the population (F:M = 4:1). These lesions consist of collections of large vascular channels containing slow-moving blood. The principal reason

Figure 4–49. A 72-year-old man with a history of alcoholic cirrhosis presented with abdominal pain and increased liver function tests. (**A**) An axial image from an abdominal ultrasound examination reveals a 3 cm hypoechoic mass in the right lobe of the liver (arrow), which demonstrates a somewhat hypoechoic rim, thought to represent tumor invasion into the surrounding parenchyma. (**B**) An axial image from a contrast-enhanced abdominal computed tomography examination in the arterial phase demonstrates the enhancing mass (arrow), as well as a slightly hypointense rim. Biopsy revealed hepatocellular carcinoma. The lifetime risk that a cirrhotic patient will develop hepatocellular carcinoma is approximately 5%.

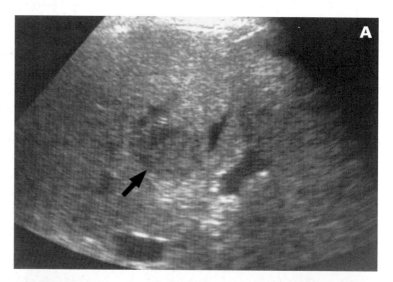

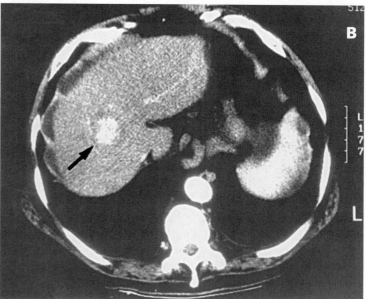

to be concerned about the presence of a hemangioma, which is nearly always asymptomatic, is to distinguish it from a more sinister process such as a hepatocellular carcinoma. By ultrasound, hemangiomas are usually uniformly hyperechoic but demonstrate posterior acoustic enhancement. By CT with contrast infusion and dynamic scanning (scanning the lesion multiple times over several minutes), they characteristically exhibit a pattern of enhancement that moves from the periphery to the center, eventually filling in completely (Fig. 4–50). On MRI, hemangiomas demonstrate marked hyperintensity on heavily T2-weighted images (the "light bulb" sign).

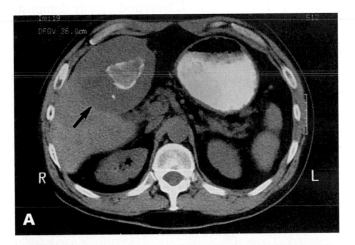

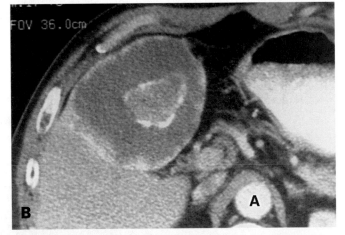

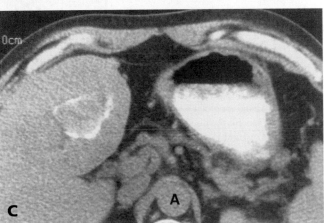

Figure 4–50. A series of axial computed tomography sections were obtained through the liver both before and after contrast infusion to characterize an incidentally discovered lesion. (A) Before contrast, this large, hypodense lesion in the inferior aspect of the liver (arrow) contains a central calcified region, and is suspicious for a cavernous hemangioma. On bolus contrast infusion, the lesion at first enhances peripherally (B), before eventually filling in centrally several minutes later (C), by which time the aorta (A) is no longer brightly enhanced. This centripetal pattern of dynamic enhancement reflects the fact that these vascular lesions exhibit very slow blood flow. Up to 20% of cavernous hemangiomas contain calcifications.

INFECTIOUS

From an imaging standpoint, infections of the liver usually take the form of abscesses. Enteric organisms such as *Escherichia coli* produce the most common pyogenic abscesses, and many are iatrogenic. On CT they often appear hypodense with peripheral enhancement, but do not fill in over time. Many contain pockets of gas. Interventionalists are often called upon to drain pockets of pus percutaneously. In combination with antibiotic therapy, drainage often produces complete resolution.

PANCREAS

CONGENITAL

The two most frequent congenital pancreatic anomalies are pancreas divisum and annular pancreas. Pancreas divisum results from lack of normal fusion of the dorsal and ventral pancreatic buds during embryogenesis, with the result that the main pancreatic drainage occurs through the minor papilla (located proximal to the papilla of Vater). It is thought that this orifice is often too small to accommodate the full volume of pancreatic secretions, resulting in obstruction and recurrent pancreatitis. Annular pancreas results from abnormal migration of the ventral pancreas, causing pancreatic encirclement of the duodenum, which can result in duodenal obstruction. Both of these conditions are best imaged with endoscopic retrograde cholangiopancreatography, in which the pancreatic duct(s) is cannulated and contrast injected under fluoroscopic monitoring (Fig. 4–51).

INFLAMMATORY

A discussion of pancreatitis is found in Chapter 6.

TUMOROUS

Ninety-five percent of all pancreatic malignancies are adenocarcinomas. The prognosis tends to be dismal, due to the common presence of metastases at the time of diagnosis,

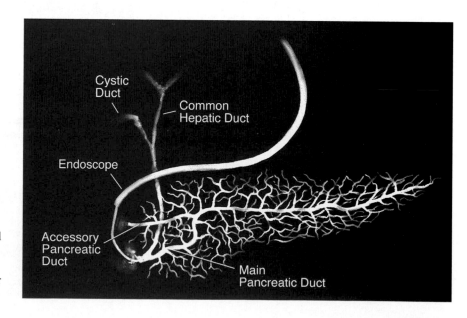

Figure 4–51. Illustration of an endoscopic retrograde cholangiopancreatogram, with endoscope passing through the distal esophagus, stomach, and into the second portion of the duodenum, with injection of contrast via a cannula into the common bile duct, and filling of the biliary and pancreatic ductal systems. Under normal conditions, the pancreatic ductal system would not be filled so extensively with contrast, for fear of inciting or exacerbating pancreatitis.

resulting in approximately 29,000 deaths per year. Pancreatic malignancy is the fourth leading cause of cancer death among both men and women. Presenting signs and symptoms include jaundice, weight loss, and Courvoisier's sign (a palpable, nontender gallbladder). Imaging usually consists of contrast-enhanced CT or ultrasound, with CT demonstrating a hypodense mass, which on ultrasound appears hypoechoic (Fig. 4–52). Cure is possible only with surgical resection, but involvement of major vessels such as

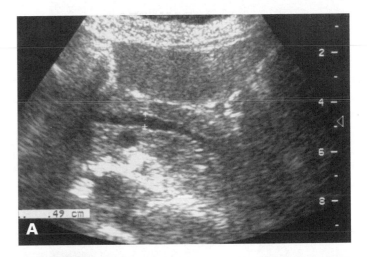

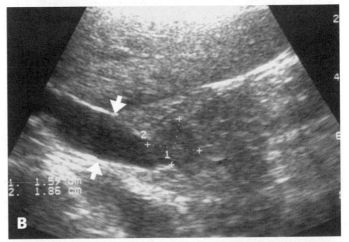

Figure 4–52. A 50-year-old woman presented with painless jaundice. (A) A transverse ultrasound image through the pancreatic body demonstrates dilation of the pancreatic duct, which measures 5 mm (3 mm is the upper limit of normal in a patient of this age). (B) A sagittal sonogram through the pancreatic head demonstrates a 1.8 × 1.6 cm hypoechoic mass (cursors) that is obstructing the distal common bile duct (CBD) (arrows), which is dilated to approximately 2 cm. (C) A transverse sonogram of the liver demonstrates multiple branching, tubular structures that demonstrated no color flow (and hence were not blood vessels), indicating intrahepatic biliary dilation. Endoscopic retrograde cholangiopancreatography (ERCP) was performed, in order to place an endoluminal stent through the region of obstruction.

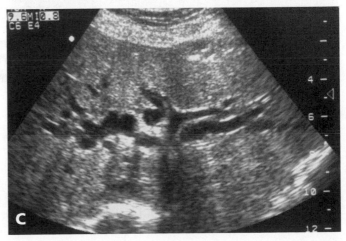

(continued)

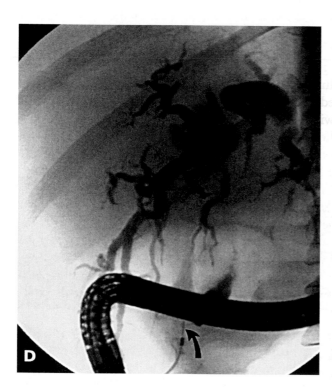

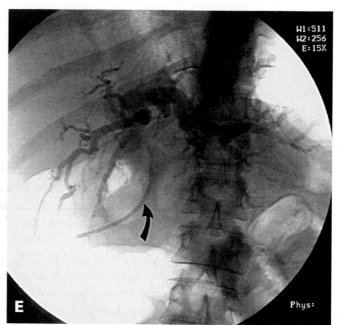

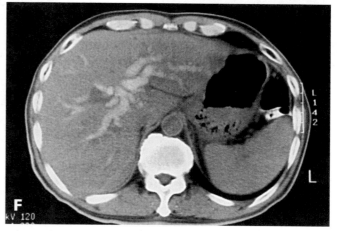

Figure 4–52. *(continued)* **(D)** A preliminary view demonstrates the endoscopic cannula extending into the distal CBD (arrow), with prominent intrahepatic biliary dilatation. **(E)** A final view after removal of the endoscope shows the radiopaque stent in the distal CBD (arrow). The patient's hyperbilirubinemia resolved over the next few days. **(F)** An axial image from a contrast-enhanced computed tomography scan of the abdomen in another patient who had just undergone an ERCP reveals contrast material in dilated and somewhat serpiginous intrahepatic biliary ducts.

the celiac artery or SMA renders the tumor nonresectable. Other pancreatic neoplasms include endocrine tumors such as insulinoma (most common) and gastrinoma, as well as cystic neoplasms such as macro- and microcystic adenomas.

ABDOMINAL TRAUMA

Trauma is the third leading cause of death in the United States, accounting for nearly 200,000 deaths per year. Because trauma constitutes the leading cause of death in persons under the age of 40 years, it exacts a particularly heavy toll in years of life lost. It also results in several million nonfatal injuries annually, many of which leave victims permanently disabled or disfigured.

Diagnosis

DIAGNOSTIC PERITONEAL LAVAGE

While diagnostic peritoneal lavage (DPL) once represented the preferred technique for detecting and evaluating free fluid, CT scanning has now largely replaced this technique at most centers. Performed by inserting a catheter into the peritoneal space and first infusing and then withdrawing sterile fluid, peritoneal lavage is a highly sensitive technique for the detection of hemoperitoneum. Occasionally, peritoneal lavage provides more specific information than CT, as when bile or a high amylase content is detected in the fluid (indicating biliary and pancreatic injury, respectively). DPL may also exhibit advantages over CT in the detection of bowel and mesenteric injury.

However, DPL is also highly nonspecific, providing no information about the source of hemorrhage. Moreover, DPL cannot distinguish between inconsequential and serious injuries. Prior to the advent of CT scanning, laparotomy represented the only means of ascertaining the location and extent of the injury. Another difficulty with DPL is the fact that it cannot evaluate the retroperitoneum. Though not as sensitive in the detection of minute amounts of free fluid, CT yields highly specific information in a noninvasive fashion.

COMPUTED TOMOGRAPHY

CT evaluation of abdominal trauma begins with the search for free intraperitoneal air (pneumoperitoneum), which tends to accumulate in the nondependent portion of the peritoneal cavity (in a supine patient, beneath the anterior abdominal wall). It is seen as a collection or rim of air attenuation appearing completely black. In the absence of penetrating trauma, free air indicates rupture of a viscus. A second critical finding is that of free fluid. Free fluid tends to accumulate in the pelvis, the most dependent portion of the peritoneal cavity in both the upright and supine positions. Such fluid is most likely to represent extravasated blood, urine, bile, or enteric contents, or transudate or exudate secondary to post-traumatic inflammation. It is important to recall that several important organs are in fact retroperitoneal, including the duodenum, the pancreas, the kidneys, and the great vessels. Fluid originating from these organs must therefore be sought in a retroperitoneal location.

As a general principle, there is a linear relationship between the hematocrit of blood and its attenuation value, as hemoglobin accounts for approximately 80% of total blood X-ray absorption. Consequently, hemorrhage in a severely anemic patient may appear surprisingly hypodense. The attenuation value of extravasated blood varies depending on the time at which it is imaged. In the first few hours after hemorrhage, a hematoma will demonstrate attenuation values equivalent to intravascular blood, approximately 50 HU. With time, however, diffusion of serum into surrounding tissues and retraction of the fibrin clot results in an increase in attenuation, with values in the neighborhood of 80 HU. Over the ensuing days and weeks, hemoglobin is broken down, with a gradual decline in attenuation eventually approaching that of water, 0 HU.

Other general signs of abdominal injury include an increase in the size of a normally shaped organ, reflecting hemorrhage or edema; intrinsic deformity of an organ

Figure 4–53. This contrast-enhanced computed tomography scan of the abdomen reveals low density subcapsular blood along the posterior aspect of the contrast-enhanced splenic parenchyma, indicating a subcapsular splenic hemorrhage.

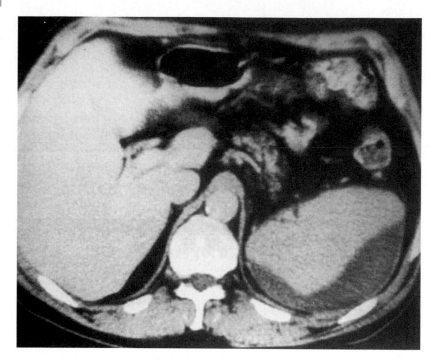

due to direct impact or swelling; displacement or deformity of an organ due to extrinsic mass effect, as from a hematoma; and discontinuity in the contour of an organ, due to laceration or rupture. To optimize the detection of injury, intravenous contrast infusion is critical, and oral contrast administration is indicated in most cases. Intravenous contrast improves lesion detection by delineating perfused and nonperfused tissues, which can be otherwise difficult to differentiate due to the isointensity of hyperacute blood (Fig. 4–53). Nonperfused areas within an organ indicate vascular injury, as in a laceration or fracture, and carry prognostic significance regarding the organ's viability. The focal accumulation of contrast suggests ongoing extravasation.

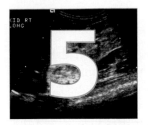

The Urinary Tract

ANATOMY AND PHYSIOLOGY

The kidneys are paired retroperitoneal structures contained within the anterior and posterior renal (from the Latin *renes,* "kidneys") fasciae, also known as Gerota's fascia. Between the anterior and posterior renal fasciae lies not only the kidney itself, but the adrenal gland, the proximal portion of the collecting system and ureter, and the renal pedicle, including the renal artery, the renal vein, and lymphatics. Only approximately two-thirds of kidneys are supplied by a single renal artery, and multiple renal veins are also seen in approximately one-third of cases. Because the left renal vein must cross the midline to reach the inferior vena cava (IVC), it is approximately three times longer than the right renal vein, which makes the left kidney the preferred organ for renal transplantation. Moreover, because the left renal vein receives the left gonadal vein, a left renal cell carcinoma with ipsilateral renal vein thrombosis will commonly present with left scrotal swelling. The right renal vein typically drains directly into the IVC.

The kidneys normally measure approximately 3.5 lumbar vertebral body heights, or about 12 cm, in length. Plain radiography routinely overestimates their length due to magnification, while ultrasound often underestimates their length due to difficulties in imaging the kidney in its longest plane. The left kidney is normally positioned 1 to 2 cm higher than the right. The renal axes parallel those of the psoas muscles, with the lower poles positioned more laterally than the upper poles.

The formation of urine involves three processes: filtration, secretion, and reabsorption. These processes are performed by the nephron, the functional unit of the kidney (Fig. 5–1). Each kidney contains approximately 1 million nephrons. The nephron begins in the glomerulus (from the Latin *glomerule,* "a round knot"), a spherical tuft of capillaries 100 times more permeable than capillaries elsewhere, across which fluid is filtered into Bowman's capsule. From there, the filtrate passes through the proximal convoluted tubule, Henle's loop, the distal convoluted tubule, and into the collecting duct. The juxtaglomerular apparatus secretes renin in response to a fall in blood pressure, activating the renin-angiotensin-aldosterone system, which in turn increases sodium reabsorption in the distal tubules. This system is further discussed later in this chapter in the nuclear medicine imaging section.

Critical structures evaluated on imaging studies include the renal vasculature, the cortical and medullary portions of the parenchyma, the pyramids, the calyces, the pelvis, the ureters, the bladder, and the urethra (Fig. 5–2). The outer renal cortex (from the Latin for "bark of a tree") consists of the glomeruli and the proximal and distal convoluted tubules. The inner medulla (Latin for "marrow") consists of the collecting tubules and Henle's loops. The medulla is made up of a number of medullary pyramids, which are cradled by the cup-shaped calyces (Latin for "outer covering" or "pod") of the collecting system. Each kidney contains approximately 12 calyces. The calyces join together to form infundibula (Latin for "funnel"), which drain into the renal pelvis (Latin for "basin").

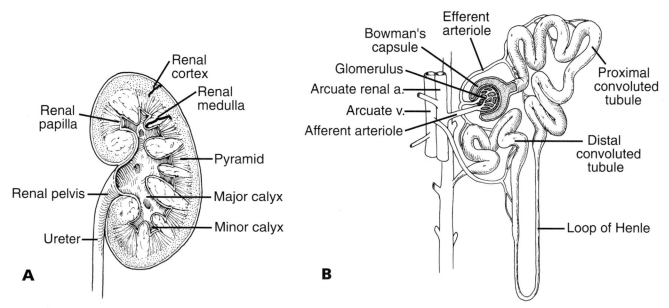

Figure 5–1. (A) The major structures of the kidney that are assessed on imaging studies. (B) Major structures of the nephron.

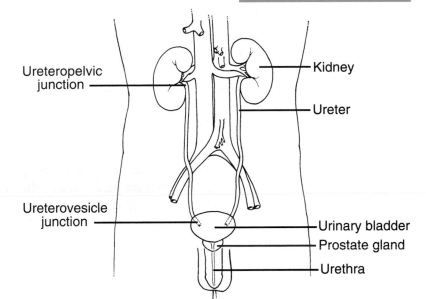

Figure 5–2. The major structures of the urinary system.

The pelvis joins the ureter (from the Greek *ourein,* "to urinate") at the ureteropelvic junction (UPJ), a common site of obstruction. The ureters contain circular and longitudinal layers of smooth muscle that actively propel urine toward the bladder by peristalsis. The bladder can accommodate between 250 and 400 mL in the normal adult. It is bounded posteriorly by the uterus in females and by the rectum in males. The bladder and urethera meet at the trigone, a triangle formed at the bladder floor by the two ureteral orifices and the urethral orifice. The reproductive and urinary tracts are completely separate in the female, but become joined at the base of the prostate gland in the male, where the ejaculatory ducts empty into the urethra. The female urethra is embedded in the anterior wall of the vagina and measures approximately 3 cm in length. The higher incidence of urinary tract infections (UTIs) in girls and young women is often attributed to the relatively short female urethra, which may facilitate retrograde passage of bacteria.

The kidneys perform a number of vital physiologic functions, including regulation of water balance, precise maintenance of electrolyte concentrations and acid-base balance, excretion of toxic metabolites such as urea, regulation of blood pressure via the renin-angiotensin system, production of erythropoietin, and conversion of vitamin D to its active form. Further discussion of renal physiology is found in the nuclear medicine section later in this chapter. Consequences of renal failure include uremia, metabolic acidosis, hyperkalemia, disordered regulation of sodium, phosphate, and calcium balance, hypertension, anemia, and immune compromise.

IMAGING

Intravenous Urography

Urography was born of syphilology. The first urogram was performed in 1923 by physicians at the Mayo Clinic, who discovered that the sodium iodide they were investigating to treat syphilis possessed two intriguing properties: (1) it was excreted via the urinary system, and therefore passed through the kidneys, ureters, bladder, and urethra; and (2) the compound was radiopaque. However, sodium iodide produced relatively poor opacification and displayed other shortcomings as well. The next crucial innovation occurred when German chemists, seeking to synthesize the "magic bullet" for syphilis, linked iodine to a pyridine ring. Although their invention proved not to be the magic bullet, their organic iodine compounds created a magic window on the urinary tract. By the early 1930s, physicians were relying on excretory urography to provide previously unimaginable images of the structure and function of the urinary system.

The intravenous urogram (IVU; often called an intravenous pyelogram, or IVP, a misnomer) is performed as follows (Fig. 5–3): First, a preliminary frontal radiograph of the abdomen is obtained. This view may demonstrate stones or soft tissue masses, and provides a limited assessment of the morphology of the kidneys. Additional tomographic views of the kidneys are obtained to ensure that the technique will be optimal for obtaining nephrotomograms after contrast injection (Fig. 5–4). After verifying that the patient has no risk factors for an adverse contrast reaction, the physician

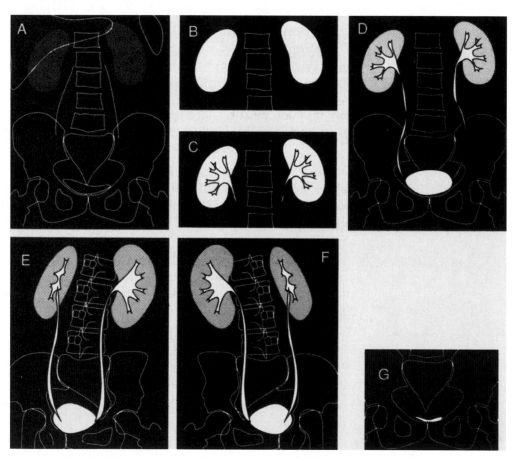

Figure 5–3. The intravenous urogram. Usual filming sequence for urography. (**A**) "Scout." (**B**) Early nephrogram phase when parenchyma is most radiopaque. (**C**) Five minute radiograph to detect differential in function. (**D**) Large abdominal radiograph to visualize kidneys, ureters, and bladder obtained at 10 to 15 minutes. (**E, F**) Two oblique projections may be obtained over the kidneys only, or may include ureter and bladder. (**G**) Postvoid radiograph may disclose unsuspected pathology in addition to providing information about residual urine. This sequence is by no means a rule and should be tailored to suit the individual patient.

injects approximately 100 to 150 cc of iodinated contrast material into a peripheral vein, and films are obtained at several minute intervals until kidneys, ureters, and bladder have been well visualized. Tomographic views of the kidneys are also obtained, which provide optimal assessment of the morphology of the renal parenchyma. The study should be monitored by a physician, who can adapt the examination to various findings.

To understand the excretory urogram, it is necessary to view it in light of renal physiology. Let us explore some potential findings on the urogram and attempt to understand their physiologic etiologies. First, suppose the patient is injected, but initial films demonstrate no renal opacification. Several explanations are possible. The concentration of contrast material in the urine, or the urographic density achieved by the examination, can be analyzed according to the following formula:

$$[U] = ([P] \times GFR)/U_{vol}$$

where $[U]$ is urographic density; $[P]$ is the plasma concentration of contrast; GFR is glomerular filtration rate; and U_{vol} is the volume of urine produced. (The formula holds because nearly 99% of the contrast is filtered by the glomerulus, and there is virtually no distal tubular excretion or reabsorption.) If the kidneys are not seen at all, this formula indicates that there is either no contrast or no blood flow. The former would raise suspicion for extravasation of contrast at the injection site, which is why every injection must be monitored. The latter would suggest either that the blood is not circulating or that the glomeruli are not filtering (Fig. 5–5).

If the blood is not circulating, the patient requires urgent attention, as a full-blown contrast reaction with hypotension or even cardiopulmonary arrest may be underway, another reason why qualified personnel must be present while a patient is undergoing an excretory urogram. If the glomeruli are not filtering, it is likely that the renal tubular pressure distal to the glomeruli is elevated, as in acute obstruction (which would

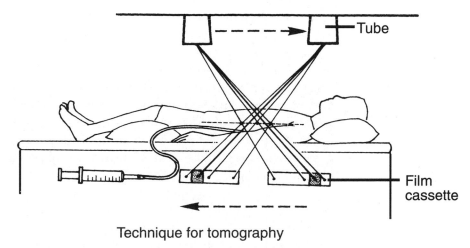

Technique for tomography

Figure 5–4. How tomograms are obtained during the intravenous urogram. The X-ray tube and film pivot around a focal plane in the abdomen centered on the kidneys, which produces clear images of the kidneys with other abdominal structures anterior and posterior to them "blurred out" by motion.

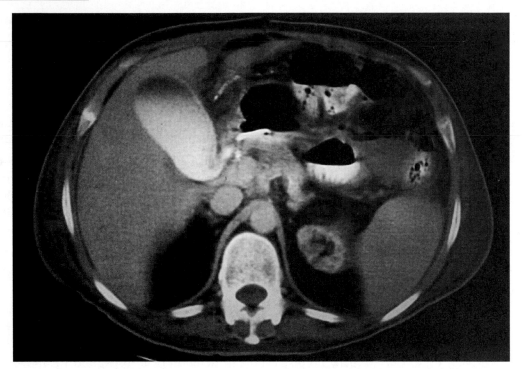

Figure 5–5. An axial image from a contrast-enhanced abdominal computed tomography scan demonstrates a small, cyst-containing, atrophic left kidney in a patient with bilateral chronic medical renal disease from hypertension. Moreover, there is prominent opacification of the gallbladder, with a bile-contrast level visible within its lumen. This illustrates the fact that the liver is also capable of excreting iodinated contrast material, which appears in the bile through a process known as "vicarious" hepatobiliary excretion in patients with impaired renal function. Why was a patient with known chronic renal failure given intravenous contrast? Not because the liver could be relied upon to excrete it, but because the patient was to receive hemodialysis the next day, at which point the contrast material would be artificially "excreted."

have to be bilateral), or the kidneys are no longer functional, as from chronic infarction, in which case the patient would be in renal failure, and a urogram should not have been ordered.

A more likely scenario would be unilateral nonvisualization, failure to identify one of the two kidneys. What could account for this? Again, obstruction, as from a stone in the ipsilateral ureter, would be the single most likely explanation, depending on the clinical situation. Other possibilities would include unilateral renal agenesis, which is rare, or ectopia, such as a kidney unexpectedly located in the pelvis; complete renal artery obstruction due to thrombosis, embolus, or stenosis, which blocks inflow to the glomerulus; acute renal vein thrombosis, which blocks outflow from the glomerulus; or a disease process in the renal parenchyma, a congenital dysplasia, polycystic disease, or a tumor.

The change in the nephrogram over time is another valuable source of information. Normally, a peak plasma concentration of contrast is rapidly reached after contrast injection. Thereafter, both the plasma concentration and, soon thereafter, the density of the nephrogram, fall linearly, with a half-time of approximately 1 hour. Hence the normal nephrogram exhibits a rapid peak in intensity followed by a linear decrease. The opposite pattern to this is the faint but gradually increasing nephrogram. Actually, the vascular causes of an "absent" nephrogram mentioned earlier typically produce not an absent nephrogram but a delayed nephrogram, which becomes increasingly dense over time. What appears initially to represent an absent nephrogram at 3 minutes postinjection usually turns out to be a delayed nephrogram, as the kidney slowly opacifies at 5, 15, or 60 minutes. This stems from the fact that, in vascular obstruction, GFR, though low, is not zero. The nephrogram becomes increasingly dense with time because what little iodine does make it into the renal tubule becomes increasingly concentrated as salt and water are reabsorbed. This same situation, the delayed but increasingly dense nephrogram, also typically occurs in the case of acute extrarenal obstruction (such as a ureteral stone), where again, GFR is unlikely to be zero (Fig. 5–6).

Another key nephrographic parameter is the parenchymal pattern. Suppose there is a single filling defect in the renal parenchma; what might be the cause? A defect indicates a focal absence of functioning nephrons. Possible explanations would include a cyst, a space-occupying collection of fluid displacing adjacent nephrons; a tumor, such as a renal cell carcinoma; an abscess, which is sometimes surrounded by a rim of hypervascular granulation tissue; or trauma, such as a renal contusion (Fig. 5–7).

In the case of multiple filling defects, likely explanations would include multiple idiopathic cysts (50% of patients older than 50 years of age have at least one); polycystic kidney disease; or multifocal pyelonephritis. A simple cyst will typically appear as a circular or oval defect occupying only a partial thickness of the renal parenchyma. Pyelonephritis, on the other hand, extends from the innermost margin of the parenchyma, the papilla, to the outermost edge of the cortex, since it typically involves the infection of an entire lobe or lobule of the kidney.

The next phase of the urogram is the excretory phase, involving opacification of the pelvocalyceal system and the descending urinary pathways, including the bladder. Among the most important filling defects that may be detected in the excretory phase are stones, blood clots, cancer (especially transitional cell carcinoma), fungus, and papillary necrosis with sloughing of an infarcted papilla.

Another commonly encountered abnormality is a stricture, which is likely either postinflammatory, as from previous impaction of a stone; infectious, most commonly

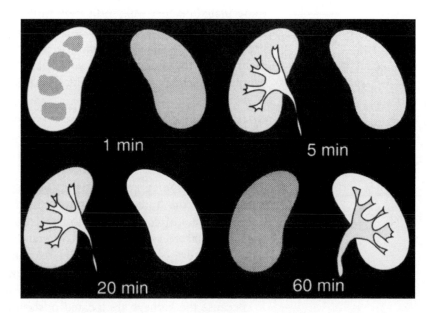

Figure 5–6. The expected urographic pattern in an acute left-sided ureteral obstruction. Note that while the right kidney passes almost completely through the nephrographic and excretory phases, the left kidney only becomes increasingly dense, with the eventual appearance of some contrast in the collecting system at 1 hour.

Figure 5–7. A left renal tomogram from an intravenous urogram demonstrates a large filling defect just below the left ureteropelvic junction, which is exerting considerable mass effect on the collecting system. The differential diagnosis of this lesion would include a cyst, a tumor, and an abscess. In this case, the lesion represented an abscess.

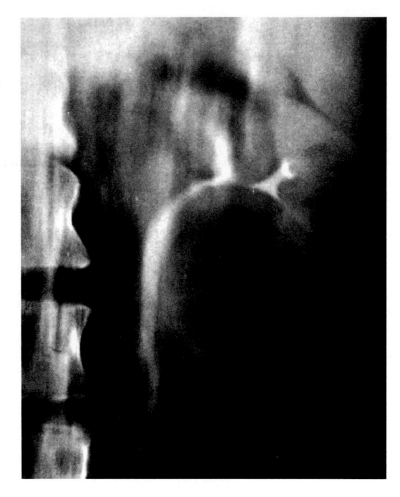

from tuberculosis or schistosomiasis; or tumorous, either intrinsic (transitional cell carcinoma) or extrinsic (such as cervical cancer, with encasement of the ureter).

A common finding in the bladder aside from a filling defect is a thickened and/or trabeculated bladder wall, indicating muscular hypertrophy or inflammation. Benign prostatic hypertrophy is the most common cause, which leads to compression of the prostatic urethra at the bladder base and resultant partial obstruction. Other causes include cystitis, which may be secondary to infection (most commonly bacterial), drugs (especially cyclophosphamide), and radiation.

Nuclear Medicine

While ultrasound, computed tomography (CT), and magnetic resonance imaging (MRI) have assumed an increasing role in the anatomic evaluation of the kidneys, nuclear medicine studies remain preeminent in the imaging evaluation of renal function. Examples of common clinical situations in which radionuclide imaging is utilized are renal artery stenosis, vesicoureteral reflux (discussed in Chapter 10), and collecting system obstruction. The four major renal parameters evaluated by radionuclide studies include renal blood flow, glomerular filtration, tubular function, and collecting system drainage.

Because the kidneys are located posteriorly within the abdomen, imaging is performed with the patient supine and the detector beneath the patient, so that renal images are in the "posterior" projection. An exception is the post-transplant patient, whose kidney is typically located anteriorly within the pelvis and is therefore better evaluated with the detector positioned anteriorly. If ureteral drainage is of special concern, the patient may be imaged upright. In every case, immobilization of the patient is critical, because count acquisition takes place not over a period of milliseconds, but over seconds or even minutes. Over a period of 20 to 30 minutes, the movement of tracer from the blood to the renal cortex, from the renal cortex to the collecting system, and from the collecting system to the bladder, can be assessed.

BLOOD FLOW

An indication of the kidney's relative physiologic importance is the fact that at rest, the kidneys receive approximately 20% of the cardiac output, despite the fact that they represent only about 3% of body weight. The ideal agent for measuring renal blood flow (or plasma flow) would be one that is completely cleared from the blood during its passage through the kidney. In the laboratory, this is accomplished by the use of para-amino hippuric acid, the use of which yields an effective renal plasma flow of 500 to 600 mL/min. The agents currently in use in nuclear medicine yield somewhat lower values of renal plasma flow and include technetium (Tc)-99m-DTPA and Tc-99m-MAG3. The measurement of renal plasma flow is based on the rate of disappearance of radiotracer from the blood. Typically, activity appears in the kidneys within several seconds of the time when the injected bolus of radiotracer reaches the abdominal aorta.

Renal plasma flow can be assessed using one of two fundamentally different techniques: the nonimaging serial quantitative assessment of radioactivity in the dose and plasma or by imaging methods. The former involves simply determining how much of the radioactivity has disappeared from the blood over a specified time interval. The latter involves the assessment of peak cortical activity, which can be compared from side to side to determine if one kidney is receiving more blood flow than the other. Such a determination is often critical, for example, in determining whether a patient with unilateral renal disease should undergo a nephrectomy. The greater the proportion of the patient's renal function supplied by the diseased kidney, the less attractive is nephrectomy.

GLOMERULAR FILTRATION

Of the liter or so of blood flowing into the kidneys each minute, approximately 20% of the plasma (which constitutes 60% of the blood by volume) is filtered through the semipermeable membrane of the glomerulus, yielding an expected GFR of approximately 125 mL/min. Filtration is not an active process, but occurs passively, based on differences in hydrostatic and oncotic pressures between the glomerular capillaries and the surrounding Bowman's capsule. Small molecular weight solutes pass freely across the glomerular basement membrane. Desirable agents for the assessment of glomerular filtration must be small enough to pass through the basement membrane, but not significantly protein bound (as plasma protein molecules are too large to be filtered). Tc-99m-DTPA is an excellent agent for the assessment of GFR, because it is small, only slightly protein bound, and undergoes no significant tubular reabsorption or secretion; thus, it only reaches the urine via glomerular filtration and virtually all of the tracer that is filtered remains in the urine (Fig. 5–8).

Figure 5–8. The expected distribution of radiotracer as a function of time elapsed after injection. Note that activity is first seen in the aorta, then the renal parenchyma, the renal collecting system, and finally in the bladder.

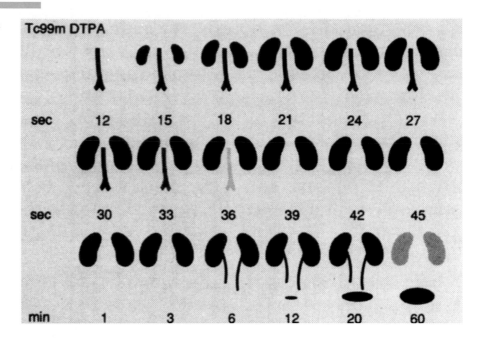

Diseases that cause prerenal reductions in GFR include heart failure (with decreased cardiac output) and renal artery stenosis. Heart failure would be expected to cause bilaterally symmetrical reductions in GFR, while renal artery stenosis is usually asymmetrical in distribution. Causes of intrarenal reductions in GFR include chronic inflammatory conditions of the glomerulus, such as systemic lupus erythematosus, and hypertensive nephropathy. Examples of postrenal causes of decreased GFR include obstruction of the collecting system or descending urinary pathways.

RENOVASCULAR HYPERTENSION

A specific application of glomerular filtration imaging is the assessment of renovascular hypertension. Over 90% of cases of hypertension are primary or idiopathic, therefore they cannot be traced to any anatomic abnormality. However, in a small percentage of cases, hypertension is secondary to diminished renal perfusion pressure, which causes production of renin by the cells of the juxtaglomerular apparatus. In the patient with renovascular hypertension, stenosis of one of the renal arteries results in diminished perfusion of the afferent arterioles, increased renin production, and resultant contraction of the smooth muscle cells surrounding the efferent arterioles, reducing the outflow of blood from the glomerulus and increasing intraglomerular hydrostatic pressure. Renin causes conversion of hepatically produced angiotensinogen to angiotensin I, which is then converted in the pulmonary capillaries to its active form, angiotensin II. Aside from causing constriction of the efferent arterioles, the active form of angiotensin also causes increased secretion of aldosterone by the adrenal cortex, promoting increased systemic blood pressure, and thereby further augmenting renal perfusion (Fig. 5–9).

To determine whether one of the kidneys is affected by renal artery stenosis, renal perfusion can be assessed with and without the injection of an angiotensin-converting enzyme (ACE) inhibitor, such as captopril. Absent ACE inhibitor injection, glomerular filtration in the affected kidney is relatively preserved, due to the increased glomerular

Figure 5–9. The renin-angiotensin axis, which provides the physiologic rationale for the use of an angiotensin-converting enzyme inhibitor in the diagnosis of renovascular hypertension.

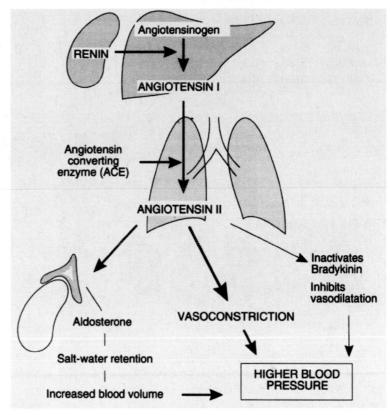

hydrostatic pressure produced by efferent arteriolar constriction. However, when the ACE inhibitor is administered, glomerular filtration is reduced, due to a drop in glomerular perfusion pressure. Such a drop in the perfusion pressure of a kidney with ACE inhibitor administration is diagnostic of renal artery stenosis, which in many cases can be successfully treated by surgery.

COLLECTING SYSTEM DRAINAGE

Occasionally, the collecting system of a kidney is found to be dilated, but it is uncertain whether this represents obstruction. If attempts to drain the affected kidney by placing the patient upright are unsuccessful, a diuretic renogram may be performed. After the standard nuclear medicine renogram is performed, a dose of furosemide is administered. If activity promptly washes out of the dilated system, the dilatation of the collecting system is likely of little or no physiologic significance. On the other hand, if there is little or no washout of activity, the dilatation of the collecting system indicates a functionally significant obstruction (Fig. 5–10).

Other Modalities

Renal imaging was dramatically enhanced by the introduction of the cross-sectional imaging modalities of ultrasound, CT, and MRI, which provide superior evaluation of the renal parenchyma compared to that of IVU and nuclear medicine. Ultrasound is the preferred modality to assess for urinary tract obstruction and evaluate

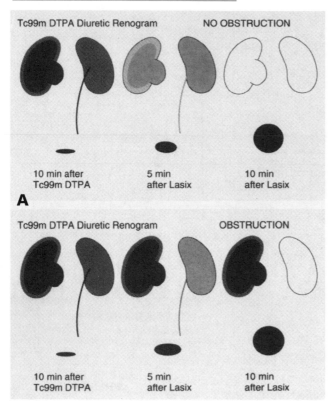

A

Tc99m DTPA Diuretic Renogram   NO OBSTRUCTION

10 min after
Tc99m DTPA   5 min
after Lasix   10 min
after Lasix

B

Tc99m DTPA Diuretic Renogram   OBSTRUCTION

10 min after
Tc99m DTPA   5 min
after Lasix   10 min
after Lasix

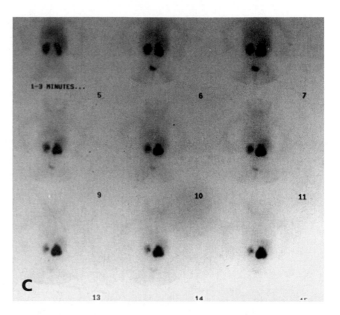

C

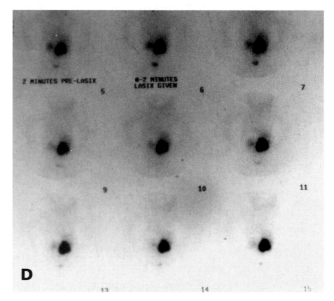

D

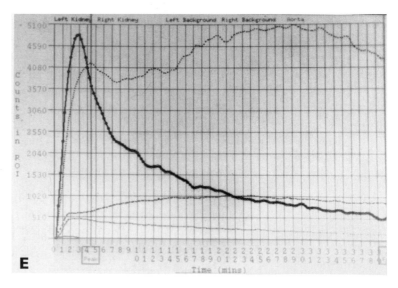

E

Figure 5–10. Diuretic renograms in two different patients demonstrate the expected appearance of a dilated collecting system (**A**) without obstruction and (**B**) with functionally significant obstruction of the left kidney. (**C**) These posterior images from an actual diuretic renogram demonstrate progressive uptake and clearance of radiotracer from the left kidney, but marked dilatation of the right renal collecting system with no discernible radiotracer clearance. (**D**) The second set of images was obtained after the injection of furosemide, which exhibits complete clearance from the left kidney, but continued dilatation on the right, with no clearance. (**E**) A graph of activity versus time for each kidney shows a progressive reduction in activity in the left kidney (bold line), but no decrease in the counts from the right kidney. These results indicate a physiologically significant obstruction to outflow from the right renal collecting system.

the renal vasculature, while contrast-enhanced CT is best in detecting and evaluating renal tumors. MRI is a good substitute for CT in patients who cannot tolerate iodinated contrast. Both CT and ultrasound are commonly employed to guide renal biopsies.

Excretory urography remains the preferred method for evaluating the collecting system and ureters, although obstruction may prevent sufficient opacification due to decreased renal contrast excretion. Pyelography (imaging of the collecting system and ureters) can be performed by either antegrade or retrograde techniques. Antegrade pyelography involves the placement of a nephrostomy catheter through the abdominal wall and into the renal pelvis, followed by the injection of iodinated contrast. The collecting system is often localized for puncture using ultrasound guidance. Retrograde pyelography is a urologic procedure and is performed by cystoscopic catheterization of the ureteral orifice, followed by retrograde contrast injection. CT also offers excellent visualization of the collecting system and ureters.

The bladder is most commonly imaged during excretory urography, utilizing both pre- and postvoid views. Superior evaluation is provided by cystography, in which a Foley catheter is used to instill iodinated contrast into the bladder lumen. Voiding cystourethrography evaluates the bladder outlet and urethra, as well as reflux into the ureters. Often, reflux may occur only during voiding, provoked by contraction of the bladder musculature and altered dynamics at the ureteral orifices. CT and MRI do not represent preferred modalities to detect bladder neoplasms, but are commonly employed in staging. The urethra can be evaluated either by retrograde urethrography (after insertion of a catheter into the distal urethra) or during the voiding phase of a cystourethrogram—both utilize iodinated contrast.

PATHOLOGY

Kidney

CONGENITAL

One of the most common congenital renal anomalies is a horseshoe kidney, so named because the lower poles of the kidneys are fused across the midline by an isthmus that may contain functional renal parenchyma or mere fibrous tissue (Fig. 5–11). It occurs in approximately 1 in 400 births and results from fusion of the inferior portions of the metanephric blastemas during embryogenesis. The isthmus causes incomplete ascent of the kidneys as it reaches the inferior mesenteric artery and also results in rotational abnormalities, with the collecting systems located anteriorly instead of medially. The isthmus often interferes with normal urinary drainage, resulting in an increased risk of hydronephrosis and complications of stasis, such as infection and stone formation. The risk of renal malignancies is also increased. In general, the probability of finding reproductive tract anomalies in patients with congenital renal anomalies is relatively high. Imaging findings include an abnormal renal axis with the inferior poles located more medially than the upper poles, an abnormally anteroinferior location of the kidneys (predisposing to injury in abdominal trauma), and demonstration of the isthmus, which may enhance with contrast administration.

Polycystic kidney disease comes in two forms: autosomal recessive (infantile) and autosomal dominant (adult). Autosomal recessive polycystic kidney disease occurs in

Figure 5–11. This overhead film from an intravenous urogram reveals fusion of the lower poles of the kidneys by contrast-enhancing renal tissue, indicative of a so-called horseshoe kidney.

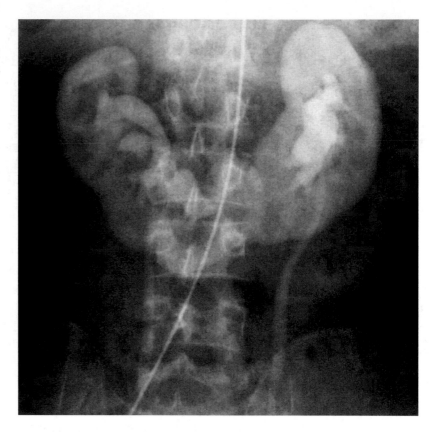

approximately 1:20,000 births and usually presents in the neonate or infant with enlarged and hyperechoic kidneys on ultrasound. Death results from renal failure or hepatobiliary fibrosis. Autosomal dominant polycystic kidney disease has an incidence of 1:1000 and accounts for approximately 10% of patients on chronic hemodialysis. It results from cystic dilatation of the nephrons, and usually presents around the fourth decade with renal failure and enlarged kidneys. It is associated with hepatic cysts (75%) and intracranial berry aneurysms (10%). Common imaging findings include enlarged kidneys with a lobulated contour, innumerable renal cysts, some of which are usually calcified, and stretching and deformity of the collecting system (Fig. 5–12).

INFECTIOUS

Pyelonephritis is the most common type of major UTI and *Escherichia coli*, *Proteus*, and *Klebsiella* are the most prevalent offending organisms. Pyelonephritis presents with the abrupt onset of fever, chills, and flank pain, with a predominantly neutrophilic leukocytosis. Urinalysis may show white cell casts, and culture typically grows out the responsible organism. Xanthogranulomatous pyelonephritis is a more indolent form of renal infection that typically occurs in older women and simmers for months or even years prior to diagnosis. Patients may complain of low-grade constitutional symptoms such as fever and malaise, and urinalysis is typically positive for white cells and proteinuria. There is a high incidence of large, branching "staghorn" calculi, and cultures usually grow out *E. coli* or *Proteus*.

Most patients with uncomplicated pyelonephritis do not require imaging studies, and are treated with antibiotics based on their clinical presentation and laboratory

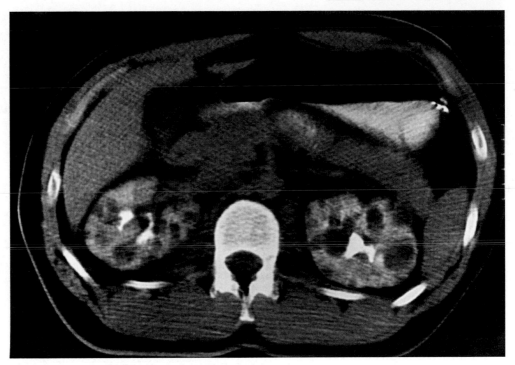

Figure 5–12. A 27-year-old man presented to the emergency room complaining of abdominal pain after a motor vehicle accident. A contrast-enhanced abdominal computed tomography scan was performed. An axial image from that examination reveals multiple small, bilateral hypodense lesions in both kidneys, some of which give the renal contour a lobulated appearance. This finding is diagnostic of adult polycystic kidney disease, which at this point had not yet progressed to the point of renal failure.

findings. However, if a patient fails to respond within 3 days, or if an underlying condition such as diabetes or a known urinary tract stone is present, an imaging study is often indicated to rule out obstruction and abscess. Imaging studies are normal in three-quarters of patients, although an especially suggestive finding is a striated nephrogram on IVU or CT (Fig. 5–13). Contrast-enhanced CT is more sensitive than ultrasound in the detection of parenchymal inflammation, although sensitivity is approximately equal for the detection of abscesses, and ultrasound has the advantage that it requires no contrast.

Other than simple hydronephrosis indicating obstruction, a key finding is the presence of pyonephrosis, which manifests as a pus-urine level in the collecting system on CT or ultrasound. Another key finding is the presence of gas within the renal parenchyma, emphysematous pyelonephritis, which occurs with an especially high frequency in diabetic patients (90%) and women (70%) (Fig. 5–14). Emphysematous pyelonephritis represents a surgical emergency, due to its high mortality rate when untreated.

TUMOROUS

EPIDEMIOLOGY

Approximately 20,000 cases of renal cell carcinoma are diagnosed each year in the United States, accounting for 9000 deaths. The peak age of incidence is the sixth

Figure 5–13. These axial images from a contrast-enhanced computed tomography scan demonstrate several important findings in renal infection. (**A**) A typical appearance of the "striated nephrogram" is seen in the left kidney at the level of the central kidneys. Note the alternating bands of hypodense (double white arrows) and enhancing tissue in the renal cortex. In addition, there is an incidental finding of marked thickening of the gallbladder wall (white and black arrows), which contains a number of poorly visualized cystic structures, representing Rokitansky-Aschoff sinuses and diagnostic of adenomyomatosis of the gallbladder. (**B**) An image at a slightly lower level demonstrates several bubbles of gas within the left renal collecting system, as well as a calculus at the ureteropelvic junction (arrow). This suggests obstruction as a contributing factor in the infection and indicates that removal of the calculus is likely to be necessary for successful treatment. (**C**) A third image at an intermediate level demonstrates another incidental finding; namely, a calcified aneurysm (A) of the right renal artery. Common etiologies of renal artery aneurysms include atherosclerotic disease and fibromuscular dysplasia.

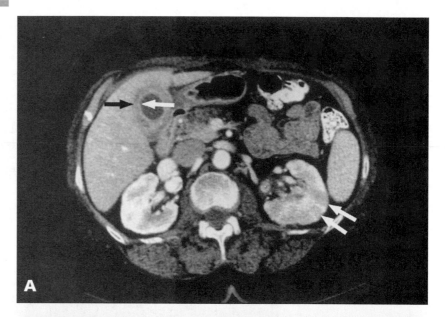

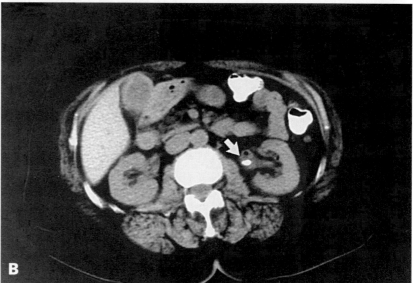

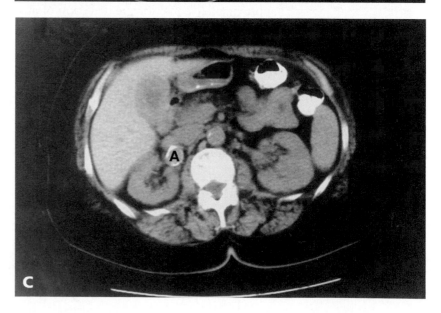

Figure 5–14. An abdominal radiograph in this elderly diabetic woman in septic shock demonstrates gas permeating the renal parenchyma and subcapsular regions, indicating the presence of emphysematous pyelonephritis, a surgical emergency. Note also a crescent of air lateral to the renal gas, likely representing gas within an associated abscess, as well as gas within the proximal ureter.

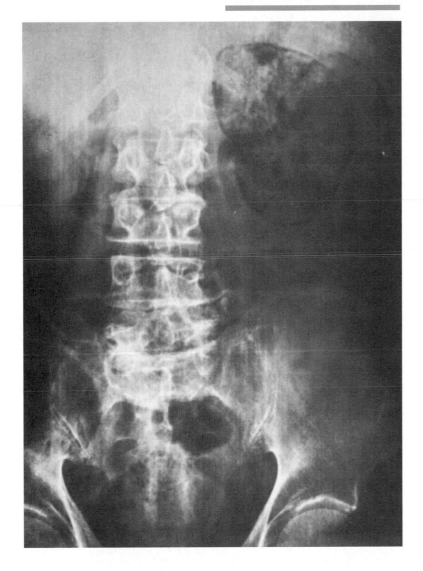

decade, and there is a male-to-female preponderance of 3:1. Most cases are idiopathic, but known risk factors include cigarette smoking, end-stage renal disease, and hereditary conditions such as von Hippel-Lindau disease. The latter, inherited as an autosomal dominant trait, includes cerebellar hemangioblastomas, retinal angiomas, and, in approximately 50% of patients, multiple renal cysts. The lifetime risk of developing renal cell carcinoma in these patients ranges up to 75%.

PATHOPHYSIOLOGY

Renal cell carcinomas are adenocarcinomas, most often of clear cell histology. They are usually hypervascular, and hemorrhage is a relatively frequent finding. Renal cell carcinoma, therefore, should be included in the differential diagnosis of hemorrhagic metastases elsewhere in the body. Typical sites of metastatic spread include the lungs, the skeleton (where lesions are characteristically lytic, with no blastic component), the liver, and the brain. Central necrosis is also relatively common. One characteristic feature of renal cell carcinoma is its propensity to invade the renal veins, from which it may spread into the IVC, which is seen in approximately 5% of cases. The tumor thrombus may even extend up the

IVC and into the right atrium (Fig. 5–15). This is an important preoperative finding, because it would require an operative approach that includes both the abdomen and the thorax.

CLINICAL PRESENTATION

A minority of patients with renal cell carcinoma present with the classic triad of flank pain, gross hematuria, and a flank mass. Such a presentation implies advanced disease. Aside from hematuria, other common presenting symptoms and signs include constitutional complaints such as weight loss and fatigue, and more specific indications of renal pathology such as hypertension, secondary to hyperreninemia induced by vascular obstruction within the kidney. A small number of patients present with an enlarging scrotal varicocele. Why? The left spermatic vein empties into the left renal vein, and when the carcinoma invades the renal vein and causes thrombosis, the normal

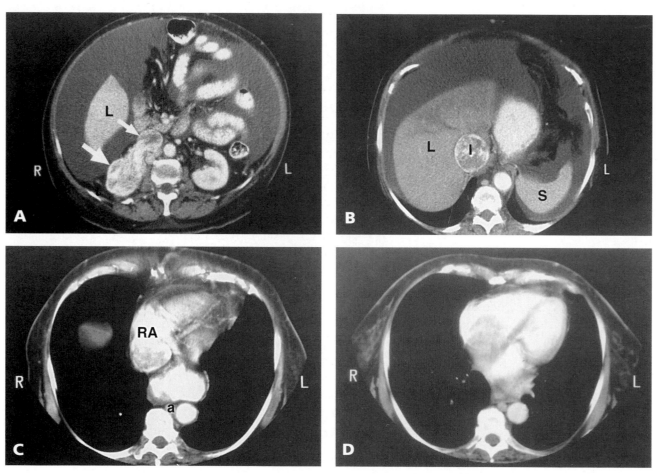

Figure 5–15. A 63-year-old woman presented with hematuria, ascites, and bilateral lower extremity swelling. These are axial images from a contrast-enhanced computed tomography scan of the chest and abdomen. (A) A heterogeneously enhancing mass replaces the right kidney (large arrow), with low-density tumor thrombus extending through the right renal vein and filling the inferior vena cava (IVC) (small arrow). Massive ascites surrounding the inferior tip of the liver and multiple small bowel loops resulted from occlusion of the IVC. (B) The tumor thrombus extends cephalad, with essentially complete occlusion of the IVC (I). L, liver; S, spleen. (C) The tumor thrombus reaches the junction of the IVC and right atrium (RA). Note the enlargement of the azygous vein (a), which has been recruited as a collateral for the obstructed IVC. (D) Low density tumor thrombus filling much of the RA.

Figure 5–16. Bilateral varicoceles (palpable distention of the pampiniform venous plexus around the testis) and the venous drainage of each hemiscrotum. The fact that the left spermatic vein empties into the left renal vein, while the right empties directly into the inferior vena cava, explains the special tendency of left renal carcinomas with renal vein thrombosis to present with new-onset left-sided varicoceles.

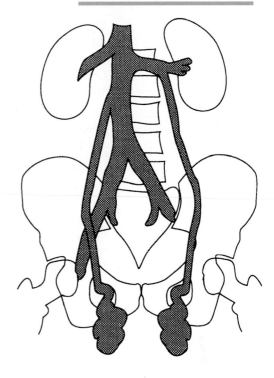

venous drainage of the left testicle is disrupted (Fig. 5–16). At least 30% of patients in whom renal cell carcinoma is detected are asymptomatic and are diagnosed based on incidental findings from an ultrasound or CT performed for another reason. On laboratory evaluation, some patients may exhibit polycythemia secondary to increased erythropoietin production (again due to vascular obstruction by the tumor).

IMAGING

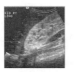

Imaging plays a critical role in the detection and staging of these tumors. IVU remains a mainstay in the evaluation of hematuria, and thus constitutes a major gateway to the diagnosis of renal cell carcinoma. Diagnosis is based on the direct finding of a mass, which is often hypervascular, or based on indirect findings such as a mass effect, with displacement of the pelvocalyceal system. CT is the most sensitive modality for the detection and staging of renal cell carcinoma. The mass is often hypervascular on postinfusion images, and may also demonstrate areas of necrosis and hemorrhage. Sonography also detects many tumors, but its primary role is in the differentiation of solid from cystic masses. Ultrasound also provides good assessment of vascular invasion. Key staging criteria include the size of the mass, the presence or absence of extension beyond the renal capsule, lymph node involvement, vascular invasion, and the presence or absence of distant metastases.

The differential diagnosis of a renal mass is long. Aside from renal cell carcinoma, the diagnosis to be excluded in every case, several other masses merit brief discussion. The most common renal mass is a simple renal cyst. On CT, simple cysts should have an attenuation value near 0 Hounsfield units (HU) (the attenuation value of water). Characteristics of a simple cyst on ultrasound include anechoic luminal contents, an imperceptible wall, a distinct posterior border, and posterior acoustic enhancement.

Posterior acoustic enhancement refers to the fact that the "water" in the cyst does not attenuate the beam, causing structures posterior to it to produce stronger echoes, and that the spherical shape of the cyst actually focuses the beam posterior to the cyst; both of these factors cause structures behind the cyst to appear more echogenic or "brighter" than they otherwise would. Many cysts will contain blood or debris secondary to hemorrhage, in which case the diagnosis becomes more problematic. The situation is further complicated by the fact that a small percentage of renal cell carcinomas are cystic. The presence of a mural nodule within a cyst is suggestive of a malignancy. When imaging criteria of a benign cyst are not satisfied, ultrasound or CT guidance may be used to perform aspiration and core needle biopsy for tissue diagnosis, especially if the suspicion of malignancy is high.

Other lesions presenting as renal masses also usually require biopsy or nephrectomy for diagnosis. Lesions typically undergoing nephrectomy include multilocular cystic nephroma, which presents as an intraparenchymal mass with multiple variably sized internal cysts, and oncocytoma, which often demonstrates a central scar on ultrasound or CT. Although both of these lesions are benign, nephrectomy remains the usual management due to the inability to differentiate them from a malignant tumor.

An exception to the general rule that tissue diagnosis is necessary is an angiomyolipoma, which, as its name implies, consists of vascular, muscular, and adipose tissue. It probably represents a hamartoma rather than a true neoplasm. These lesions are most commonly found in middle-aged females, as well as in 80% of patients with tuberous sclerosis. Tuberous sclerosis is a hereditary condition, inherited on an autosomal dominant basis, and is associated with a classic triad of mental retardation, seizures, and cutaneous lesions called adenoma sebaceum (a misnomer). Central nervous system lesions include subependymal giant cell astrocytomas and cortical hamartomas. The vast majority of patients have renal involvement, with bilateral angiomyolipomas and perhaps cysts. The angiomyolipoma is of interest because CT can definitively establish the diagnosis, based on the finding of fat attenuation tissue within the lesion (approximately -100 to -50 HU for fat; recall that water's attenuation value is 0 HU). The absence of fat does not prove that the lesion is not an angiomyolipoma, but its presence is highly reassuring. However, a rare renal cell carcinoma may entrap renal sinus fat and lead to an erroneous diagnosis of benignity.

Another important type of renal malignancy is a neoplasm arising in the collecting system, most often a transitional cell carcinoma. While these account for only about 10% of renal malignancies, they often present with a distinctive imaging appearance, confined to the lumen of the collecting system. Moreover, it is important to establish that a renal tumor is a transitional cell carcinoma, due to the greatly increased risk of malignancy in the distal urinary tract. Often referred to as field carcinogenesis, this effect means that all portions of the urothelium are at increased risk of malignancy. Up to 80% of patients with transitional cell carcinomas will develop transitional cell carcinoma elsewhere in the urinary tract. Hence once a transitional cell carcinoma is detected, the remainder of the urinary tract must be carefully examined. The differential diagnosis of a filling defect in the renal collecting system on excretory urography includes a transitional cell carcinoma, a blood clot, and a radiolucent calculus, although many other lesions, such as a sloughed renal papilla, are also possible (Fig. 5–17).

INFLAMMATORY

A wide variety of insults can, by the final common pathway of inflammation, produce the commonly encountered sonographic finding of diffusely hyperechoic kidneys.

Figure 5–17. Postinfusion abdominal computed tomography scan demonstrating a filling defect in the left renal collecting system, representing a transitional cell carcinoma. This mandates careful evaluation of the remainder of the urinary tract, due to the increased risk of another uroepithelial malignancy.

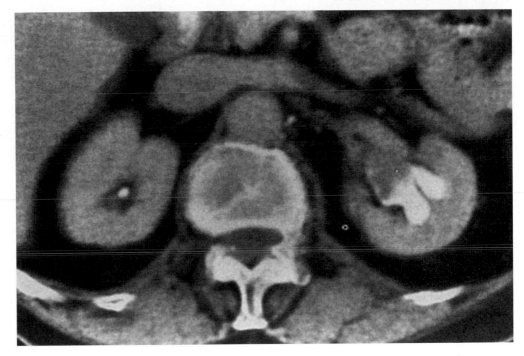

Common etiologies include glomerulosclerosis from hypertension or diabetes, infectious glomerulonephritis, infantile polycystic kidney disease, and acquired immunodeficiency syndrome (AIDS)-related nephropathy. When the kidneys are not only echogenic but shrunken, the disease process can be assumed to be chronic in nature, and the patient will invariably suffer from some degree of chronic renal insufficiency.

TRAUMATIC

Renal trauma is being managed in an increasingly conservative fashion. Imaging plays a crucial role in identifying the 80 to 90% of patients whose injuries do not require surgery. Minor injuries include hematomas, small lacerations, and small infarctions. Major injuries include renal rupture or masceration, vascular thrombosis, and renal pedicle avulsion. In the severely traumatized, unstable patient, a "one-shot" IVU is sometimes performed in the emergency room; contrast opacification of both kidneys rules out arterial thrombosis and pedicle avulsion. The study of choice is a contrast-enhanced CT scan, which evaluates not only the renal parenchyma and vasculature, but also the integrity of the collecting system and ureter (Fig. 5–18).

VASCULAR

A number of renovascular disorders have been discussed in the nuclear medicine imaging section. Renal papillary necrosis is an additional vascular disorder that is frequently seen on IVU in patients with histories of flank pain, obstruction, or UTIs. Papillary necrosis results when focal ischemia occurs in the papillary portions of the renal pyramids, a region of relatively tenuous arterial supply. Common etiologic factors include diabetes mellitus, sickle-cell disease, infection, and analgesic use. Central cavitation within the papillary tip may produce a so-called ball on tee appearance, while sloughed papillae may produce filling defects within the collecting system (Fig. 5–19).

Figure 5–18. An abdominal computed tomography scan with oral contrast only was obtained to evaluate a sudden drop in hematocrit in this patient who had just undergone extracorporeal shock-wave lithotripsy for nephrolithiasis. An axial image demonstrates a large, high-density fluid collection (large arrows) displacing the left kidney (small arrow) anteriorly and inferiorly. This fluid collection represents a perinephric hematoma. Stone fragments are visible in the renal collecting system.

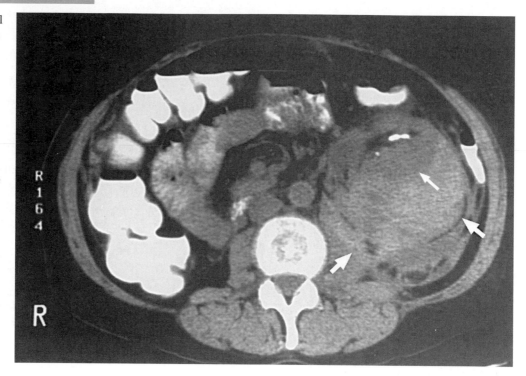

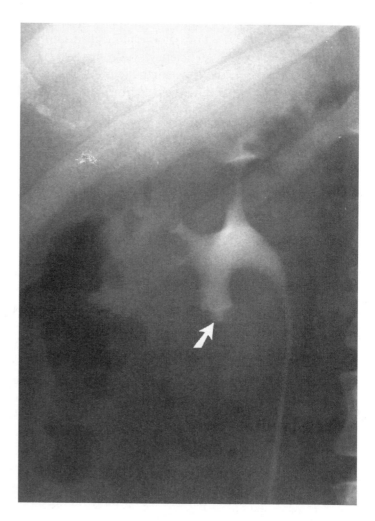

Figure 5–19. A 30-year-old woman with a history of repeated urinary tract infections was referred for an intravenous urogram. A magnified view of the right kidney during the excretory phase demonstrates evidence of papillary necrosis, with a "ball-shaped" collection of contrast in the expected location of the renal papilla (arrow).

Ureter

CONGENITAL

Ureteral duplication and congenital megaureter are two relatively common anomalies often detected in the adult. Ureteral duplication has an incidence of 1:200, and may be complete or incomplete (i.e., the two ipsilateral ureters fuse before reaching the bladder) (Fig. 5–20). In complete duplication, the ureter arising from the lower pole joins the bladder at its normal location, while the upper pole ureter enters the bladder more inferomedially (ectopically), often resulting in obstruction and hydronephrosis. The incidence of ectopic ureter is approximately six times greater in females than males. Congenital megaureter results from a functional (not mechanical) obstruction of the distal ureter, somewhat analogous to achalasia in the esophagus. Both disorders are readily diagnosed by IVU.

Bladder

INFECTIOUS

Run-of-the-mill acute cystitis most often results from infection by *E. coli* or *Staphylococcus*. Risk factors include instrumentation (commonly an indwelling Foley catheter), bladder outlet obstruction (commonly benign prostatic hypertrophy), calculi, and tumor. Patients present with complaints of abdominal pain, dysuria, and hematuria. Findings include air within the bladder lumen (which can be a normal finding in patients with an indwelling bladder catheter), irregular bladder wall thickening, and stranding in the fat around the bladder. Gas within the bladder lumen may also indi-

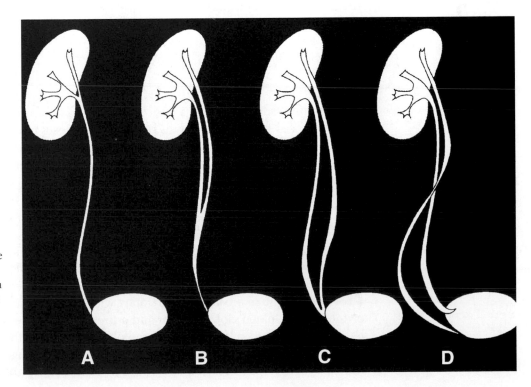

Figure 5–20. (A) Bifid renal pelvis. (B) Incomplete duplication, or "Y" ureter. (C) Incomplete duplication where two ureters join into single ureteral orifice. (D) Complete duplication where both ureters have a separate insertion into bladder.

cate the presence of a fistula, commonly connecting to the vagina or rectum in patients who have undergone radiation therapy for cervical carcinoma. Emphysematous cystitis is a more dramatic form of cystitis, which causes gas within the bladder wall, and, like emphysematous pyelonephritis, is most commonly seen in diabetic women. Fortunately, this condition responds readily to antibiotics and is not associated with significant mortality (in contrast to emphysematous pyelonephritis).

TUMOROUS

EPIDEMIOLOGY

Bladder carcinoma is the fifth most common cancer diagnosis in the United States, with more than 50,000 cases detected each year.

PATHOPHYSIOLOGY

 Over 90% of bladder carcinoma is of the transitional cell type, with squamous cell carcinoma representing most of the remaining 10%. Recall that the normal epithelium of the bladder and ureter exhibits a transitional histology. Because transitional cell carcinoma is by far the most common type, this discussion will focus on it. Most patients who develop carcinoma of the bladder are in the sixth or seventh decade of life, with 90% of patients older than 50 years of age at the time of diagnosis. Most patients are men.

Risk factors for transitional cell carcinoma include cigarette smoking (which increases risk five times), employment in the plastics industry, aniline dye exposure, previous pelvic radiation, cyclophosphamide therapy, and chronic infection. A patient with a history of previous transitional cell carcinoma of the upper urinary tract has an 80% probability of developing a tumor in the bladder, indicating that the carcinogenic effect is distributed throughout the urinary epithelium. The recurrence rate of the disease is at least 50%.

CLINICAL PRESENTATION

Patients present with hematuria, increased urinary frequency (due in part to the reduction in bladder capacity produced by the space-occupying lesion), obstruction, and metastases. Laboratory analysis commonly discloses not only red cells, but malignant cells in the urine. The definitive diagnosis of bladder carcinoma is established via cystoscopy and biopsy, but radiology plays a major role in determining the presence or absence of a morphologic abnormality.

IMAGING

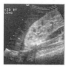 Key imaging findings, whether on IVU, CT, ultrasound, or MRI, include a filling defect in the bladder lumen or irregularity of the bladder wall (Fig. 5–21). When a filling defect is seen, other diagnostic possibilities include prostatic hypertrophy with a prominent impression on the base of the bladder, blood clot, calculus, and a ureterocele. Once the histologic diagnosis has been established, a key role of the radiologist is to stage the tumor. Aside from CT assessment of metastatic deposits in the lymph nodes, lung, liver, and bones, local tumor extent can be assessed according to tumor morphology. For example, the

Figure 5–21. A 64-year-old male cigarette smoker presented to his urologist with a complaint of hematuria. An intravenous urogram (not shown) demonstrated a filling defect in the bladder lumen, which was biopsied cystoscopically and found to represent transitional cell carcinoma. A postinfusion staging computed tomography examination was performed. (A) An axial image from the study demonstrates a prominent right-sided soft tissue mass (large arrow), which extends exophytically into the bladder lumen and is associated with irregular bladder wall thickening and extension into the perivesical tissues. Note also a small left-sided bladder diverticulum (small arrow). (B) A second image at the level of the kidneys reveals right hydronephrosis and cortical thinning (arrow), due to chronic right ureterovesicle junction obstruction by the tumor.

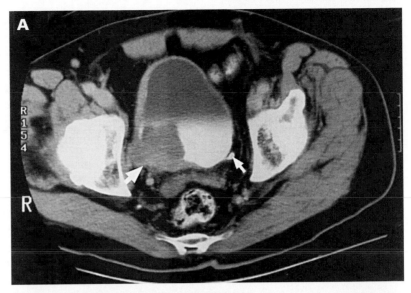

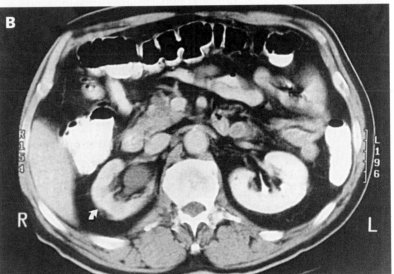

tumor may be pedunculated (on a stalk), which generally indicates a lower probability of bladder invasion. On the other hand, a sessile tumor associated with adjacent wall thickening is likely to have penetrated deep into the bladder wall. If the tumor is confined to the bladder, the integrity of the perivesicle fat planes should be preserved.

COMMON CLINICAL PROBLEMS

Hematuria

EPIDEMIOLOGY

Microscopic hematuria is a common clinical problem, found in 10 to 15% of men older than 35 years of age and women older than 55 years of age. Microscopic hematuria is defined as at least three to five red blood cells per high power field. From a strictly physiologic point of view, the finding of any red cells in the urine represents an abnormality, inasmuch as the vascular and urinary pathways should be completely separate. However, it is well known that vigorous exercise alone is sufficient to produce at least microscopic hematuria in otherwise healthy patients. As a screening test, chemical assays for hemoglobin are often substituted for microscopic examination, and more precise quantitation of the number of red blood cells per high power field is reserved for patients with chemical abnormalities.

PATHOPHYSIOLOGY

The distinction between gross and microscopic hematuria proves clinically useful, in that the frequency of various diseases varies between the two, as does the probability of serious disease. Gross hematuria is generally more serious than its microscopic counterpart, and nearly two-thirds of patients will have a source in the bladder or prostate. Cystitis, bladder neoplasm, prostatic hypertrophy, prostatitis, and renal pathologies, including neoplasm, constitute the most common diagnoses. Almost 60% of patients with gross hematuria have marked abnormalities, and 20% have life-threatening disorders, such as carcinoma.

In the setting of microscopic hematuria, bladder disease is relatively less common, accounting for only 10% of cases. The prostate gland is the most common source, with the urethra (especially urethritis) second. In microscopic hematuria, no cause is found in over one-third of patients, and only 20% of patients have a marked abnormality. The incidence of life-threatening pathology is only about 4%. Hence the key distinction between gross and microscopic hematuria is that a kidney or bladder neoplasm is many times more likely to be the source in gross hematuria.

CLINICAL PRESENTATION

A variety of laboratory tests can assist in the workup of hematuria. The finding of protein in the urine suggests glomerulonephritis with inflammation-associated increased capillary permeability as the etiology. Urine culture and microscopic examination for leukocytes may reveal a UTI. In concert with hematuria, pyuria often indicates hemorrhagic cystitis. Urine cytology may demonstrate sloughed malignant uroepithelial cells. Cystoscopy and retrograde endoscopic examination of the ureter and renal collecting system enable direct visualization and biopsy of lesions.

IMAGING

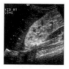

A young woman whose symptoms of hemorrhagic cystitis resolve after appropriate antibiotic therapy generally requires no further evaluation. In the workup of older patients with unexplained hematuria, imaging is a logical first step, because the pretest probability of a serious disorder such as malignancy is elevated. As a general rule, in patients younger than 40 years of age, the incidental finding of microscopic hematuria probably does not warrant further urologic investigation. However, by age 65 years, when the incidence of a disease such as bladder cancer has increased nearly 100 times, a more aggressive approach to diagnostic evaluation is warranted. When imaging is undertaken, its principle goal is to detect, localize, and if possible, characterize any morphologic abnormality. Many abnormalities, such as urinary tract calculi and simple cysts, can be characterized as benign based on imaging criteria alone. When a lesion's features are equivocal in terms of benignity, imaging localization may direct further urologic examination (such as cystoscopy) and also provide guidance for biopsy.

The two preferred tests in the radiologic evaluation of hematuria, discussed earlier, are ultrasound and IVU. In general, ultrasound will be preferred in patients in whom the use of intravenous contrast material is contraindicated due to renal disease, heart disease, a history of adverse contrast reactions, or other factors.

Acute Renal Failure

EPIDEMIOLOGY

Classically, acute renal failure is divided into three categories: prerenal causes, renal causes, and postrenal causes.

PATHOPHYSIOLOGY

Prerenal causes of acute renal failure center on a diminished flow of blood to the nephron, and include decreased circulating blood volume due to hemorrhage, congestive heart failure (CHF), hypotension, and renal artery stenosis. A clue to the prerenal nature of the failure is contained in the ratio of serum blood-urea nitrogen (BUN) to creatinine. Both substances, major metabolic waste products excreted by the nephron, are freely filtered at the glomerulus, but urea is reabsorbed by the peritubular capillaries. Decreased peritubular perfusion causes impaired urea reabsorption, and BUN increases disproportionately to creatinine. Generally, it is possible to determine if a patient is suffering from prerenal causes of acute renal failure based on clinical grounds, including not only the BUN/creatinine ratio, but a history of CHF or hypotension, accumulation of excess fluid within body tissues, and blood pressure.

Intrinsic renal causes of acute renal failure include acute tubular necrosis (ATN) and acute glomerulonephritis. In hospitalized patients, ATN is relatively more common and accounts for the majority of cases. In community-acquired acute renal failure, acute glomerulonephritis is relatively more common. In all types of intrinsic renal disease, there will be a loss in the kidney's ability to concentrate urine, and the patient with intrinsic renal acute renal failure will excrete a relatively dilute urine, while the patient with prerenal disease (whose concentrating ability is relatively unimpaired) will excrete a highly concentrated urine.

From the point of view of diagnostic imaging, the most important causes of acute renal failure are postrenal. Up to 25% of patients with acute renal failure suffer from urinary tract obstruction. To cause a significant alteration in BUN and creatinine, the output of both kidneys must be obstructed. In rare cases, this may result from bilateral ureteral obstruction, as seen in diffuse retroperitoneal processes such as lymphoma or retroperitoneal fibrosis. However, a far more common cause is urethral obstruction, especially that secondary to prostatic enlargement. This diagnosis can be readily confirmed by ultrasound examination to determine if the bladder is distended, or even more readily, by passing a Foley catheter into the bladder, which should promptly restore normal urine output. In the case of a patient with an indwelling bladder catheter who becomes anuric, the hypothesis should be entertained that the catheter has become obstructed, often secondary to blood clot, and patency of the catheter should be verified.

CLINICAL PRESENTATION

Acute renal failure typically manifests first by oliguria (the production of < 400 mL of urine per day), followed by a rise in the BUN and creatinine. It should be noted, however, that patients in renal failure may continue to produce normal or even increased volumes of urine; however, they will have lost the ability to concentrate urine to the normal degree.

IMAGING

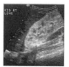

The principal reason that ultrasound examinations are routinely obtained in patients presenting in acute renal failure is to exclude the possibility of a postrenal (obstructive) cause. Ruling out obstruction is critical for two reasons. First, obstruction, as distinct from prerenal and intrinsic renal disorders, is generally a surgical problem, as opposed to a medical problem. Moreover, postrenal pathologies are often readily and completely reversible through relief or correction of the anatomic lesion. In all cases of postrenal acute renal failure of sufficient duration, ultrasound examination should reveal signs of hydronephrosis, dilatation of the renal collecting system secondary to increased pressure proximal to the obstruction.

The sonographic finding of echogenic kidneys tends to indicate intrinsic renal disease (Fig. 5–22). The size of the kidneys is also important. Normal-sized or enlarged kidneys indicate a good probability that the disorder may still be reversible. On the other hand, if the kidneys are small and echogenic, the condition is likely to be irreversible.

Figure 5–22. A longitudinal image of the right kidney in this 25-year-old human immunodeficiency virus-positive man demonstrates markedly increased renal echogenicity (arrow), as compared to that of the adjacent liver. The renal cortex is normally slightly less echogenic than the parenchyma of the liver and spleen. Common causes of diffusely increased renal echogenicity include glomerulonephritis, acquired immunodeficiency syndrome-related nephropathy, acute tubular necrosis, and end-stage renal disease.

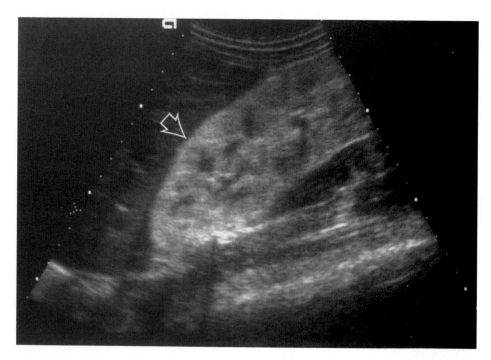

Acute Flank Pain

The patient presenting with acute flank pain is generally evaluated for the presence of urolithiasis and pyelonephritis. However, one of the most common causes of acute flank pain is lumbosacral pathology, including muscle strain and degenerative disease of the spine. Additional differential diagnostic considerations include appendicitis, dissecting or ruptured aortic aneurysm, bowel obstruction or ischemia, and retroperitoneal fibrosis, among numerous other possibilities. True urinary tract pain is generally associated with symptoms such as dysuria, urinary frequency, and urgency. The key to differentiating true renal pain from other causes of abdominal and back pain is the urinalysis. If hematuria and pyuria (at least several red blood and/or white blood cells per high power field) are not present, the pain is unlikely to be of urinary tract origin.

UROLITHIASIS

EPIDEMIOLOGY

The formation of renal calculi is an extremely common problem in the United States, affecting at least 1 of every 20 persons at some time during their lives. There is a definite male preponderance, and the condition becomes more prevalent with age. Once a patient has suffered a bout of urolithiasis, the lifetime probability of recurrence is 50 to 70%, making a prior diagnosis of stone one of the most important elements in a good history of the suspected stone patient. Conditions predisposing to stone formation include infection, hypercalcemia, renal tubular acidosis, and hyperoxaluria, among others.

PATHOPHYSIOLOGY

Approximately 70% of kidney stones are formed of calcium oxalate, 15% of struvite (magnesium ammonium phosphate), 10% of uric acid, and 5% of calcium phosphate. The vast majority of calcium oxalate stones are considered idiopathic. Crohn's disease is an example of a condition that predisposes patients to form oxalate stones. Dietary oxalate is normally complexed with calcium in the gut, but the fat malabsorption associated with Crohn's disease causes lipid saponification of calcium, meaning that oxalate passes unbound into the colon, where it is absorbed into the blood. The oxalate is then eliminated in high amounts in the urine, where it causes stone formation.

Any condition that increases urinary calcium concentration will contribute to calcium stone formation. An example is type I renal tubular acidosis, in which urine pH remains fixed above 5.5 and there is a leak of calcium into the urine with an associated deficiency of one of the most important stone inhibitors, citrate. Struvite stones are associated with infection by urea-splitting organisms such as *Proteus* and *Pseudomonas,* with an increase in urine pH. Struvite stones may become particularly large, forming a cast of the collecting system, and are then referred to as staghorn calculi. As distinct from the other major types of stones, uric acid stones are often radiolucent (Fig. 5–23). They are associated with low urine pH, which decreases the solubility of uric acid. Common predisposing conditions include gout, hemolytic anemia, and myeloproliferative disorders, the latter two secondary to cell lysis.

The management of urolithiasis begins with adequate hydration and analgesia,

Figure 5–23. This film of the left kidney from an excretory urogram demonstrates a radiolucent filling defect within the contrast-opacified collecting system, representing a uric acid stone.

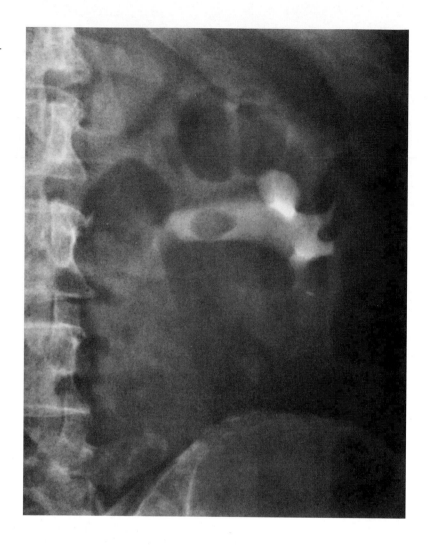

generally employing narcotics. At least 80% of stones will pass spontaneously, and no further intervention is required. Virtually all stones less than 0.5 cm in diameter pass without any medical or surgical assistance. Those larger than 1 cm usually require surgical removal. This is often accomplished via ureteroscopically guided crushing and extraction of the stone. Extracorporeal shock-wave lithotripsy relies on the use of focused shock waves to pulverize stones without surgery. Complications include infection due to stasis, calyceal perforation, and the development of chronic obstruction with associated loss of nephrons and irreversible loss of renal function.

CLINICAL PRESENTATION

Urolithiasis is the most common cause of both acute urinary tract obstruction and acute flank pain. Renal colic refers to spasms of intense pain that begin in the region of the flank and radiate into the groin. The pain results from spasms of ureteral smooth muscle, generated by the ureter's attempt to overcome the distention and increased intraluminal pressure caused by obstruction. Other common presenting symptoms include urinary urgency and frequency. The differential diagnosis of an obstructing lesion in the urinary tract includes—in addition to stone—blood clot, tumor, sloughed papilla, and extrinsic compression.

IMAGING

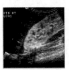 Imaging begins with a high-quality abdominal plain film, which will reveal a calculus in up to 90% of cases (Fig. 5–24). Stones must generally measure at least 2 mm in diameter and contain some calcium to be visible by plain film. Ureteral calculi tend to lodge at one of three positions, the UPJ, the pelvic brim, and the ureterovesical junction (UVJ), the latter being the most frequent. In the appropriate clinical setting, the finding of a calculus in the distribution of the urinary tract, particularly at one of these locations, is strongly suggestive of urolithiasis. Mimics of calculi include gallstones, phleboliths, and calcified mesenteric lymph nodes.

Intravenous urography is still widely employed in the evaluation of stones, and many stones are first detected on the "scout" film (precontrast administration) of an IVU. A scout film should be obtained at the beginning of every urogram to optimize patient positioning and radiographic technique, to detect calculi (which will become invisible once surrounded by contrast material), and to determine if bowel preparation is adequate. Indirect signs of a radiolucent obstructing calculus include an ipsilateral delayed nephrogram, delayed excretion, and dilatation of the collecting system. A contrast-filled, dilated ureter may eventually be followed down to the level of the obstruction.

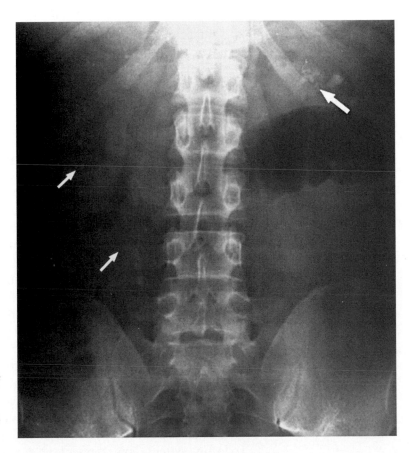

Figure 5–24. A 26-year-old previously healthy man presented with the acute onset of right flank pain and microscopic hematuria. A supine radiograph of the abdomen demonstrates a row of calculi in the mid-right ureter (large arrow), the so-called *steinstrasse* (German for "street of stones"). In addition, there are bilateral renal calcifications in the distribution of the medullary pyramids (small arrows). These findings strongly suggest a diagnosis of medullary sponge kidney, which results from cystic dilation of the renal collecting tubules, followed by stasis and the development of medullary calcifications.

Figure 5–25. This longitudinal ultrasound image of the right kidney demonstrates marked dilatation of the collecting system, termed *pelvicaliectasis*, but no evidence of cortical thinning. These findings are most consistent with a diagnosis of acute hydronephrosis. The combination of hydronephrosis and cortical thinning would suggest that the process has been present long enough to produce tissue loss.

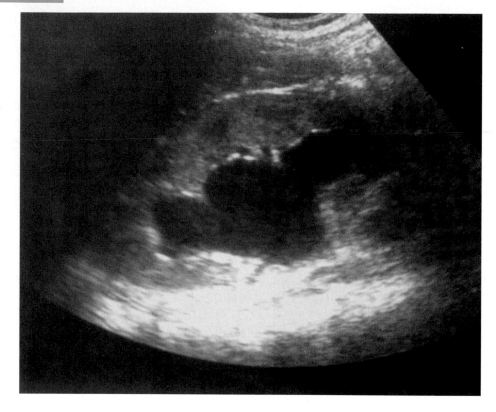

Ultrasound is particularly useful in the evaluation of patients with mild or repetitive attacks, pregnant women, and patients with a contraindication to IVU. Stones are seen as hyperechoic, often shadowing foci within the collecting system or ureter. The uterovesicle junctions can be visualized using the urinary bladder as an acoustic window. The presence of a ureteral jet on the affected side argues against the presence of a complete obstruction. If the patient is well hydrated and the uterovesical junction is continuously monitored for a sufficient length of time, the absence of a jet is essentially diagnostic of complete obstruction. If obstruction has been present for a sufficient length of time to produce hydronephrosis, ultrasound is quite sensitive in its detection (Fig. 5–25). Mild hydronephrosis refers to slight distention of the collecting system, with multiple anechoic spaces that conform to the expected configuration of the renal collecting system and communicate with a dilated renal pelvis. Severe hydronephrosis includes not only greater dilatation, but thinning of the renal cortex as well.

Recently, thin-section (approximately 0.5 mm) noncontrast CT examination has begun to supplant IVU as the study of choice in many cases of urolithiasis. This study possesses several important advantages. First, the lack of contrast administration eliminates any risk of adverse reaction. Second, the patient requires no bowel preparation to eliminate overlying fecal material and gas. Third, the superior contrast sensitivity of CT over plain radiography means that even noncalcified calculi, such as uric acid stones, are usually visible. Other findings on CT include hydronephrosis and hydroureter. By using a collimation that is narrower than the usual 1 cm, such as 5 mm, even small stones can be reliably detected. A major role of interventional radiology in the management of obstruction is the placement of percutaneous nephrostomy and nephroureterostomy catheters (Fig. 5–26) to provide drainage of an obstructed collecting system. This represents an emergent procedure in a patient with urosepsis.

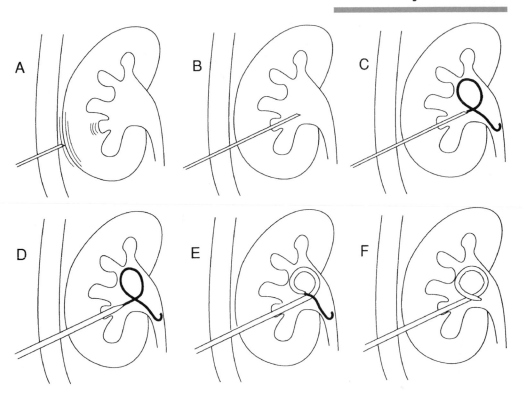

Figure 5–26. Permanent nephrostomy tube (PNT) placement. (**A**) After local anesthesia is instilled, the introductory needle is directed toward the kidney. Slight deflecting motion of the kidney assures the operator that he or she is in the appropriate plane. (**B**) Puncture is made into the posterior calyx. (**C**) Proper position is confirmed by obtaining urine. Needle obdurator is exchanged for a guidewire. (**D**) Tract is dilated using progressively larger dilators. (**E**) Finally, PNT is placed over the guidewire, coiled in the collecting system, and (**F**) locked in place.

ADRENAL GLANDS

Anatomy and Physiology

Although the adrenal glands belong to the endocrine system and not the excretory system, they are often discussed in conjunction with the kidneys. In fact, the adrenal glands are named for their close renal proximity (*ad-*, "near," and *renal*, "kidney"). The adrenal glands are paired structures lying within the perirenal space, superior or anteromedial to the upper poles of the kidneys. On axial cross-sectional images, they appear as inverted Y- or V-shaped structures with limbs measuring less than 1 cm in width.

About 80% of the mass of the adrenal gland is composed of adrenal cortex, which consists of three layers or zones (Fig. 5–27). These zones produce steroid hormones from a cholesterol precursor. The outer zona glomerulosa produces the mineralocorticoid aldosterone, which acts on the distal convoluted tubules of the nephrons to enhance sodium retention and potassium excretion. Aldosterone is absolutely essential for life, and its absence rapidly produces a state of circulatory shock due to hypovolemia. The glucocorticoids such as cortisol are produced in the middle zona fasciculata and the

Figure 5–27. The anatomic relationship between the kidneys and adrenal glands, as well as the structure of the adrenal cortex and medulla.

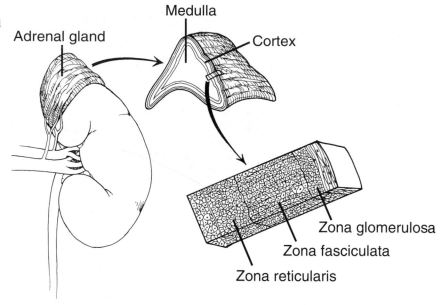

inner zona reticularis. Cortisol functions in gluconeogenesis, and stress adaptation, and in suppressing the inflammatory and immune responses. The adrenal cortex also produces sex hormones, including the androgens that are responsible for the growth of pubic and axillary hair, enhancement of the pubertal growth spurt, and sex drive in women.

Global adrenal cortical hypofunction is called Addison's disease and is associated with hyperkalemia and hyponatremia, hypoglycemia, and poor response to stress. Most cases are thought to be autoimmune in etiology, although bilateral infarction or hemorrhage may also be responsible. Conn's syndrome refers to hyperaldosteronism. It manifests with hypertension and hypokalemia, and most often results from an isolated, hormonally active adrenal adenoma. Cushing's syndrome refers to excess glucocorticoid secretion and manifests with truncal obesity, hypertension, muscle atrophy, cutaneous striae, and amenorrhea. Most cases result from bilateral adrenal hyperplasia, which in 90% of cases is due to a corticotropin-secreting pituitary adenoma (Cushing's disease); 10% of cases are due to an adrenocortical carcinoma (Fig. 5–28).

The adrenal medulla is composed of modified postganglionic sympathetic neurons, which release their "neurotransmitter" directly into the circulation under sympathetic stimulation. Its greatest product is epinephrine. Levels of epinephrine in the blood may rise by as much as 300 times under severe stess, preparing the organism for the so-called fight-or-flight response.

Pathology

By far the most important role of imaging in the evaluation of the adrenal glands lies in the detection, characterization, and staging of adrenal tumors.

TUMOROUS

Adrenal cortical tumors include both benign and malignant varieties. A benign adrenal adenoma is the most prevalent tumor, frequently detected as an incidental

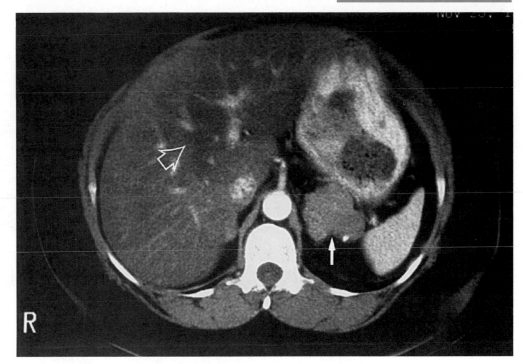

Figure 5–28. A 53-year-old woman presented with Cushing's syndrome. An axial image from a contrast-enhanced abdominal computed tomography examination reveals a 5.5 cm lobulated left adrenal mass, which contains some calcifications (white arrow). Note also decreased attenuation in the left lobe of the liver (open arrow), indicating fatty infiltration, for which hypercortisolism is always one differential diagnostic consideration. At surgery, an adrenal adenocarcinoma was resected. Approximately 50% of adrenocortical carcinomas are hormonally active, and Cushing's syndrome is the most common presentation.

finding on imaging studies performed for other reasons. These tumors characteristically produce no endocrine abnormalities, measure 3 cm or less in diameter, exhibit slight uniform enhancement, and have a CT attenuation value of less than 10 HU, due to the presence of a considerable amount of lipid material. This lipid material can also prove useful in characterizing these lesions by MRI, where fat suppression techniques will demonstrate a dramatic drop-off in signal intensity in an adenoma.

The most prevalent adrenal cortical malignancy is a metastasis, found at autopsy in approximately one-quarter of patients who die from malignancy. Common sources of adrenal metastases include lung cancer (especially small cell carcinoma), breast cancer, and melanoma, among others. Unfortunately, small metastases often appear homogeneous and well-defined on CT, proving indistinguishable from adenomas. On MRI, however, metastases will be hyperintense on T2-weighted images. CT or ultrasound-guided needle biopsy can easily resolve equivocal cases.

Adrenocortical carcinoma is the most common primary adrenal cortical malignancy. Approximately 50% of these tumors exhibit clinically significant endocrine function, usually Cushing's syndrome. The masses are usually 5 cm or greater in size, demonstrate areas of necrosis, hemorrhage, or calcification, and typically have a poor prognosis due to their large size (and high probability of metastasis) at the time of diagnosis.

Pheochromocytoma is the most important adrenal medullary tumor. These tumors follow the so-called rule of 10s: 10% are extradrenal, 10% are bilateral, and 10% are malignant. Pheochromocytomas are associated with the multiple endocrine neoplasia syndrome type II (medullary thyroid cancer, pheochromocytoma, and

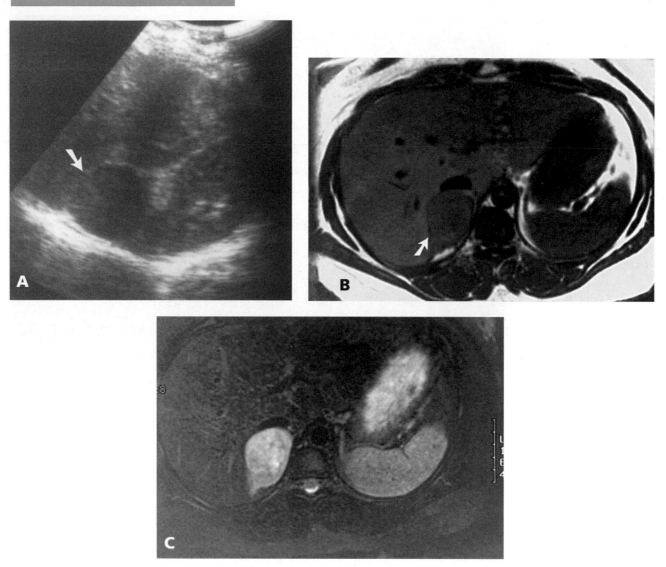

Figure 5–29. A 20-week pregnant woman presented with new-onset hypertension. (A) A longitudinal ultrasound view of the right adrenal bed demonstrates a 4 cm round, homogeneously hypoechoic adrenal mass (arrow). A magnetic resonance imaging examination was requested to better characterize the lesion and to rule out metastatic disease. (B) An axial image from a T1-weighted sequence demonstrates a well-circumscribed, slightly hypointense right adrenal mass (arrow). (C) On a heavily T2-weighted image, the lesion appears very bright, consistent with the diagnosis of pheochromocytoma. The study revealed no evidence of malignancy or associated conditions such as multiple endocrine neoplasia or von Hippel-Lindau disease (the other adrenal was normal, and the kidneys and pancreas contained no cysts).

parathyroid or other soft tissue tumors). Patients often present with symptoms of sustained or episodic catecholamine excess, including hypertension, tachycardia, and headaches. Imaging studies include nuclear medicine radioactive iodine labeled metaiodobenzylguanidine scans (especially useful for localizing extraadrenal tumors or metastatic lesions), ultrasound, and CT or MRI. Pheochromocytomas enhance strongly and demonstrate extremely high signal on T2-weighted MR images (Fig. 5–29). Because manipulation of these tumors can precipitate a hypertensive crisis, pharmacologic prophylaxis is warranted before biopsy.

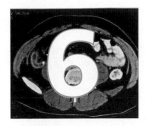

6 The Acute Abdomen

Acute abdominal pain is one of the three or four most common complaints of patients presenting to emergency rooms and admitted to hospitals. The goal of this chapter is not to provide a comprehensive review of this complex topic, but to present a general imaging approach to the problem and to discuss seven of the most frequently encountered and illustrative etiologies. The single most common etiology of acute abdominal pain is functional and has no specific therapy. However, other conditions do warrant urgent or emergent medical and surgical therapy; these include peptic ulcer disease, gallbladder disease, pancreatitis, intestinal obstruction, appendicitis, diverticular disease, urinary tract infection (considered in Chapter 5), and diseases of the female reproductive tract (considered in Chapter 7). Before discussing these entities, let us briefly examine several general radiographic signs that must be sought out in every acute abdomen.

CRITICAL RADIOGRAPHIC SIGNS

Pneumoperitoneum

A key finding to rule out on every abdominal plain film is pneumoperitoneum, or free intraperitoneal air (Fig. 6–1). In the nontraumatic setting, free air most often indicates perforation of a duodenal or gastric ulcer, although rupture of any hollow viscus may produce this sign. In the setting of obstruction, free air generally indicates a bowel perforation. The most prevalent cause in hospitalized patients is iatrogenic, secondary to

Figure 6–1. This "black bone" digital fluoroscopic image demonstrates massive gas collections under each hemidiaphragm and constitutes as dramatic a case of pneumoperitoneum as one could expect to see. This degree of intraperitoneal gas produces a tense abdomen, with centralization of abdominal contents, and also exerts upward pressure on the diaphragm (arrows), interfering with normal lung ventilation.

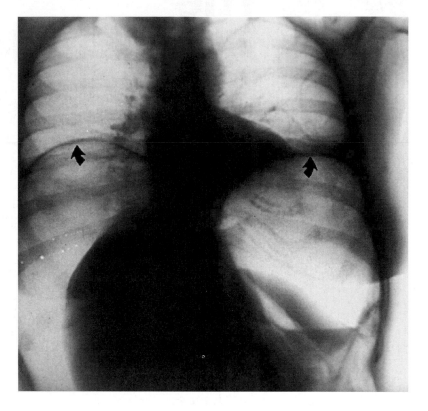

surgery or peritoneal dialysis. In the postsurgical setting, most free air should resolve within 3 to 6 days, and failure to resolve or an increase in the amount of gas should prompt evaluation for a leak at the surgical site. Pneumoperitoneum generally resolves more slowly in thin patients than in obese patients. Air may also be introduced into the peritoneal cavity via the female genital tract. Free air in a patient with an acute abdomen warrants emergent surgical consultation.

Free air is best detected on upright chest radiographs, where it will be seen as a rim of lucency immediately below the diaphragm. In the patient who cannot be placed upright, a left-side-down decubitus view will allow air to appear between the liver and the lateral abdominal wall. On supine films, often the only films obtained in patients in the intensive care unit, free air may manifest as Rigler's sign (gas on both sides of the bowel wall, causing unusually good visualization) or the "football sign," which appears as a large central lucency in the abdomen (Fig. 6–2).

Pneumatosis Intestinalis

Another finding to be ruled out on every abdominal radiograph is pneumotosis intestinalis, or gas within the bowel wall, which usually signifies severely ischemic bowel. It appears as linear gas, either encircling the bowel when viewed on end, or paralleling the bowel lumen when viewed from the side (Fig. 6–3). Pneumatosis must be distinguished from the normal layering out of air over luminal contents in the nondependent portion of the bowel. The former appears as gas that extends around the dependent portion of the bowel wall as well. Every case of pneumatosis does not herald an abdominal catastrophe, and many cases turn out to be benign, related to such factors as obstruction, ileus, and medications. In the setting of an acute abdomen, however, it naturally heightens concern.

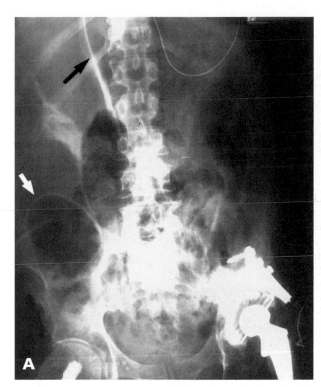

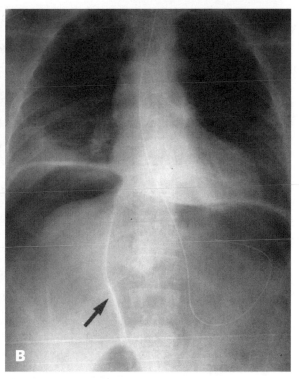

Figure 6–2. A 62-year-old man with a history of peptic ulcer disease had just undergone pinning of a right femoral neck fracture when the orthopedic surgeon noted that the patient had developed a tense abdomen and signs of hemodynamic instability. (A) A stat portable abdominal radiograph reveals evidence of massive free intraperitoneal air, including air outlining the falciform ligament (black arrow) and clear visualization of both sides of the bowel wall (known as Rigler's sign; white arrow). Note not only the pinning of the right femoral neck, but a left total hip arthroplasty with superior acetabular reconstruction using a metallic plate and screws. (B) An upright film corroborates these findings, with a massive amount of air underneath both hemidiaphragms and air outlining the falciform ligament (arrow). A nasogastric tube is coiled in the stomach. At emergent surgical exploration, a ruptured duodenal ulcer was found.

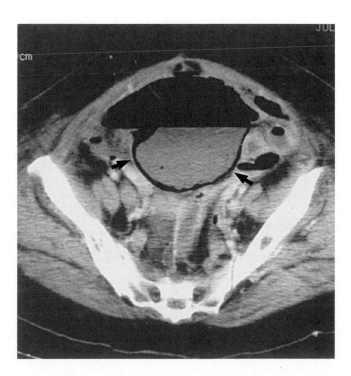

Figure 6–3. This 72-year-old woman, who had recently undergone a modified Whipple's procedure for duodenal carcinoma, complained of increased abdominal pain and went into shock. An axial image from an abdominal and pelvic computed tomography scan demonstrates gas throughout the wall of a dilated cecum (arrows). We can confidently assert that the gas is intramural rather than merely intraluminal because it is present even along the dependent aspect of the bowel wall.

Hepatic Gas

The finding of gas collections over the liver shadow, particularly if they exhibit a linear, branching pattern, should arouse suspicion for one of two processes: portal venous gas (pneumoportia) or gas within the biliary tree (pneumobilia). Portal venous gas usually results from severe intestinal ischemia, and gas can be tracked up through the superior or inferior mesenteric arteries into the portal venous system. Portal venous gas is usually peripheral within the liver, tracking out from the main

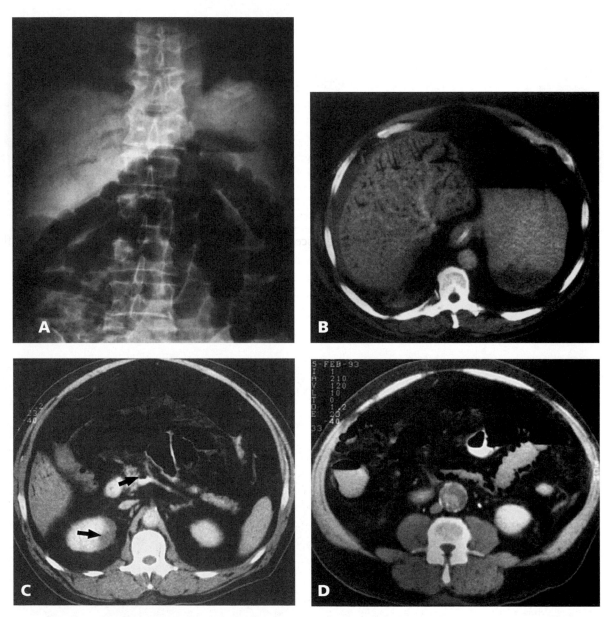

Figure 6–4. (A) An upright plain radiograph of the abdomen reveals multiple air-fluid levels in dilated segments of small and large bowel, as well as linear gas collections over the liver. (B) An axial image from a contrast-enhanced computed tomography scan in the same patient reveals multiple linear gas collections in the periphery of the liver, representing gas in the portal veins. (C) A lower axial section reveals gas in the superior mesenteric vein (short arrow). Note also evidence of an infarction of the upper pole of the right kidney (long arrow). (D) Another image reveals gas within the wall of the small bowel (pneumatosis intestinalis).

portal vein into its smaller branches (Fig. 6–4). Biliary gas, on the other hand, is usually located within the central biliary ducts at the porta hepatis. The most common cause of pneumobilia is previous surgery, such as a papillotomy to relieve obstruction at the sphincter of Oddi or choledochojejunostomy performed in conjunction with a Billroth II procedure for pancreatic cancer. Other causes include a fistula from the gallbladder into the bowel, as in gallstone ileus, or a peptic ulcer eroding into the common bile duct.

PATHOLOGY

Abscess

Over three-quarters of abdominal abscesses occur in postoperative patients, but other causes include perforated peptic ulcer, diverticulitis, and inflammatory bowel disease. Abdominal abscesses can be difficult to diagnose by plain film, but should be suspected whenever an abnormal gas collection is seen outside the expected distribution of the gastrointestinal (GI) tract in a patient with fever and leukocytosis. Other signs of abdominal abscess include a soft tissue mass displacing adjacent structures such as air-filled bowel (which will often exhibit a focal ileus), pleural effusion (especially when the abscess involves the subdiaphragmatic space), and effacement of normal tissue planes, such as the psoas muscle shadow. On computed tomography (CT), it is much easier to definitively ascertain the presence of a gas-containing, loculated fluid collection outside the alimentary canal, which may demonstrate a rim of enhancement (Fig. 6–5). Recently, the role of the radiologist has extended beyond the diagnosis of abscesses to include their treatment; a discussion of percutaneous catheter drainage is found in Chapter 1.

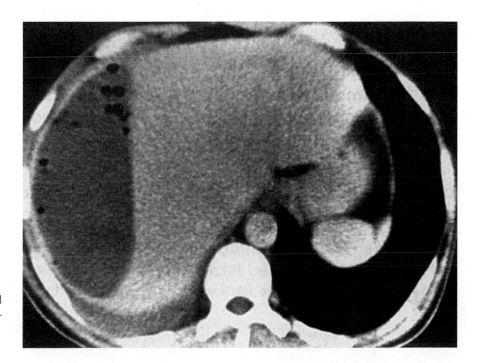

Figure 6–5. This axial section from a contrast-enhanced abdominal computed tomography scan reveals a low-density fluid collection within the lateral aspect of the liver, which contains multiple tiny collections of gas. This represented a pyogenic hepatic abscess.

Peptic Ulcer Disease

EPIDEMIOLOGY

It is estimated that between 200,000 and 300,000 Americans suffer from peptic ulcer disease each year, which may involve the stomach or the duodenum. Risk factors for peptic ulcer disease include male gender (M:F = 3:1), use of nonsteroidal anti-inflammatory drugs or steroids, severe illness, and bacterial infection.

PATHOPHYSIOLOGY

Duodenal ulcers are much more common than gastric ulcers (discussed in Chapter 4), but each represents a manifestation of the same disease, which is characterized by a breakdown in intrinsic protective mechanisms of the mucosa, with subsequent acid-induced mucosal and submucosal erosions. Recently, an important role in the pathogenesis of peptic ulcer disease has been attributed to the spiral gram-negative bacterium *Helicobacter pylori.* This bacterium is present in approximately one-quarter of the general population and has been found to inhabit the gastric mucosal epithelium of most (85 to 100%) patients with duodenal ulcers; its eradication is associated with a dramatic reduction in ulcer recurrence. The presence of *H. pylori* can be diagnosed by endoscopic biopsy or breath test, due to the organism's urea-splitting capabilities. In contrast to gastric ulcers, duodenal ulcers are virtually never malignant.

CLINICAL PRESENTATION

The uncomplicated ulcer patient presents with burning or gnawing epigastric pain that tends to occur before meals and is relieved with food. When peptic ulcer disease presents acutely, it is due to deeper penetration of the ulcer crater into the duodenal mucosa, which may result in perforation and an abdominal catastrophe (Fig. 6–6). Perforated duodenal ulcers present with severe abdominal pain that often radiates to the back and right shoulder, and loss of enteric fluid into the peritoneal cavity may cause hypotension, peritonitis, and shock. Nearly all perforations involve the posterior aspect of the duodenum.

IMAGING

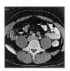

In young patients with uncomplicated symptoms, the initial diagnostic study for peptic ulcer disease should consist of an empirical trial of antisecretory therapy that includes type II histamine receptor blocking agents such as cimetidine or ranitidine.

UNCOMPLICATED ULCER

Both younger patients in whom empirical therapy is not successful and older patients in whom the possibility of a gastric malignancy must be considered should undergo imaging. While endoscopy is more sensitive and specific than barium studies in detecting small or superficial ulcers, a barium study is a significantly more comfortable and less costly procedure for the patient (between one-quarter and one-third the

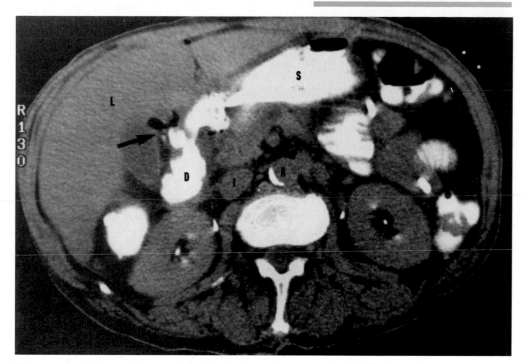

Figure 6–6. A 69-year-old man admitted to the intensive care unit in shock had complained of severe right upper quadrant and back pain. An abdominal computed tomography scan without intravenous contrast (due to acute renal failure) was obtained to rule out a ruptured aortic aneurysm. An axial image shows orally administered contrast material throughout the stomach and portions of the bowel. In the second portion of the duodenum is a barium-filled crater along the lateral wall, with extraluminal gas, representing a perforated duodenal peptic ulcer (arrow). There is no evidence of aneurysm. Note the partially calcific rim of the aorta, indicating atherosclerotic disease. A, aorta; I, inferior vena cava; D, duodenum; S, stomach; L, liver.

cost). Endoscopy may be reserved for the small percentage of patients in whom radiology is equivocal or tissue biopsy is required (e.g., when an ulcer has failed to heal completely with 6 weeks of antisecretory therapy or when an underlying malignancy must be excluded).

Findings of peptic ulcer disease on upper GI examination include an ulcer crater (a fixed pocket of barium) and associated deformities, such as an edematous collar around the ulcer, radiating folds of mucosa, and scarring (Fig. 6–7).

Patients whose duodenal ulcers are refractory to therapy should be evaluated for Zollinger-Ellison syndrome, which is related to the presence of a gastrinoma (Fig. 6–8). Serum gastrin levels should be obtained for diagnosis. Unfortunately, a high percentage of these lesions are malignant (60%), and surgery offers the only hope for cure. Formerly, symptomatic relief could often be achieved only by gastrectomy, but now many patients can be palliated by the use of omeprazole, a medication that blocks the proton pump of the parietal cell responsible for gastric acid secretion. Because the typical gastrinoma is a relatively small tumor, with a mean size of 3 cm, detection can be difficult. Techniques include ultrasound, CT, and nuclear medicine studies. The nuclear medicine I-131 metaiodobenzylguanidine (MIBG) study relies on the fact that pancreatic islet cell tumors such as gastrinomas arise from cells in the amine precursor uptake and decarboxylation (APUD) system. These cells selectively take up this norep-

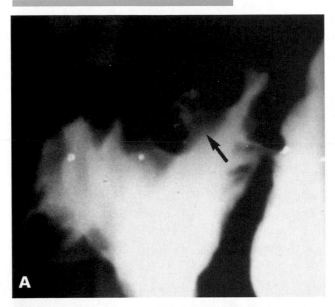
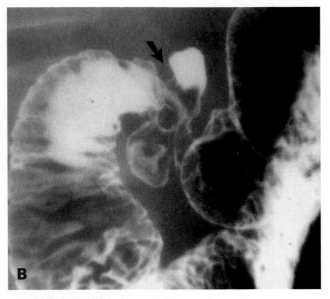

Figure 6–7. (A) A magnified spot film of the duodenal bulb from an upper gastrointestinal examination demonstrates a filling defect in the superior aspect of the duodenal bulb associated with a central collection of barium (arrow). This represents a duodenal bulb ulcer, with a central crater of barium surrounded by a prominent mound of mucosal edema. (B) A spot film of the duodenum in another patient demonstrates a severely deformed and contracted duodenal bulb, in a so-called cloverleaf pattern (arrow). This deformity results from scarring and fibrosis associated with healing of multiple previous peptic ulcers. In contrast to gastric ulcers, duodenal ulcers are virtually never found in an underlying malignancy.

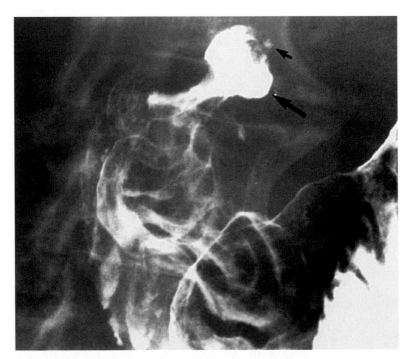

Figure 6–8. An 82-year-old woman presented with epigastric pain and melena. An upper gastrointestinal examination was ordered. This spot film, centered on the pyloric region, demonstrates a large, persistent collection of barium extending superiorly and posteriorly from the duodenal bulb, representing a giant ulcer (large arrow). Interestingly, a smaller collection of barium extends outward from the ulcer crater, consistent with a more acute ulceration (small arrow). Note the long neck of the ulcer, implying a large collar of soft tissue. Unfortunately, soon after this study, the patient became hypotensive and expired. Autopsy revealed a small gastrinoma within the pancreatic head.

inephrine-like compound, and neoplasms comprised of such cells appear "hot" on MIBG scintigraphy.

SUSPECTED PERFORATION

In contrast to the patient with symptoms of an uncomplicated duodenal ulcer, the first study in every case of suspected perforation should be plain films of the abdomen. These are obtained to look for evidence of free air under the diaphragm on upright views or adjacent to the liver on left-side-down decubitus views. If perforation is suspected but no free air is seen, an upper GI examination with water soluble contrast agents should be performed, looking for evidence of extravasation of contrast. Endoscopy is contraindicated, because the large amounts of air insufflation required to adequately open the lumen for visualization are likely to exacerbate the problem. Definitive treatment consists of surgical repair.

Acute Cholecystitis

EPIDEMIOLOGY

Gallstones are present in approximately 15% of persons between the ages of 40 and 60 years, four of five of whom are asymptomatic (Fig. 6–9). There is an extremely high incidence of gallstones among the Navaho and other groups of Native American Indians. Cholecystitis constitutes the most common cause of acute abdominal surgery in women, and the second most common cause in men, resulting in approximately one-half million operations per year in the United States.

There are two types of gallstones: cholesterol stones (85%) and bilirubin stones (15%). Risk factors for the formation of bilirubin stones relate to hemolytic anemia, and include hemoglobinopathies, especially sickle-cell disease, a prosthetic heart valve,

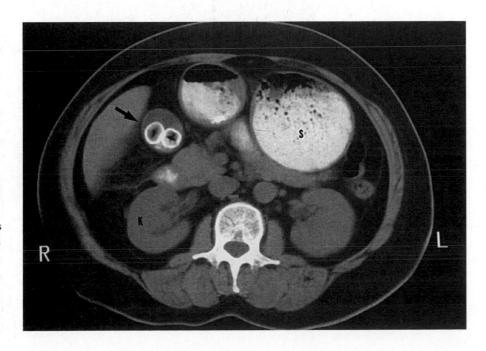

Figure 6–9. This axial image from an abdominal computed tomography scan demonstrates two calcified stones in the gallbladder (arrow). The central gas-containing cracks within the stones are thought to result from dehydration, with subsequent filling by nitrogen gas, often producing the so-called crow foot sign. K, right kidney; S, stomach.

and hypersplenism, while the risk factors for the more common cholesterol stones include female gender (F:M = 4:1), diabetes, and cirrhosis. Ileal disease, such as Crohn's disease, is another risk factor, as it disrupts the normal enterohepatic circulation of bile salts.

PATHOPHYSIOLOGY

 Gallstones as such are harmless, but they become symptomatic when they obstruct some portion of the biliary tree, most commonly the cystic duct, resulting in acute cholecystitis (Fig. 6–10). Obstruction of the cystic duct produces bile stasis within the gallbladder, which may permit the proliferation of bacteria, or may produce inflammation due to direct irritation by the bile salts themselves.

CLINICAL PRESENTATION

The typical patient with biliary colic presents with the acute onset of right upper quadrant or epigastric pain that increases in intensity over minutes to hours and then persists for 6 or more hours. Some patients experience nausea and vomiting. Acute

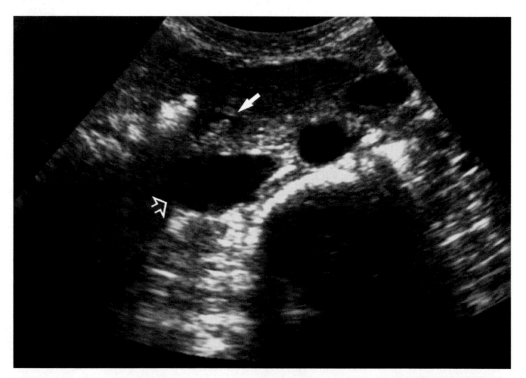

Figure 6–10. A 36-year-old mildly obese woman with four children presented with a history of intermittent right upper quadrant pain that had acutely worsened over the last 24 hours, as well as elevated serum levels of bilirubin and alkaline phophatase. This transverse image from an abdominal ultrasound examination, taken just above the level of the pancreatic head, demonstrates two hyperechoic stones within a mildly dilated (8 mm) common bile duct (choledocholithiasis; arrow). While the stones are not large enough to cause complete obstruction of the bile duct at this level, it is possible that they (or others like them) were responsible for obstruction of the bile duct as it narrows more distally. Note also the inferior vena cava (open arrow).

cholecystitis is suspected once the pain has persisted beyond 6 hours, indicating persistent biliary tract obstruction. The pain of acute cholecystitis often radiates to the right shoulder and is associated with nausea, vomiting, low-grade fever, and chills. Laboratory analysis may demonstrate leukocytosis.

Laboratory analysis is often helpful in the diagnosis of acute cholecystitis. Alkaline phosphatase, which is also produced in bone and other tissues, derives primarily from the biliary tract. Hence a normal alkaline phosphatase level usually excludes biliary tract disease, and high levels are classically associated with extrahepatic biliary obstruction. Hepatitis may also produce increased alkaline phosphatase levels, but these are typically not as high as in biliary obstruction and are accompanied by elevated transaminases (aspartate aminotransferase [AST] and alanine aminotransferase), which are produced by the hepatocytes themselves. Pancreatitis usually produces an elevation of pancreatic amylase and lipase. In suspected pyelonephritis, white blood cells and bacteria should be sought in the urine.

A potentially worrisome sign in a patient with acute or chronic cholecystitis is the sudden resolution of pain. If the patient develops peritoneal signs such as guarding and rebound tenderness shortly thereafter, perforation of the gallbladder is suggested, which may prove rapidly fatal. Although there is a risk of perforation in every patient, surgeons typically prefer to delay surgery for several days in cases of acute cholecystitis, to give antibiotics an opportunity to calm the inflammation. The patient is treated with narcotic analgesia (*not* morphine, which induces spasm of the sphincter of Oddi, but meperidine). However, if there is evidence of perforation, or the patient does not respond within hours to medical management, urgent surgery is required. Patients at highest risk of perforation include diabetic patients and patients with debilitating illnesses.

IMAGING

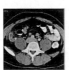 Only approximately one-third of patients presenting with acute right upper quadrant pain suffer from acute cholecystitis. A patient with right upper quadrant pain and a history consistent with acute cholecystitis may be suffering from any one of several common conditions. The differential diagnosis includes hepatitis, pancreatitis, peptic ulcer disease, and even pyelonephritis or pneumonia. It is important to ascertain the source of the patient's pain because, while acute cholecystitis is often managed surgically, the usual treatments for these other conditions are nonsurgical.

Plain films of the chest and abdomen are often helpful. First, they help to rule out pneumonia or evidence of free intraperitoneal air, which would indicate perforation of a viscus and a surgical emergency. Second, the plain film will demonstrate gallstones in approximately 15% of cases (the inverse of renal stones, 85% of which are radiopaque), and when stones are found, the probability of a biliary etiology increases.

ULTRASOUND

The imaging study of first choice in suspected acute cholecystitis is ultrasonography, which is more than 95% sensitive and specific for the presence of gallstones. Stones are found in 90 to 95% of patients with acute cholecystitis. While the presence of gallstones does not prove that the patient has inflammation secondary to obstruction, the absence of stones is strong evidence against it. Stones appear as rounded, echogenic structures in the gallbladder that cast acoustic shadows and move with a change in patient position (because they are suspended in bile) (Fig. 6–11). Another corroborative finding is biliary dilatation, either intra- or extrahepatic, which occurs once the biliary tract has been obstructed for a period of hours. The combination of an impacted stone in a dilated cystic duct or common bile duct virtually assures the diagnosis.

To increase the specificity of ultrasound for the detection of acute cholecystitis, in

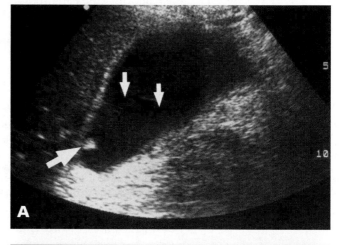

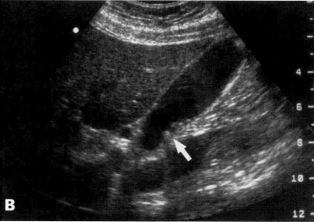

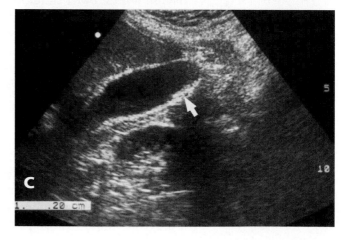

Figure 6–11. (A) This longitudinal plane gallbladder ultrasound image in a supine patient demonstrates an echogenic focus within the gallbladder lumen (large arrow). Is it a stone? Probably not, for two reasons: (1) it demonstrates no posterior acoustic shadowing, and (2) it adheres to the nondependent wall and did not move with changes in the patient's position. The lesion most likely represents a cholesterol polyp. Note also the slightly echogenic sludge (concentrated bile) layering in the dependent portion of the lumen (small arrows), likely because the patient had not eaten for some time prior to the examination. By contrast, (B) supine and (C) upright ultrasound images of the gallbladder in another patient clearly demonstrate echogenic, shadowing foci in the dependent portion of the gallbladder lumen (arrows) that move from near the neck of the gallbladder when the patient is supine down to the fundus when the patient assumes an upright position, the so-called rolling stones sign.

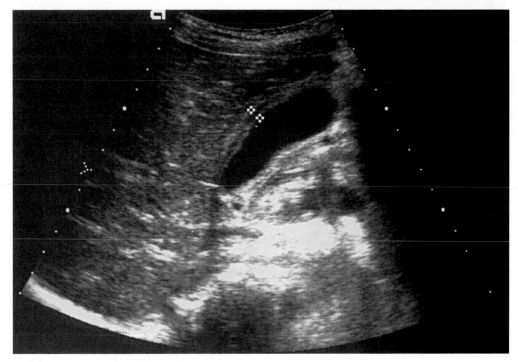

Figure 6–12. A longitudinal ultrasound image of the gallbladder demonstrates gallbladder wall thickening, which measured 8 mm (cursors). Causes of diffuse wall thickening other than cholecystitis include portal venous hypertension and congestive heart failure (both increasing hydrostatic pressure within the cystic vein), hypoalbuminemia, hepatitis, and acquired immunodeficiency syndrome (AIDS). This patient had AIDS, and the gallbladder wall thickening may have reflected infection with cytomegalovirus or mycobacterium avium intracellulare complex.

addition to stones, the following two findings should be present: a positive sonographic Murphy's sign (maximum tenderness is elicited directly over the gallbladder) and thickening of the gallbladder wall with intramural sonolucency, indicating edema. The thickness of the wall of a normal gallbladder should measure 3 mm or less (Fig. 6–12).

Additional findings that further increase the specificity of ultrasound in the diagnosis of acute cholecystitis relate to its complications. If fluid is visible around the gallbladder in the gallbladder fossa (pericholecystic fluid), this likely indicates perforation of the gallbladder, with bile extravasation. A discrete, heterogeneous fluid collection in the region of the gallbladder may represent an abscess, also secondary to perforation. When such a collection contains gas, it is almost certainly an abscess. Similarly, air within the gallbladder lumen or its wall (emphysematous cholecystitis) strongly suggests complicated cholecystitis (Fig. 6–13).

NUCLEAR MEDICINE

A second test that is equally sensitive for the detection of acute cholecystitis, and actually demonstrates physiologically the cystic duct obstruction, is cholescintigraphy. The most important disadvantage of cholescintigraphy as compared to ultrasound (and CT) is the latter's ability to evaluate other right upper quadrant sources of pain. The cholescintigram is at least as good as any other imaging modality in

Figure 6–13. This upright abdominal radiograph reveals both air layering out above fluid within the gallbladder lumen, as well as gas within the gallbladder wall, indicating emphysematous cholecystitis.

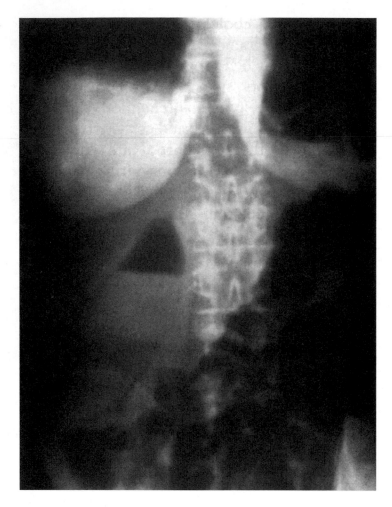

detecting acute cholecystitis, but if the patient's pain has some other etiology, the cholescintigram is far less likely than other studies to reveal it. In an era when laparoscopy has become the preferred means of surgically removing the gallbladder, ultrasound's ability to provide preoperative information about the size and position of the gallbladder, the presence or absence of wall thickening and pericholecystic fluid, and the size, number, and location of stones is especially beneficial to the surgeon.

Mechanism of localization

The cholescintigram relies on the avid hepatic uptake and biliary excretion of technetium (Tc)-99m-labeled iminodiacetic acid compounds into the biliary system by the liver, even in the presence of an elevated serum bilirubin. Normally, the radiopharmaceutical begins to accumulate in the liver promptly after injection, and activity appears within minutes in the gallbladder, and soon thereafter in the small bowel, as bile is ejected out the common bile duct through the ampulla of Vater. Acute cholecystitis is diagnosed when there is no activity in the gallbladder 30 minutes after injection (Fig. 6–14). The absence of activity in the small bowel indicates a common duct obstruction, which would eventually produce jaundice and perhaps pancreatitis.

Figure 6–14. (A) These sequential images from a nuclear medicine hepatobiliary scan obtained after the intravenous injection of technetium-99m mebrofenin demonstrate the appearance of homogeneous radiotracer activity throughout the liver in early images (arrow). With time (9 minutes), radiotracer appears in the gallbladder (curved arrow), ruling out cystic duct obstruction and acute cholecystitis. Activity is also seen in the common bile duct and the small bowel, ruling out obstruction. (B) Four scintigraphic images in another patient with right upper quadrant pain demonstrate excretion of radiotracer into the biliary system and into the small bowel. However, no activity is seen in the gallbladder (the expected location of which is indicated by the curved arrow). Morphine administration and reinjection of additional radiotracer (not shown) still produced no activity in the gallbladder. A diagnosis of acute cholecystitis was made and later confirmed at surgery.

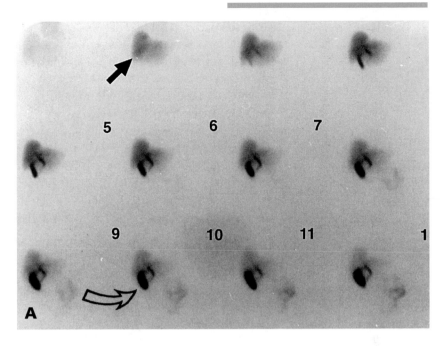

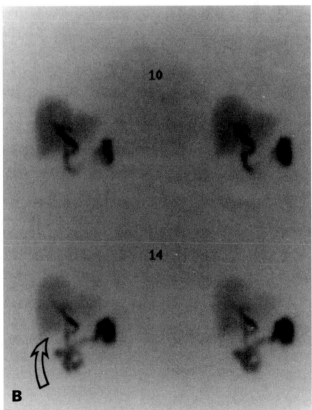

Pharmacologic maneuvers

Two pharmacologic maneuvers may be employed to enhance the specificity of the hepatobiliary scan. The first involves the administration of morphine, which causes contraction of the sphincter of Oddi, and thereby tends to shunt bile into the gallbladder. If the patient's gallbladder was contracting at the time of the study, perhaps under influence of a recent meal, bile might not enter the gallbladder. However, morphine-induced sphincter of Oddi contraction helps to ensure that excreted bile is shunted into the gallbladder.

The second pharmacologic maneuver is the administration of cholecystokinin analogue. Cholecystokinin is the hormone secreted by the duodenal epithelium in response to intraluminal protein and lipid content, which causes contraction of the gallbladder and ejection of bile. In a patient who has been fasting for a long period of time, the gallbladder may be full, and thus not fill during the examination. In this case, an injection of cholecystokinin can be administered, followed by repeat radiopharmaceutical injection. The absence of gallbladder filling after one or both of these maneuvers further increases the radiologist's confidence in the diagnosis of acute cholecystitis.

Perhaps 5 to 10% of patients with acute cholecystitis may exhibit no stones and no evidence of biliary obstruction. These patients suffer from a condition termed acalculous cholecystitis, which may be caused by ischemia or infection of static bile. Patients at risk include patients on total parenteral nutrition (who may be given periodic cholecystokinin injections prophylactically to empty the gallbladder), burn patients, patients who have suffered severe trauma, or acquired immunodeficiency syndrome patients. While ultrasound will demonstrate no stones in these cases, the hepatobiliary scan will still demonstrate nonfilling of the gallbladder in the vast majority of cases, although specificity is much lower than in the typical "calculous" cholecystitis.

INTERVENTIONAL PROCEDURES

The interventional radiologist may be called upon to treat acute biliary obstruction. In severely ill patients who are poor surgical candidates, the gallbladder may be decompressed percutaneously under ultrasound guidance, with a drainage catheter left in place, in a procedure known as percutaneous cholecystostomy (Fig. 6–15). The biliary system may be directly visualized by percutaneous transhepatic cholangiography, in which a catheter is placed into the biliary tree and contrast injected. If an obstruction in the common duct is found, a stent can be placed across it, typically extending from the common hepatic duct into the small bowel, permitting internal drainage of the biliary system. The latter procedure is most commonly performed in patients with neoplasms obstructing the bile duct, such as cholangiocarcinoma or carcinoma of the pancreas.

Pancreatitis

Pancreatitis comes in two presentations: acute and chronic. Acute pancreatitis is defined as inflammation of the pancreas with the potential for complete healing, while chronic pancreatitis is associated with permanent sequelae including altered structure and impaired function. In chronic pancreatitis, the loss of both endocrine function (insulin and glucagon secretion) and exocrine function (secretion of digestive enzymes, including amylases, proteases, and lipases) may play a role in the clinical course. It should be emphasized that chronic pancreatitis is not equivalent to repeated episodes of acute pancreatitis, and both types may be associated with episodes of acute exacerbation.

Figure 6–15. An 85-year-old woman presented with chronic abdominal pain and mental status changes. The plain film of the abdomen (not shown) demonstrated a large right-sided soft tissue mass displacing bowel loops into the left side of the abdomen. (A) A longitudinal sonogram of the right side of the abdomen demonstrates a large hydropic gallbladder (white arrows) with a dilated cystic duct (curved arrow) containing an echogenic, shadowing focus—an obstructive stone (straight black arrow). (B) An axial computed tomography image demonstrates the hydropic gallbladder displacing bowel into the left hemiabdomen. The patient was a poor surgical candidate, and the gallbladder was drained via percutaneous cholecystostomy. Note the severely calcific superior mesenteric artery (white arrow). G, gallbladder.

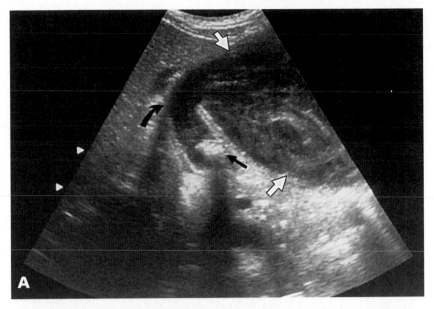

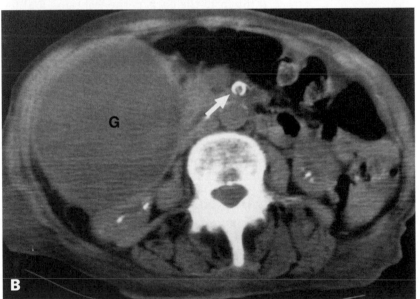

EPIDEMIOLOGY

The annual incidence of acute pancreatitis is approximately 1 case per 10,000 persons, with a peak age of incidence in the sixth decade. The two most important risk factors for the development of acute pancreatitis are, in order of frequency in the United States, cholelithiasis and alcoholism.

PATHOPHYSIOLOGY

The pathophysiology of pancreatitis is multifaceted and complex, but all mechanisms probably have in common the end point of pancreatic autodigestion, with activated pancreatic enzymes escaping from the ductal system and lysing the tissue of the pancreas and adjacent structures.

The fact that the pancreas lacks a capsule tends to facilitate the spread of the inflammatory process.

In the United States, by far the two most prevalent causes of acute pancreatitis are binge alcohol ingestion and cholelithiasis. Alcohol ingestion is more common in men, while gallstones are more common in women. Gallstone pancreatitis presumably results from impaction of a gallstone in the distal common bile duct, after the point of entry of the pancreatic duct, with resultant obstruction of pancreatic secretion. Alcoholic pancreatitis may stem from inspissation of secretions in the pancreatic ductal system, secondary to the increased concentration of secretions associated with alcohol consumption. It is also known that alcohol causes activation of intracellular digestive enzymes in the pancreatic acini. Other causes include pancreas divisum, trauma (including iatrogenic), penetrating ulcer, hyperlipoproteinemia, and various drugs. Alcoholism is the most prominent cause of chronic pancreatitis.

CLINICAL PRESENTATION

Patients experiencing an acute attack present with severe abdominal pain that radiates through to the back, peritoneal signs, and fever. Patients may exhibit respiratory distress with atelectasis and effusions, subcutaneous fat necrosis (manifesting as purple skin lesions), and saponification of serum calcium, with resultant symptoms of hypocalcemia such as Chvostek's sign. In severe cases, patients present in shock, with renal failure and disseminated intravascular coagulation.

The diagnosis of acute pancreatitis is best made clinically, based on the constellation of history, physical signs, and laboratory findings, especially an increase in serum lipase. Classic laboratory findings include elevations of serum amylase and lipase, with the latter being the more specific of the two, because the salivary glands, fallopian tubes, and lungs also synthesize amylase.

IMAGING

ACUTE PANCREATITIS

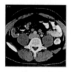 Imaging is usually performed in cases where the diagnosis is uncertain or to detect complications and assess prognosis. In the acute setting, CT is the study of choice, providing a comprehensive assessment of the gland itself and the surrounding tissues. In many cases, the gland appears normal, which does not exclude the diagnosis. Common findings include diffuse or focal swelling of the gland, inhomogeneity, poor definition, fluid collections, and thickening of the pararenal fascia.

One of the most important complications of acute pancreatitis, seen in 10% of cases, is a pancreatic pseudocyst. A pancreatic pseudocyst is a fluid collection surrounded by a fibrous capsule, but is not a true cyst because it does not have an epithelial lining (Fig. 6–16). A significant percentage of pseudocysts will not resolve spontaneously. Pseudocysts are often seen not only within the pancreas, but in the lesser sac (between the pancreas and stomach) and in the left pararenal space, potential spaces with which the gland itself is continuous.

Abscess, a rarer but more threatening condition, develops in approximately 1 in 20 cases and is fatal up to three-quarters of the time. Abscesses are often recognized by the presence of gas and require urgent drainage. Patients whose hematocrits are falling

Figure 6–16. This axial image from a contrast-enhanced computed tomography scan of the abdomen demonstrates a huge pancreatic pseudocyst with an enhancing rim filling virtually the entire abdomen at this level. These cysts result from perforation of the pancreatic duct, with leakage of pancreatic secretions into the surrounding tissues. Note the surrounding capsule, which demonstrates contrast enhancement, a somewhat atypical finding. A pseudocyst of this size would be a good candidate for percutaneous drainage, with a high rate of success and a relatively low rate of complications such as infection.

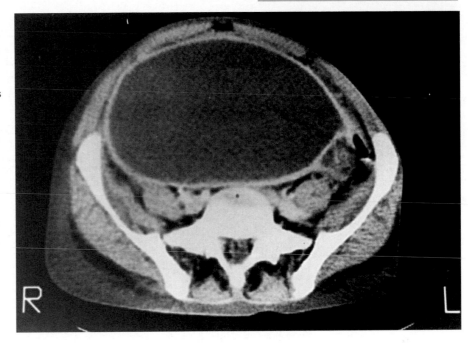

should be suspected of an even rarer condition, hemorrhagic pancreatitis. Pseudoaneurysm formation or rupture may present in a similar way. Ultrasound is useful in following up on complications and in guiding therapeutic interventions, such as the drainage of fluid collections.

CHRONIC PANCREATITIS

Chronic pancreatitis more often requires imaging to confirm the diagnosis, as symptoms may be vague. Some of the most common manifestations of chronic pancreatitis are the presence of calcifications in the pancreatic parenchyma (which are often visible on plain films), a dilated or irregular appearing pancreatic duct, and generalized atrophy of the gland (Fig. 6–17). The presence of calcification is not an indicator of disease severity, whereas ductal abnormalities usually indicate more severe insufficiency. It is not possible to state with certainty that a pancreatic mass represents inflammatory tissues, and a small percentage of patients with chronic pancreatitis will also harbor a carcinoma. Frequently, image-directed biopsy (with CT or ultrasound guidance) is necessary, although it must be borne in mind that biopsy may itself provoke a flare-up of inflammation.

Diverticular Disease

EPIDEMIOLOGY

Nearly 50% of Americans over the age of 50 years have colonic diverticula, and the condition becomes increasingly common with advancing age. While the majority of patients will never suffer symptoms, up to one-quarter will suffer at least one episode of diverticular inflammation during their lifetime. The spectrum of diverticular dis-

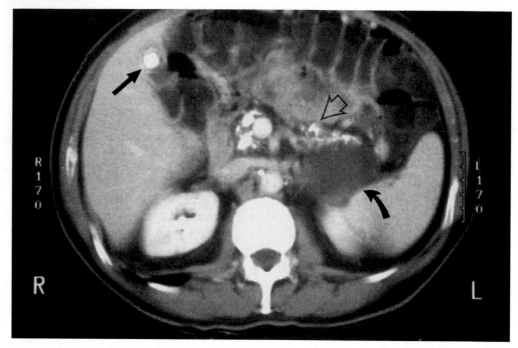

Figure 6–17. A 66-year-old man with squamous cell carcinoma of the floor of the mouth underwent a contrast-enhanced computed tomography scan to rule out the presence of distant metastases. An axial image from the study at the level of the liver and spleen reveals an atrophic, calcific pancreas (open arrow), with a fluid collection arising from the pancreatic tail (curved arrow). This fluid collection represented a pancreatic pseudocyst. Two possible etiologies of the patient's pancreatitis are suggested. First, many patients with squamous cell carcinomas of the head and neck are cigarette and alcohol users, and the pancreatitis may have been alcoholic-related. Second, in the right upper quadrant is a striking gallstone (arrow), with a central calcific nidus surrounded by a lobulated rim of calcification, suggesting the possibility that another gallstone may have produced gallstone pancreatitis.

ease ranges from simple diverticulosis (the presence of one or more diverticula) to diverticular disease (multiple diverticula and evidence of colonic muscular hypertrophy), to frank diverticulitis (perforation and peridiverticular abscess formation) (Fig. 6–18). Nearly 0.1% of Americans are admitted to the hospital each year for this disease, and nearly one-fifth of these require an emergency operation.

PATHOPHYSIOLOGY

 Diverticula are thought to result from decreased stool bulk, with impaired colonic motility, overactivity of the bowel musculature, and herniation of mucosa through defects in the muscle layers. While this is by far the most common condition of the colon in the United States, it is virtually unheard of in many developing nations, which consume diets much higher in dietary fiber. As one would expect, the distribution of diverticula within the colon is highest in the sigmoid region, which is the narrowest segment and generates the highest pressures. The outpouchings of the wall are often associated with hypertrophy of the longitudinal and circular smooth muscle layers, which causes the mucosal folds to become bunched together and limits luminal distensibility, diagnosed on barium enema as diverticular disease.

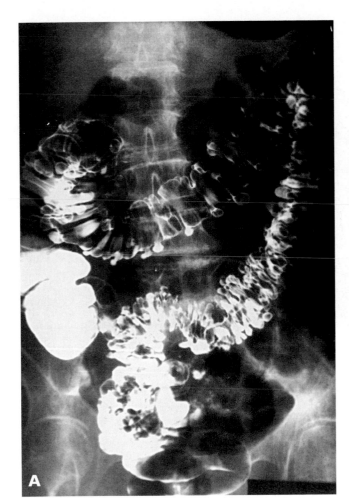

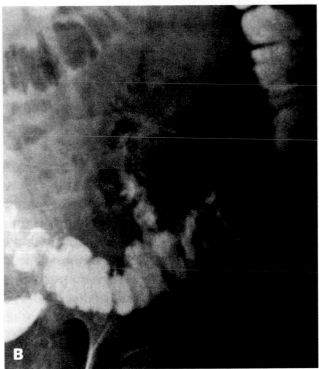

Figure 6–18. (A) This overhead film from a double-contrast barium enema reveals marked colonic diverticulosis, with the most severe involvement in the sigmoid and descending portions of the colon. The sigmoid colon also reveals evidence of diverticular disease, with narrowing of the lumen due to prominent circular muscle hypertrophy. (B) This radiograph from a single-contrast barium enema in another patient reveals diverticulosis, diverticular perforation, and formation of a diverticular abscess, manifesting as a gas and contrast-containing mass adjacent to the bowel.

Diverticulitis results from inspissation of luminal contents within a diverticulum, which may abrade the mucosa and incite inflammation. As the inflammatory process within the thin wall of the diverticulum progresses, it may cause tiny perforations, with extraluminal leakage of contents (including feces and bacteria) into the surrounding fat, and result in the formation of an abscess within the wall or external to the wall of the colon.

CLINICAL PRESENTATION

Patients with uncomplicated diverticulosis may experience spasmodic pain and mild rectal bleeding. Once diverticulitis develops, patients typically present with pain, tenderness, and/or a mass in the left lower quadrant. Fever is also present in many patients, as is leukocytosis.

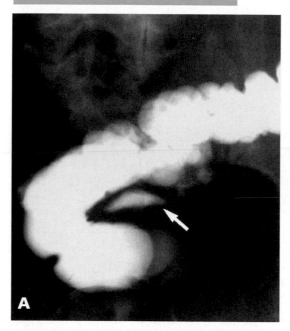
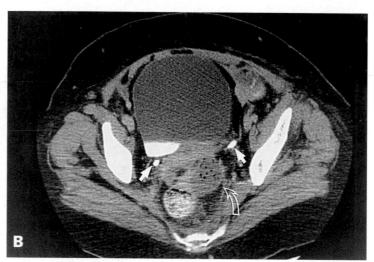

Figure 6–19. A 73-year-old woman with a clinical diagnosis of diverticulitis was sent to the radiology department for a water-soluble contrast enema to rule out the presence of extravasation and abscess. (**A**) A frontal spot film from the contrast enema examination reveals a pocket of extravasated contrast extending from the most distal sigmoid colon into the perirectal soft tissues (arrow). (**B**) To better define the extent of this process, a pelvic computed tomography examination was performed, which shows the collection of mixed fluid and gas immediately to the left of the rectum (open arrow) and associated with stranding in the perirectal fat, indicative of inflammation. Note also the contrast-filled distal ureters (arrows). The patient subsequently underwent surgical resection of the diseased portion of the bowel, as well as incision and drainage of the abscess.

IMAGING

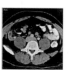 The radiologist has several roles in the diagnostic process. First, the diagnosis must be made: is there or is there not imaging evidence of diverticulitis? Second, the extent of the disease must be assessed: is the process largely confined to the wall of the bowel, or how far has the inflammatory process spread within the abdomen? Third is the role for radiologic intervention: is percutaneous or transrectal drainage of an abscess necessary? If the disease is mild, the patient is likely to be managed with antibiotics. If inflammation is more widespread, or an abscess is formed, surgical or radiologic intervention is likely to be required. The radiologic approach to percutaneous abscess drainage is discussed in the interventional section of Chapter 1. The definitive treatment, typically delayed if possible until the inflammatory process has subsided, is resection of the diseased segment of the bowel.

Radiologic findings vary by modality. Plain films of the abdomen may demonstrate a left lower quadrant soft tissue mass, a focal ileus, or even a gas collection suggestive of an abscess. One of the main functions of the plain film is to rule out free air, which would indicate perforation. If there is no evidence of perforation, a water soluble contrast enema may be performed to look for evidence of an abscess and extravasation of contrast through a fistula, which virtually establishes the diagnosis (Fig. 6–19). In advanced cases, fistulae may develop to the bladder, vagina, and small bowel. Infused CT is the examination of choice and should be performed with oral and, if necessary, rectal contrast to ensure good bowel opacification. Findings include diverticulosis, inflammation in the pericolic fat, a pericolic fluid collection that may contain air (indicating abscess), and perhaps fistula. The possibility of a perforated colonic neoplasm cannot be absolutely ruled out on the basis of any of these studies.

Appendicitis

EPIDEMIOLOGY

Acute appendicitis constitutes the most common abdominal surgical emergency, affecting approximately 1 in 14 Americans at some point in their lives, and 0.1% of the U.S. population per year. Approximately 250,000 appendectomies are performed each year, of which approximately 20% disclose a normal appendix.

PATHOPHYSIOLOGY

 The appendix arises from the cecum 1 to 2 cm below the ileocecal valve and demonstrates considerable lymphoid tissue when sectioned. While highly variable in size, it typically measures approximately 8 cm in length and its diameter is 6 mm or less. Acute appendicitis results from obstruction of the appendiceal lumen, which is secondary to lymphoid hyperplasia in the majority of cases, and secondary to a fecalith in approximately one-third of cases (Fig. 6–20). Continued mucosal secretion results in increased intraluminal pressure, which may eventually compromise venous drainage, resulting in ischemia and breakdown of

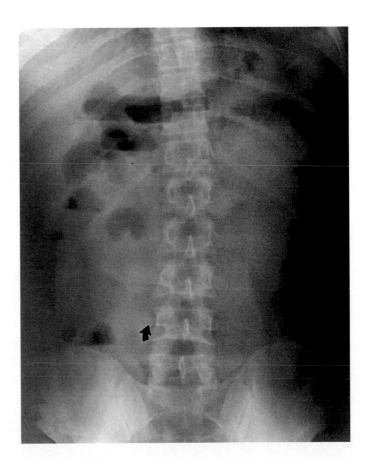

Figure 6–20. An upright radiograph of the abdomen in a patient with abdominal pain reveals multiple small bowel air-fluid levels, as well as a subtle 1 cm oval radiodensity superimposed over the right transverse process of the L4 vertebral body (arrow). This represented a surgically confirmed fecalith, also known as an appendicolith. Appendicoliths represent an insensitive but highly specific sign of appendicitis in the appropriate clinical setting.

the mucosa. Bacterial superinfection may also result. The major danger in appendicitis is perforation, which occurs in approximately one-quarter of patients, and can result in abscess formation, peritonitis, and life-threatening sepsis. The hazards associated with these complications render acute appendicitis a surgical emergency.

CLINICAL PRESENTATION

The typical patient presents with right lower quadrant pain and tenderness. Additional findings in many patients include fever, nausea and vomiting, and leukocytosis, which is present in nearly 90% of patients. In the majority of patients, the clinical diagnosis is relatively straightforward. However, acute appendicitis presents atypically in approximately one in four patients, and even in the best of hands, appendectomy discloses a normal appendix approximately 20% of the time. The single most difficult clinical situation is a young woman, in whom a ruptured ovarian cyst, ectopic pregnancy, or pelvic inflammatory disease could produce virtually identical symptoms and signs. Judicious use of imaging resources should make it possible to reduce the rate of negative appendectomy in the subgroup of patients in whom the diagnosis is uncertain.

IMAGING

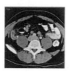 The first radiologic studies to obtain in suspected appendicitis are supine and upright radiographs of the abdomen. These are abnormal in most patients, although the findings may be nonspecific. The only specific finding is a calcified appendicolith, which is only seen 10% of the time but is associated with a nearly 50% probability of perforation. An appendicolith is usually approximately 1 cm in diameter, is round or oval in shape, and demonstrates concentric rings of calcification, so-called lamellation. If an appendicolith is detected, appendectomy is warranted. Nonspecific plain film findings in the right lower quadrant include a soft-tissue mass, a dilated loop of bowel with an air-fluid level, and loss of the psoas muscle margin.

The barium enema is used less frequently today than several decades ago, but still possesses a high degree of accuracy in ruling out the disease. Obviously, bowel preparation is impossible, and the examination will be performed in single-contrast fashion. The single most helpful finding in excluding the disease is filling of the entire appendix with barium, which will not occur if the appendiceal lumen is obstructed. If the appendix does not fill and there is evidence of mass effect on the cecum and terminal ileum, with evidence of mucosal inflammation in these regions, the probability of appendicitis is high. However, the appendix does not fill in 20% of normals, and a number of other processes may produce a right lower quadrant mass effect.

Ultrasound has recently received considerable attention as a means of diagnosing appendicitis. In skilled hands, it has a sensitivity over 90%, and an even higher specificity. The examination is performed by gradually pressing the transducer down on the skin of the right lower quadrant, thereby displacing gas-filled bowel loops and minimizing the distance between the transducer and the appendix. The diagnosis is made when the diseased appendix is identified as a tubular, noncompressible structure measuring 6 mm or more in diameter and demonstrating no peristalsis. Confidence is further increased when an appendicolith, an echogenic focus with posterior shadowing seen in approximately one-third of patients, is identified (Fig. 6–21). Difficulties

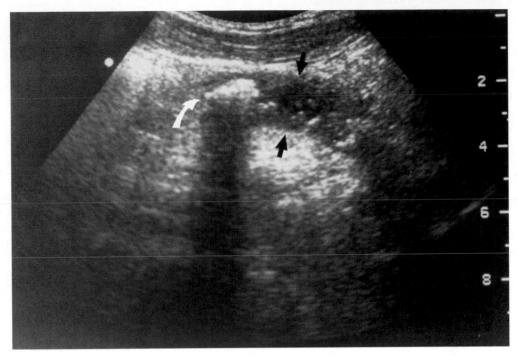

Figure 6–21. A 22-year-old man presented with right lower quadrant pain and mild leukocytosis. The patient was referred from the emergency department for an ultrasound examination to rule out appendicitis. The patient was placed supine on the examination table and asked to point to the site of pain. The ultrasound transducer was placed over this area and immediately revealed a tubular, noncompressible, fluid-filled structure measuring 1.1 cm in diameter (arrows). In addition, this structure contained an echogenic, shadowing focus at one end (curved arrow). These findings are virtually diagnostic of an appendicolith within the proximal end of a dilated, inflamed appendix. These findings were confirmed at appendectomy.

with the ultrasonographic approach include a retrocecal appendix and obese or uncooperative patients. Moreover, the examination is highly operator dependent.

CT represents perhaps the best radiologic modality, because it not only directly visualizes the appendix and surrounding structures, but also provides the most help in assessing the presence of other abdominal and pelvic pathologies. Accuracy is well over 95% in the diagnosis of acute appendicitis. Noncontrast scanning offers improved visualization of appendicoliths, but both intravenous and oral contrast should be administered to enhance differentiation of the bowel from other structures and to assess enhancement patterns. The inflamed appendix appears as a fluid-filled tube with wall thickening of several millimeters, and is surrounded by periappendiceal inflammation that appears as ill-defined stranding in the fat, which may extend to involve adjacent bowel (Fig. 6–22). If perforation has occurred, an abscess may be seen.

Bowel Obstruction

EPIDEMIOLOGY

At least three-quarters of small bowel obstructions in the United States and other industrialized nations result from postsurgical adhesions, making prior surgery one of the most common reasons for acute abdominal surgery. Other causes of small bowel

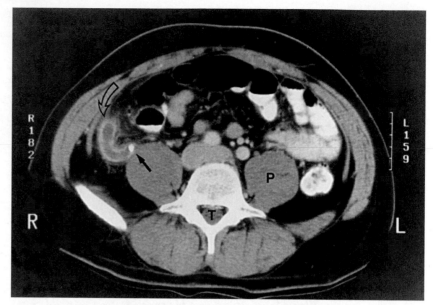

Figure 6–22. A 35-year-old man presented with right lower quadrant pain and mild fever. However, the clinical examination was not classic for appendicitis, so a computed tomography scan of the abdomen and pelvis was requested for further evaluation. An axial image at the level of the proximal common iliac vessels demonstrates a dilated, fluid-filled appendix (curved arrow) with enhancing walls and a stone lodged in its neck (arrow), which is accompanied by stranding in the periappendiceal fat. The radiologic diagnosis of appendicitis was confirmed at surgery. Up to one-quarter of patients with suspected appendicitis present with indeterminate symptoms and signs, and the picture can be especially confusing in young women, in whom several reproductive tract abnormalities can easily mimic appendicitis. It is in these cases that imaging makes the greatest contribution to management. P, left psoas muscle; T, thecal sac containing spinal cord and/or nerve roots.

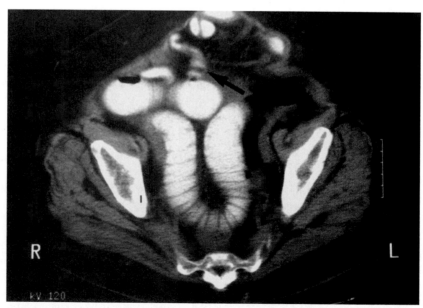

Figure 6–23. An 87-year-old woman presented with a 24-hour history of severe abdominal pain, fever, and leukocytosis. This axial image from an oral-contrast only pelvic computed tomography scan demonstrates dilated, contrast-filled segments of small bowel leading up to a point of herniation of bowel beyond the abdomen (arrow), into a hernia sac containing largely collapsed bowel. This represented a hypogastric (below the umbilicus) ventral hernia. No contrast was seen in the colon. At surgery, ischemic bowel was found in the ventral hernia. I, right ilium.

obstruction in adults include incarcerated hernia, malignancy, intussusception, and volvulus (Fig. 6–23).

PATHOPHYSIOLOGY

In general, bowel obstruction results from one of three causes: an endoluminal mass, thickening or inflammation of the bowel wall, or extraluminal compression. Small bowel obstructions account for approximately four of five cases of adult GI tract obstruction.

While it is obvious why a bowel obstruction will produce serious consequences over a period of days to weeks, the reasons why suspected obstructions warrant urgent diagnostic evaluation may be less clear. One reason for urgency is the effects of obstruction on the bowel proximal to it. Swallowed air, saliva, and GI secretions (succus entericus) progressively accumulate proximal to the point of obstruction, and stasis allows bacterial proliferation and the production of toxins that directly injure the bowel.

Moreover, increasing distention of the bowel increases intramural tension, as described by the law of LaPlace, which states that for a constant intraluminal pressure, increasing the radius of a viscus by a factor of two will double its intramural tension. This increased intramural tension may eventually overcome capillary perfusion pressure and result in ischemic injury, with subsequent tissue necrosis, perforation, and peritonitis. The law of LaPlace also explains why the cecum is the segment of colon most likely to perforate. The cecum is relatively thin walled and has the greatest initial luminal diameter; thus, for a given colonic pressure, it will experience the greatest intramural tension and hence distend the most.

For these reasons—stasis and distention—one of the first and most important therapeutic interventions in suspected obstruction is to make the patient NPO (nothing by mouth) and to pass a nasogastric tube with suction, in an attempt to prevent the accumulation of intraluminal contents.

Mechanical obstruction may be classified according to several categories. The first is simple obstruction, which simply refers to blockage of the intestinal lumen without compromise of mural blood supply. A closed-loop obstruction refers to blockage of both afferent and efferent limbs of an obstructed segment, with a higher risk of bowel ischemia, which is often seen in volvulus or incarcerated hernias (Fig. 6–24). A strangulated obstruction refers to obstruction with impairment of blood supply, which usually occurs first in the venous outflow.

CLINICAL PRESENTATION

Clinical indicators of small bowel obstruction include nausea and vomiting, hyperactive followed by absent bowel sounds, progressive abdominal distention and pain, and absence of flatus and bowel movements.

IMAGING

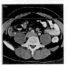

Radiology plays a major role in the evaluation of intestinal obstruction. Because radiographs often detect obstruction many hours before the clinical diagnosis can be made with confidence, they can delineate the level and often the etiology of obstruction, and they can be used to follow the course of obstruction over time.

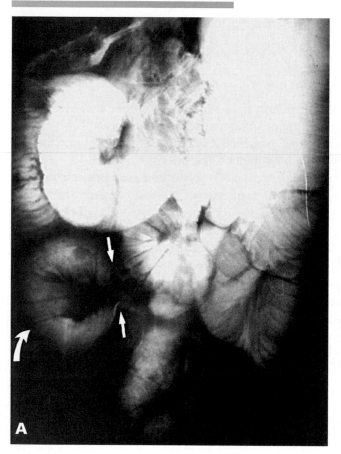
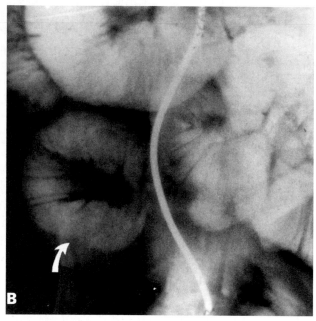

Figure 6–24. These films from a barium examination of the small bowel demonstrate two critical radiographic findings in small bowel obstruction. (**A**) The first, is a C-shaped segment of bowel (curved arrow), with tapering of both ends of the "C" (arrows), indicating a closed loop obstruction. (**B**) A spot film of the same area was obtained after placing a radiopaque marker over the course of an abdominal surgical scar, which convincingly demonstrates that the obstruction resulted from the protrusion of a loop of bowel (curved arrow) through the inlet of a surgical adhesion.

SMALL BOWEL OBSTRUCTION

The most common radiographic sign of small bowel obstruction is distention, which is visualized as dilated, air-filled segments of small bowel (measuring 3 cm or greater in diameter), with or without air-fluid levels. Air-fluid levels are sometimes divided into adynamic and dynamic varieties. Dynamic air-fluid levels appear as unequal heights of the fluid columns within the same loop of bowel. Dynamic air-fluid levels tend to indicate the presence of a mechanical obstruction (secondary to a distal point of luminal narrowing) (Fig. 6–25). By contrast, adynamic air-fluid levels are equal in height and tend to suggest the presence of an ileus, bowel distention secondary to reduced peristalsis. The most common causes of ileus include medication (opiate analgesics and anticholinergics), metabolic derangements (diabetes mellitus, hypokalemia, and hypercalcemia), and the postoperative state (which usually resolves within several days to a week). However, the distinction between dynamic and adynamic air-fluid levels is not a hard and fast one, and these findings should be regarded as merely suggestive in distinguishing between mechanical and nonmechanical obstructions.

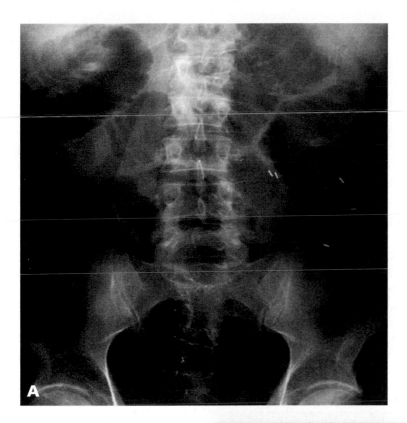

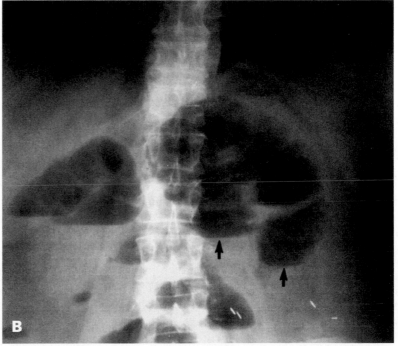

Figure 6–25. (A) Supine and (B) upright abdominal radiographs in a 58-year-old man who presented with vomiting and abdominal distention demonstrate multiple gas-distended, abnormally dilated segments of small bowel in the upper abdomen, with multiple dynamic air-fluid levels. The dynamic character of the air-fluid levels stems from the fact that individual loops contain fluid at different levels (arrows), and tends to suggest a mechanical obstruction. The etiology is revealed on the film, with multiple surgical clips and sutures. We can be confident that the dilated bowel is the small bowel and not the colon because we see valvulae conniventes completely traversing the lumen, and because the patient is status post near-total colectomy for ulcerative colitis. At surgery, obstructive postsurgical adhesions were lysed.

The level of obstruction can be estimated by assessing the number of dilated segments of bowel and the location at which the dilated segments terminate (Fig. 6–26). A proximal small bowel obstruction will produce relatively few dilated loops, which will be located predominately in the left upper quadrant. A distal small bowel obstruction will produce a greater number of dilated loops, extending down into the right lower quadrant. How does one determine whether loops of air-filled bowel are enteric or colonic? Generally, small bowel loops will exhibit valvulae conniventes extending all the way across their lumen, whereas the haustral markings of large bowel do not extend all the way to the luminal midline (Fig. 6–27).

A common cause of small bowel obstruction in elderly women is gallstone ileus, caused by erosion of a large gallstone through the gallbladder wall and into the duodenum, with passage into the distal small bowel and eventual impaction, usually in the ileocecal region. In the majority of cases, gallstone ileus will manifest radiographically as one or more of the findings of Rigler's triad, including dilated small bowel loops, air in the biliary tree (secondary to choledochoduodenal fistula), and a calcified gallstone outside the gallbladder fossa (Fig. 6–28).

Signs of intestinal ischemia include bowel wall thickening, effacement of folds, and, eventually, the appearance of intramural air (pneumatosis intestinalis), which may travel via the portal vein into the biliary tree. For the latter, frank necrosis has usually occurred (Fig. 6–29).

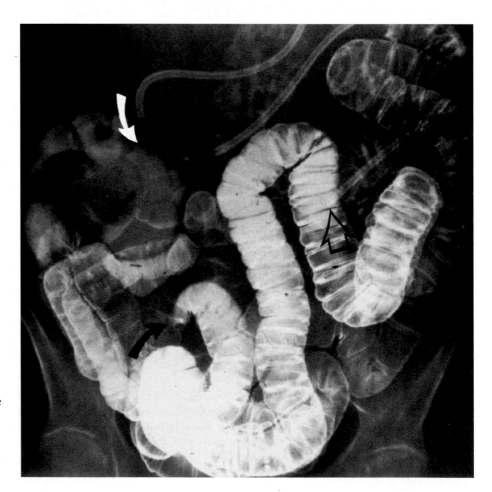

Figure 6–26. A technique such as enteroclysis removes all doubt about the level of intestinal obstruction. In this overhead view, the point of a partial small bowel obstruction secondary to an adhesive band is revealed by the gradual increase in barium density as it approaches the lesion and by the abrupt cut-off in the contrast column at the point of obstruction (curved arrow). Note the distal tip of the enteroclysis catheter (open arrow), which passes through the stomach, the duodenal "C" loop (white arrow), and into the proximal jejunum.

Figure 6–27. (A) Characteristic appearance of the fold patterns of the small bowel (including jejunal and ileal valvulae conniventes) and large bowel (haustrations). (B) Fold patterns on double contrast radiology.

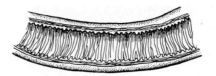

Small bowel w/valvulae conniventes

A

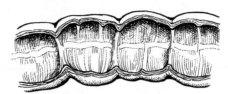

Large bowel w/haustrations

B

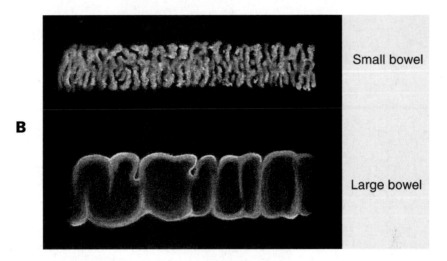

Small bowel

Large bowel

LARGE BOWEL OBSTRUCTION

Large bowel obstructions are generally more ominous than small bowel obstructions, because they tend to occur in older age groups and reflect more serious pathologies, such as malignancy. Nearly two-thirds of adult large bowel obstructions reflect the presence of a colon carcinoma, and pelvic malignancies such as cervical and ovarian carcinoma constitute the second most frequent offender (Fig. 6–30). A more benign process, diverticulitis, is the third most common cause. Other causes include sigmoid volvulus, in which the colon twists around its mesentery, fecal impaction, and ischemia.

The findings in colonic obstruction depend on whether the ileocecal valve is incompetent. If it is competent, distention will be confined to the colon, which cannot decompress into the small bowel, while if it is not competent, reflux of luminal contents into the small bowel will produce both colonic and distal small bowel distention. Regardless of the level of colonic obstruction, the cecum is the segment that dilates most, and when its diameter exceeds 10 cm, it is at risk for perforation. While plain films are often diagnostic, barium enema may be used to precisely localize and characterize the obstructing lesion prior to surgery.

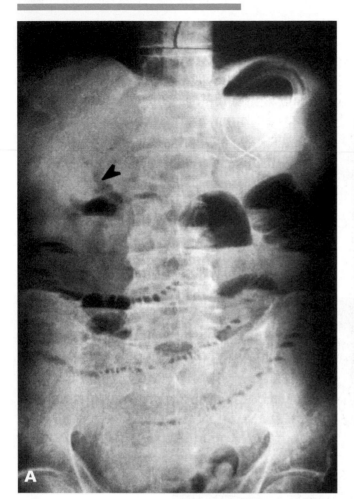

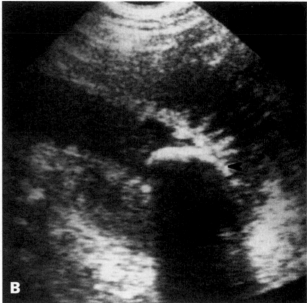

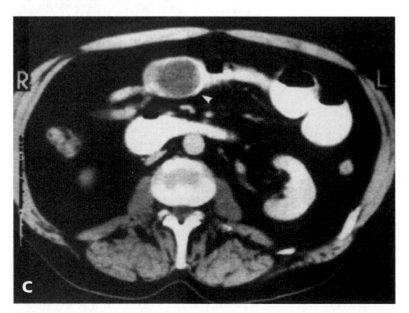

Figure 6–28. (A) An upright abdominal radiograph reveals multiple air-fluid levels within dilated segments of small bowel, as well as gas within the biliary tree (arrowhead). (B) A transabdominal ultrasound image from the left lower quadrant demonstrates a fluid-filled, distended segment of bowel containing a shadowing, echogenic focus at one end (a gallstone; arrowhead). (C) A transverse computed tomography image reveals the peripherally calcified stone impacted in a segment of small bowel (arrowhead). These findings are diagnostic of gallstone ileus.

Figure 6–29. (A) This frontal overhead film from a single-contrast barium enema demonstrates prominent fold thickening of the descending colon (arrows). In addition, there appears to be gas within the wall of a portion of this bowel (curved arrow). (B) A coned-down view of this region corroborates the presence of pneumotosis intestinalis (arrows). The differential diagnosis of fold thickening includes submucosal edema (as in ischemia or inflammatory bowel disease), submucosal hemorrhage (as in anticoagulation), and submucosal tumor (such as lymphoma). In this case, ischemia was the culprit. In what arterial distribution is this lesion? Distal to the splenic flexure, the blood supply to the colon is via the inferior mesenteric artery. In inferior mesenteric artery ischemia, occlusion due to thrombus or embolus is only rarely responsible, and most cases result from general hypoperfusion. Patients generally present with a diverticulitis-type picture, and most cases respond well to nonsurgical management. In contrast, patients with superior mesenteric artery ischemia are often very sick and require emergent surgery.

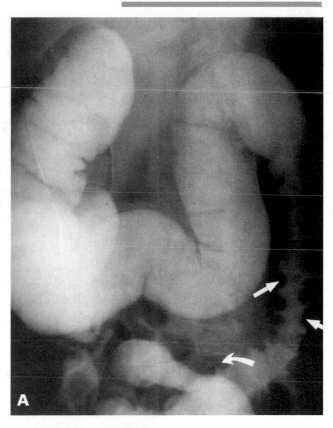

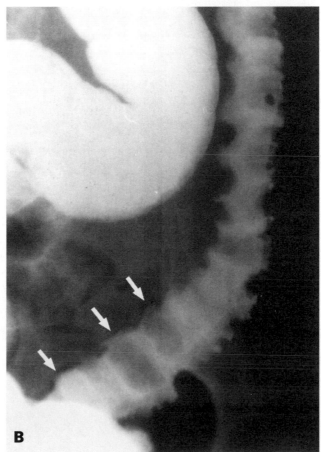

Figure 6–30. This supine abdominal radiograph reveals marked colonic distention, most
marked in the cecum. This obstruction resulted
from invasion of the sigmoid colon by metastatic ovarian carcinoma. The presence of multiple
gas-filled loops of small bowel indicates an
incompetent ileocecal valve, through which the
obstructed colon was able to decompress.

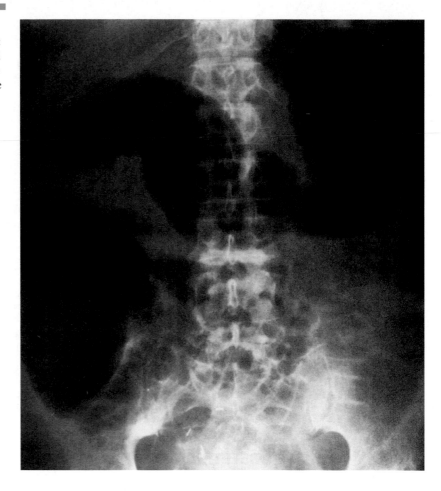

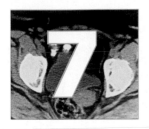

7 The Reproductive System

BREAST IMAGING

Anatomy and Physiology

Anatomically, the breast is a relatively simple structure, consisting primarily of skin, supportive elements (Cooper's ligaments), fat, the nipple-areolar complex, and ductal and lobular tissue (Fig. 7–1). The network of lactiferous (from the Latin *lac,* "milk") ducts branches out from the nipple and terminates in lobules, each of which is made up of sac-like alveoli, where milk production occurs. The duct system remains rudimentary in the nongravid breast, but proliferates under the stimulation of high levels of estrogen (from the Latin *oestrus,* "frenzy") during pregnancy.

Mammary gland function depends on the secretion of prolactin-releasing hormone by the hypothalamus, which induces secretion of prolactin by the anterior lobe of the pituitary gland, as well as the secretion of oxytocin (from the Greek *oxys,* "quick," and *tokos,* "birth") from the hypothalamus, by way of the posterior pituitary. The word *mammary* is derived from the Latin, *mamma* (breast), from which the term *mammal* is derived. Prolactin stimulates milk production, while oxytocin stimulates

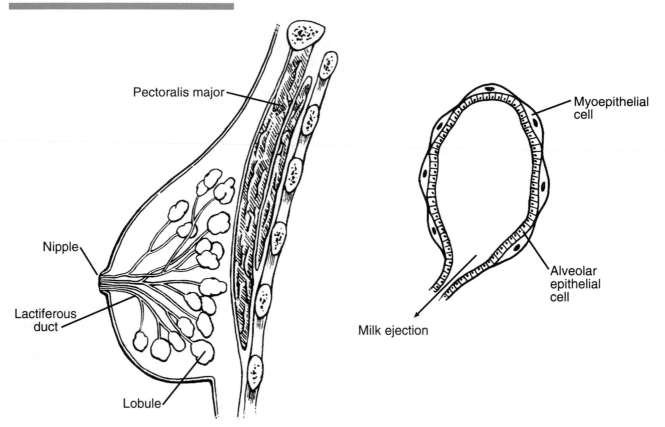

Figure 7–1. Anatomy of the breast and the terminal lobule. The lobule and its duct constitute the terminal lobular-ductular unit, from which the vast majority of breast cancers arise.

milk letdown, by inducing contraction of the myoepithelial cells surrounding the alveoli. Recall that oxytocin also stimulates uterine contractions during labor. Both prolactin and oxytocin are secreted in response to the nipple stimulation of suckling. The estrogen-dependent proliferation of tissue in the nonlactating breast also functions in sexual dimorphism, conferring a distinctively female appearance.

Pathology

BREAST CANCER

While all categories of pathology may manifest in the breast, the imaging diagnosis of breast disease is almost completely focused on a single pathologic entity: breast cancer. Interest in other types of lesions, including a variety of benign processes, stems largely from their ability to mimic cancer and the need to reliably distinguish benign from malignant disease.

EPIDEMIOLOGY

The importance of breast imaging is conveyed by the fact that breast cancer is the most common cancer of U.S. women, with approximately 185,000 new cases per year. It is second only to lung cancer as a cause of cancer death among women, resulting in

45,000 deaths annually. It has been estimated that as many as one in nine U.S. women will develop the disease during her lifetime, should she live long enough. The risk of breast cancer increases with age; very few cases are diagnosed in women under age 30 years, and the vast majority of patients are over age 50 years. Female gender is the greatest risk factor for breast carcinoma, as only 1% of cancers occur in men. In women, the single strongest risk factor for the development of breast cancer is a personal history of previous breast cancer. Additional risk factors include a first-degree relative with the disease, nulliparity or late parity, and exposure to large amounts of ionizing radiation, as in radiotherapy for lymphoma. However, approximately 70% of women diagnosed with breast cancer have no significant risk factors.

PATHOPHYSIOLOGY

 Infiltrating ductal carcinoma, accounting for approximately 80% of cases, is the most common type of breast cancer. These cancers arise from the epithelial cells that line the breast ducts (Fig. 7–2). Approximately 10% of breast cancers arise from the terminal lobules and are called lobular carcinomas. Medullary breast carcinoma arises from the supporting stromal cells of the breast, while mucinous carcinoma is associated with large amounts of cytoplasmic mucin. The latter two are generally larger than ductal and lobular carcinomas at the time of diagnosis, but enjoy a better prognosis, due to their lower propensity to metastasize. Paget's disease, a ductal carcinoma that has invaded the skin of the nipple, tends to be detected early and therefore also has a somewhat better prognosis. A prognostically less favorable type of breast cancer is inflammatory carcinoma, which represents an aggressive tumor that has invaded the dermal lymphatics, and presents clinically with prominent breast inflammation.

An important prognostic indicator in breast cancer is the level of estrogen and progesterone receptors expressed by the tumor. Tumors expressing higher levels of hormone receptors tend to be both more differentiated and more responsive to hormone deprivation. This explains the widespread use of tamoxifen (an anti-estrogen agent) in this disease, which is generally used in postmenopausal patients whose tumors express estrogen receptors.

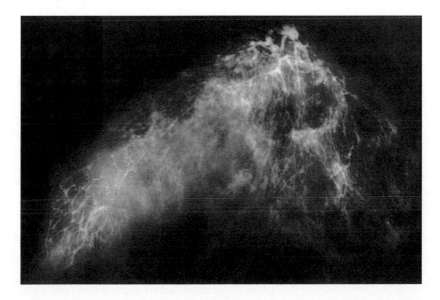

Figure 7–2. This normal galactogram demonstrates the ductal system of the breast. The examination is performed by cannulating the lactiferous sinuses at the nipple and injecting iodinated contrast material. This procedure is part of the workup for patients presenting with a nonmilky or bloody discharge, which can result from an intraductal mass.

A ductal carcinoma in situ is a tumor whose cells have not yet penetrated the basement membrane of the ducts. It is thought that nearly all breast cancers arise in the terminal duct-lobular unit, beginning as ductal or lobular carcinoma in situ, which at some point becomes invasive. When a carcinoma in situ is detected, local treatment to the breast is generally considered adequate. In contrast, local therapy generally does not suffice for invasive ductal carcinoma, which has a propensity to metastasize hematogenously and via the lymphatics. Invasive carcinoma is treated with a combination of local and systemic therapy.

Local therapy may consist of mastectomy alone or lumpectomy with radiation. Both generally involve an axillary nodal dissection for staging. In patients with large tumors and small breasts, conservative therapy (lumpectomy) is less likely to produce an acceptable cosmetic result. Adjuvant therapy is intended to irradicate micrometastases and is employed in most premenopausal patients and in those postmenopausal patients whose tumors do not exhibit estrogen receptors.

CLINICAL PRESENTATION

The goal of breast cancer screening is to diagnose breast cancer in patients who have not yet developed clinical signs or symptoms of the disease. By the time symptoms and signs have developed, the tumor has usually become invasive and the prognosis is less favorable. The most typical clinical presentation of breast cancer is a painless breast mass. Many women feel soft lumps within their breasts, which are sometimes painful and may wax and wane with the menstrual cycle; such findings are almost always benign. On the other hand, a hard, nontender, unchanging or slowly growing mass is of concern. Other clinical findings of breast cancer include changes in the contour of the breast, skin thickening, a new bloody nipple discharge, and axillary or supraclavicular adenopathy.

The trend toward conservative therapy has increased the importance of the radiologist in the detection and management of breast cancer, for two reasons. First, this option is only available when the disease is detected at an early stage (Fig. 7–3). Second, prior to therapy, the remainder of the involved breast and the contralateral breast must be exonerated. A patient with multicentric breast cancer (multiple lesions more than 2 cm apart) is a poor candidate for conservative therapy.

IMAGING

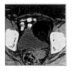 While no effective means of preventing breast cancer is at hand, the prospects for patient survival can be dramatically improved by detecting the disease early in its course through screening. Ten-year survival rates in women whose lesions are small (> 2 cm), and therefore likely not to have spread at the time of diagnosis, are better than 90%, while larger cancers, which are more likely to have metastasized, fare more poorly. The number of cells in a breast cancer has a typical doubling time of approximately 3 to 6 months.

Mammography

Mammography consists of highly tailored plain radiographs of the breast. It detects more than 90% of breast cancers, many before they become palpable. By far the most important role of mammography is to screen asymptomatic patients for breast cancer at an early stage, when most lesions are curable. Large trials of annual screening mam-

Figure 7–3. This coned down view of a mediolateral oblique mammogram demonstrates a very obvious spiculated mass that measures 5 cm in diameter and is associated with thickening of the areola and retraction of the nipple. While mammography easily demonstrates this infiltrating carcinoma, this does not represent the optimal use of the mammogram. The lesion has been detected far too late, when it should be easily detectable on physical examination, and is beyond the point at which it would likely be curable.

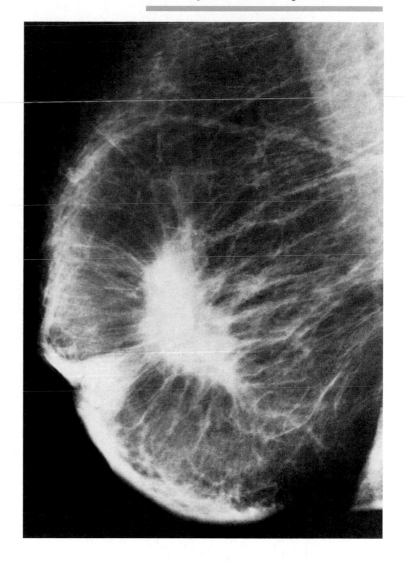

mography indicate that breast cancer mortality can be decreased by as much as 70%. Current guidelines call for women between the ages of 40 and 49 years to receive a mammogram every 1 to 2 years, and for women age 50 years and older to receive annual mammograms. Because the lead time to detect cancer at a curable stage tends to be shorter in younger patients, another sensible approach would be annual mammography between the ages of 40 and 70 years, with mammograms every 2 years thereafter. Nearly 10% of breast cancers are detected not by mammography but by palpation; hence, monthly self-examination and annual physician examination are also recommended. Lesions must be at least 1.5 to 2 cm in diameter to be palpable.

Mammography is also indicated in patients presenting with a bloody nipple discharge or a palpable mass, to find and characterize the responsible lesion. In addition, it is important to search both breasts for other lesions. Conservative therapy is contraindicated, for example, in patients with cancers in multiple quadrants of the breast.

The risk of cancer due to the ionizing radiation dose to the breast in mammography appears to be negligible in women over the age of 40 years. It is estimated that the risk of breast cancer death from a mammogram may be as high as 1 to 2 per million, while the risk of death from spontaneous breast cancer is between 700 and 1000 per million. The risk of radiation-induced breast cancer is inversely correlated with age, while the risk of death from spontaneous breast cancer is directly correlated with age—hence, the recommendation that annual screening commence between the ages of 40 and 50 years.

The standard screening mammogram includes two views of each breast: the craniocaudal view and the mediolateral oblique (MLO) view (Fig. 7–4). In both cases, the name of the view describes the course of the X-ray beam through the breast; for example, the MLO view is angled from superomedial to inferolateral. To obtain optimal visualization, the technologist must mobilize, elevate, and pull the breast forward to place as much of the breast as possible over the film cassette; any portions of the

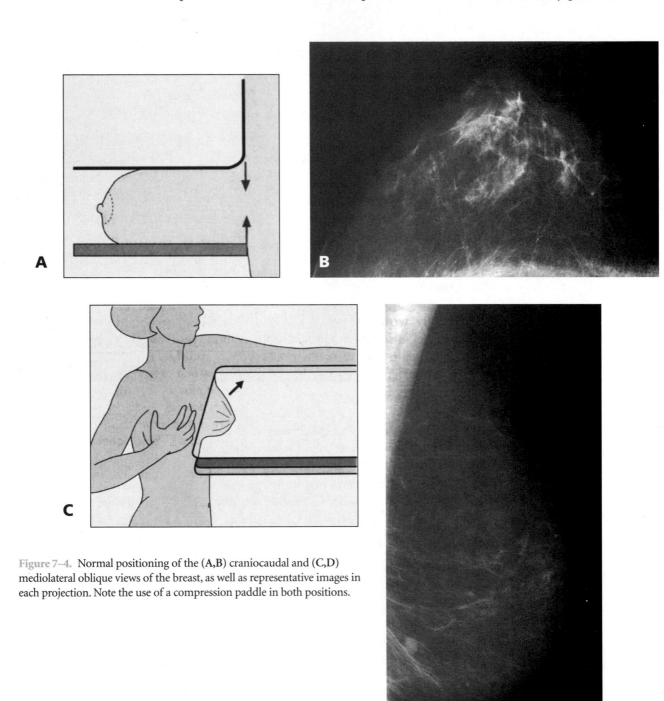

Figure 7–4. Normal positioning of the (A,B) craniocaudal and (C,D) mediolateral oblique views of the breast, as well as representative images in each projection. Note the use of a compression paddle in both positions.

breast not visualized on the film constitute "blind spots" for cancer detection. Compression of the breast spreads apart otherwise overlapping structures, reduces motion artifact (produced when the patient moves during the 1- to 2-second interval during which the film is exposed), minimizes unsharpness by placing breast structures as close as possible to the film, and minimizes radiation dose.

Once a possible abnormality is detected, additional views, including other projections (such as a lateral view), spot compression views, and magnification views, may be obtained. Palpable abnormalities are often marked with a radiopaque BB to facilitate correlation with the physical findings. Comparison with previous films is highly valuable, because stability tends to imply benignity, while lesions that increase in size or the aggressiveness of their appearance are generally worrisome. The principles of mammographic interpretation are relatively straightforward, although practice is considerably more complex. The mammographer seeks to identify such abnormalities as masses, calcifications, architectural distortions, and adenopathy.

Signs of malignancy

While the size and number of masses is important, the critical characteristic of a mass is its margins, which represent the radiologic signature of a lesion's biologic behavior. Ill-defined and irregular margins indicate infiltrative behavior and likely represent malignancy, while well-defined, regular margins suggest benignity. The margins of a classic breast cancer are spiculated, meaning that strands of tissue are seen to radiate outward in a stellate (star-like) pattern from the mass (Fig. 7–5). Histologically, spiculation represents a combination of tumor cells infiltrating out into surrounding tissue

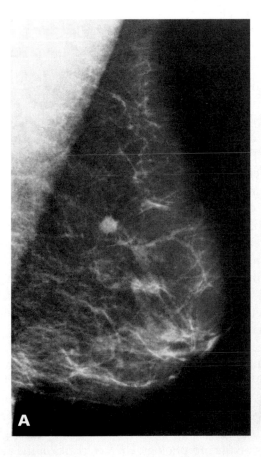
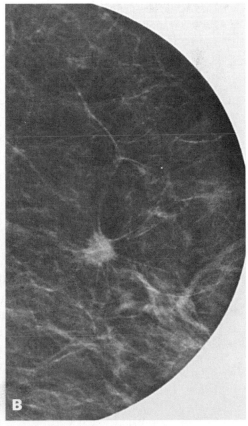

Figure 7–5. (A) A mediolateral oblique mammogram in this asymptomatic patient demonstrates a small mass in the upper inner quadrant of the left breast. (B) A magnified view demonstrates a stellate appearance, with a solid center and radiating spicules. Histology was infiltrating ductal carcinoma.

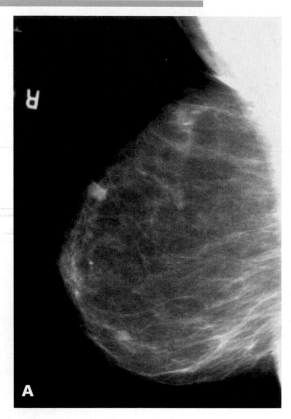 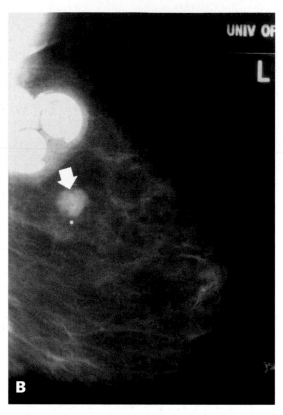

Figure 7–6. A 63-year-old woman being treated for multiple myeloma was found on a routine chest radiograph to have developed multiple pulmonary nodules (not shown). Her clinician palpated a mass in the left breast and suspected a primary breast carcinoma. The palpable lesion was marked with a BB (arrow on lesion). Mediolateral oblique views of the (**A**) right and (**B**) left breasts demonstrate multiple bilateral well-circumscribed nodules. Biopsy of the palpable lesion revealed multiple myeloma. Note the double-lumen chemotherapy infusion port in the left chest wall.

and fibrotic reaction to the tumor's presence. However, all spiculated masses are not malignant, and this appearance may also be seen in areas of scarring due to previous trauma or surgery. Before films are taken, sites of previous biopsies or lumpectomies should be marked with radiopaque BBs. In young and middle-aged patients, multiplicity of masses tends to indicate benignity (either cysts or fibroadenomas), while in older patients, metastases must be considered (Fig. 7–6).

The other primary mammographic sign of malignancy is calcification, and approximately one-half of all mammographically detected malignancies are found through the presence of suspicious microcalcifications. Calcification as such is not usually worrisome. Most breasts contain some type of calcification, and only certain types of microcalcifications tend to suggest malignancy (Fig. 7–7). Microcalcifications associated with carcinoma form a "cast" of the inner walls of the ductules and lobules of the tumor. The most worrisome types of calcification are fine, granular or branching, and pleiomorphic (heterogeneous) in morphology (Fig. 7–8). They invariably measure less than 2 mm in diameter and most are less than 0.5 mm. This is why mammographic technique has been developed to provide the highest spatial resolution of any radiologic examination, up to 20 or more line pairs per millimeter. When a suspicious cluster of microcalcifications is identified on standard views, additional spot magnification views are often obtained to provide better assessment of their number and morphology. In general, a mass containing suspicious microcalcifications has a 25 to 30% chance on biopsy of proving to be malignant, although the probability varies widely depending on the morphologic characteristics of the particular lesion.

Figure 7–7. The types of microcalcifications commonly seen on mammographic studies. Of these types, only linear and branching or pleiomorphic are strongly suggestive of malignancy.

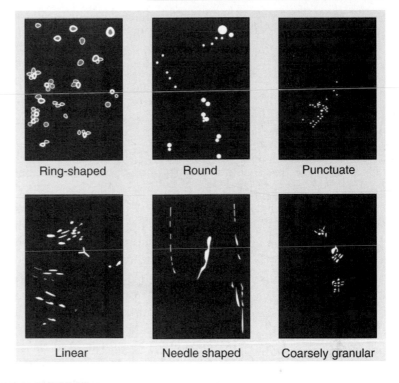

Ring-shaped   Round   Punctuate

Linear   Needle shaped   Coarsely granular

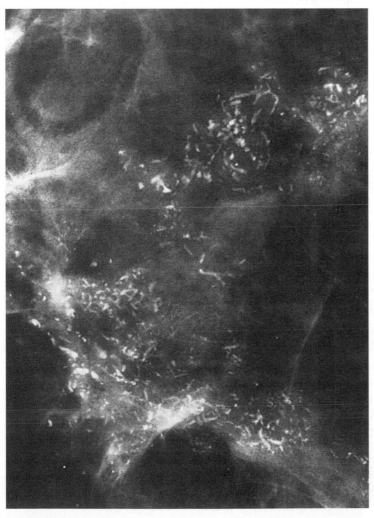

Figure 7–8. This magnified view demonstrates a dramatic appearance of malignant microcalcifications, with innumerable pleiomorphic linear and branching forms.

Secondary signs of malignancy include distortion of breast architecture, thickening or retraction of the skin or nipple, and asymmetry of breast tissue. Other than malignancy, a common cause of architectural distortion is previous trauma or surgery. Skin thickening and nipple retraction may be caused by tumor-related fibrosis, but can also be seen in benign conditions such as infection or disorders associated with edema such as congestive heart failure. Asymmetric dense tissue is seen in up to 5% of breasts. What is the difference between a mass and an asymmetric density? A mass does not change shape on different views, while an asymmetric density does. An asymmetry generally raises concern only if it is associated with a palpable abnormality or other mammographic abnormalities, especially if they are progressing over time.

Benign lesions

The relatively simple structures within the breast can give rise to numerous benign abnormalities, whose benignity can sometimes be proved only by tissue biopsy. The most common benign lesion is a simple cyst, which may be seen in up to one-half of examinations. These appear as rounded, sometimes lobulated lesions, and are usually multiple in number. When a worrisome lesion that could represent a cyst is identified mammographically, the diagnosis of simple cyst usually can be definitively established by ultrasound. As elsewhere in the body, a simple cyst will appear as an anechoic structure with sharply defined margins, round or oval in shape, and will demonstrate posterior acoustic enhancement (tissue directly behind it will appear somewhat brighter than adjacent tissue) (Fig. 7–9). If the appearance of the cyst is not classic, it may be aspirated under ultrasound guidance; complete disappearance with aspiration is also diagnostic, because it indicates that no solid tissue was present.

The most common solid benign lesion of the breast is a fibroadenoma, which probably represents estrogen-induced proliferation of normal lobular connective tissue. These masses occur during the reproductive years, often enlarging during pregnancy and involuting after menopause. In contrast to malignancies, fibroadenomas usually exhibit smooth, regular margins and are often round or oval in shape. One classic mammographic sign of a fibroadenoma is the presence of internal "popcorn" dystrophic calcification.

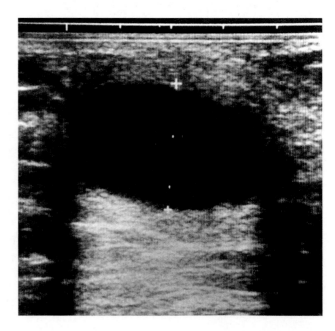

Figure 7–9. A 48-year-old woman had noticed enlargement of a mass in her left breast, which was readily palpable on physical examination. This sonographic image of the palpable lesion demonstrates the sonographic characteristics of a simple cyst, with no internal echoes, a smooth, oval shape, sharp margins, and posterior acoustic enhancement. The lesion was undetectable after aspiration, which yielded clear fluid.

Biopsy and staging

Once a suspicious mass is identified and a tissue diagnosis is needed, the radiologist plays several additional roles. First, mammographically or ultrasonographically guided fine needle aspiration and/or core needle biopsy can be performed to obtain tissue for pathologic analysis. These procedures offer a high rate of success, low cost, and low rate of complications. When a surgical approach to biopsy is chosen, the radiologist may perform a needle localization to guide the surgeon to nonpalpable lesions such as a suspicious cluster of microcalcifications. In the needle localization procedure, mammographic or ultrasonographic guidance is used to place a hooked wire within the lesion, which the surgeon then follows by palpation to locate the area of breast tissue to excise (Fig. 7–10).

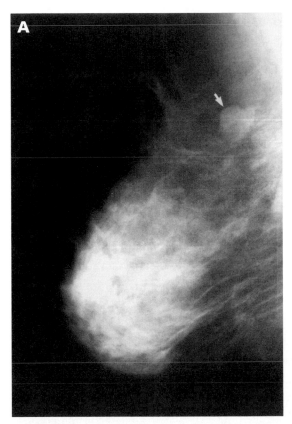

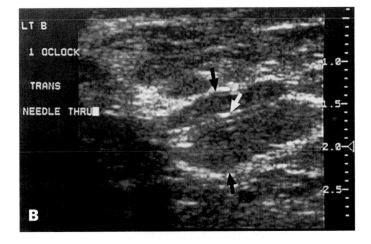

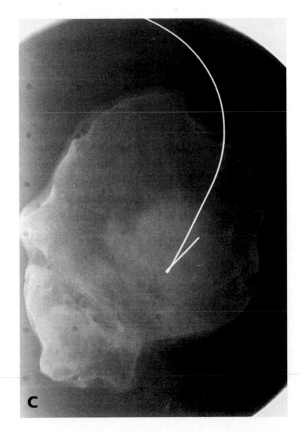

Figure 7–10. A middle-aged woman was found on screening mammography to have a new mass in the axillary tail of her right breast. (A) The right mediolateral oblique mammogram demonstrates the lobulated mass in the axillary tail (arrow). Because it had appeared since the previous examination 3 years earlier, the decision was made to excise the lesion. Since it was not palpable, needle localization was requested. (B) A sonographic image of the lesion (black arrows) demonstrates that a needle (white arrow) has been advanced through its center, through which a wire was advanced and left in place. The needle localized tissue was then surgically excised, and a (C) specimen radiograph was taken to ensure that the lesion had been removed. The specimen radiograph verifies that the lesion was included in the surgical specimen.

Once a cancer is discovered, several factors affect prognosis. These include not only size, but evidence of lymph node spread (especially involving the axilla) and distant metastases (often involving the lung, liver, skeleton, or central nervous system [CNS]). One of imaging's most important roles in the management of breast cancer lies in the staging of disease (looking for metastases in organs such as the liver, lungs, and skeleton), and in monitoring response to therapy (e.g., assessing the change in size of metastatic lesions after a course of chemotherapy). Plain radiographs of the chest and bones, nuclear medicine bone scans, and computed tomography (CT) of the head, chest, and abdomen constitute the most frequently employed modalities. Magnetic resonance imaging (MRI) may play a greater role in cancer detection and staging in the future and is currently employed in the evaluation of breast implants.

FEMALE PELVIS

Any time an imaging study of the pelvis is reviewed, it is important to follow an ordered search pattern to ensure that all major structures are dependably evaluated. The aortic bifurcation and iliac vessels should be traced out to rule out aneurysms, and their accompanying nodal chains should be inspected for adenopathy. Their venous counterparts should be inspected for the presence of thrombus. The distal gastrointestinal (GI) tract should be inspected for masses and mural abnormalities, as well as for the presence of surrounding ascites. The urinary tract, including the distal ureters and bladder, should be evaluated for masses, mural abnormalities, and evidence of obstruction. As always, bones and soft tissues should be inspected. In a male patient, special areas of attention include the size, shape, and brightness of the prostate gland, as well as the condition of periprostatic tissues. In a female patient, attention should be directed to the size, shape, and position of the uterus, cervix, and adnexa (from the Latin for "appended to") (Fig. 7–11).

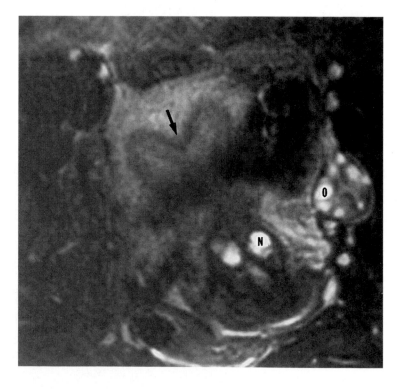

Figure 7–11. A 29-year-old woman presented with a history of infertility. A T2-weighted fast spin echo oblique coronal image from a pelvic magnetic resonance imaging examination demonstrates a septum partially dividing the endometrium into two canals (arrow), the result of a failure of resorption of the median septum during uterine development. In addition, two high signal intensity nabothian cysts (retention cysts) are seen in the cervix. Note the multiple high signal intensity follicles in the left ovary. N, nabothian cyst; O, ovarian follicle.

Anatomy and Physiology

The female pelvis contains the vagina, the cervix, the uterus, and the paired oviducts and ovaries (Fig. 7–12). The muscular, expansile vagina (from the Latin for "sheath") serves both as the female organ of copulation and the birth canal. The cervix (from the Latin for "neck") is the distal portion of the uterus that projects into the vagina and represents the site from which cells are scraped in a "Pap smear" (after George Papanicolaou) in an effort to detect cervical cancer at an early stage. The muscular, thick-walled uterus is responsible both for housing the developing embryo/fetus during gestation and for expelling it during parturition (from the Latin, *parere,* "to bring forth," from which the term *parity* is derived). The oviducts function to collect the ovum (from the Latin for "egg") from the ovary at ovulation, as the site of fertilization, and as the conveyors of the fertilized egg to the uterus. The ovaries perform the two expected gonadal (from the Greek *gone,* "seed") functions, gametogenesis (ovum production) and the secretion of sex hormones.

The female reproductive tract performs a greater variety of functions than its male counterpart. These include gametogenesis; receiving sperm; transporting both sperm and ova to the site of fertilization; transporting the fertilized ovum (zygote) to its endometrial site of implantation; sheltering and nourishing the developing fetus (with the aid of the placenta) until it can survive outside the mother's body; and parturition.

Female reproductive anatomy and physiology exhibit a notable cyclicity. In the male, gonadotropin secretion and spermatogenesis are pulsatile over hours but otherwise essentially constant, whereas female sex hormones display wide swings, and only one ovum is produced each menstrual cycle. In the first half of the menstrual cycle, the ovarian follicle secretes estrogens and low levels of progesterone, while in the second half, after a surge in leutinizing hormone levels stimulates ovulation, the corpus luteum (Latin for "yellow body") secretes estrogen and high amounts of progesterone to prepare the uterus for implantation. If fertilization does not occur, the corpus luteum involutes and the thickened uterine lining is sloughed at menstruation. Imaging findings such as the number and size of follicles in the ovaries, the presence of free fluid in the pelvic cul-de-sac (the peritoneal extension into the space between the uterus and rectum), and the thickness of the endometrial stripe are all hormonally mediated and markedly variable, depending on the phase of the menstrual cycle.

Pathology

Rather than attempt to review all categories of disease that may afflict each of the female pelvic organs in turn, this section focuses on several common clinical presentations and the role of imaging in their evaluation.

PELVIC MASSES

CLINICAL DATA

Palpable pelvic masses are a common clinical problem. In hospitalized patients of both genders, a distended urinary bladder is the most common culprit. In women, the most common cause of a pelvic mass is an enlarged uterus. In women of reproductive age, pregnancy is the most likely explanation, while leiomyomata are the most prevalent when postmenopausal patients are included. The next most common cause of a mass in the female pelvis is an ovarian cyst.

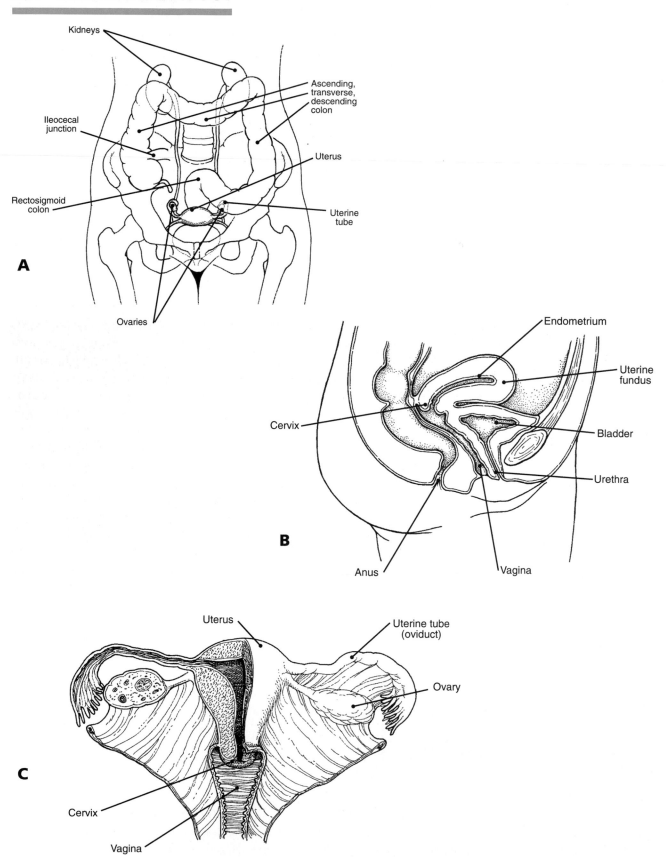

Figure 7–12. (**A**) Diagram depicting the close proximity of other physiologic systems (e. g., urinary and digestive systems) to the female reproductive organs. Multiple systems must be borne in mind when a patient presents with pelvic symptoms. (**B**) Sagittal and (**C**) coronal views of the key anatomic structures of the female reproductive system.

In order to evaluate a pelvic mass, certain aspects of the clinical history are crucial. The first question to be answered is simply whether the patient is pregnant. Pregnancy constitutes the single most common cause of pelvic masses in women under the age of 35 years. The second crucial bit of clinical data is the patient's age, because the likelihood of various lesions, both malignant and benign, varies dramatically depending on the age at presentation. Additional data that must be available if a pelvic mass is to be adequately evaluated include the date of the last menstrual period, hormone use, previous surgery, and any symptoms the patient is experiencing.

IMAGING

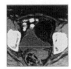

Ultrasound is by far the most important radiologic modality in the evaluation of the pelvis, and alone is adequate to characterize more than 90% of lesions (Fig. 7–13). The crucial questions to be addressed by the sonographer include the following: Which anatomic structure is involved?

Figure 7–13. These (**A**) longitudinal and (**B**) transverse ultrasound images of the pelvis demonstrate the normal sonographic appearance of the pelvic structures. A: 1, filled urinary bladder; 2, uterus; 3, cervix; 4, vagina; 5, rectum. B: 1, filled urinary bladder; 2, uterus; 3, right ovary; 4, left ovary; 5, colon. (**C**) The planes in which images are normally obtained. Image A was obtained in plane I and image B was obtained in plane V.

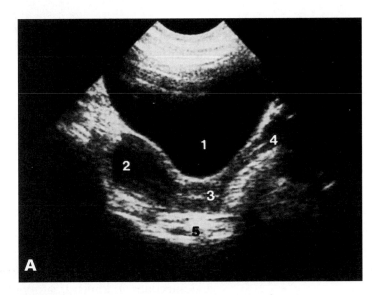

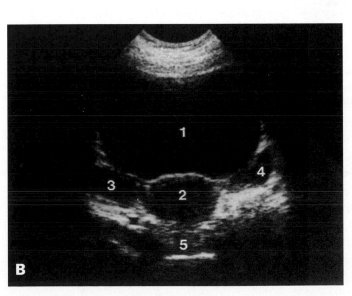

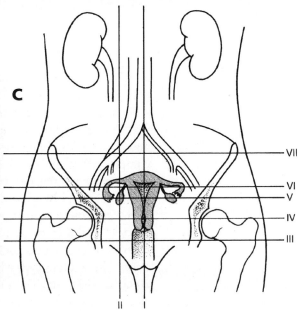

Figure 7–14. This frontal radiograph of the pelvis in a middle-aged woman demonstrates the classic "popcorn" appearance of cacifications within large uterine leiomyomata (arrows).

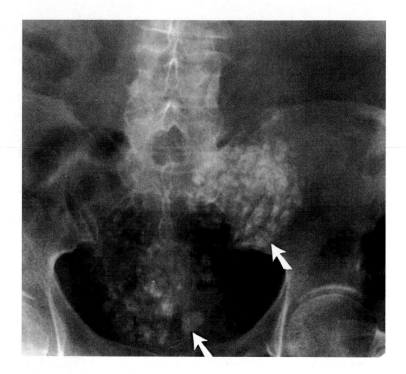

What are the imaging characteristics of the lesion? How is it changing over time? The most common pelvic masses, aside from pregnancy, include uterine leiomyomata ("fibroids"), ovarian cysts, pelvic inflammatory disease, endometriosis, and cancers of the ovary and uterus (Fig. 7–14). This discussion is organized around the different anatomic points of origin of pelvic masses.

Adnexal masses

A variety of benign processes may produce adnexal masses. The two most important categories of disease are "medical" (nonsurgical) conditions such as physiologic cysts and infectious and inflammatory processes and "surgical" processes, for which urgent surgical intervention should be considered.

"Medical" adnexal masses

Among the physiologic cysts, the most common are the follicular cysts. These typically arise either from failure of a follicle to involute after ovulation or an anovulatory cycle. Follicular cysts also represent the most common cause of an ovarian mass in the neonate and can be traced to maternal estrogen stimulation. In most cases, they appear round and anechoic, fulfilling the sonographic criteria of a simple cyst. However, they may be complicated at any age by hemorrhage, and commonly present with pain. The presence of internal hemorrhage gives them a heterogeneous echotexture on ultrasound. The next most prevalent physiologic cyst is a corpus luteum cyst, typically formed by hemorrhage into the corpus luteum after ovulation (Fig. 7–15). These are usually larger than follicular cysts and often measure 5 to 10 cm in diameter. They are most common in the first months of pregnancy. High levels of human chorionic gonadotropin (HCG) may produce a theca lutein cyst, which is the largest of all ovarian cysts and may measure up to 20 cm in diameter. The finding of a theca lutein cyst should raise suspicion for either

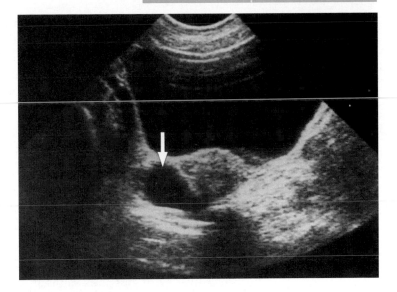

Figure 7–15. This transverse sonographic image of the pelvis demonstrates a nearly anechoic 2.4 cm cyst of the right adnexa, representing a corpus luteum cyst (arrow).

multiple gestations or gestational trophoblastic disease (hydatidiform mole or choriocarcinoma). Each of these lesions may have the appearance of a simple or complex cyst, and the differentiation must be based on clinical grounds.

Infectious causes of pelvic masses include nongynecologic processes such as appendicitis and diverticulitis, which can sometimes be distinguished from gynecologic processes on the basis of absence of cervical motion tenderness and purulent vaginal discharge. Pelvic inflammatory disease is the most common gynecologic cause. Risk factors include young age, history of previous salpingitis, and use of an intrauterine device. Patients may present with pain, vaginal discharge, abnormal bleeding, or peritoneal signs, depending on the stage of infection. Ultrasound is used primarily in assessing for signs of advanced disease. Visible oviducts are abnormal, and in hydrosalpinx one or both oviducts have a characteristic folded, tubular shape (Fig. 7–16). A tuboovarian abscess usually appears as an ill-defined mass with heterogeneous echotexture. Fluid is often seen in the cul-de-sac. The most common organisms are *Neisseria gonorrhoreae* and *Chlamydia trachomatis*.

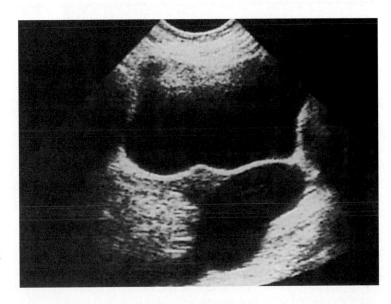

Figure 7–16. This transverse sonogram demonstrates behind the bladder a sausage-shaped, dilated, fluid-filled left oviduct, indicating the presence of a hydrosalpinx in association with pelvic inflammatory disease.

By far the most common inflammatory condition causing an adnexal mass is endometriosis, the presence of functional endometrial tissue outside the uterine cavity. Seen in 5% of premenopausal women, the incidence is much higher in series of infertility patients. The endometrial implants undergo expected changes with the menstrual cycle, with hemorrhage producing local inflammation and adhesions. Endometriosis usually presents with dysmenorrhea, chronic pelvic pain, dyspareunia, or infertility. In patients with minor disease, the lesions are often undetectable by imaging. In more severe cases, the ultrasound appearance is typically that of a cystic, hyperechoic mass, and it often proves indistinguishable from a hemorrhagic ovarian cyst.

"Surgical" adnexal masses

Ectopic pregnancy, the implantation of the fertilized egg outside the uterine cavity, occurs in approximately 1% of all pregnancies, with a peak incidence in the teens and twenties. Approximately 75,000 cases are diagnosed each year. The principal risk factor is a history of previous salpingitis, and 95% of ectopic pregnancies occur in the oviducts. Ectopic pregnancy has a 10% risk of recurrence. It accounts for 15% of all maternal deaths, and the risk of maternal death in ectopic pregnancy is 10 times greater than that of natural childbirth. Death results from massive hemorrhage following tubal rupture. Patients present with a classic picture of abnormal vaginal bleeding, pelvic pain, amenorrhea, and a palpable adnexal mass in only a minority of cases. Diagnostically, two critical questions must be answered, one clinical and one ultrasonographic: (1) Is the patient pregnant? (2) Is there an intrauterine pregnancy? If the answer to (1) is yes, and to (2) no, then the diagnosis of ectopic pregnancy must be strongly considered, and emergent surgery may be indicated.

Another important diagnostic tool in suspected ectopic pregnancy is the levels of HCG. Low levels of HCG are strongly suggestive of an ectopic pregnancy, which is corroborated on ultrasound by such features as a normal uterus with no gestational sac, free fluid in the cul-de-sac (from tubal bleeding), a complex adnexal mass, and the finding of a live embryo outside the uterus (diagnostic) (Fig. 7–17). A live extrauterine embryo is seen in approximately 25% of cases. If an intrauterine pregnancy is seen,

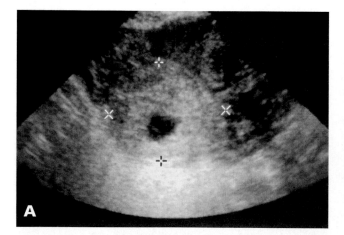
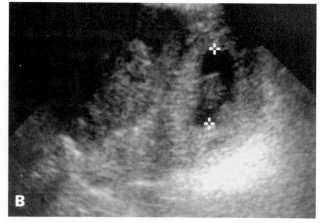

Figure 7–17. A 19-year-old woman with a positive pregnancy test presented complaining of pelvic pain and vaginal bleeding. Multiple transabdominal and transvaginal images of the uterus (not shown) demonstrated no intrauterine pregnancy. However, (**A**) transvaginal examination of the left adnexa in the coronal plane disclosed a thick echogenic ring of tissue surrounding a central fluid collection (delineated by measurement cursors), the so-called donut sign (marked by cursors). Color Doppler interrogation (not shown) revealed intense color flow within this annular tissue, the so-called ring of fire sign. (**B**) A magnified view of the central fluid collection demonstrated a fetal pole within a gestational sac (marked by cursors), with regular fetal heart tones (not shown; 180 beats per minute). The diagnosis is tubal pregnancy.

and the patient is not on fertility drugs (which increase the probability of multiple gestations), the diagnosis of ectopic pregnancy is essentially excluded, because concomitant intra- and extrauterine pregnancies are seen in only 1 in 7000 cases, even in patients at risk for multiple gestation.

Ovarian torsion may occur in a normal ovary, but more often occurs in an ovary enlarged by the presence of a cystic or solid mass. Torsion results from rotation of the ovary on its vascular pedicle, with venous and then arterial obstruction. It most commonly occurs in children and adolescents, and presents with pain and a palpable mass in half of patients. Ultrasound demonstrates an enlarged, heterogeneous ovary, and free fluid is often seen in the cul-de-sac. As in suspected testicular torsion, Doppler examination may be useful in demonstrating decreased or absent blood flow on the affected side.

Benign versus malignant neoplasms

Pregnancy excluded, the essential distinction to be made in the diagnostic workup of most adult adnexal masses is whether they are likely to represent malignancy. The case in which this question can be answered firmly in the negative is that of the simple cyst. Physiologic cysts may measure up to 3 cm in diameter, and demonstrate cyclical change in size with the menstrual cycle. No follow-up is required, so long as the cyst measures less than 3 cm and the patient is premenopausal. If the patient is postmenopausal, follow-up in 2 to 3 months is indicated. The premenopausal patient requires such follow-up only for cysts measuring between 3 and 5 cm. When the finding represents a cyst measuring more than 5 cm, or a solid mass of any size, tissue will need to be obtained. Many of these lesions will turn out to be pedunculated benign uterine leiomyomata simulating an adnexal mass, but there is no way to make this determination without histology. Tissue is obtained surgically, either by laparoscopy or, if the probability of malignancy is considered higher, by laparotomy.

At least 80% of adnexal tumors are benign and usually present in women between the third and fifth decades. While numerous types of lesions are known, the most interesting from a radiologic point of view is the dermoid cyst, also sometimes referred to as a benign cystic teratoma. These tumors generally appear in a somewhat lower age range, in the teens and twenties. Fortunately, they represent the most common ovarian neoplasm in the reproductive years. Strictly speaking, a teratoma represents a tumor containing all three cell types—ectoderm, mesoderm, and endoderm—while a dermoid contains only ectodermal elements. Depending on the maturity of the ectodermal elements in these tumors, they often contain structures such as hair, bone, and teeth. Calcified elements including teeth are sometimes visible on abdominal plain films, and the finding of fat within the lesion on CT is also virtually diagnostic (Fig. 7–18). A common ultrasound appearance is that of a cystic lesion with a mural nodule, which often contains fluid–fluid levels.

Ovarian carcinoma is the fifth leading cause of cancer death among American women, resulting in approximately 25,000 new cases and 15,000 deaths per year. This translates to a lifetime risk of approximately 1 in 70 women, although the risk is increased in patients with a positive family history or a history of prior breast cancer. Symptoms are relatively uncommon prior to dissemination, rendering regular pelvic examination with palpation of the adnexa a key to early diagnosis. Because epithelial cells on the surface of the ovary are the source of 90% of malignant ovarian tumors, and these cells are readily shed into the peritoneal cavity, approximately three-quarters of patients present with disseminated disease. Symptoms and signs of dissemination include constipation, edema, invasion of adjacent structures such as the uterus or rec-

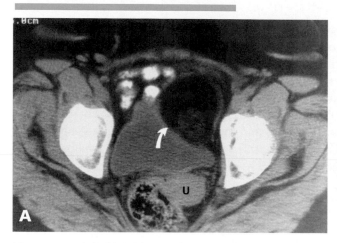
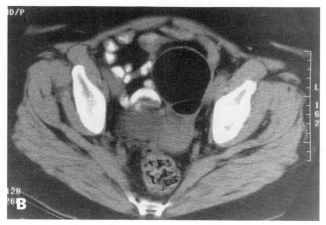

Figure 7–18. **(A)** This axial image from a computed tomography scan of the pelvis reveals a large, well-circumscribed mass indenting the anterolateral aspect of the urinary bladder on the left (arrow). The mass has a clearly defined, regular soft tissue capsule and contains mainly fat-density tissue (–80 Hounsfield units), with a slightly higher density central component. **(B)** Another image at a slightly more inferior level demonstrates an exclusively fat-density lesion containing a single septation. These findings are diagnostic of an ovarian dermoid, and effectively rule out the possibility of malignancy.

tum, ascites, and pleural effusions. CA 125 levels are elevated in approximately 80% of patients.

Common types of epithelial ovarian malignancies include mucinous and serous cystadenocarcinomas. The principal roles of imaging are to identify lesions warranting surgery for histologic characterization and to stage known carcinoma. On ultrasound, carcinomas typically exhibit a cystic appearance, ranging from simple unilocular cysts to complex multilocular cystic lesions containing considerable solid elements (Fig. 7–19). In general, the more solid tissue visualized, the more likely the lesion is to prove malignant. A significant percentage of tumors are bilateral. The primary route of spread is peritoneal seeding, with implants on the omentum producing a characteristic pattern of "omental caking." Ascites argues strongly in favor of implants on the

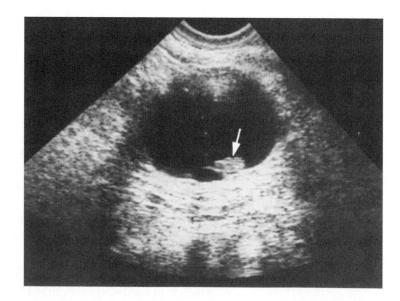

Figure 7–19. This sonographic image of the left ovary demonstrates a predominantly cystic mass of the left ovary, which contains a central septation. However, it also contains a mural nodule of solid tissue (arrow). At surgery, a proliferating serous cystadenoma was found, which likely represents a premalignant lesion.

omentum, bowel mesentery, or peritoneal membrane. Hematogenous spread to lungs and liver tends to occur late.

Uterine masses

The three most important masses involving the uterus are leiomyomata, endometrial carcinoma, and cervical carcinoma. Leiomyomata ("fibroids") represent the most common uterine tumors, seen in more than one-quarter of women over the age of 35 years. Most are located within the myometrium, although they may also arise from the submucosa (in which case they are very likely to produce symptoms) or the subserosa (which often results in a pedunculated tumor). Due to their estrogen sensitivity, they often enlarge during pregnancy and tend to regress at menopause. Most lesions are asymptomatic, although patients may present with abnormal bleeding, pain, and infertility. On ultrasound, most leiomyomata tend to be hypoechoic, multiple, and may deform the uterine contour. On plain film and CT, they often contain coarse calcifications. On MRI, they tend to be hypodense relative to the uterus on T2-weighted images, although cystic degeneration may produce areas of hyperintensity (Fig. 7–20).

Endometrial hyperplasia is a precursor to endometrial carcinoma. Hyperplasia occurs with unopposed estrogen stimulation, as seen in exogenous estrogen therapy, anovulation, and estrogen-producing tumors. Tamoxifen, which is often employed in breast cancer therapy, possesses weak estrogenic activity and is therefore associated with endometrial hyperplasia. Risk factors for endometrial carcinoma are similar to those of breast cancer, and include nulliparity, early menarche and late menopause, and ovulatory failure. The histology of endometrial carcinoma is adenocarcinoma. On

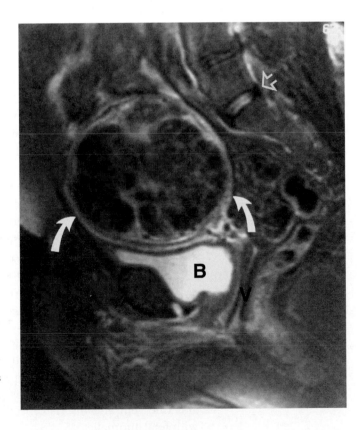

Figure 7–20. A 50-year-old woman presented with a large pelvic mass. A T2-weighted sagittal magnetic resonance image of the pelvis demonstrates a large, round, well-circumscribed, predominately hypointense but heterogeneous mass arising from the uterus (curved arrows). Note the high-intensity signal of the urine in the bladder (B) inferiorly and intervertebral discs posteriorly (open arrow). Hysterectomy confirmed a large fibroid uterus. v = vagina.

ultrasound, endometrial hyperplasia appears as thickening of the echogenic endometrial stripe. In a premenopausal women, a thickness of 15 mm is sufficient to warrant biopsy, while in the postmenopausal patient, the same recommendation would follow for a thickness greater than 5 mm. Findings of endometrial carcinoma include a thickened endometrial stripe, and the presence of fluid within the endometrial cavity (hydrometria) due to cervical obstruction.

Deaths due to cervical carcinoma have been dramatically reduced due to the widespread practice of annual Pap tests. Risk factors include multiple sex partners and a history of sexually transmitted diseases. Human papilloma virus is implicated as an etiologic factor. In contrast to endometrial carcinoma, cervical carcinoma is of squamous cell histology. Findings include endometrial fluid collections and masses arising from the cervix. CT is commonly employed in staging.

OBSTETRICAL IMAGING

Anatomy and Physiology of Pregnancy

After ovulation, an egg requires approximately 4 to 5 days to travel through the oviduct into the uterine cavity. It remains fertile for only 24 hours, meaning that fertilization must take place in the ampullary (most lateral) portion of the tube. Once fertilized, the zygote begins to divide, reaching the blastocyst stage by the time it implants in the endometrial lining of the uterus, approximately 7 days after ovulation. During this time, the ruptured graafian follicle in the ovary gives rise to the corpus luteum, which produces the estrogen and progesterone (from the Latin *pro*, "before," *gestatio*, "carry," and the chemical terms *sterol*, "from cholesterol," and *one*, "ketone"), necessary for the maintenance of pregnancy during the first 10 weeks. The corpus luteum requires the stimulation of HCG, which is synthesized by the chorion. HCG is the hormone detected by most pregnancy tests, and its levels double approximately every 2 to 3 days. After 10 weeks, the placenta (from the Greek *plakos*, "flat cake") takes over the production of estrogens and progesterones, and the corpus luteum involutes. After that point, castration is compatible with a normal pregnancy outcome.

At implantation, the outermost layer of the blastocyst, the trophoblast, releases proteolytic enzymes that allow it to burrow into the endometrium. In response, the surrounding endometrial tissue becomes increasingly vascular (corresponding to increased echogenicity on ultrasound), and is called the decidua (Fig. 7–21). The digestion of decidual cells by the trophoblast supplies energy to the growing embryo until the formation of the placenta. Important membranes in the developing products of conception include the amnion, the fluid-filled cavity that cushions the embryo; the chorion, with which the enlarging amnion eventually fuses; and the yolk sac, which is located outside the amniotic cavity but within the chorionic cavity and is connected to the primitive gut by the omphalomesenteric duct (which may persist into postnatal life as a Meckel's diverticulum). The yolk sac is involved in early hematopoiesis, and a portion of it is incorporated into the primitive gut. The placenta becomes well established and operational by approximately 5 weeks after implantation, interlocking the fetal (chorionic) and maternal (decidual) circulations, and allowing for the exchange of nutrients and waste products. The umbilical cord normally contains two arteries and one vein and inserts centrally on the placenta. Two-vessel cords are associated with fetal anomalies.

Figure 7–21. The state of the embryo, membranes, and uterus at the 7th week of gestation.

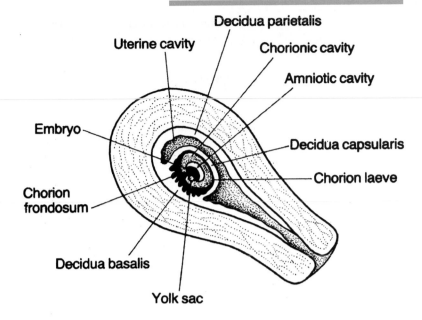

Uterine cavity

Decidua parietalis

Chorionic cavity

Amniotic cavity

Embryo

Decidua capsularis

Chorion laeve

Chorion frondosum

Decidua basalis

Yolk sac

Imaging

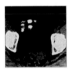

Because ultrasound involves no ionizing radiation and allows real-time assessment of a number of obstetrical parameters, it constitutes the preferred imaging technique of pregnancy (Fig. 7–22). Most patients can be examined transabdominally. Patients early in pregnancy are encouraged to drink several glasses of water prior to the examination to fill the urinary bladder, which provides an excellent acoustic window on the pelvis. In patients with a retroverted uterus, a transvaginal approach may be necessary, at least early in pregnancy.

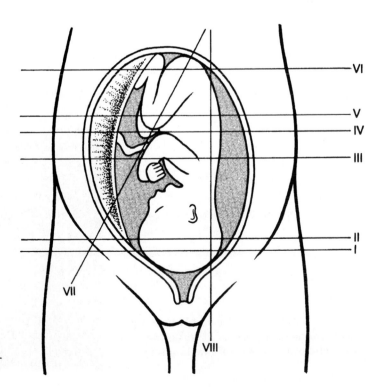

Figure 7–22. The scan planes for evaluating various parameters of a fetus in cephalic presentation. I, lateral ventricles; II, head circumference; III, chest circumference; IV, abdominal circumference; V, fetal kidneys; VI, urinary bladder; VII, femur length; VIII, spine.

Generally, the rationale for the examination differs depending on whether it is performed in the first trimester of pregnancy or thereafter.

FIRST TRIMESTER

Indications for imaging in the first trimester include: to confirm an intrauterine pregnancy; to evaluate a suspected ectopic pregnancy; to define the cause of vaginal bleeding of uncertain etiology; to estimate gestational age; to assess the number of gestations; to confirm embryonic life; to aid in the performance of chorionic villus sampling or amniocentesis; and to evaluate the uterus and any pelvic masses. The key determination to be made in the first trimester is the presence or absence of an intrauterine pregnancy. The determination of gestational age is another important consideration, in part because up to one-quarter of patients are uncertain about the date of their last menstrual period, especially those with irregular menstrual cycles. In general, the embryo should be detectable by transabdominal scanning by the sixth or seventh week of gestation. If the embryo is seen, it should be possible to detect heart motion, which indicates viability.

The earliest finding of pregnancy on prenatal ultrasound is the presence of a gestational sac, which normally becomes visible by ultrasound when it is 2 mm in diameter, at about 28 to 30 days of pregnancy. Though not as accurate as the crown–rump length, the length of pregnancy can be approximated by the mean sac diameter (MSD). The number of days of pregnancy roughly equals the MSD plus 30 days. The yolk sac and fetal heart beat both become visible near week 5.

The key questions to be answered in every first trimester examination include the location of the gestational sac, the presence of an embryo, and the crown–rump length, which allows the most accurate estimation of gestational age. When the embryo is first detectable, it is not possible to determine which end is the crown and which the rump, but the measurement of the longest axis is sufficient. The first-trimester crown–rump length measurement provides an accurate measure of gestational age to within 5 to 7 days and is used in conjunction with the last menstrual period to calculate the expected date of confinement (Fig. 7–23). It can be compared to the diameter of the gestational

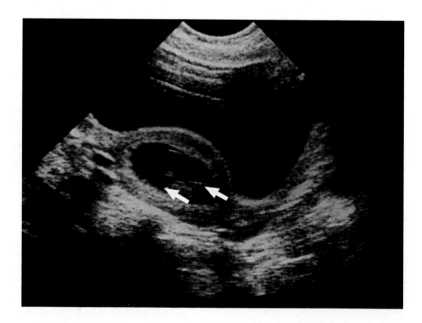

Figure 7–23. This longitudinal sonogram demonstrates a crown–rump length of 2.5 cm (arrows), which corresponds to a fetus of 9 weeks gestation.

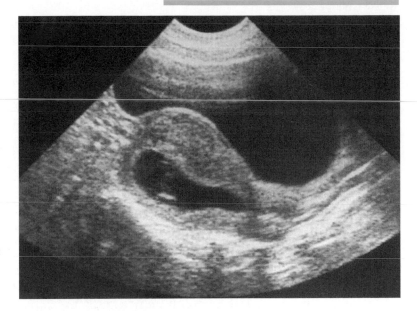

Figure 7–24. This longitudinal sonogram of the pelvis in an 11 week pregnancy demonstrates descent of the gestational sac and abnormal dilatation of the internal cervical os, indicating a threatened abortion progressing to an inevitable abortion.

sac, which can be identified by 5 weeks. Other important data include the number of gestations and the presence or absence of heart activity. The maternal pelvis should also be examined, including the size of any uterine fibroids or other pelvic masses. Extensive fibroids may contribute to spontaneous abortion.

VAGINAL BLEEDING

An important indication for prenatal ultrasound is vaginal bleeding. Threatened abortion refers to vaginal bleeding in the presence of a closed cervical os during the first 20 weeks of pregnancy. Approximately one-half of these pregnancies will end in spontaneous abortion. Spontaneous abortion refers to vaginal bleeding with the passage of tissue; in a high percentage of cases, the fetal tissues are found to harbor chromosomal abnormalities. An inevitable abortion is diagnosed when there is vaginal bleeding and an open cervical os (Fig. 7–24). Incomplete abortion refers to continued vaginal bleeding due to retained products of conception and is often an indication for dilation and curettage. Finally, missed abortion refers to embryonic death with no spontaneous abortion. The most important criterion of fetal death is the absence of cardiac activity in an embryo of at least 5 mm crown–rump length (Fig. 7–25).

The differential diagnosis of vaginal bleeding includes a number of possibilities. By far the most important diagnosis to exclude in threatened abortion is ectopic pregnancy, which has been discussed in the section on pelvic masses. It is worth reiterating that a normal (nongravid) transvaginal ultrasound does not exclude the diagnosis of ectopic pregnancy, but the finding of a normal intrauterine pregnancy virtually does, unless the mother is taking fertility drugs. Other differential possibilities in vaginal bleeding include inevitable abortion, incomplete abortion, and missed abortion, as well as a blighted ovum (an anembryonic pregnancy).

GENETIC SCREENING

Under certain circumstances, imaging may be employed to assist in the acquisition of tissue for genetic screening. Indications include maternal age over 35 years, a history of other children with genetic defects, certain metabolic disorders such as diabetes,

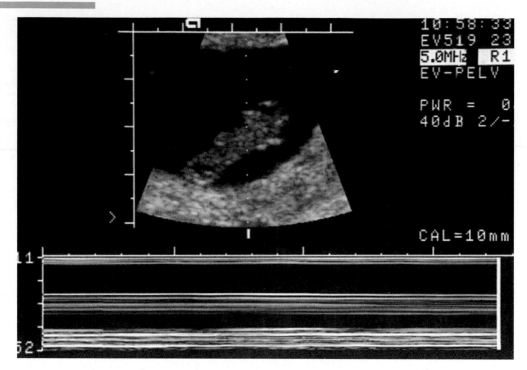

Figure 7–25. This patient's menstrual dating indicated a gestational age of approximately 12 weeks. However, the crown–rump length of this fetus indicated an age of only 8 weeks. Moreover, despite repeated attempts, no fetal heart activity could be detected, as indicated by the "flat line" tracing below. These findings indicate fetal demise and a missed abortion.

and exposure to teratogens or toxins. Another indication for genetic screening is an abnormality in maternal serum alpha-fetoprotein (AFP) levels. AFP is formed by the fetal liver, and levels in the maternal blood may be elevated when there is increased diffusion of AFP into the maternal blood, as in an open neural tube defect. Tissue can be obtained via amniocentesis (aspiration of amniotic fluid and culture of desquamated fetal cells), transcervical chorionic villus sampling, and fetal blood sampling, which allows the most rapid analysis of the fetal karyotype. Ultrasound is used to guide the biopsy needle.

Genetic screening may also be indicated by certain findings on obstetrical ultrasound. For example, the finding of a cystic hygroma in the cervical region has a high association with a variety of chromosomal abnormalities, including Turner's syndrome, trisomies 13, 18, and 21, and Noonan's syndrome ("male Turner's syndrome"). Cystic hygroma is found in 1 in 6000 pregnancies, and carries a poor prognosis (Fig. 7–26).

SECOND AND THIRD TRIMESTERS

In the second and third trimesters, assessment of fetal viability and number of gestations remain important, but new parameters come into play as well. An assessment of fetal presentation is helpful to the obstetrician, a cephalic (head down) presentation being the most common and most favorable for vaginal delivery. However, it must be borne in mind that many breech and transverse presentations will correct themselves by the time of delivery, at which point such lies are seen in only a few percent of cases.

The amount of amniotic fluid can be an important parameter of fetal well-being. Amniotic fluid volume is a dynamic quantity, with complete turnover every 3 to 4

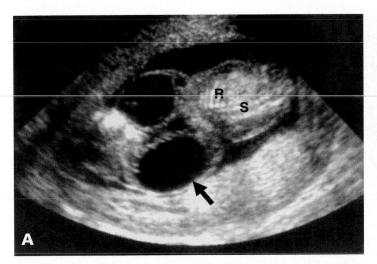 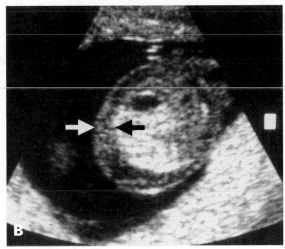

Figure 7–26. Routine obstetrical ultrasound examination in this 25-year-old woman with a gestational age of 20 weeks demonstrates evidence of fetal lymphatic obstruction and lymphedema. (A) A coronal image through the fetal thorax and head demonstrates large bilateral cervical cysts (arrow), representing cystic hygromas, which are caused by obstruction of flow in the jugular lymphatics. R, ribs; S, spine. In addition, (B) an axial image at the level of the stomach demonstrates considerable body wall thickening due to edema (arrows), measuring 1 cm in width. These findings are most commonly associated with Turner's syndrome, and amniocentesis confirmed an XO karyotype in this fetus. The constellation of cystic hygroma and fetal hydrops in a Turner's fetus is uniformly fatal.

hours, in part because the fetus can swallow up to one-half liter per day. One means of determining the amount of amniotic fluid is the so-called four-quadrant method, in which the largest fluid pocket in each of the four uterine quadrants is measured; a total between 5 and 20 cm is generally regarded as within normal limits (Fig. 7–27). An excess of amniotic fluid is called polyhydramnios, and is associated with fetal conditions that interfere with normal swallowing and absorption of amniotic fluid, such as CNS abnormalities and GI atresias. Additional and more common associations include maternal diabetes and hypertension. Oligohydramnios, too little amniotic fluid, is associated with decreased fetal urine output, as seen in renal agenesis, multicystic dysplastic kidney, and urinary tract obstruction. Obstruction of the urinary tract is seen most commonly at the ureteropelvic junction, although ureterovesical junction obstruction and posterior urethral valves are also important differential considerations (the latter in males). Oligohydramnios is associated with the Potter sequence, in which the paucity of amniotic fluid causes pulmonary hypoplasia and a characteristic facies (low-set ears, beaked nose, receding chin, etc.). Other causes of oligohydramnios include fetal demise, IUGR, and premature rupture of membranes.

The character of the placenta must be noted. The finding of a retroplacental hemorrhage represents a significant threat to fetal well-being, and proliferation of trophoblastic tissue beyond the normal endometrium can be associated with severe maternal hemorrhage at delivery. The location of the placenta must be determined, particularly as regards its relationship to the internal cervical os. When the placenta overlies the os, a placenta previa may be diagnosed. Placenta previa is associated with an increased risk of hemorrhage and fetal demise. However, such a diagnosis should not be entertained prior to 20-weeks gestation, as many apparent previas resolve spontaneously prior to that time. In some cases, emptying the bladder will reveal that an apparent placenta previa is in fact merely a low-lying placenta, which is not as hazardous.

Figure 7–27. This sonogram from a 22-week pregnancy demonstrates a normal amount of amniotic fluid separating the fetus on the viewer's left from the placenta on the right.

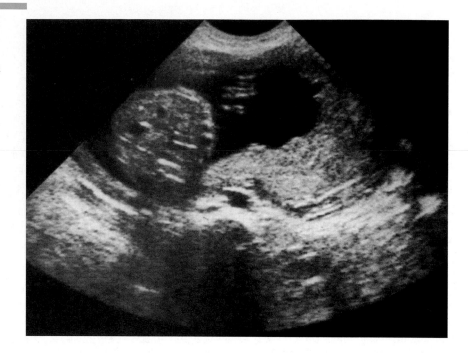

CENTRAL NERVOUS SYSTEM

The assessment of the fetal CNS begins with a search for neural tube defects, seen in 1 in 600 U.S. births. The two most common neural tube defects are anencephaly and myelomeningocele. Anencephaly (Latin, "without head"), absence of the cranial vault, is an invariably lethal condition, and is recognized as an absence of the cranium above the level of the orbits (Fig. 7–28). Myelomeningocele is more common in the British Isles and in women over 35 years of age. Like anencephaly, it is associated with increased maternal serum AFP. Failure of closure of the caudal neuropore most often results in separation of the posterior lamina of the lumbosacral spine, with a dorsally protruding leptomeningeal sac containing cerebrospinal fluid (CSF; meningocele) and neural tissue (myelomeningocele). It is associated with mental retardation, incontinence, and motor impairment.

Another important parameter of the CNS assessment is the size of the lateral ventricles. Ventriculomegaly (> 10 mm in the coronal plane) is associated with hydrocephalus, the most common CNS abnormality. Hydrocephalus ("water head") is called obstructive when there is a blockage of normal flow of CSF from the choroid plexus in the lateral and third ventricles, through the cerebral aqueduct, into the fourth ventricle, and out through the foramina of Magendie and Luschka into the subarachnoid space over the brain and spinal cord. Myelomeningocele is a common cause of blockage, as is congenital aqueductal stenosis. A less common nonobstructive cause is prenatal hemorrhage, in which intraventricular blood degradation products may interfere with the absorption of CSF by the arachnoid granulations in the region of the superior sagittal sinus. It is important to bear in mind that ventriculomegaly is not the same entity as hydrocephalus, because cerebral atrophy secondary to in utero vascular insult or infection (particularly TORCH [toxoplasmosis, rubella, cytomegalovirus, and herpes simplex] infections) may result in ex vacuo dilatation of the ventricles.

In practical terms, the triad of a normal cavum septum pellucidum, normal-sized lateral ventricular atria (< 10 mm), and a normal-sized cisterna magna (2 to 11 mm) virtually excludes a CNS anomaly.

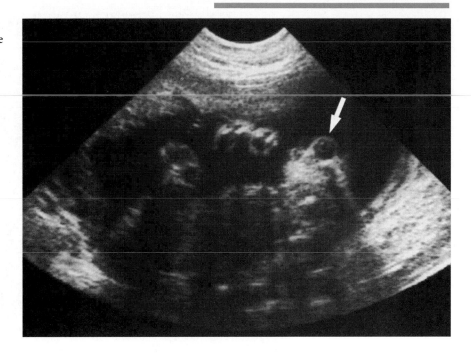

Figure 7–28. This longitudinal scan in a 22-week pregnancy demonstrates absence of the cranial vault above the level of the fetal eye (arrow), indicating anencephaly.

THORAX

Evaluation of the fetal thorax includes primarily the heart and lungs. The prenatal detection of congenital heart disease is difficult due to the small size and rapid beating of the heart. Abnormalities visible on the four-chamber view include endocardial cushion defects, commonly seen in Down's syndrome, and hypoplastic left heart syndrome, which manifests as absence of the left ventricle, with mitral and aortic atresia. The tetralogy of Fallot, the most salient feature of which is pulmonary stenosis, manifests as a large aorta and a small pulmonary artery on views of the outflow tracts. Important thoracic disorders that may be detected include congenital diaphragmatic hernia, with bowel present in the thorax; cystic adenomatoid malformation, characterized by a solid or cystic pulmonary mass; and masses in the mediastinum, including cystic hygromas (lymphangiomas) and neurogenic tumors.

ABDOMEN

Assessment of the fetal abdomen includes the search for normal anatomic structures. Failure to visualize the stomach suggests such disorders as oligohydramnios (a paucity of fluid available to fill the gastric lumen), esophageal atresia, and a CNS defect with impaired swallowing (the latter two associated with polyhydramnios). Duodenal atresia classically presents with a combination of polyhydramnios and a "double bubble" sign, representing the dilated, fluid-filled gastric and proximal duodenal lumens (Fig. 7–29). Abnormalities of the abdominal wall include gastroschisis and omphalocele. Gastroschisis ("split stomach") involves a defect in all three layers of the wall, with herniation of abdominal contents through a small paraumbilical defect (Fig. 7–30). It is invariably associated with abnormalities of bowel rotation. Omphalocele (from the Greek *omphalos,* "navel," and *kele,* "hernia") involves a midline abdominal defect covered by peritoneum, with the umbilical cord inserting centrally into the hernia sac. Although gastroschisis is the more serious defect, omphalo-

Figure 7–29. This transverse sonogram in a 27-week pregnancy demonstrates the classic "double bubble" sign of duodenal atresia. 1, stomach; 2, duodenum.

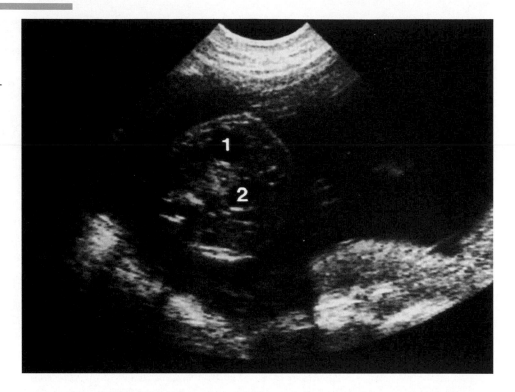

Figure 7–30. This transverse scan in a 35-week pregnancy demonstrates multiple ring-like fluid-filled loops of bowel floating in the amniotic cavity in a case of gastroschisis.

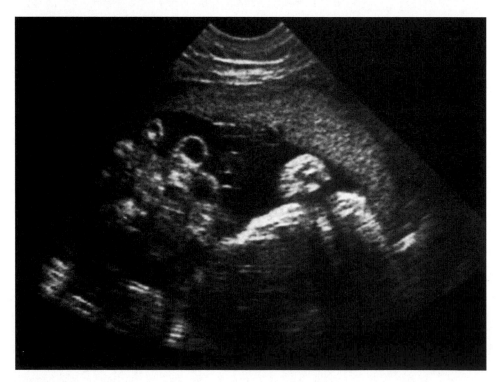

cele carries a graver prognosis, due to a 70% association with other malformations. One of the most important abnormalities of the urinary tract is obstruction, most prevalent at the level of the ureteropelvic junction. Multicystic dysplastic kidney is the most common renal mass and appears as a mass in the renal bed containing numerous cysts.

GESTATIONAL AGE

Gestational age can be assessed using a combination of biparietal diameter and femur length. Fetal growth is assessed primarily by measurement of abdominal circumference, which is especially important in detecting intrauterine growth retardation (IUGR). IUGR is best diagnosed around the 34th week of gestation. The most important cause is uteroplacental insufficiency, most commonly of maternal etiology. Other causes include malnutrition, hypertension, and alcohol or tobacco use. IUGR is associated with a 5- to 10-fold increase in the risk of prenatal or neonatal death. Macrosomia is associated with maternal diabetes and increases the risk of prolonged labor and meconium aspiration.

MALE REPRODUCTIVE TRACT

Anatomy and Physiology

The male gonads are suspended extra-abdominally within the scrotum, into which the testes (from the Greek for "witness," perhaps because a man testifying in court was required to place one hand on his scrotum) descend in the 7th month of intrauterine life (Fig. 7–31). Spermatogenesis takes place beginning at puberty within the seminiferous tubules, which account for 80% of the testicular mass. These highly coiled tubules measure approximately 250 m long and contain both the sperm-producing spermatogonia and the supporting Sertoli cells. The seminiferous tubules converge on the rete (from the Latin for "net") testis, which empties into the epididymis (from the Greek for "upon" and "testicle"). The epididymis is another highly coiled tube that measures 6 m long and is located along the posterosuperior aspect of the testis. The epididymis empties into the vas deferens, which conveys sperm into the abdominal cavity and becomes the ejaculatory ducts at the base of the bladder. The secretions of the secondary sex glands, the seminal vesicles and prostate gland, empty their secre-

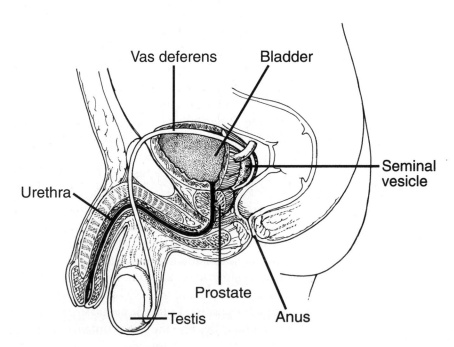

Figure 7–31. Sagittal view of the major structures of the male reproductive system.

tions into the ejaculatory ducts. The ejaculatory ducts empty into the urethra, at which point the reproductive and urinary systems share a common pathway in the male. The penis contains cylinders of erectile tissue, the paired corpora cavernosa and the single corpora spongiosum, with the urethra traveling in the latter.

As in the female, the gonads perform the functions of gametogenesis and sex hormone production. In contrast to the female, the male hypothalamic gonadotropin-releasing hormone occurs in bursts every few hours, but otherwise does not exhibit the wide cycles that characterize female reproductive structure and function. The Leydig cells, located within the testicular interstitium between the seminiferous tubules, produce testosterone. Testosterone is necessary for the normal in utero differentiation of the male reproductive tract and is also responsible for male secondary sexual characteristics such as growth of the beard, deepening of the voice, and broadening of the shoulders. A healthy young man produces several hundred million sperm per day, which are contained at ejaculation in approximately 3 mL of ejaculated semen. Produced by the accessory sex glands, the semen (from the Latin for "seed") contains fructose, an energy source for sperm; prostaglandins, which stimulate the smooth muscle of the female reproductive tract to aid in sperm transit; and alkaline secretions, which help to neutralize vaginal acidity.

Pathology

SCROTUM

The most important scrotal pathologies may be divided into several categories, including tumors, inflammation, fluid collections, and vascular insult. In each case, the first and often only imaging study to be performed is ultrasound, because the scrotum and its contents are superficial structures containing no air or bone and are therefore readily accessible sonographically. Moreover, ultrasound does not subject the gonads to ionizing radiation.

Scrotal ultrasound embodies a key radiologic principle; namely, the use of the normal side for comparison. The bilateral symmetry of the vertebrate body plan constitutes one of nature's greatest boons to clinical imaging. Whether comparing testes, breasts, lungs, or hemispheres of the brain, the radiologist's eyes move back and forth from side to side, looking for asymmetries. In the case of the testes, key points of comparison include size, echotexture, and blood flow. When performing scrotal ultrasound, it is advisable to begin with the unaffected side. Not only is the unaffected side less tender, thereby enabling the examiner to put the patient somewhat at ease, but it provides a baseline against which to assess possible abnormalities on the symptomatic side.

TUMOR

Primary testicular neoplasms constitute 1% of all male malignancies, most commonly occurring in the 25 to 35 year age group. Ninety percent are germ cell neoplasms, with mixed tumors being the most common histologic type, followed by pure seminomas. Useful clinical adjuncts in diagnosis include the serum AFP and HCG; both are typically negative in seminomas, while the AFP will be elevated in a tumor with a yolk sac cell component and the HCG will be elevated in choriocarcinoma (the tumor with the worst prognosis). Testicular neoplasms often present as painless masses.

Perhaps because the testis contains innumerable seminiferous tubules, each representing an acoustic interface, the normal testis is a relatively echogenic structure.

Therefore, tumors tend to demonstrate a relatively hypoechoic appearance. Seminomas exhibit well-defined margins and homogeneous hypoechogenicity, while nonseminomas tend to appear less well-defined with a more heterogeneous echotexture (Fig. 7–32). Determining the cell type of a testicular neoplasm radiologically is not necessary, because the probability of malignancy in an intratesticular mass is high, and orchiectomy with definitive histologic diagnosis constitutes typical management.

The tunica albuginea, a tough membrane covering the testis, usually prevents local extension of neoplasms. Hence lymphatic and hematogenous routes of spread are most frequent, and it is not uncommon for a patient with testicular malignancy to present with massive retroperitoneal adenopathy. Overall, the prognosis is good, with stage I or II disease (confined to the scrotum or extension into the retroperitoneal lymph nodes, respectively) enjoying a better than 95% 5-year survival. Even stage III disease, which involves metastases beyond the retroperitoneum (especially the lungs) carries a 5-year survival rate of better than 70%. The most common metastatic malignancies to involve the testes are lymphoma and leukemia, which are only very rarely diagnosed on the basis of testicular involvement.

EPIDIDYMITIS

The two most common testicular pathologies to present acutely are epididymitis and torsion. Epididymitis typically involves the spread of lower urinary tract pathogens into the epididymis via the vas deferens. The most important pathogens in young men are the expected venereal organisms chlamydia and gonococci. In about one-quarter of cases, there is associated orchitis, or inflammation of the testis itself. Viral orchitis is most commonly associated with mumps. Findings on ultrasound examination include an enlarged, hypoechoic epididymis, which appears hyperemic as compared to the unaffected side on Doppler examination (Fig. 7–33).

TESTICULAR TORSION

The key differential consideration in the acutely painful and swollen testis is epididymitis versus torsion, and the determination of whether torsion is present must be

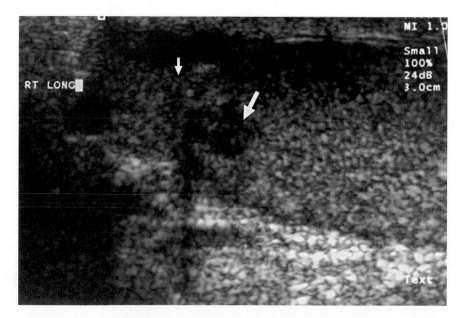

Figure 7–32. This longitudinal image from a testicular ultrasound examination shows a small, hypoechoic mass within the superior pole of the testis (large arrows), which at surgery was found to represent a seminoma. The small arrow indicates the boundary between the testis and the epididymis.

Figure 7–33. This patient experienced scrotal pain after a vasectomy. A longitudinal image from an ultrasound examination of the testis demonstrates a predominately hypoechoic lesion (arrow) occupying much of the epididymis at the inferior pole of the testis, which represented a granuloma. Such lesions are sometimes seen in patients who have undergone vasectomy, and are thought to arise from the blockage of testicular outflow.

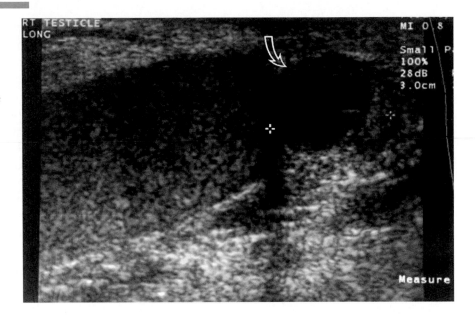

made immediately. The rate of salvage of torsed testes drops precipitously after the patient has been symptomatic for more than 6 hours, with a worse than 20% salvage rate after 12 hours. Torsion occurs secondary to trauma, sexual activity, or physical exertion, when the spermatic cord twists around its axis, impairing both venous drainage via the pampiniform plexus and arterial inflow via the testicular, deferential, and external spermatic arteries. Patients present with torsion most frequently in the newborn and teenage years. Certain individuals are predisposed to torsion because at least one of their testes is completely enveloped by the peritoneal membrane, called the tunica vaginalis, which prevents secure anchoring of the testis to the scrotal sac. More than one-half of patients exhibit this abnormality bilaterally, rendering bilateral orchipexy standard surgical therapy when the affected testis is salvageable.

The key sonographic findings in testicular torsion can be visualized on color Doppler imaging. In complete torsion, the affected testis will demonstrate absence of flow, while an incomplete torsion may demonstrate markedly diminished flow. Additional findings of torsion on gray-scale imaging may include increased size and decreased echogenicity of the testis, as compared to the normal side. Nuclear medicine imaging is less frequently employed today, but remains a useful substitute when sonography is not available. After peripheral injection of technetium (Tc)-99m-pertechnetate, a "cold" or photopenic area will be seen in the region of the affected testis, manifesting its lack of perfusion.

VARICOCELE

The most common fluid collection within the testis is a varicocele, a dilated and serpiginous pampiniform venous plexus. This condition is clinically important because it may be associated with infertility, and varicoceles in fact constitute the most frequent correctable cause of infertility in the male. At least 95% of varicoceles are left-sided and probably result from incompetence of the valves in the internal spermatic vein. One hypothesis regarding the left-sided predominance of varicoceles is that the left-sided gonadal vein drains into the renal vein, while the right gonadal vein drains directly into the inferior vena cava. The finding of a new varicocele in a patient over age 40 years is of special significance, because it may herald the development of a neoplasm causing obstruction of the gonadal or renal vein (most often a renal cell carcinoma).

PROSTATE

EPIDEMIOLOGY

Approximately 200,000 cases of prostate cancer are diagnosed each year in the United States, and this number has been increasing rapidly, primarily due to the aging of the population. Another factor in this increase is the detection of clinically occult disease through screening programs. Prostate cancer is the second leading cause of cancer death in men, resulting in approximately 43,000 deaths per year, second only to lung cancer. However, the toll of prostate cancer in years of life lost is much less than that of breast cancer, due to the fact that it typically kills at a much later age; in the United States, breast cancer is responsible for over 100 years of life lost per 100,000 people under the age of 65 years, while prostate cancer is responsible for less than 10.

PATHOPHYSIOLOGY

 An understanding of the anatomy of the prostate gland is critical in interpreting imaging studies, because different pathologic processes tend to arise in different portions of the gland (Fig. 7–34). The prostate gland surrounds the urethra at the base of the bladder and contains the junction point between the urethra and ejaculatory ducts. Approximately three-fourths of the gland is located in the peripheral zone, which surrounds the remainder of the gland posterolaterally. Most prostate cancers arise here, and 95% of these malignancies are adenocarcinomas. The transitional zone, which surrounds the urethra, constitutes only 5% of the gland, but represents the site of benign prostatic hyperplasia (BPH), and hence may enlarge markedly.

The workup of a newly diagnosed patient generally includes measurements of serum alkaline phosphatase and liver function tests, as well as chest radiographs, bone scan, and abdominal and pelvic CT. MRI or transrectal ultrasound is more accurate than CT in assessing local extension of the disease. In patients presenting with an elevated prostate-specific antigen (PSA), transrectal ultrasound is often employed to guide biopsy of the gland.

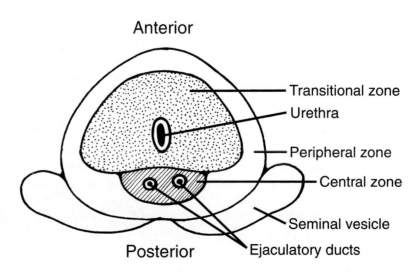

Figure 7–34. The key zones of the prostate gland seen on imaging studies such as ultrasound and magnetic resonance imaging.

CLINICAL PRESENTATION

The clinical presentation of prostate cancer includes symptoms such as urinary frequency, nocturia, and urinary urgency. Unfortunately, these same symptoms are associated with BPH, which is seen to some degree in most men as they age. A distinguishing feature that tends to favor malignancy is a relatively abrupt change in symptoms. The two most widely employed screening methods are serum assays for PSA and digital rectal examination. PSA levels below 5 µg/dL are considered normal, while levels greater than 10 µg/dL suggest prostate cancer. Digital rectal examination, performed by inserting a gloved finger into the rectum and palpating the prostate gland along the anterior rectal wall, is relatively sensitive but nonspecific. Findings worrisome for malignancy include a firm, asymmetrical mass or an irregularly enlarged gland.

Benign processes in the differential diagnosis of prostate carcinoma include BPH, which involves the transitional zone, and prostatitis, which generally causes the entire gland to become boggy, swollen, and edematous. The most common organism is *Escherichia coli.*

It is not uncommon for patients to present with metastatic disease, which manifests with such symptoms as impotence (due to disruption of neurovascular structures), as well as back pain and bone pain (due to skeletal metastases). Approximately 80% of patients with metastatic disease exhibit only bone involvement, but other sites include lymph nodes, liver, and lung.

IMAGING

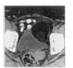

Imaging findings that support the diagnosis of prostate carcinoma depend on the modality employed. Transrectal ultrasound findings include one or more hypoechoic nodules in the peripheral zone, mass effect on surrounding tissues, and asymmetric enlargement of the gland (Fig. 7–35). On T2-weighted MR images, cancers typically appear as hypointense (dark) lesions amid the relatively bright parenchyma of the peripheral zone. Ultimately, the diagnosis is established by biopsy, and ultrasound has the advantage that it readily guides biopsy of suspicious lesions via a transrectal route.

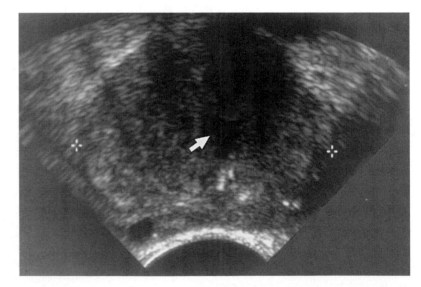

Figure 7–35. A 60-year-old man presented with an elevated prostate-specific antigen. A transrectal ultrasound image of the prostate gland demonstrates a hypoechoic lesion within the peripheral zone (arrow). A core needle biopsy of this lesion yielded a pathologic diagnosis of prostatic carcinoma.

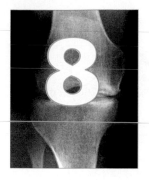

The Musculoskeletal System

ANATOMY AND PHYSIOLOGY

Bone is living tissue, consisting of a combination of cells and an extracellular organic matrix laid down by those cells. The extracellular matrix (osteoid) consists of a combination of collagen fibers and a mucopolysaccharide-rich gel, referred to as ground substance. This ground substance or osteoid gives the bone a somewhat rubbery consistency that is responsible for its tensile strength. Precipitation of hydroxyapatite crystals (primarily calcium phosphate) within this matrix renders the bone hard, providing compressional strength. Cartilage is similar to bone, although it is unmineralized. The parts of a long bone include the epiphysis, the physis or growth plate, the metaphysis, and the diaphysis (Fig. 8–1).

Bone growth is growth hormone mediated. Bones grow in length through the addition of new chondrocytes at the epiphyseal end of the growth plate. These carti-

Figure 8–1. The principal parts of a long bone, in this case the femur.

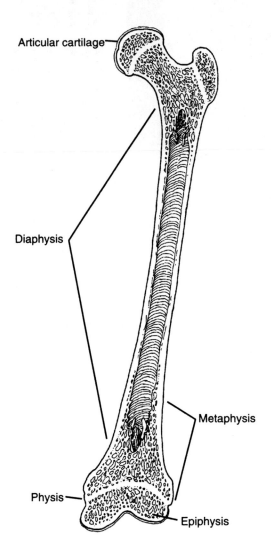

Articular cartilage

Diaphysis

Metaphysis

Physis

Epiphysis

lage cells have no blood vessels and receive nutrients by diffusion through the ground substance. As the cartilage cells become mineralized toward the metaphyseal end, their tenuous blood supply is interrupted, and they die. Osteoclasts move in to clear out the dead chondrocytes, and osteoblasts move in to lay down bone in the remnants of the cartilage. Osteoblasts are literally bone formers, whereas osteoclasts are bone destroyers, which secrete acids that dissolve the hydroxyapatite crystals and enzymes that break down the organic matrix. Although the osteoblasts become entrapped in bone, and are then called osteocytes, they do not die due to the network of nutrient-conveying canaliculi to which they are connected. Long bones grow in diameter through the action of osteoblasts within the periosteum, the connective tissue sheath that covers the outer surface of the bone. Osteoclasts simultaneously dissolve away the inner cortex of the bone, allowing the marrow cavity to expand apace.

The skeleton performs a number of functions. First, it provides the mechanical scaffolding necessary to support the body and allow for movement through the lever action of skeletal muscles. Second, it protects vital internal organs such as the brain, spinal cord, heart, and lungs. Third, blood cells are manufactured in the bone marrow. Fourth, the skeleton serves as a storage reservoir for calcium and phosphate; 99% of the calcium in the body is found in the bones. The key regulator of serum calcium levels is parathyroid hormone (PTH), produced by the four parathyroid glands found posterior to the thyroid gland in the neck. Absence of PTH is incompatible with life, and a patient typically dies within several days when hypocalcemia-induced repiratory muscle spasm results in asphyxiation.

To understand the myriad pathologic processes to which bone is subject, it is first necessary to understand normal bone anatomy and physiology. Consider the following example. It is often observed that patients with severe neurologic impairment that confines them to bed develop articular deformities, involving such joints as the hip and knee joints. Why? Part of the answer lies in the normal physiology of articular cartilage. The cartilage of the hip and knee joints receives its nutrients not from blood vessels, but from the synovial fluid within the joint space itself. The cartilage and synovial fluid function rather like a sponge and water, respectively. When we place weight on the joint, the cartilage is compressed and some of the synovial fluid is squeezed out. When mechanical force is removed, the cartilage expands slightly and draws in fresh fluid, from which it extracts nutrients. Hence the maintenance of normal joint morphology is dependent on regular joint function, a principle that applies more broadly to the whole of the skeleton.

The structure of bone is of a more dynamic nature than the structure of any other adult organ. Bone undergoes continual remodeling throughout life. Both the mass of bone and the three-dimensional orientation of bone elements respond to the functional demands placed on the skeleton, a principle that applies in both health and disease. Therefore, individuals who exercise regularly tend to have stronger bones than those who do not.

The observation that exercise increases bone mass is especially notable in light of the fact that maximum bone mass is attained early in the third decade of life. In order to avoid the ravages of osteoporosis, exercise during young adult life is therefore critical, as bone mass usually increases no further after that time. A person's bone mass at that age constitutes the point of departure for a subsequent inexorable decline after age 40 years, which becomes more rapid in women after menopause. An example of the rapidity with which bone loss may occur is seen in astronauts, who tend to undergo very rapid loss of bone mass due to the lack of mechanical stress in a weightless environment. Early astronauts lost 20% of their bone mass during only a short time in orbit, and resistance exercises are now a routine part of life in space. The adage "use it or lose it" is an especially apt description of bone physiology.

Osteoporosis does not represent the death of bone or a decline in bone function; in fact, truly dead or devascularized bone cannot become osteoporotic in the first place, because it lacks not only osteoblastic but also osteoclastic activity. Rather, osteoporosis represents a change in the balance of osteoblastic and osteoclastic activity. Living bone is anything but a static structure. The term *osteoporosis*, which refers to decreased density of bone, should be distinguished from the more general term osteopenia (from "bone" and "poor"), which simply means an increased radiolucency of bone. Aside from osteoporosis, another cause of osteopenia is osteomalacia, which results from abnormal bone mineralization.

Another graphic example of the dynamic nature of bone is seen in the bone's response to osseous lesions. If the lesion is slow growing enough to give the bone a chance to react, it will tend to have sclerotic (dense) margins, representing in part an attempt by the remaining intact bone to compensate for the lack of mechanical

Figure 8–2. A radiograph of the arm in this battered child reveals healing fractures of the humerus, radius, and ulna, as manifested by sclerosis and periosteal reaction. Note the exuberant callus formation around the mid-diaphyseal humeral fracture, which represents a kind of "physiologic splinting." With time, such fractures may heal without a trace, a dramatic testimony to the bone's prodigious powers of remodeling. Of course, the urgent medical mission is to extract the child from the hostile environment in which the abuse is taking place.

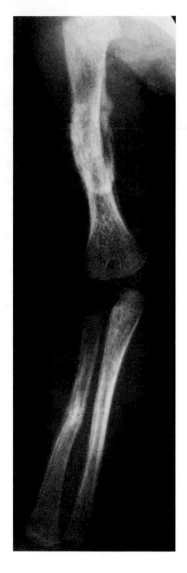

support provided by the abnormal bone. So, too, in cases of traumatic fracture, the formation of callus can be regarded as a process of physiologic casting, with the callus temporarily assuming the burden of weight-bearing while the underlying bone heals (Fig. 8–2). Highly aggressive bone malignancies, on the other hand, tend to destroy surrounding bone at such a rapid pace that no osseous response can be mounted, and thus tend to manifest a lytic appearance. The stress fractures that occur in individuals who undertake rigorous exercise programs likewise reflect the fact that the bone must first become weaker before it can be made stronger; the attempt to remodel the bone for greater strength entails an initial loss of osteoid and mineral.

While many factors are involved, the primary players in the dynamic remodeling of bone are the osteoblasts and osteoclasts. Osteoblastic activity is stimulated by compressive forces on the bone, by the thyroid hormone calcitonin, and by low local pO_2, or passive hyperemia. Osteoclastic activity, on the other hand, is stimulated by tensile forces on the bone, by parathormone, and by high local pO_2, or active hyperemia. Because the osteoclasts are more efficient than the osteoblasts—a single osteoclast working at maximum capacity would require over 100 osteoblasts to counterbalance it—negative bone balance is an ever-present possibility.

IMAGING MODALITIES

The modalities employed in musculoskeletal imaging include magnetic resonance imaging (MRI), computed tomography (CT), nuclear medicine, ultrasound, and plain radiography. MRI plays an increasing role in the evaluation of joints, soft tissues, and the spine because of its unique strengths in assessing tissue composition, imaging lesions in multiple planes, and accurately delineating geographic relationships. CT provides accurate assessment of lesions in the axial plane and is especially useful in evaluating calcification, although its capabilities in evaluating the soft tissues are considerably inferior to MRI. Radionuclide bone scans provide physiologic information on cell turnover and generally constitute the best means of screening for lesions throughout the skeleton. Ultrasound has played a more limited role in the assessment of joint effusions, blood flow, and the presence of foreign bodies within the soft tissues, although it is being used increasingly to assess soft tissue structures such as tendons. Despite the important contributions of other modalities, plain radiography stands out as the single most useful skeletal diagnostic study in most situations.

PATHOLOGY
Congenital

Congenital or developmental dysplasias exert their effects at the physis (growth plate), impacting such processes as cartilage cell proliferation (achondroplasia), cartilage matrix production (mucopolysaccharidoses), or the mineralization of cartilage matrix with calcium hydroxyapatite (rickets). Ricketts, which usually represents an acquired metabolic disorder, is discussed in Chapter 10. A variety of noxious agents, including infections such as syphilis and toxins such as alcohol, may also interfere with this process.

ACHONDROPLASIA

Achondroplasia is the most common nonlethal skeletal dysplasia and the most prevalent form of short-limbed dwarfism. It is characterized by rhizomelic (proximal segment) limb shortening and is inherited in an autosomal dominant fashion, although most cases are sporadic. The fundamental abnormality is a defect in enchondral bone formation. Characteristic findings on clinical examination include short, stubby fingers, extremities that are disproportionately short in relation to the trunk, and a prominent calvarium with frontal bossing.

Radiographic findings include a small foramen magnum and short and narrowing interpediculate distances as one moves from cephalad to caudad down the spine (Fig. 8–3). As a result, patients are predisposed to spinal stenosis, with neurologic complaints secondary to compression of the spinal cord and nerve roots.

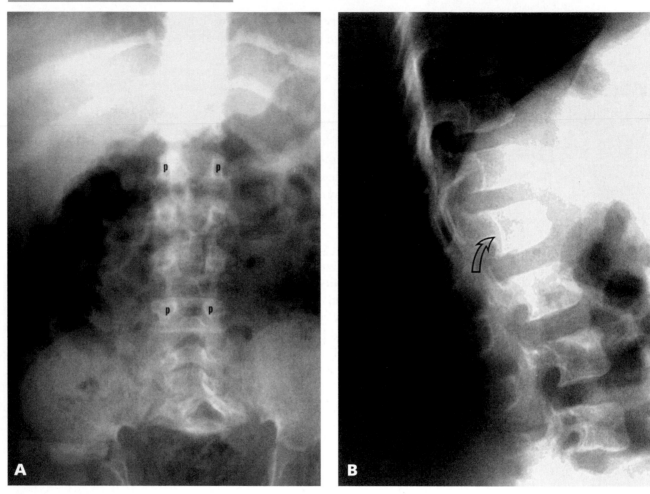

Figure 8–3. A 1-year-old boy demonstrates two characteristic radiographic stigmata of achondroplasia. (A) The frontal film demonstrates decreasing interpediculate distances as one moves caudally through the lumbar spine. Normally, the distances between vertebral pedicles increase caudally. p, pedicle. (B) The lateral film demonstrates posterior vertebral body scalloping. Normally, the posterior margins of the vertebral bodies are essentially straight, but in this case they are convex toward the front (arrow).

OSTEOPETROSIS

Osteopetrosis is a rare but edifying disease that illustrates some of the essential principles of bone pathophysiology. It is transmitted in both autosomal recessive (fatal) and autosomal dominant forms and is caused by an enzymatic abnormality that results in impaired osteoclastic function. As a result, bone remodeling, which is critical in both bone's growth and its response to mechanical stress, occurs abnormally. Patients with the nonlethal form of this disease present with frequent fractures and anemia, among other problems. The fractures stem from the fact that bone cannot adapt to mechanical stresses by remodeling normally. The anemia results from a lack of normal bone tubulation, with diminution or even obliteration of the marrow space, and resultant decreased hematopoeisis.

Radiographic findings are predictable and include generalized osteosclerosis (dense bones), the so-called Erlenmeyer flask deformity of the distal femur (due to abnormal remodeling of the metaphysis with growth), and frequently, pathologic fractures (Fig. 8–4).

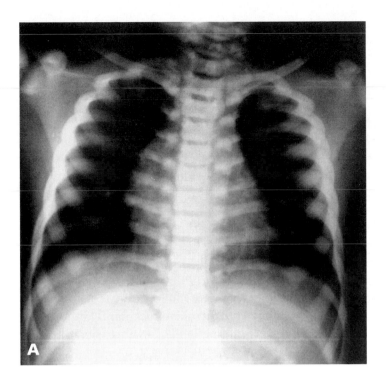

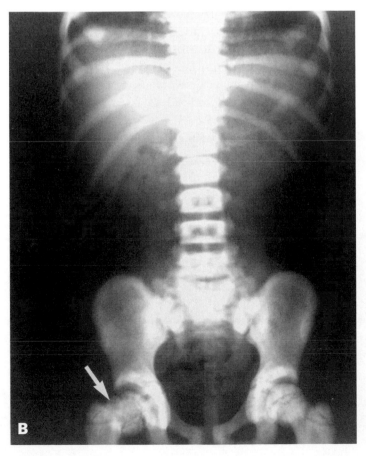

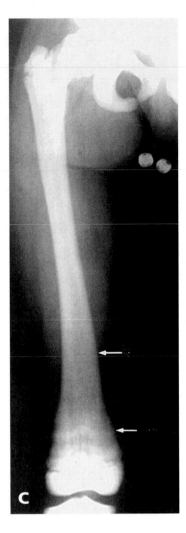

Figure 8–4. A 7-year-old girl presented with a painful right-sided limp and was found to be anemic. Plain films of the (**A**) chest, (**B**) abdomen, and (**C**) right femur demonstrate a marked, diffuse increase in bone density. The slight increase in the cardiothoracic ratio reflects the heart's attempt to compensate for the anemia. The dramatic elongation and flaring of the distal femoral metaphysis (C, small arrows), known as an Erlenmeyer flask deformity, results from abnormal bone remodeling. Can you find the etiology of the patient's limp? It can be difficult to find on the femur film, but compare the appearance of the proximal femurs at the bottom of the abdomen film. Note that the right femoral neck appears shortened and forms a more acute angle relative to the femoral diaphysis as compared to the left (B, large arrow). The metabolic defect in bone remodeling has produced one of its characteristic complications in this patient—a pathologic fracture of the femoral neck.

Infectious

OSTEOMYELITIS

EPIDEMIOLOGY

Osteomyelitis typically refers to pyogenic infection of the medullary canal of bone. It results from two principal routes of infection: hematogenous spread and local extension from soft tissues. Hematogenous spread is the most frequent, often from a source in the urinary tract, lungs, or skin. Hematogenous osteomyelitis tends to occur in the young and old, generally sparing patients between 20 and 50 years of age. Local spread may occur at any age and tends to occur in patients with circulatory or immune disorders, such as diabetic patients, who often suffer infected skin ulcers.

Pathogens can often be predicted according to the clinical circumstances. After the newborn period, *Staphylococcus aureus* is the most likely organism. Salmonella is relatively more common in sickle-cell disease patients, and *Pseudomonas* deserves special consideration in intravenous drug abusers and patients with a history of a puncture wound to the foot, especially through a shoe. Polymicrobial infection is common in situations such as diabetic foot ulcers. Numerous other etiologies, including tuberculosis, are also possible (Fig. 8–5).

PATHOPHYSIOLOGY

The damage to bone in osteomyelitis results from a vicious cycle of infection and host response. Initially, an inoculum of bacteria is deposited hematogenously, which then begins to colonize the perivascular space. The host inflammatory response produces local inflammation and edema, which often extends into the surrounding soft tissues (Fig. 8–6). The associated increase in local tissue pressure, related to both hemostatic and oncotic factors, has four potential consequences. First, there is wider dissemination of the infection, as

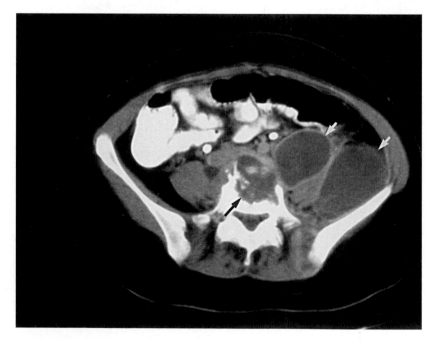

Figure 8–5. A 26-year-old woman presented with a 1-year history of progressively worsening back pain. An axial computed tomography image at the lumbosacral level demonstrates prominent destruction of the fifth lumbar vertebral body (black arrow), with paraspinal fluid collections involving the iliacus and psoas muscles on the left (white arrows) and, to a lesser degree, the psoas on the right. The indolent clinical course, prominent spinal destruction, and large paraspinal abscesses are all typical of tuberculosis, which is called Pott's disease when it involves the spine. A pyogenic infection involving an organism such as *Staphylococcus aureus* would exhibit a more acute course.

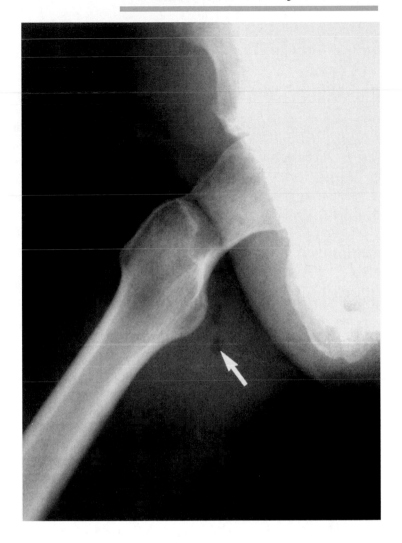

Figure 8–6. A 60-year-old woman with a history of pelvic irradiation developed pain and decreased mobility of the right hip. A plain film of the hip demonstrates tiny gas collections in the soft tissues medial to the lesser trochanter (arrow), indicating cellulitis due to gas-forming organisms.

cells are forced out into the lower pressure trabecular spaces surrounding the infectious focus. Next, there results a reduction in the blood supply to the region, which both impairs the delivery of immune cells (and antibiotics) and eventually produces a rim of infarction. Thereafter, an abscess forms in an effort to contain the infection, which unfortunately renders eradication of the infectious focus more difficult. Eventually, there results a sequestrum, an area of osseous infection completely cut off from the rest of the bone.

Two forces produce the characteristic bone destruction seen both pathologically and radiographically. The first is a hyperemically stimulated increase in osteoclastic activity surrounding the focus of infection. The second is frank marrow necrosis.

The distribution of the focus of infection within long bones varies according to the age of the patient. Infectious organisms tend to deposit in the regions of most sluggish blood flow, the most distal arterioles and capillaries. In patients younger than 1 to 2 years of age, in whom arteries coming from the metaphyseal side of the physis cross over into the epiphysis, infections often involve the epiphysis. After about 2 years of age, the transphyseal supply is eliminated, and most infections occur in the metaphysis. In the adult, closure of the growth plate again allows metaphyseal vessels to reach the epiphysis, which again becomes a prime site of inoculation. In the adult, the most frequently involved sites are the tibia, femur, and humerus, as well as the vertebrae.

CLINICAL PRESENTATION

Patients of any age tend to present with an increased white blood cell count, fever, and other systemic evidence of infection, which may be accompanied by local symptoms such as pain and swelling. However, neonatal osteomyelitis, typically secondary to group B streptococcus, *Escherichia coli,* or staphylococcal infection, often presents with little symptomatology. In older pediatric age groups, there is often a history of refusal to bear weight or to use the affected limb. Additional pediatric signs include fever, irritability, and lethargy. Many adults will complain of vague extremity or back pain. At every age of presentation, physical examination may disclose point tenderness, muscle spasm, or even a draining sinus (the so-called cloaca, which may be thought of as nature's way of draining an abscess). A common but nonspecific laboratory finding is an elevated erythrocyte sedimentation rate.

IMAGING

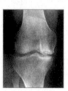 Blood cultures should be obtained in every patient in whom osteomyelitis is a consideration, because they identify an organism in approximately 50% of cases, and antimicrobial therapy can be tailored accordingly. One reason that osteomyelitis requires weeks of antibiotic therapy is that the conduits of local antibiotic delivery, the capillaries, are compromised, and only with time can adequate antibiotic concentrations within the focus of infection be attained.

Plain radiography is not as sensitive as bone scan or MRI, but is routinely obtained. In the first week of infection, there is likely to be little or no discernible change. The first sign of infection is swelling of the surrounding soft tissues, a nonspecific finding that can be seen in cellulitis or deep soft tissue infection. The first finding in the bone is osteoporosis, which results from the local active hyperemia produced by the inflammatory response. At about 2 weeks, periosteal reaction may be seen. Eventually, signs such as sequestrum and cloaca formation may be seen, although today it is rare for osteomyelitis to progress to these points.

A more sensitive study, likely to be positive within the first 2 days of infection, is a radionuclide bone scan utilizing technetium (Tc)-99m-MDP, which will usually demonstrate increased uptake at the site of infection (Fig. 8–7). Even more sensitive and specific are radionuclide-labeled white blood cell (WBC) scans, utilizing indium-111 or Tc-99m, which demonstrate the site of acute infection after 24 hours. MRI is also quite sensitive for acute infection, demonstrating low signal in the marrow on T1-weighted images and high signal on T2-weighted images, secondary to the increased edema associated with infection. Adjacent soft tissues also become hyperintense on T2-weighted images early in the infection.

SEPTIC ARTHRITIS

EPIDEMIOLOGY

Septic arthritis is often associated with osteomyelitis, but it frequently occurs alone. From the Greek *sepsis,* meaning "putrefaction," *arthron,* meaning "joint" (related to *arti*culation), and *-itis,* meaning "inflammation," septic arthritis is a rapidly progressive pyogenic infection of the joint space, which, if untreated, results in loss of joint function. Patients at increased risk include those with preexisting arthritis, diabetes,

Figure 8–7. This child refused to bear weight on his left leg. (A) A frontal radiograph of both lower extremities reveals no discernible bony abnormality, although there is notable swelling and increased density of the soft tissues of the left calf as compared to the right. (B) A bone scan was performed. The most remarkable finding on this frontal scintigraphic image is not a focal area of increased activity, but rather the relative photopenia (decreased activity) in the proximal left tibial growth plate and diaphysis (arrow), relative to the right tibia. The lack of radiotracer uptake in such a case reflects severe bone marrow edema secondary to infection and concomitant inflammation. The hydrostatic pressure within the marrow cavity rises to such a degree that it overcomes capillary perfusion pressure, resulting in infarction and necrosis. (C) A lateral radiograph obtained weeks later

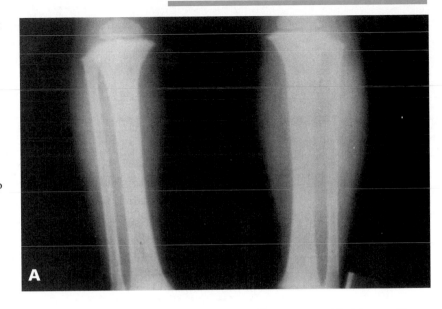

demonstrates the severity of the process, with prominent destruction of much of the tibia. This case illustrates two critical themes. First, when interpreting plain films in suspected osteomyelitis, it is important to pay close attention to the soft tissues as well as the bones, as they are the first indicators of infection. Second, in interpreting bone scans, it is vital that one understand both the mechanism of radiotracer uptake and the pathophysiology of the disease. One cannot always assume that osteomyelitis will manifest by increased radiotracer activity. In the most severe cases, characterized by the most severe bone marrow edema, the typical pattern will be the exact opposite.

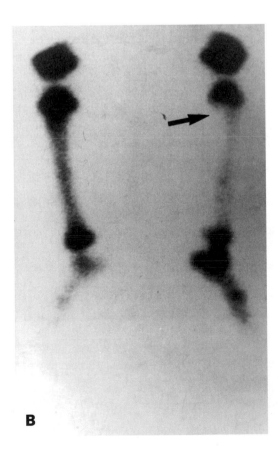

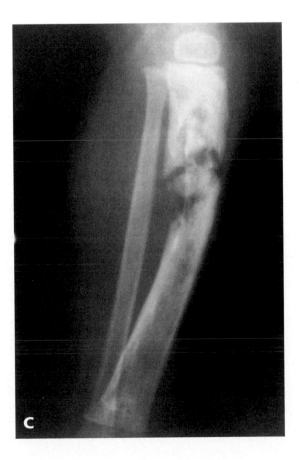

alcoholism, and immunocompromising disorders. Septic arthritis with osteomyelitis most often results from trauma, such as animal or human bites, puncture wounds, and surgery. The most common organism is *S. aureus,* although *Neisseria gonorrhoeae* is more prevalent in the sexually active young population. Intravenous drug abusers and diabetic patients are at increased risk for gram-negative organisms.

PATHOPHYSIOLOGY

 The pathophysiology of septic arthritis includes synovial hyperemia with exudation of fluid. Because of this fluid's high fibrin content and the rapid consumption of nutrients in the synovial fluid due to bacterial proliferation, cartilage nutrition is inhibited. Once cartilage cells are lost, they cannot be replaced. The release of cytotoxic enzymes by inflammatory cells also produces tissue destruction. Septic arthritis is treated similarly to osteomyelitis, with intravenous antibiotics over a period of weeks, as well as repeated joint aspirations and immobilization.

CLINICAL PRESENTATION

Patients present with the classic signs of local inflammation: *rubor, tumor, calor,* and *dolor* (redness, swelling, warmth, and pain) and with systemic signs of infection including fever and leukocytosis.

IMAGING

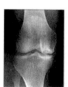 Septic arthritis is not a radiologic diagnosis. By the time radiographic signs of infection appear, irreversible joint damage has already occurred. The key to diagnosis is joint aspiration, which in some cases may require ultrasonographic or fluoroscopic guidance. Joint fluid is opaque, demonstrates a low glucose, and has a WBC count greater than 100,000. Radiographic findings include soft tissue swelling extending to the joint, joint space loss, and periarticular osteopenia, as well as the findings of periosteal reaction and cortical destruction associated with osteomyelitis.

Tumorous

Bone tumors can be classified based on many criteria, including benign versus malignant and primary versus metastatic. Let us begin by considering the distinction between primary and metastatic lesions.

METASTASES

EPIDEMIOLOGY

Bone metastases are approximately 50 to 100 times more frequent than primary bone malignancies. The finding of even a single skeletal metastatic lesion is of immense clinical significance, because it indicates that the primary tumor cannot be surgically resected for cure.

PATHOPHYSIOLOGY

 Hematogenous dissemination is the most frequent route by which metastatic cells reach the skeleton. Most metastatic lesions appear in multiples, because multiple cells from the primary tumor tend to gain access to the bloodstream. A solitary bone lesion has only a 1-in-10 chance of representing a metastatic process.

What percentage of cancer patients develop bone metastases? The lung and the liver, and not the skeleton, are in fact the two most common sites of metastatic spread. Yet the rich blood supply of the skeleton's hematopoietic tissues explains why approximately one-third of all cancer patients eventually develop bone metastases. The rich sinusoidal bed of the marrow capillaries, with its large gaps between endothelial cells, presents a very hospitable environment for wayward tumor cells. This explains why metastatic lesions are much more common in bone than in, for example, the soft tissues surrounding the bone, such as muscle, tendons, ligaments, and fat.

Of all skeletal metastases in adults, more than 80% can be traced to one of five primary malignant sources: prostate, breast, lung, kidney, and thyroid. Prostate carcinoma accounts for more than one-half of all skeletal metastases in men, as does breast carcinoma in women. Of these, prostate carcinoma has a special anatomic propensity to metastasize to bone. Its venous drainage through Batson's plexus renders the lumbar spine, pelvis, and proximal femur the first capillary beds reached by blood-borne tumor cells (Fig. 8–8).

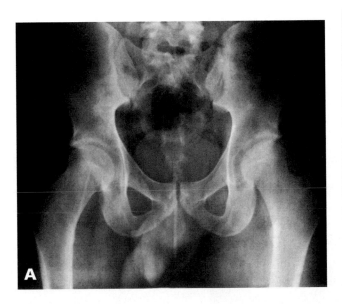

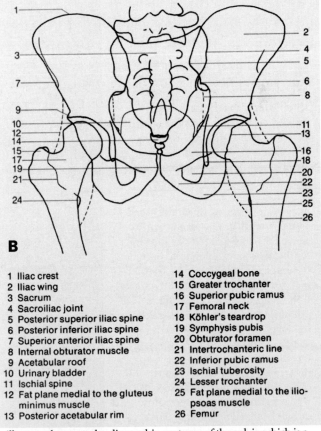

1 Iliac crest	14 Coccygeal bone
2 Iliac wing	15 Greater trochanter
3 Sacrum	16 Superior pubic ramus
4 Sacroiliac joint	17 Femoral neck
5 Posterior superior iliac spine	18 Köhler's teardrop
6 Posterior inferior iliac spine	19 Symphysis pubis
7 Superior anterior iliac spine	20 Obturator foramen
8 Internal obturator muscle	21 Intertrochanteric line
9 Acetabular roof	22 Inferior pubic ramus
10 Urinary bladder	23 Ischial tuberosity
11 Ischial spine	24 Lesser trochanter
12 Fat plane medial to the gluteus minimus muscle	25 Fat plane medial to the iliopsoas muscle
13 Posterior acetabular rim	26 Femur

Figure 8–8. (A) This frontal radiograph and (B) accompanying diagram illustrate the normal radiographic anatomy of the pelvis, which is a favored site of metastatic disease from prostate carcinoma.

Although the most frequent carcinomas may metastasize to virtually any location, certain sites tend to suggest particular types of primary lesions. When metastatic lesions are found in the distal extremities, particularly the hands and feet, bronchogenic carcinoma is the most likely culprit. The most common tumors to affect the skull are multiple myeloma, and carcinomas of the lung and breast. Breast cancer is also the most likely culprit when metastatic lesions are found in the axial skeleton, and accounts for approximately three-quarters of spine metastases.

CLINICAL PRESENTATION

Clinically speaking, bone metastases may represent the first indication of a malignancy, although the vast majority of patients in whom metastatic skeletal lesions are found have known primary tumors. Clinical signs of skeletal metastases include hypercalcemia and the syndrome known as hypertrophic pulmonary osteoarthropathy (HPO). HPO consists of clubbing of the digits, periosteal reaction, and pain. Approximately 1 in 20 patients with bronchogenic carcinoma develops the syndrome (Fig. 8–9).

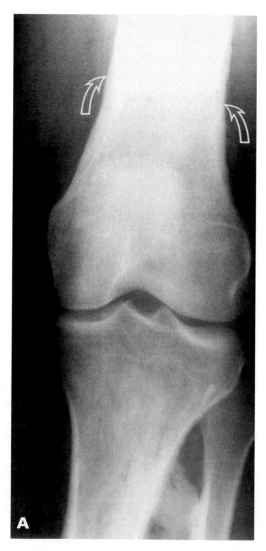
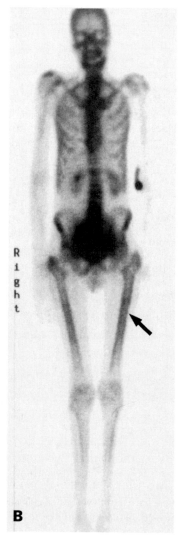

Figure 8–9. A 51-year-old man presented with bilateral knee pain and clubbed digits. (**A**) A frontal view of the left knee demonstrates dense, chronic periosteal reaction of the distal femur (arrows), which was also present on the right. On the basis of this finding, a thoracic computed tomographic examination was obtained, which elucidated a small bronchogenic carcinoma. Also seen on the knee film is ossification of the interosseous membrane between the tibia and fibula, likely post-traumatic in origin. (**B**) A bone scan image from another patient demonstrates prominent periosteal radiotracer activity along both femoral diaphyses in a so-called tram-track pattern, which is typical of hypertrophic osteoarthropathy (arrow). Aside from bronchogenic carcinoma, other processes associated with hypertrophic osteoarthropathy include benign fibrous tumor of the pleura, mesothelioma, inflammatory bowel disease, and cyanotic heart disease. The pathophysiology is unknown.

Bone metastases typically present in one of two ways. Pain is the most common presentation, seen in most patients, while the other is pathologic fracture. While from one point of view all fractures are by definition "pathologic," the term refers to fractures that take place through preexisting bone lesions, which weaken the bone and predispose it to mechanical disruption. Obviously, the bone lesions most likely to develop pathologic fractures are those in the weight-bearing skeleton, and the most prevalent sites are the spine and the femur. Approximately 5 to 10% of all patients with skeletal metastases eventually develop a pathologic fracture. One key role of the radiologist, once metastatic lesions have been detected, is to determine which lesions are at significant risk for fracture, so that prophylactic measures can be instituted, such as radiating the lesion or decreasing the mechanical load on the bone.

IMAGING

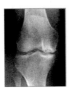

Radiologic indicators of an increased risk of pathologic fracture include destruction of more than 50% of bone cortex (with a 60 to 70% risk of fracture), lesions of 3 cm or greater in the proximal femur, or an appropriately positioned lesion that continues to cause pain even after radiotherapy (Fig. 8–10). Lesions that involve substantially less than 50% of the cortex produce pathologic fractures in less than 20% of cases. While every

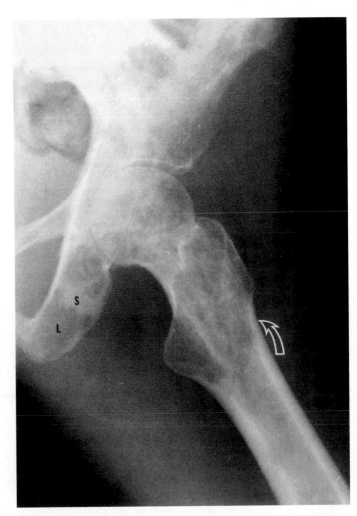

Figure 8–10. A 28-year-old woman with metastatic breast carcinoma presented with left hip pain. The frontal radiograph of the left hip demonstrates a mixed lytic and sclerotic pattern of metastatic disease throughout the innominate bone and femur. The intertrochanteric region of the femur is virtually replaced by a tumor (arrow), indicating a high risk of pathologic fracture. Because such fractures heal very poorly (due to the absence of bone-forming cells, which have been replaced by tumor), it is important to recognize potential fractures before they occur, so that prophylactic treatment such as radiation can be instituted. L, lytic lesion; S, sclerotic lesion.

metastatic lesion would, in theory, eventually become large enough to cause a fracture, most patients with metastatic disease will die of other consequences of their malignancy before this occurs.

Lytic versus blastic

While metastases can have virtually any appearance, certain metastatic lesions tend to exhibit characteristic radiographic patterns. For example, breast and prostate carcinoma should be at the top of any differential for blastic (sclerotic) lesions, while renal cell and thyroid carcinoma characteristically exhibit a lytic appearance. Breast, lung, and gastrointestinal metastases often exhibit a mixed lytic and blastic appearance.

Hidden in these figures is an important principle—less common presentations of common diseases are usually more common than common presentations of uncommon diseases. Most metastases from breast carcinoma are lytic (two-thirds) and only 10% present with a blastic appearance. Why then should one think "breast" when a blastic lesion is encountered in a woman? The answer is that breast carcinoma is the single most prevalent source of skeletal metastases, and even its less common presentations will be seen more often than the typical presentations of much less common malignancies, such as thyroid carcinoma (Fig. 8–11).

It should be noted again that a lytic appearance generally suggests an aggressive lesion, while a blastic appearance indicates a more indolent process. The latter implies that the surrounding bone has had sufficient time to mount an osteoblastic response. The typically lytic appearance of renal cell carcinoma and thyroid carcinoma can be explained on the basis of the extreme hypervascularity of these tumors, with associated hyperemia and increased osteoclastic activity.

Aside from pathologic fracture and the presence of a lytic or blastic lesion, other radiographic indicators of metastatic disease include destruction of a vertebral pedi-

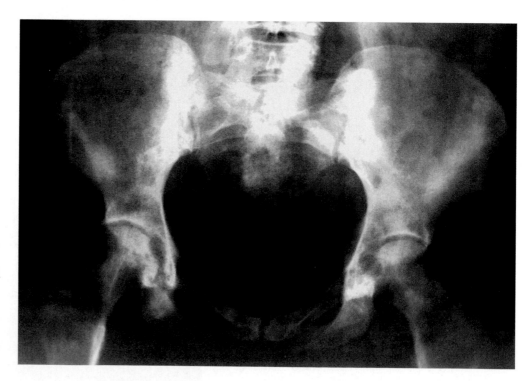

Figure 8–11. This frontal radiograph of the pelvis demonstrates bilateral sclerotic metastases throughout the pelvis and proximal femurs in a 32-year-old woman with treated breast carcinoma. Other sources of sclerotic metastases include prostate carcinoma and, less likely, lymphoma.

Figure 8–12. This coned-down frontal radiograph of the lumbar spine demonstrates an extremely sclerotic L4 vertebral body, due to metastatic prostate carcinoma.

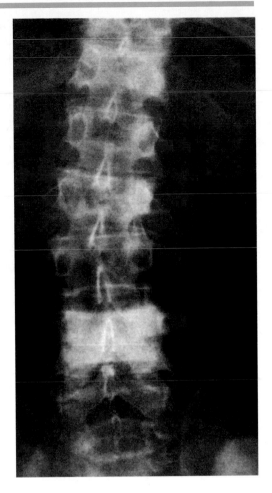

cle, the presence of a soft tissue mass, periosteal reaction, compression fracture of a vertebral body (another type of pathologic fracture), and an "ivory" or unusually dense (and hence white) vertebra. When an ivory vertebra is seen, metastatic disease is a strong possibility, although two other processes are more likely culprits—Paget's disease and Hodgkin's lymphoma (Fig. 8–12).

Bone scan

In a patient with a primary malignancy in whom skeletal metastases need to be ruled out, the optimal study is generally the nuclear medicine bone scan, which efficiently and relatively inexpensively screens the entire skeleton (Fig. 8–13). The bone scan employs Tc-99m-labeled diphosphonate compounds. Tc-99m is an excellent radiolabel, due to its ready availability, low cost, 140 keV principal photon (meaning that it is easily detected by conventional scintigraphic detectors), and 6 hour half-life, which limits the patient's absorbed radiation dose.

Perfusion and osteoblastic activity

The distribution of radiotracer within bone is dependent on two factors: regional blood flow and osteoblastic activity. A change in either can cause an abnormal pattern of activity on bone scan. In the case of blood flow, an increase in perfusion will tend to cause increased radiotracer activity, while oligemia will tend to cause decreased activity. Similarly, an increase in osteoblastic activity results in the incorporation of more of the diphosphonate molecule into the mineral matrix of bone, causing it to appear "hot" or "dark," while absence of osteoblastic activity produces a "cold" or photopenic ("photon poor") area, due to decreased radiotracer localization and photon emission. Examples of photopenic lesions on bone scan would include bone infarcts (no blood flow) and bone destruction (no osteoblasts), while lesions that appear hot on bone scan include healing fractures and osteoblastic tumors, such as osteogenic sarcoma.

Technique

The bone scan is probably the most frequently performed nuclear medicine study in the United States. Hence some familiarity with its technique is desirable. Because Tc-99m is excreted via the kidneys, the urinary bladder represents the critical organ; that is, the bladder is the organ that typically receives the highest radiation dose. A typical bladder dose for the study would be approximately 3 rads. In an effort to minimize absorbed dose, patients are kept well hydrated and encouraged to void frequently after the procedure, which lasts approximately 3 hours (by which time 50% of the injected dose will have been taken up by bone). Images are obtained using whole body scintillation detectors, in both anterior and posterior projections.

Even when clinical concern is focused only on a particular region, whole body images are obtained. Why? The answer lies in the fact that, once the radiotracer is injected, the whole body has been "dosed," and therefore it makes sense to obtain at least survey views of the entire skeleton. Of course, in the case of a search for bone metastases, such whole body views are the purpose of the study. When an abnormality is detected on whole body views or a specific region is of particular clinical concern, spot views are obtained, which provide significantly better resolution of the area in question.

Findings

Multiple areas of increased activity can be predicted in the normal patient. In children and adolescents, whose growth plates have not yet closed, increased activity will be seen in these regions. The "hottest" areas are those undergoing the most rapid growth, including the distal femur, the proximal tibia, and proximal humerus. In the adult, greater activity is seen in the axial skeleton than in the appendicular skeleton (i.e., the spine and pelvis are hotter than the limbs), and the kidneys are routinely visualized.

Greater than normal activity in the kidneys is most commonly due to urinary tract obstruction, while bilaterally decreased activity most often reflects renal failure. An important exception to the latter is the absence of renal activity in the so-called superscan, in which diffuse skeletal uptake is so avid that renal uptake is undercut. A common condition producing a superscan is diffusely metastatic prostate carcinoma (Fig. 8–14).

When bone scanning is employed in the search for skeletal metastatic disease, the likely skeletal sites of metastasis should be noted. Because the vast majority of bone metastases are deposited hematogenously, metastatic disease is most frequently found in bones that receive the greatest blood supply. By far the most richly perfused bone is that which contains red (hematopoietic) marrow, which in adults is found in the axial skeleton (spine and pelvis), as well as the cranium and the proximal humeri and femurs.

Figure 8–13. These anterior (left) and posterior (right) whole body images from a bone scan demonstrate multiple abnormal foci of increased radiotracer activity. The study was performed to rule out metastatic disease. The activity in the lumbar spine proved on plain radiographs to be secondary to degenerative change. The activity in the left humerus and the lateral aspect of an adjacent rib was post-traumatic, as the patient reported a history of a fall some months before. The diffusely increased activity in the right femur is characteristic of Paget's disease. The single focus of increased activity in the right ilium was a solitary metastasis, as proved by plain films and biopsy. The ability of the bone scan to screen the entire skeleton often produces multiple findings.

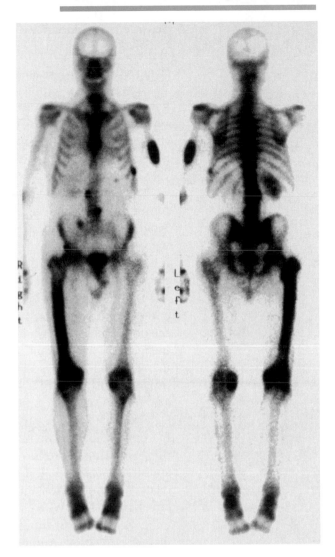

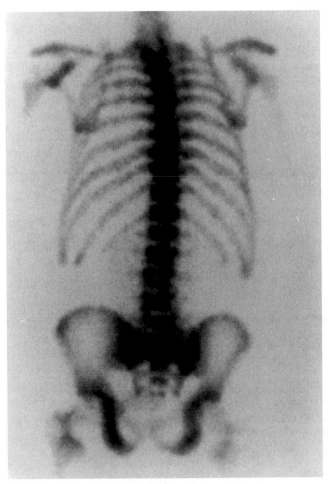

Figure 8–14. A 79-year-old man underwent bone scan to stage his known gastric carcinoma. This posterior view demonstrates diffuse uptake of radiotracer throughout the axial and proximal appendicular skeleton, with no renal activity. These findings represent a "superscan," in which bone uptake is so stimulated by extensive marrow metastatic disease that little tracer remains for excretion by the kidneys.

Sensitivity and specificity

Bone scan is much more sensitive than plain radiography in the detection of metastatic lesions, because the latter requires at least a 30 to 50% alteration in bone density before a lesion becomes detectable, while the former can detect much smaller alterations in local bone metabolism. These alterations result from the bone remodeling stimulated by tumor growth. The amount of osteoblastic remodeling may not be enough to produce a blastic appearance on plain radiography, but it will generally be more than sufficient to cause increased radiotracer uptake on bone scan (Fig. 8–15).

The site of increased activity is not the tumor per se, but the interface between the tumor and the remodeling bone; thus, many larger lesions will manifest as a central "cold" area (representing "pure" tumor) surrounded by a rim of tumor-bone interface, where remodeling is taking place. MRI is actually superior to bone scanning in detecting the earliest lesions, due to its ability to display alterations in marrow signal accompanying tumor invasion. Moreover, both MRI and plain films are much more effective at characterizing individual lesions. However, despite these advantages, to screen the entire skeleton by these modalities proves relatively time-consuming and costly, and the bone scan is nearly always the study of choice. The most important exception to this general rule is multiple myeloma, the lesions of which typically do not exhibit increased radiotracer accumulation, and thus may be missed. In the case of multiple myeloma, the plain film skeletal survey, including both the axial and appendicular skeleton, is usually the preferred study.

The bone scan is a highly sensitive but nonspecific study, as many processes other than metastatic disease may produce multiple foci of radiotracer accumulation. One process that may produce multiple "hot" areas is osteoarthritis (OA). However, the appearance is not typical of metastatic disease because the abnormalities tend to be bilaterally symmetrical and found in locations very unusual for metastases, such as the knees and ankles. When suspicious hot spots are seen in the spine or involving such joints as the hips or shoulders, it may be necessary to obtain plain films or MRI for further evaluation. Another prevalent cause of multiple hot spots is trauma, which tends not to be bilaterally symmetrical. Trauma often enters the differential diagnosis in the ribs, and obtaining a good history from the patient often proves critical in sorting out whether metastatic disease or trauma is responsible (Fig. 8–16).

In the setting of a known primary tumor with a tendency to metastasize to bone, however, multiple abnormal areas of increased radiotracer activity are virtually diagnostic of metastatic disease. Of course, the ultimate means of discriminating between benign and malignant etiologies of increased bone agent uptake is tissue biopsy, for which imaging guidance is often used.

PRIMARY BONE TUMORS

EPIDEMIOLOGY

Depending on how one defines primary malignant bone tumor, the incidence of these lesions is relatively low, with only about 3000 new cases diagnosed each year in the United States (not counting multiple myetoma). In decreasing order of frequency, the most important primary malignant lesions of bone include multiple myeloma, osteogenic sarcoma, chondrosarcoma, lymphoma, and Ewing's sarcoma (Fig. 8–17).

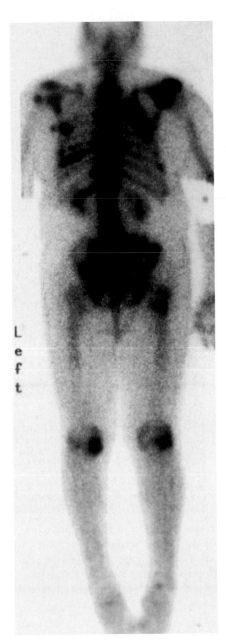

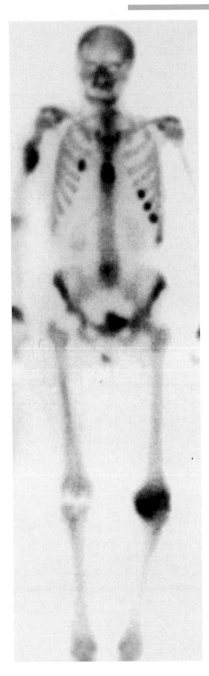

Figure 8–16. This anterior whole body image from a bone scan demonstrates multiple abnormal foci of increased radiotracer uptake in the ribs. Is this likely due to metastatic disease? In fact, questioning of the patient revealed that she had been involved in an auto accident several weeks previously and had developed rib pain thereafter. Was she sitting in the driver's seat or passenger's seat? The pattern of the abnormality suggests that she was sitting in the passenger's seat, with a shoulder belt extending across her chest from the right shoulder to the left hip. Even if it were impossible to question the patient, such a pattern of activity would make metastatic disease extremely unlikely. Note also the increased activity in the left knee, due to osteoarthritis. The increased activity in the right humerus was due to a fracture that stemmed from her accident.

Figure 8–15. Despite negative plain films, this patient's whole body bone scan (posterior image) demonstrates multiple abnormal foci of increased radiotracer activity throughout scapulae, ribs, spine, pelvis, and right femur. These were due to metastatic lung carcinoma.

Benign primary tumors are much more common; for example, it is estimated that as many as 40% of children harbor at least one benign fibrous cortical defect or nonossifying fibroma somewhere in their skeletons. At the opposite end of the life cycle, evidence of Paget's disease can be found in 4% of persons older than age 50 and 10% of persons older than 80 years of age (Fig. 8–18).

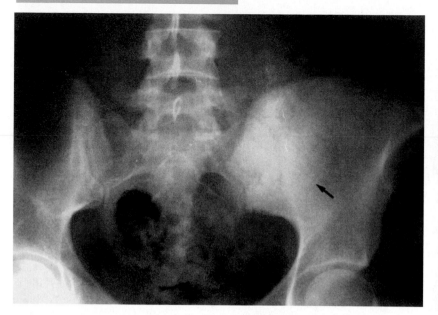

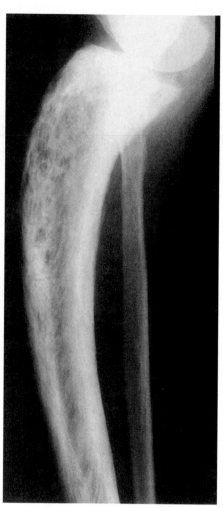

Figure 8–17. A 23-year-old women presented with left lower back and hip pain. The frontal radiograph of the sacral area demonstrates sclerosis and cloud-like ossification in and around the left ilium (arrow), indicating the presence of an osteogenic sarcoma. Osteogenic sarcomas represent the second most common malignant bone tumor after multiple myeloma, and are typically found in patients aged between 10 and 30 years. The most prevalent type has a 5-year survival rate of approximately 20%, although the prognosis tends to be worse when the tumor involves flat bones such as the pelvis, as in this case.

Figure 8–18. A 77-year-old man presented with a long history of right knee pain. The lateral view of the tibia and fibula demonstrates a mixed lytic and sclerotic coarsening of the tibial trabecular pattern, with a "woven" appearance classic for Paget's disease. Complications of Paget's disease include bowing deformity (seen here) and pathologic fractures due to weakening of the bone, as well as malignant transformation to osteogenic sarcoma in perhaps 1 in 10,000 patients. Bone scan, in which the lesions appear "hot," is the most efficient means of determining the extent of disease throughout the skeleton.

PATHOPHYSIOLOGY

Predictably, primary bone tumors tend to occur in certain locations in the skeleton, with the highest incidence of both benign and malignant tumors in the regions of the most rapid and prolonged bone growth. These include the metaphyseal regions of the distal femur and the proximal tibia. When in doubt about the most frequent site of any particular primary bone tumor, the distal femur, the site of greatest growth, represents the best guess.

Primary bone tumors are classified according to the pattern of their cellular differentiation, meaning the cell type of which they most remind the pathologist. Among the principal cell types are bone cells (as in osteogenic sarcoma), cartilage cells (chondrosarcoma), primitive mesenchymal cells (Ewing's sarcoma), lipid cells (liposarcoma), neural cells (neurofibroma), and fibroblasts (fibrosarcoma). A variety of hematopoietic cell types may be seen, the most prominent of which is the plasmacytoma, the isolated harbinger of multiple myeloma. Tumor grading, which tends to correlate directly with the aggressiveness of the lesion and inversely with prognosis, is based on the degree of cellular anaplasia or dedifferentiation.

CLINICAL PRESENTATION

Many bone tumors are identified incidentally on radiologic studies undertaken for other purposes, but others are evaluated on the basis of their clinical presentation. The principal presenting symptoms include mass, pain, and impairment of function.

IMAGING

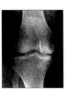 A key distinction to be made in the evaluation of bone tumors, whether benign or malignant, is between single and multiple lesions. As we have seen, myeloma and metastases are the malignant lesions by far most likely to be multiple at the time of diagnosis. The most prevalent benign polyostotic lesions include Paget's disease (most likely due to a chronic paramyxovirus infection of bone), fibrous dysplasia, and eosinophilic granuloma. In the remainder of this discussion, we will concern ourselves primarily with the radiographic evaluation of isolated lesions.

One of the most difficult tasks of the radiologist is simply to detect lesions, which may exhibit a quite subtle appearance. In some cases, lesions on radiographs are detected only in retrospect, after they have undergone additional growth and development. Once a solitary bone lesion is identified, a variety of factors go into its analysis.

Age

Even if one knows little about the particular radiologic characteristics of bone tumors, the correct diagnosis can often be predicted merely on the basis of the incidence of different tumors at various ages. In the case of malignant tumors, most tumors in the first two decades will be either Ewing's sarcoma or osteosarcoma, with the former tending to occur earlier than the latter. After the age of 40 years, solitary metastases, multiple myeloma, and chondrosarcoma are the most likely diagnoses. If the patient has a known primary tumor that generally metastasizes to bone, metastasis will usually become the primary suspect at any age.

Lesion margins

How does the radiologist determine if the lesion is likely to be malignant? The single most useful criterion is the radiographic appearance of the lesion's margins, which more than any other characteristic reflects its biologic behavior (Fig. 8–19). Lesions with narrow, well-defined zones of transition with adjacent normal bone tend to be benign, whereas lesions with wide, ill-defined zones of transition tend to be malignant. Radiologists often describe the margins of bone lesions as either geographic, implying a clear demarcation between the normal and abnormal regions due to a slow rate of growth, usually indicating benignity; motheaten, implying a less well-defined margin with a wider zone of transition and indicating a more rapid rate of growth; and permeative, denoting a very rapidly growing lesion that merges imperceptibly with normal bone (Fig. 8–20). Certain processes, such simple bone cyst, characteristically exhibit geographic borders, while others, such as Ewing's sarcoma and metastatic neuroblastoma, have characteristically permeative borders (Fig. 8–21). Still other processes, such as infection or metastases, may exhibit any type of border.

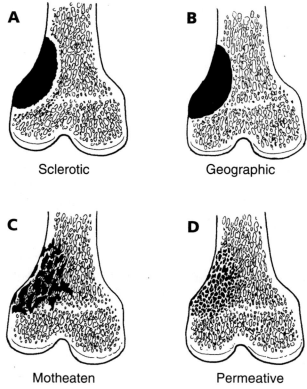

Sclerotic | Geographic

Motheaten | Permeative

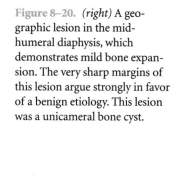

Figure 8–20. *(right)* A geographic lesion in the mid-humeral diaphysis, which demonstrates mild bone expansion. The very sharp margins of this lesion argue strongly in favor of a benign etiology. This lesion was a unicameral bone cyst.

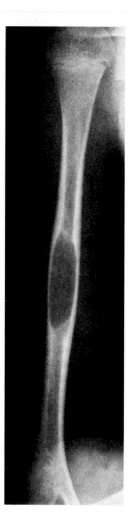

Figure 8–19. *(above)* The radiographic terms used to describe the degree of definition of a lesion's margins, varying from (**A**) extremely well defined, sclerotic margins in sclerotic lesions, to (**B**) well-defined but nonsclerotic margins in geographic lesions, to (**C**) poorly defined margins in motheaten lesions, to (**D**) margins that merge imperceptibly with normal bone in permeative lesions.

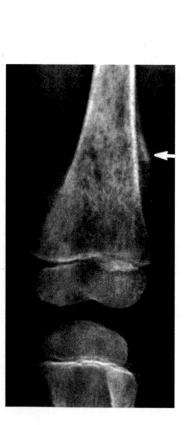

Figure 8–21. *(right)* This permeative lesion in the femoral metaphysis is associated with a Codman's triangle type of periosteal reaction (arrow). Both the permeative character of the lesion and Codman's triangle indicate an aggressive lesion, which in this case turned out to be a metastasis from neuroblastoma.

Periosteal reaction

The response of the periosteum to a contiguous lesion may also supply important information about the lesion's biologic behavior. Generally speaking, a slow-growing, benign process will give the periosteum time to lay down dense, uniform, or solid new bone, whereas a fast-growing, malignant tumor process will not allow the periosteum a chance to complete its work, and the pattern of periosteal reaction will be interrupted, with a lamellated ("onionskin"), sunburst, or amorphous appearance (Fig. 8–22). Another type of aggressive periosteal reaction is the so-called Codman's triangle, in which the periosteum is lifted progressively farther from the bone as one moves toward the center of the lesion. Again, benign lesions such as infection, eosinophilic granuloma, and osteoid osteoma may produce aggressive periosteal reaction (Fig. 8–23). However, when a benign pattern of periosteal reaction is seen, the probability of malignancy is very low.

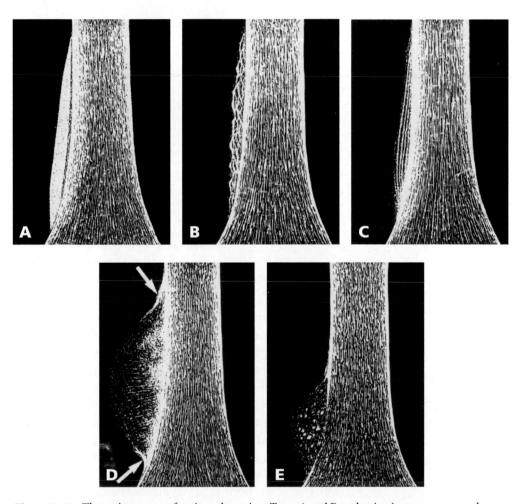

Figure 8–22. The various types of periosteal reaction. Types A and B are benign in appearance, and may be described as (A) thick and (B) undulating. Types C through E are more aggressive and more likely malignant and may be described as (C) laminated or "onion skin," (D) perpendicular or "sunburst," and (E) amorphous. Although not a perfect indicator, the pattern of periosteal reaction is one visual manifestation of a lesion's biological behavior.

Figure 8–23. A 5-year-old boy complained of night pain in his right calf. A frontal radiograph of the fibula and tibia demonstrates an "onionskin" pattern of lamellated periosteal reaction about the mid-diaphysis of the tibia, indicating the presence of considerable inflammation (arrow). However, the periosteal reaction remains well-ordered and the laminations are quite uniform. This lesion turned out to be an osteoid osteoma, a benign bone-forming tumor. The tumor is associated with prostaglandin production, which is responsible for the pain and explains why many patients characteristically experience relief with aspirin, a prostaglandin synthesis inhibitor.

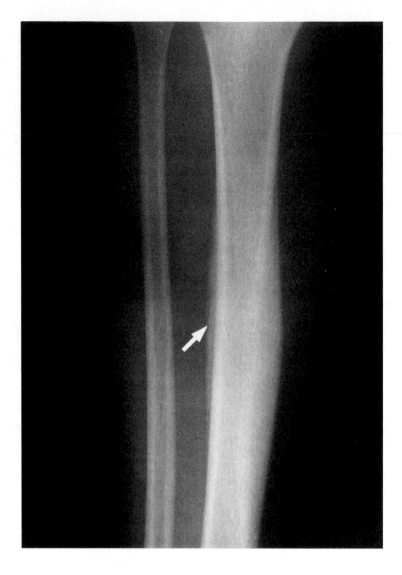

Osseous distribution

A final characteristic of note in any solitary osseous lesion is its location within the bone. This location should be described in both longitudinal and axial dimensions, with different tumors tending to occur in characteristic locations (Fig. 8–24). In the axial plane, the central medullary cavity of bone is a characteristic location for enchondroma and simple bone cysts, while osteosarcoma tends to occur in an eccentric medullary position, and benign fibrous cortical defects and osteoid osteomas are characteristically cortical. In the longitudinal plane, chondroblastoma (a benign lesion of children and young adults) and giant cell tumor are epiphyseal lesions, while osteogenic sarcoma and chondrosarcoma are characteristically metaphyseal in location, and Ewing's sarcoma and fibrous dysplasia are typically diaphyseal.

The role of the bone scan is typically less in the workup of primary bone malignancies than in metastatic disease. In the case of a primary bone tumor, the orthopedic surgeon needs to assess the extent of the lesion within bone and surrounding soft tissues, neither of which is well evaluated by the scintigram. On the other hand, bone scanning does play a role in the evaluation of tumors that often produce distant metastases, such as osteogenic sarcoma. In the case of an osteogenic sarcoma, increased tracer activity

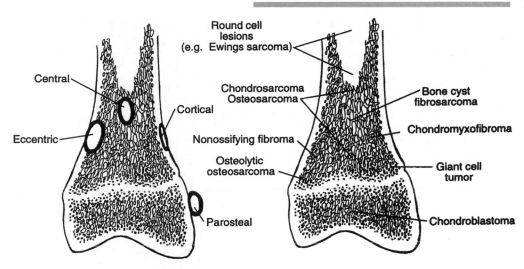

Figure 8–24. The typical location within long bones of various bone lesions, which can be very helpful in formulating a differential diagnosis.

may be detected not only in bone metastases, but in pulmonary and soft tissue metastases as well, due to the tendency of metastatic deposits to form bone matrix. Even tumors that do not produce an osteoblastic response may be detected on bone scintigraphy, due to the regional hyperemia they produce.

Multiple myeloma, a malignant tumor of B lymphocytes, arises in the hematopoietic marrow in the skull, axial skeleton, pelvis, and proximal portions of the humeri and femurs. It is associated with monoclonal protein spikes, Bence-Jones proteinuria, and other signs of a bone marrow malignancy, such as anemia, infection, increased alkaline phosphatase, and hypercalcemia. Characteristic features of multiple myeloma on plain radiography include a punched-out appearance with endosteal scalloping (implying a site of origin within the central, marrow-containing portion of the bone) or a bubbly appearance that may be associated with a soft tissue mass (Fig. 8–25).

Inflammatory

The suffix -*itis* is used to denote an inflammatory condition. In the case of OA, the inflammatory suffix is probably something of a misnomer, because the true pathophysiology of the condition likely consists instead of repeated episodes of microtrauma, with secondary inflammatory reaction. However, rheumatoid arthritis (RA), the other major form of joint pathology, is undoubtedly inflammatory in nature, and because the two represent the most important joint pathologies, both OA and RA are considered under the heading of inflammatory disease.

OSTEOARTHRITIS

EPIDEMIOLOGY

The most common joint disease of human beings, OA, also commonly referred to as degenerative joint disease, clinically afflicts more than one-half of persons older than 65 years of age. It is one of the leading causes of disability in this age group. It is estimated that at least 80% of persons harbor at least radiographic evidence of OA by the

Figure 8–25. A 57-year-old man with multiple myeloma underwent a radiographic skeletal survey to determine the extent of his disease. This frontal radiograph of his proximal right humerus demonstrates multiple "punched-out" lytic lesions with endosteal scalloping (erosion of the inner margin of the cortex), a characteristic appearance. Multiple myeloma is the principal primary skeletal malignancy, with approximately 12,000 cases per year diagnosed in the United States; 95% of patients are older than 40 years of age.

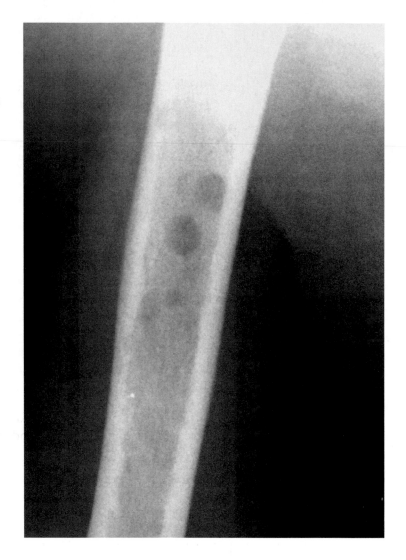

time they reach 50 years of age. While hereditary factors have been implicated in the development of OA, most cases are idiopathic, and mechanical factors are usually invoked. For example, ballet dancers suffer a higher incidence of ankle and toe OA than the general population.

PATHOPHYSIOLOGY

OA is often categorized into primary and secondary forms. Primary OA results from abnormal mechanical forces on a normal underlying joint and is age-related. Secondary OA results from normal forces on an abnormal joint and is seen in conditions such as calcium dihydrate pyrophosphate deposition disease (CPPD), rheumatoid arthritis (discussed later), trauma, and septic joint.

Strictly speaking, OA afflicts only the synovial joints. Important mechanical characteristics of synovial joints include stability during motion, joint lubrication, and uniform load distribution. The articular cartilage is vital in providing a smooth and relatively frictionless surface for joint motion and in helping to dissipate loading forces as one bone mechanically compresses another. Articular cartilage itself contains only one cell type, the chondrocyte, and an extracellular matrix. It contains no nerves or blood vessels. As noted earlier in this chapter, chondrocytes depend for their metabolism on the diffusion of nutrients and metabolites through the cartilage matrix. Despite their relatively precarious nutritional state, they maintain a level of metabolic activity similar to that of some cells in vascularized tissues.

The cyclic loading and unloading of cartilage stimulates matrix synthesis, whereas prolonged stable loading or the absence of loading and motion (as in prolonged immobilization) causes degradation of the matrix and eventually leads to joint degeneration. In addition to prolonged immobilization, another disorder that predisposes to OA is a septic joint, in which bacteria compete with chondrocytes for glucose and other nutrients in the synovial fluid.

OA is not primarily an inflammatory process. Instead, it consists of a retrogressive sequence of cell and matrix changes that result in loss of articular cartilage structure and function, accompanied by attempted cartilage repair and bone remodeling. Three phases can be discerned: cartilage damage, chondrocyte response, and over time, a gradual diminution in chondrocyte response.

The first sign of OA pathologically is softening and loss of articular cartilage. As OA progresses, cartilage thins and becomes fibrillated, with eventual uncovering of underlying bone. This causes eburnation (sclerosis), microfractures with cyst formation, and osteophyte formation. Why does the bone form osteophytes? The proliferation of these outgrowths of bone around joint surfaces may be regarded as an attempt by bone to increase the surface area of the joint and thereby distribute mechanical forces more widely (Fig. 8–26). With loss of the shock-absorbing properties of articular cartilage, fragments of cartilage or bone may break off from the articular surface and become loose intraarticular bodies, interfering with joint motion and causing sudden "locking."

CLINICAL PRESENTATION

OA usually presents with mono- or pauciarticular involvement. Patients complain of an aching pain that is aggravated by use and alleviated by rest. The pain originates not within the cartilage, which is uninnervated, but within the periosteum and subchondral bone, secondary to structural distortion and microfractures. Physical examination discloses swelling and tenderness around the involved joint, crepitus (from bone rubbing on bone), and effusion. The warmth and swelling are less than that seen in RA. Moreover, in contrast to the hour or more of morning stiffness associated with RA, that experienced by OA patients usually lasts only a period of 10 to 20 minutes.

IMAGING

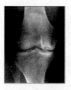 The radiographic hallmarks of OA, in contrast to RA, include normal mineralization, productive changes (osteophyte and subchondral bone formation), and nonuniform joint space loss (Fig. 8–27). In the hand, the joints most often involved by OA include the distal interphalangeal joints (producing Heberdon's nodes) and the proximal interphalangeal joints (Bouchard's nodes). The metacarpophalangeal joints are characteristically spared, whereas they are generally involved by RA. Other prominant sites of involvement by OA include the base of the thumb, the hip, the knee, and the spine.

A strong indication that OA is a mechanical disorder is the fact that the risk of OA is increased in obese patients, patients with congenitally dislocated hips, and those who have suffered prior trauma associated with cartilage disruption. In the hip, there is nonuniform loss of joint space and superolateral migration of the femoral head. In the knee, joint space loss is likewise nonuniform and more often involves the medial than lateral femoral-tibial compartment. Strictly speaking, OA of the spine refers only to degeneration of the apophyseal joints, while spondylosis is the term for degenerative disk disease. The osteophyte production associated with OA of the spine often encroaches on the neural foramina, resulting in spinal nerve root compression (see the discussion of back pain in Chapter 9).

Initial treatment of OA is primarily symptomatic, employing aspirin or acetaminophen. As the disease progresses, preservation of mobility and function become increasingly important concerns, and improvement of joint mechanics and physical therapy often prove helpful. In patients who are refractory to medical therapy, orthopedic surgery is often performed to repair or replace the damaged joint. Approximately 250,000 joint replacements are performed each year in the United States, the majority of which involve the hip or the knee. Hemiarthroplasties involve replacement of only one side of a joint, while total arthroplasties involve prosthetic components in both sides. Prosthetic components are attached to bone either with cement (methylmethacrylate) that has been made radiopaque by the addition of barium; press fitting so that there is direct contact between the prosthesis and the bone cortex; or biologic

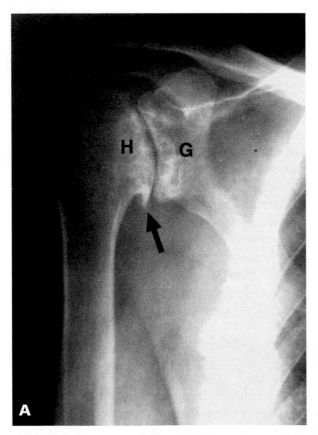
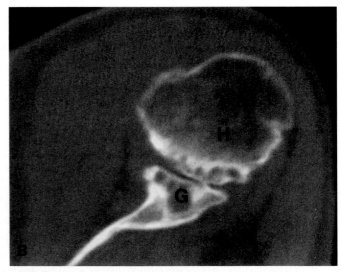

Figure 8–26. A 67-year-old man with a history of repeated shoulder trauma presented with longstanding pain and decreased mobility in his right shoulder. (A) A frontal radiograph demonstrates classic changes of severe osteoarthritis (OA), including near-obliteration of glenohumeral joint space, sclerosis, subchondral cysts, and osteophytes (arrow). One might say that the osteophytes appear to be attempting to increase the surface area of the joint. (B) An axial computed tomography image of the shoulder using bone algorithm demonstrates the same changes on both the humeral and glenoid sides of the joint. It should be noted that the shoulder is a relatively unusual location for primary OA, and this patient's disease was presumed to be secondary to trauma. G, glenoid of the scapula; H, humeral head.

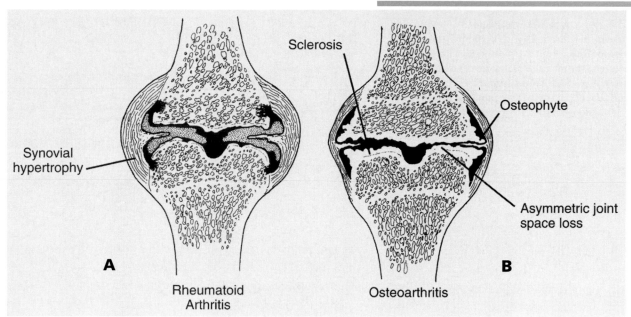

Figure 8–27. The important morphologic differences between (**A**) rheumatoid arthritis (RA) and (**B**) osteoarthritis (OA). Note that OA involves little or no loss of mineralization, osteophyte formation, and nonuniform loss of joint space. RA, on the other hand, involves juxta-articular osteoporosis, periarticular erosions, and an absence of productive changes (osteophytes).

methods, in which fenestrations are created in the prosthesis, into which new bone can grow. Another common reason for joint replacement is trauma, particularly femoral neck fracture.

Radiography is one of the most important tools available to the orthopedic surgeon in assessing joint prostheses. In the immediate postoperative period, radiographs are taken to ascertain component position and to detect intraoperative fractures or dislocation (Fig. 8–28). The most common delayed complications, which should be suspected in patients with recurrent or persistent pain, are loosening and infection. Unfortunately, the two can be difficult to differentiate radiographically. Signs especially suspicious for infection include irregular periostitis, poorly marginated lucencies, and sinus tracts. The presence of infection can be verified by needle aspiration. Signs of loosening include migration of the components (hence the importance of comparison with previous radiographs), fracture of the cement or prosthesis, and widening of the prosthesis-cement interface. Additional complications include profuse heterotopic bone formation, dislocation, and stress fractures.

RHEUMATOID ARTHRITIS

EPIDEMIOLOGY

Afflicting approximately 1% of the population, RA is a major source of disability in the United States. Women are afflicted approximately three times as often as men, and in 80% of cases the onset of symptoms occurs between the ages of 35 and 50 years. While genetic susceptibility is a definite factor, environmental factors appear also to play a role. Some patients develop only mild symptoms that spontaneously and completely remit, while others suffer profound systemic sequelae and marked joint deformities. Most patients experience a course somewhere between these two extremes. If

Figure 8–28. A frontal radiograph in a 77-year-old man who had just undergone a left hip hemiarthroplasty for osteoarthritis demonstrates a longitudinal fracture of the medial aspect of the femoral diaphysis (arrow). This fracture was immediately treated by the placement of cerclage wires around the proximal femur.

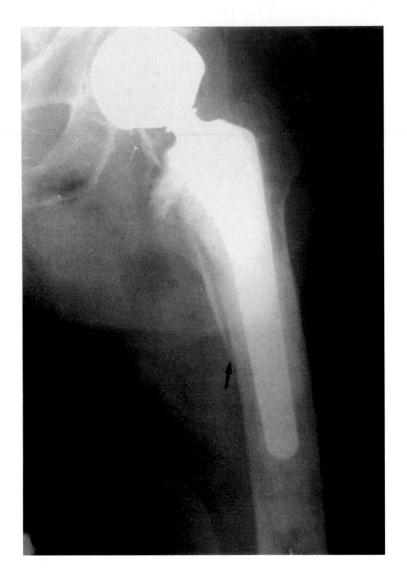

RA persists for more than a decade, more than four of five patients will have some degree of joint deformity (Fig. 8–29).

PATHOPHYSIOLOGY

 The pathophysiology of RA is the subject of debate. Immune phenomena are clearly implicated. More than two-thirds of adult RA patients exhibit circulating rheumatoid factor, which consists of autoantibodies reactive with the Fc portion of immunoglobulin G (IgG). It has been hypothesized that complexes of circulating rheumatoid factor and IgG may be the inciting factors in synovial inflammation. However, rheumatoid factor may also be present in systemic lupus erythematosus (SLE), sarcoidosis, and infectious mononucleosis, among other disorders. Early inflammatory changes of RA include synovial hypervascularity, edema, and cellular infiltration. Synovial inflammation and associated hyperemia induce osteoclastic activity, resulting in bone "wash out" around joints seen on radiographs as juxta-articular osteoporosis. With time, the synovium hypertrophies, a process called pannus formation. This synovial proliferation produces erosion of sub-

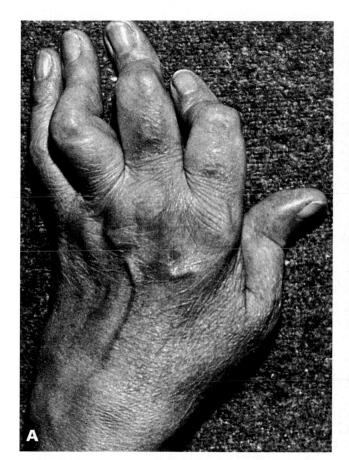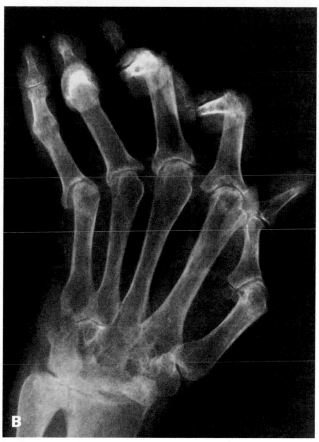

Figure 8–29. (A) Photograph and (B) radiograph of a patient with long-standing rheumatoid arthritis demonstrates the severe deformity and loss of function that may result from this disease.

chondral bone and ligamentous laxity, which may be followed by subluxation and ankylosis.

CLINICAL PRESENTATION

The onset of RA is usually insidious, with constitutional symptoms such as fatigue, anorexia, and weakness, although a number of patients will also note vague musculoskeletal symptoms. Over a period of months, more specific musculoskeletal symptoms appear, with pain, swelling, tenderness, and limitation of motion symmetrically involving the hands, wrists, knees, and/or feet. Prolonged morning stiffness (> 1 hour) helps to distinguish a truly inflammatory arthritis such as RA from noninflammatory arthritides such as OA. Because the joint capsule is richly innervated with pain fibers, swelling secondary to hyperemia, edema, and accumulation of synovial fluid, with distension of the joint capsule, can produce severe pain. As a result, patients often hold the joint in a flexed position, to maximize joint volume and minimize pressure.

The extra-articular manifestations of RA are legion. These include rheumatoid nodules, which develop in one-quarter of patients and vary in size and consistency but are usually found in periarticular locations, on extensor surfaces, or in areas subject to mechanical pressure. Pleural and pericardial manifestations include effusions and inflammation. Pulmonary fibrosis may result. Other manifestations include vasculitis, scleritis, osteoporosis, and Felty's syndrome, which consists of RA, splenomegaly, neutropenia, and anemia.

IMAGING

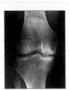 Although RA is a systemic disease, it nearly always presents with inflammation in the synovial lining of the joints. As one would expect, these inflammatory changes and the associated hypervascularity cause hyperemia-induced juxta-articular osteoporosis, which, along with soft tissue swelling, are the first radiographic signs of the disease (Fig. 8–30). The later hallmarks of RA include articular erosions, bilaterally symmetrical involvement, and absence of bone production (osteophyte formation).

The hands are the most commonly involved region where, following symmetrical soft tissue swelling and juxta-articular osteoporosis, RA produces characteristic erosions in the "bare areas" of the joints, where bone is directly exposed to the synovium

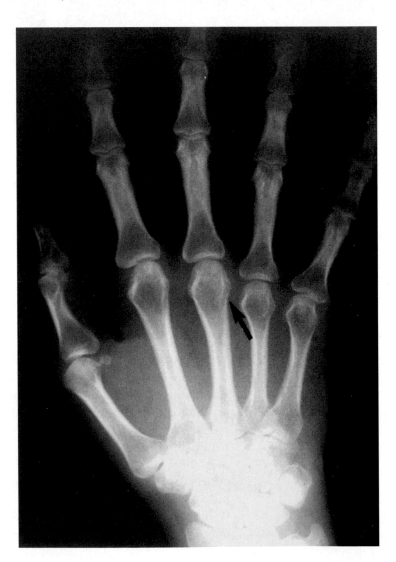

Figure 8–30. A 45-year-old woman with pain and stiffness in her hands demonstrates one of the earliest radiographic changes of rheumatoid arthritis, juxta-articular osteoporosis (arrow). This loss of bone mineral around the joints is secondary to the hyperemia associated with synovial inflammation. Note also mild narrowing of the proximal and distal interphalangeal joints, which reflects early (and unrelated) osteoarthritis.

Figure 8–31. Many of the characteristic hand deformities seen in rheumatoid arthritis. 1, hyperextension and subluxation of the distal phalanx of the thumb; 2, flexion at the proximal and extension at the distal interphalangeal joint (boutonniere deformity); 3, extension at the proximal and flexion at the distal interphalangeal joint (swan-neck deformity); 4, destruction of bone ends; 5, ulnar deviation at the metacarpophalangeal joints with subluxation; 6, dislocation of the metacarpophalangeal joints ("main en lorgnette" or "telescoping"); 7, erosion and compression of the metacarpophalangeal joints ("ball in socket"); 8, erosion, sclerosis, and partial fusion of the carpal joints; 9, tapering of the distal ulna; 10, sclerosis, narrowing, or ankylosis of joints.

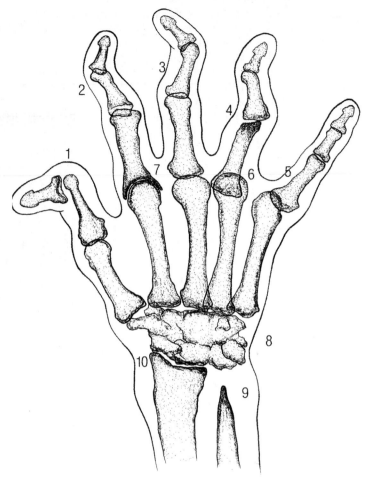

because it is not protected by articular cartilage. Characteristic locations include the entire carpal compartment, as well as the metacarpophalangeal and proximal interphalangeal joints, with sparing of the distal interphalangeal joints.

Characteristic deformities are seen clinically and radiographically in RA (Fig. 8–31). These include the swan-neck deformity, with hyperextension of the proximal interphalangeal joints and flexion of the distal interphalangeal joints; boutonniere deformity, with flexion deformity of the proximal interphalangeal joints and extension of the distal interphalangeal joints; and "Z" deformity, with radial deviation of the wrist and ulnar deviation of the digits (if ulnar deviation is seen without erosions, one should think of SLE). These can be traced to destruction or weakening of ligaments, tendons, and cartilage; muscle imbalance; and altered physical forces produced by the use of affected joints.

Other characteristic areas include the feet, hips (with axial migration of the femoral head and protrusio acetabuli deformity), knees (with tricompartment joint space narrowing, including the medial and lateral femoral-tibial compartments and the patellofemoral joint), and shoulder (with chronic rotator cuff tear and erosion of the distal clavicle). Nearly 50% of RA patients have involvement of the cervical spine, while the thoracic and lumbar spines are generally not involved (Fig. 8–32). One of the most important findings is atlanto-axial subluxation, which is best detected on flexion views.

Figure 8–32. A 54-year-old woman with long-standing rheumatoid arthritis demonstrates multiple subluxations of the cervical vertebrae secondary to the apophyseal joint erosions and ligamentous laxity often seen in this condition. Normally, a line drawn through the anterior margins of the vertebral bodies should form a gentle arc, but in this case there are step-offs or discontinuities in that imaginary line. Note also disk space narrowing from degenerative disease at C5-6, which paradoxically may have helped to stabilize this joint, as it is not subluxed.

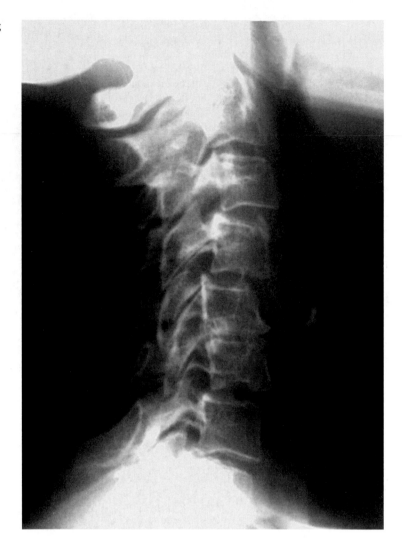

SERONEGATIVE SPONDYLOARTHROPATHIES

The seronegative spondyloarthropathies are an important class of joint diseases that are distinguished from RA in part by the fact that the rheumatoid factor is negative. These include disorders such as ankylosing spondylitis and psoriatic arthritis. Ankylosing spondylitis is far more common in men than women, and 95% of patients are HLA-B27 positive. Around the age of 20 years, patients begin to note the insidious onset of back stiffness and pain. Radiographically, the initial site of involvement is the sacroiliac joint, but the process gradually progresses to involve the entire spine. The sacroiliac joints eventually ankylose (fuse), as do the vertebral bodies. The characteristic intervertebral fusion produces the so-called bamboo spine (Fig. 8–33). Psoriasis usually manifests first with skin changes, and only 10 to 20% of patients develop psoriatic arthropathy. In contrast to ankylosing spondylitis, psoriatic arthritis tends to involve the peripheral joints as well as the axial skeleton and often produces asymmetric involvement in the spine and sacroiliac joints. Characteristic findings include a combination of erosive and proliferative changes (in contrast to RA, which is only erosive), soft tissue swelling of the digits producing a so-called sausage digit, and the presence of periosteal reaction (Fig. 8–34).

Figure 8–33. This coned-down view of a lateral lumbar spine radiograph demonstrates a classic appearance of ankylosing spondylitis, with ossification of the annulus fibrosus (the outer portion of the intervertebral disk; arrow), which will eventually progress to bony fusion of the spinal ligaments and spinal ankylosis. This appearance is often referred to as a "bamboo spine."

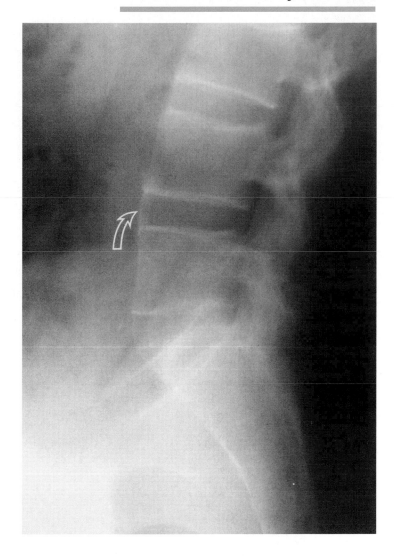

Metabolic

ACROMEGALY

Acromegaly is a classic metabolic bone disorder that usually stems from autonomous hypersecretion of pituitary somatotropin by a functional microadenoma. The excess growth hormone results in overstimulation of cartilage growth. When this occurs prior to growth plate closure, it results in gigantism. After closure of the growth plate, it results in acromegaly. The effects of acromegaly are most dramatically seen in structures with the greatest number of cartilage end plates, such as the hands, feet, skull (where sutures remain open until age 45 years), and face. Hence the inclusion of hat, glove, and shoe sizes in the endocrinologic history, as well as the value of old photographs to assess for coarsening of the facial features.

Radiographic features include widened joint spaces due to cartilage growth, which is associated with secondary osteoarthritic changes (Fig. 8–35). The osteoarthritic changes are presumed to result from impaired diffusion of nutrients from synovial fluid through the thickened cartilage. Other findings include prognathism (protrusion of the jaw), frontal bossing due to overgrowth of the frontal sinuses, and in some

Figure 8–34. This hand radiograph demonstrates classic changes of psoriasis, including prominent soft tissue swelling of the second and third digits ("sausage digits"), lamellated periosteal reaction around the metacarpals and proximal phalanges, and periarticular erosions. Both the periosteal reaction and erosions are well seen in the distal aspect of the second proximal phalanx.

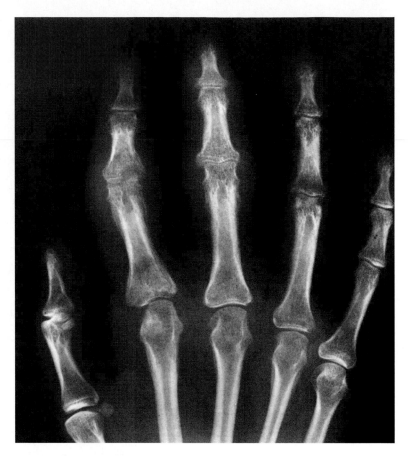

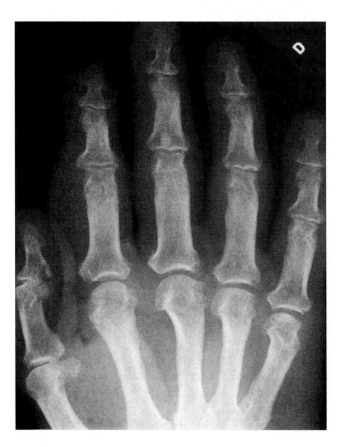

Figure 8–35. This hand radiograph demonstrates two characteristic features of acromegaly, including spade-like distal phalangeal tufts and widening of the joint spaces due to cartilaginous hypertrophy.

cases, enlargement of the sella turcica. As discussed in Chapter 9, MRI is often used to localize the pituitary lesion.

CHRONIC RENAL FAILURE

EPIDEMIOLOGY

One of the most prominant metabolic disorders of bone stems from renal dysfunction. Chronic renal failure is a relatively common condition in the United States, representing the final common pathway of a number of prevalent diseases. The most important is diabetes, which is responsible for 28% of cases and is associated pathologically with the Kimmelstiel-Wilson lesion (nodular glomerulosclerosis). The second most common is prolonged hypertension, the cause of 24% of cases, which is associated pathologically with nephrosclerosis. Other major causes include glomerulonephritis and polycystic kidney disease.

PATHOPHYSIOLOGY

 The term *chronic renal failure* encompasses decreased glomerular filtration, renal tubular dysfunction, and decreased enzymatic activity, particularly the conversion of 25-OH-vitamin D to 1,25-$(OH)_2$-vitamin D. Secondary hyperparathyroidism results from the kidney's inability to normally excrete phosphate, resulting in hyperphosphatemia, consequent hypocalcemia, and increased secretion of PTH. The hypocalcemia is exacerbated by loss of renal 1-hydroxylase activity, with a deficiency of the active form of vitamin D. Renal osteodystrophy refers to the production of bone that is deficient in mineral content, with increased liability to fractures.

Secondary hyperparathyroidism is distinguished from both primary and tertiary hyperparathyroidism. Primary hyperparathyroidism, which is especially common in middle-aged and elderly women, results in at least 80% of cases from a benign, autonomous adenoma, which causes suppression of the three remaining parathyroid glands. Other causes of primary hyperparathyroidism include hyperplasia (seen most often in the multiple endocrine neoplasia syndromes) and carcinoma. Tertiary hyperparathyroidism refers to autonomous gland function following long-standing renal failure.

Therapies employed in chronic renal failure include chronic hemodialysis, peritoneal dialysis, and renal transplantation. Transplantation now enjoys a 1-year survival rate in most centers of greater than 90%.

CLINICAL PRESENTATION

Nearly all patients with end stage renal disease will eventually develop secondary hyperparathyroidism. The clinical manifestations of secondary hyperparathyroidism include bone pain, proximal muscle weakness, pruritis, and eventually, diffuse soft tissue calcification. The latter finding is more likely when the product of the serum calcium and phosphate exceeds 50 mg/dL.

IMAGING

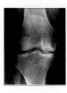 Numerous radiographic findings are possible. Osteosclerosis, the cause of which is unknown, refers to an apparent increased bone density in certain areas, especially the "rugger jersey spine" (Fig. 8–36). Bone resorption is seen in up to 70% of long-standing cases. Subperiosteal resorption is pathognomonic and characteristically involves the radial

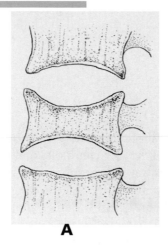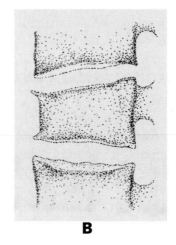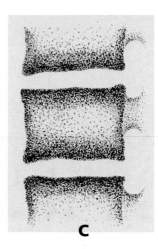

A   **B**   **C**

Figure 8–36. The characteristic differences between osteoporosis, osteomalacia, and hyperparathyroidism in the spine. (A) Osteoporosis manifests as a biconcave vertebral body with prominent vertical trabeculae. (B) Osteomalacia manifests as uniform deossification with a loss of trabecular detail and anterior wedge-shaped compression fractures. (C) The "rugger jersey" spine of secondary hyperparathyroidism manifests as increased density adjacent to the vertebral end plates.

aspects of the middle phalanges. Endosteal resorption causes a classic "salt and pepper" appearance of the calvarium (Fig. 8–37). Subchondral resorption is often seen in the hands and may simulate the erosions of inflammatory arthritis. Brown tumors are localized areas in which bone is replaced by fibrous tissue and appear as well-defined, lytic lesions, which may cause osseous expansion. Another finding is soft tissue and vascular calcifications.

CRYSTALOPATHIES: GOUT

EPIDEMIOLOGY

A disease of middle-aged and elderly men and postmenopausal women, gout afflicts approximately 3 of every 1000 people in the United States, although it is found in up to 5% of patients with clinical arthritis.

PATHOPHYSIOLOGY

 The risk of suffering an attack of gout is directly proportional to the plasma level of uric acid, and a person with a uric acid level of greater than 10 mg/dL has a greater than 90% probability of suffering an attack. The attack is thought to occur when uric acid crystals begin to precipitate in the synovial fluid and cartilage, with phagocytosis of the crystals by leukocytes, which are subsequently damaged by the "indigestible" crystals and release the toxic contents of their phagolysosomes into the joint, causing inflammation. When aspirated joint fluid is inspected microscopically, monosodium urate crystals appear as needle-like refractile bodies, which are strongly negatively birefringent (yellow when aligned parallel to the compensatory axis).

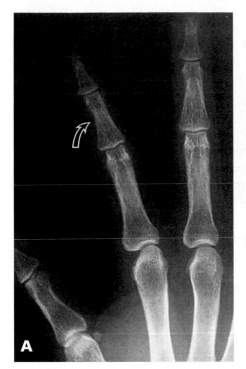
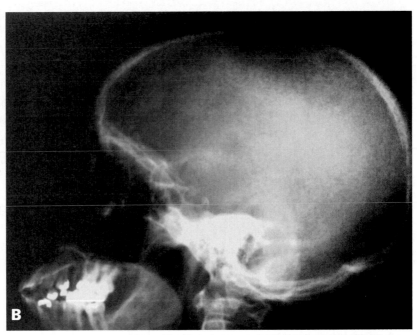

Figure 8–37. A 55-year-old woman with end-stage renal disease on chronic hemodialysis demonstrates classic changes of secondary hyperparathyroidism. (A) Frontal radiographs of the second and third digits show prominent subperiosteal resorption along the radial aspects of the second (arrow) and third middle phalanges. (B) A lateral view of the skull shows endosteal resorption, producing a "salt and pepper" appearance, best seen in the superior aspect of the calvarium.

Gout is divided into primary and secondary forms, depending on the underlying etiology of the increased uric acid levels. Primary gout is seen in patients with an underlying disorder of purine metabolism, which is heritable and predominately afflicts males, or in patients who undersecrete uric acid. Most patients with idiopathic gout fall into the latter category. Secondary gout is seen in patients with some other primary disorder that increases uric acid levels. Secondary gout may be further divided into disorders associated with increased uric acid production, such as leukemia and cytotoxic chemotherapy, and disorders associated with decreased uric acid excretion, such as renal failure. Risk factors for gout include alcoholism, which both increases uric acid production and decreases excretion, and salicylate use, which decreases excretion. Treatment of gout is directed at the acute manifestation, synovitis, as well as the underlying etiology, the increased uric acid level.

CLINICAL PRESENTATION

Only about 5% of hyperuricemic patients develop gout. The typical attack of acute gouty arthritis is that of an exquisitely painful monoarthritis, most often the first metatarsophalangeal (MTP) joint (podagra). The patient with podagra finds weight-bearing impossible, and the joint often appears red and swollen. The attack generally subsides within days to weeks, and the patient becomes asymptomatic until the next attack. Eventually, the patient may develop tophi and chronic gouty arthritis, with nodular deposits of monosodium urate involving the external ears and the ulnar surface of the forearms.

IMAGING

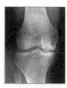 Radiographic changes of gout are seen in up to 50% of patients. The most commonly involved joint is the first MTP joint, which is the initial finding in 60% of patients (Fig. 8–38). After the first MTP joint, other common sites of gouty arthritis include other toes, ankles, hands, and the olecranon bursa, typically with sparing of the hips and shoulders. Bone mineralization is initially normal. Findings include soft-tissue tophi (containing birefringent monosodium urate crystals), punched-out erosions with sclerotic borders and overhanging edges, and preservation of the joint space. As the disease progresses and more uric acid crystals deposit in the articular cartilage, the cartilage itself is eroded away, and secondary arthritis with joint space narrowing ensues.

CRYSTALLOPATHIES: PSEUDOGOUT

EPIDEMIOLOGY

Pseudogout, better termed *calcium pyrophosphate dihydrate deposition disease,* afflicts predominately elderly patients and is found in up to 5% of the general population, rendering it much more common than gout. It is seen with increased frequency in patients with hyperparathyroidism, gout, and hemochromatosis.

PATHOPHYSIOLOGY

 CPPD is defined as calcification in the hyaline cartilage of articular surfaces and is seen as a thin rim of calcification outlining the surface of the joint. It most often involves the knees (especially the patellofemoral joint), the pubic symphysis, and the hands and wrist (especially the radial-carpal and carpal-lunate joints). These calcium deposits interfere with normal cartilage structure and function, and predispose to secondary OA (Fig. 8–39).

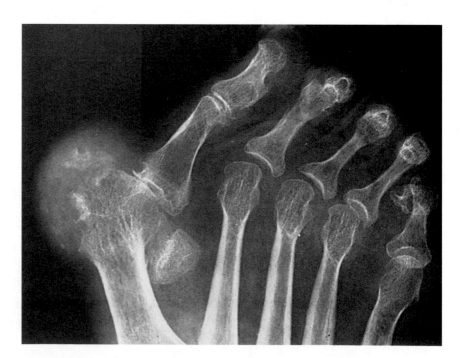

Figure 8–38. This patient with long-standing gout demonstrates characteristic destruction of the first metatarsal head, an erosion at the first proximal phalanx, and a large tophus at the first metarsophalangeal joint, all of which have produced lateral subluxation at this joint.

Figure 8–39. This elderly patient complained of knee pain. A frontal radiograph of the right knee demonstrates joint space narrowing, osteophytosis, and sclerosis of the lateral compartment of the knee joint, as well as sharpening of the (midline) tibial spines. In addition, there is calcification of the hyaline cartilage in the medial compartment (arrow), called chondrocalcinosis. These findings are typical of calcium pyrophosphate deposition disease arthropathy.

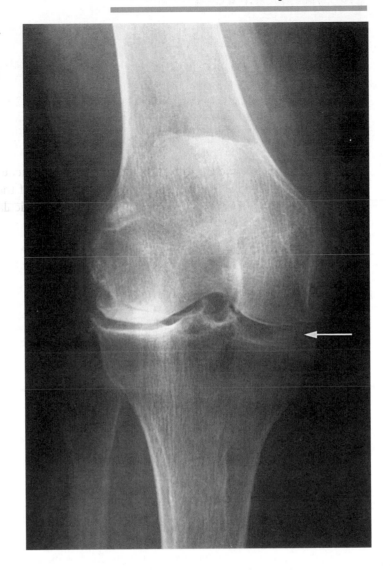

CLINICAL PRESENTATION

Only approximately 25% of patients with CPPD present with an acute pseudogout attack, most frequently involving the knee. The involved joint is red, swollen, warm, and painful. A minority of patients experience attacks involving multiple joints, which can be confused with RA.

IMAGING

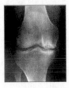 Because articular cartilage is radiolucent, the rim of surface calcification associated with CPPD appears to be "floating in space" above the end of the bone. It should be suspected when OA-like changes are seen in unusual joints, such as the elbow, shoulder, or the metacarpal-phalangeal joints of the hand, or when joints commonly involved with OA demonstrate an unusual appearance, such as a hip with uniform joint space loss (Fig. 8–40). The definitive diagnosis rests on the finding of calcium pyrophosphate crystals in synovial cells, which appear blunt and rectangular, and demonstrate slight positive birefringence, thus appearing blue.

Figure 8–40. A 62-year-old man presented with hand pain. A frontal radiograph of the left hand demonstrates narrowing of the third metacarpophalangeal joint (small arrow), an unusual location for osteoarthritis. In addition, note the beak-like osteophytes involving the distal metacarpal heads (large arrow). These findings are diagnostic of calcium pyrophosphate deposition disease arthropathy.

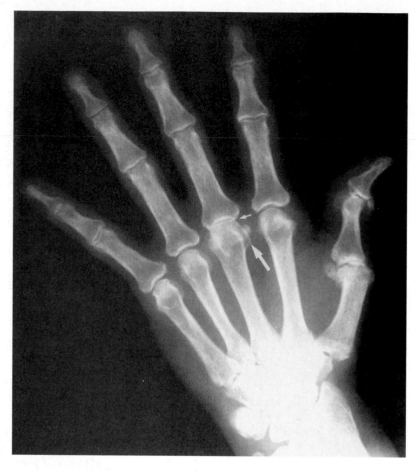

HYDROXYAPATITE DEPOSITION DISEASE

While calcium pyrophosphate deposits in articular cartilage, the form of calcium that deposits in tendons, ligaments, and bursae is calcium hydroxyapatite. This type of soft tissue calcification is seen on a secondary basis in a number of conditions, including collagen vascular diseases such as scleroderma, dermatomyositis, and lupus, as well as hyperparathyroidism and hypervitaminosis D. Hydroxyapatite deposition may also occur on an idiopathic basis, especially in the shoulder and the wrist (Fig. 8–41).

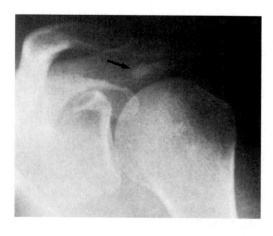

Figure 8–41. This frontal radiograph demonstrates deposition of calcium hydroxyapatite within the subacromial bursa of the shoulder (arrow).

Traumatic

JOINT INJURY

Displacement of a bone relative to another bone at a joint may be described as a dislocation, a subluxation, or a diastasis. A dislocation is diagnosed when there is complete loss of continuity of the bones at a joint surface. A subluxation, by contrast, occurs when the bones are less severely displaced and some degree of continuity at the joint surface remains (Fig. 8–42). A diastasis occurs with displacement at a slightly moveable joint, such as the sacroiliac joint, and is often associated with a fracture elsewhere.

FRACTURE: EXTREMITY TRAUMA

EPIDEMIOLOGY

The first clinical use of the X ray in the United States took place just 5 weeks after Roentgen's announcement of its discovery. On February 3, 1896, at Dartmouth University, astronomy professor Edwin Frost radiographed a young man's fractured forearm. Fracture remains one of the most common emergency room diagnoses in the

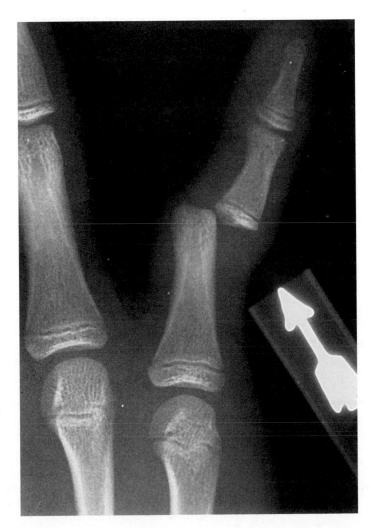

Figure 8–42. A 13-year-old boy injured his right hand playing basketball. The radiograph of the fifth digit demonstrates near-complete ulnar subluxation at the proximal interphalangeal joint (arrow). This injury rests on the cusp between a subluxation and a dislocation, as only minimal continuity at the joint is preserved. Note that the patient's growth plates are not yet closed. They would typically be closed in a girl of the same age, because the female skeleton matures more quickly than that of the male.

United States, and nearly every patient with a suspected fracture undergoes plain film radiography.

PATHOPHYSIOLOGY

Newton's laws of motion supply the physical principles vital to understanding musculoskeletal trauma. Newton's second law states that energy is neither created nor destroyed, but only changes form. This law provides the theoretical framework for understanding the events that transpire when the human body and another object collide. Suppose, for example, that in a motor vehicle accident an unrestrained passenger is thrown against the dashboard. The car is decelerated from a speed of 30 miles per hour to 0 miles per hour, as is the passenger within. In order for an object to come to a complete stop, its kinetic energy must be absorbed. In the case of the automobile, energy is absorbed by the front end of the car, as the sheet metal and frame in this region buckle. The biological analogue of the automobile's sheet metal and frame is the passenger's soft tissues and skeleton.

Two additional principles vital to understanding the physics of trauma are kinetic energy and force. In assessing the kinetic energy of an object, it is important to recall the equation, $KE = 1/2\ mv^2$. This relationship implies that velocity is relatively more important than mass in determining an object's kinetic energy. Doubling an object's velocity does not merely double, but in fact quadruples, its kinetic energy, hence four times as much energy must be absorbed in the impact. Force introduces the additional element of time, the rate at which the object's velocity reaches 0. Force is equal to the product of mass and acceleration (the rate of change in velocity). A common unit of acceleration is the "G," equivalent to the acceleration due to gravity. A high speed motor vehicle accident might produce a deceleration equivalent to 30 G, indicating that both the dashboard and the 150-lb passenger who strikes it would feel a force at impact of approximately 4,500 lb (Fig. 8–43).

Bone provides a lightweight yet strong scaffold for the soft tissues, and as such can

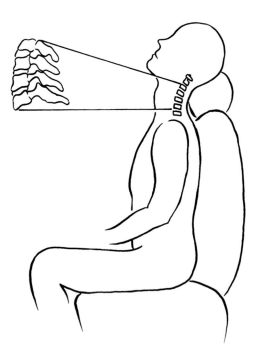

Figure 8–43. A rear-impact collision pushes forward all components of the body that are in contact with the seat. If the head restraint is not high enough to contact the posterior skull, severe angulation of the neck occurs.

support considerable loads with merely elastic deformation, not suffering any permanent deformity. Despite the fact that the 206 bones of the human skeleton support the entire weight of the body, the skeleton itself accounts for only about 18% of that weight. A general principle underlying all fractures is that of the load-deformation curve, which describes the strain that occurs with increasing stresses. The differing concentrations of calcific extracellular matrix in the bones of adults and children accounts for the different patterns of fracture seen in the two groups. The bones of children have a relatively long plastic deformation phase, during which the bone will bend without fracturing completely, because it contains relatively little rigid extracellular matrix. The bones of adults, however, contain more mineral, and are therefore stronger but more brittle.

Fractures may be classified according to the health of the underlying bone and the nature of the stresses placed upon them. The most common type of fracture is that which occurs from a single episode of major trauma to a normal bone, and these are the sorts of fractures seen many times every day in a busy hospital emergency room. A second type of fracture is the so-called fatigue fracture, which results from the application of lower magnitude, repetitive stresses to normal bone, as in military recruits subjected to a program of markedly increased physical activity, such as marching and running (Fig. 8–44). Insufficiency fractures are seen in osteopenic individuals, most notably elderly patients, in whom normal stresses surpass the weakened bone's mechanical capacity. Pathologic fractures occur in tumor-containing bone and are usually associated with normal stresses.

CLINICAL PRESENTATION

Most cases of trauma present no great challenge to the clinician, consisting of isolated extremity fractures and the like. They present with point tenderness, deformity, and

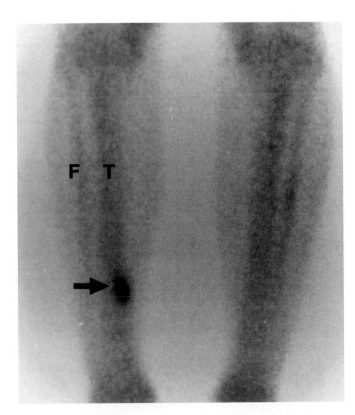

Figure 8–44. A 34-year-old runner presented with a history of 3 to 4 weeks of pain in the left shin. Routine radiographs of the left tibia and fibula (not shown) were normal. A bone scan was obtained for further evaluation. This posterior image of both lower legs demonstrates a focus of increased radiotracer activity in the medial aspect of the left distal tibial diaphysis (arrow), consistent with a fatigue-type stress fracture. The patient's symptoms resolved after a period of abstinence from running. T, tibia, F, fibula.

loss of normal function, and the patient may report having felt or even heard the bone break.

IMAGING

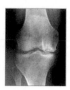

The subject of extremity trauma is vast. What follows are brief descriptions of some of the most common and illustrative osseous injuries.

Elbow

A key radiographic principle in the diagnosis of trauma about the elbow is the so-called "fat-pad sign." An anterior fat pad, detected as a subtle luceny anterior to the distal humerus on the lateral view, is seen normally. However, if this fat pad is elevated from the bone, assuming a sail-like configuration, it is abnormal. There is also a posterior fat pad behind the humerus, but it cannot normally be visualized. However, in the case of an elbow joint effusion in a trauma patient, visualization of either the posterior fat pad or an elevated anterior fat pad constitutes presumptive evidence of a fracture within the elbow joint capsule (Fig. 8–45). In a child, the most common type of fracture is a supracondylar fracture of the humerus. In an adult, a radial head fracture is most common.

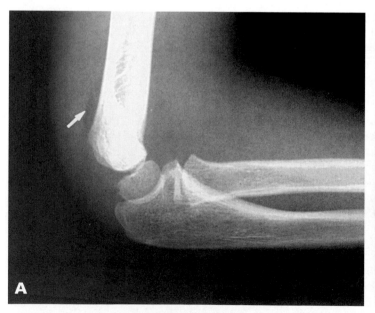

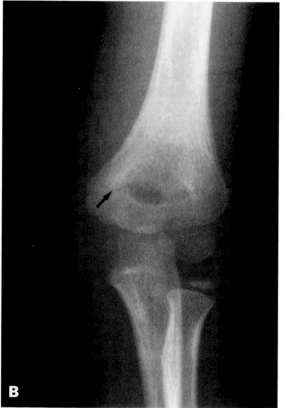

Figure 8–45. A 6-year-old fell down the steps of his front porch and presented complaining of elbow pain. (A) A lateral radiograph of the elbow demonstrates a prominent posterior fat-pad sign (arrow), which in the setting of trauma constitutes presumptive evidence of an elbow joint hemarthrosis secondary to a fracture. (B) A frontal view of the elbow demonstrates the culprit, a fracture through the supracondylar humerus (arrow).

Wrist and Hand

There are 27 bones in the human hand, including the carpals, the metacarpals, and the phalanges (Fig. 8–46). Fully 90% of carpal bone fractures involve the scaphoid. Most of these are transverse fractures across the scaphoid waist, which may not be visible on initial films and should be followed up 7 to 10 days later, if clinically indicated based on pain and point tenderness in the snuffbox. These fractures exhibit a high rate of non-union and avascular necrosis (AVN), due to the fact that the blood supply to the proximal pole comes from the more distal portion of the bone. This means that a fracture through the waist, especially proximally, is likely to compromise the proximal pole's blood supply (Fig. 8–47). The next most often seen fracture is an avulsion from the triquetrum, which is seen as a dorsal bone fragment on lateral views.

Common fractures of the metacarpals include the boxer's fracture, which typically occurs when delivering a punch with a closed fist. These are most often seen in the fourth and fifth metacarpals, with the expected volar (palmar) angulation of the distal fragment. Whenever a boxer fracture is seen, vigilance is warranted regarding a possible septic arthritis, due to inoculation of the puncher's metacarpophalangeal joint

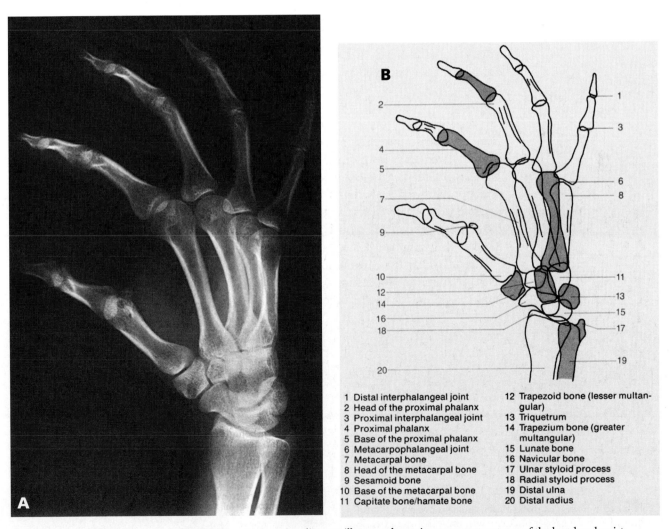

1 Distal interphalangeal joint	12 Trapezoid bone (lesser multangular)
2 Head of the proximal phalanx	
3 Proximal interphalangeal joint	13 Triquetrum
4 Proximal phalanx	14 Trapezium bone (greater multangular)
5 Base of the proximal phalanx	
6 Metacarpophalangeal joint	15 Lunate bone
7 Metacarpal bone	16 Navicular bone
8 Head of the metacarpal bone	17 Ulnar styloid process
9 Sesamoid bone	18 Radial styloid process
10 Base of the metacarpal bone	19 Distal ulna
11 Capitate bone/hamate bone	20 Distal radius

Figure 8–46. (A) Oblique radiograph and (B) accompanying diagram illustrate the major osseous structures of the hand and wrist.

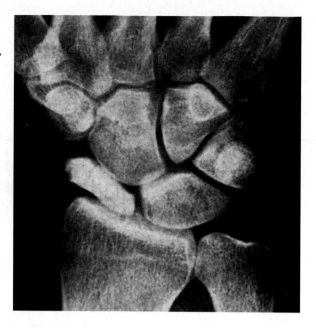

Figure 8–47. This coned-down view of the wrist demonstrates non-union of a fracture through the waist of the scaphoid, which has resulted in avascular necrosis and sclerosis of the proximal pole.

with oral flora from the victim's teeth. Infections associated with human bites are among the most difficult to eradicate with antibiotics. Fractures in the phalanges include avulsion injuries, which may involve either the flexor or extensor tendons. An extensor tendon injury is known as a "baseball" (mallet) finger, while the flexor tendon avulsion is described as a "volar plate" injury (Fig. 8–48).

Hip

Over 250,000 subcapital ("below the head") femoral fractures occur each year in the United States, the vast majority of which are secondary to osteoporosis (Fig. 8–49). They represent the single greatest source of morbidity and mortality associated with osteoporosis, with a nearly 10% mortality rate secondary to the immobilization that tends to accompany such fractures in elderly patients (with cardiac deconditioning, risk of deep venous thrombosis, etc.). By the age of 80 years, 20% of white women and 10% of white men will sustain a hip fracture.

Intracapsular fractures (above the trochanters) are associated with a high risk of AVN, because the blood supply enters the femoral neck and head from distal to proximal (Fig. 8–50). Usually such fractures are apparent on plain radiographs, but if

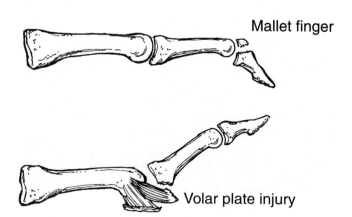

Figure 8–48. The characteristic appearances of mallet finger and volar plate injuries. The mallet finger results from a hyperflexion injury, while the volar plate injury results from excessive extension.

Figure 8–49. A 72-year-old woman presented after a fall with a shortened left leg held in external rotation. The frontal radiograph of the hip demonstrates a mildly displaced subcapital fracture of the femur (arrow). This places the fracture within the hip joint capsule (an intracapsular fracture), which carries an increased risk of avascular necrosis of the femoral head, as well as non-union, due to the relatively tenuous blood supply in this region. The male:female ratio of such fractures is approximately 4:1, reflecting the increased incidence of osteoporosis in elderly women.

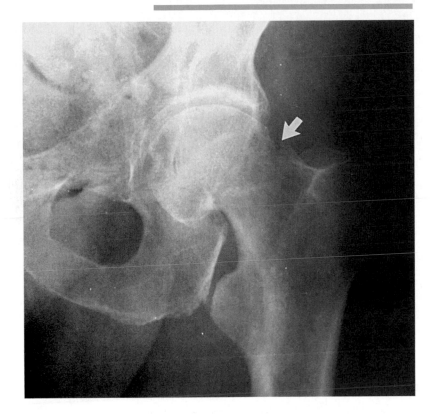

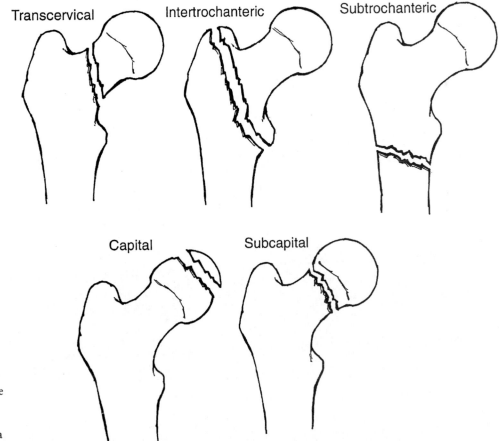

Figure 8–50. The anatomic classification of femoral fractures. The inter- and subtrochanteric fractures are outside the joint capsule, while the others are within the hip joint capsule. Subcapital fractures are common, and carry a 25% risk of avascular necrosis.

clinical suspicion of fracture is high and the diagnosis cannot be established radiographically, MRI is extremely sensitive. Fractures are seen on T1-weighted images as a transverse band of low intensity marrow replacement, with surrounding edema (high signal) on T2-weighted images. Fatigue fractures are seen in the medial femoral neck in young patients, while insufficiency fractures may also involve the acetabulum or pubic rami in the elderly.

Knee

No joint in the body is more commonly imaged by MRI than the knee. MRI offers several important advantages over other imaging modalities, including noninvasiveness, ability to evaluate soft tissue structures such as tendons, ligaments, menisci, and cartilage, and its multiplanar capabilities (Fig. 8–51). The complex anatomy of the knee as revealed by MRI makes it especially important that a systematic approach be used in every case. T1-weighted coronal sequences should be evaluated for marrow signal of the femur, tibia, and fibula, as well as osteophyte formation.

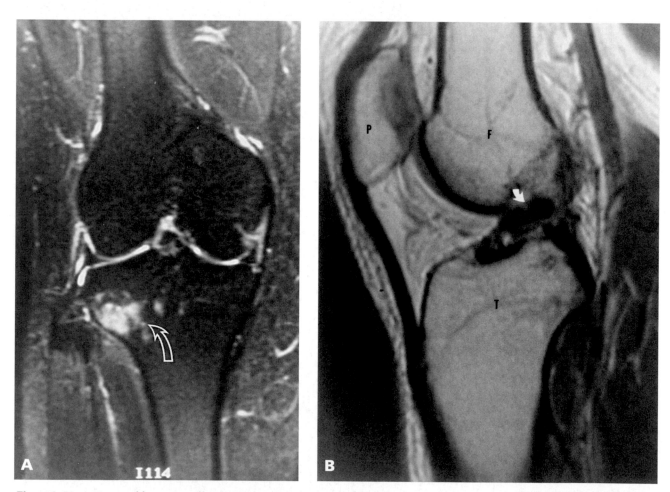

Figure 8–51. A 22-year-old woman suffered a blow to the lateral aspect of her knee 3 weeks previously. Standard radiographs of the knee were normal. (A) Using a sequence that is especially sensitive to the presence of water, a coronal image of the knee demonstrates prominent bone marrow edema in the lateral aspect of the tibial plateau, reflecting a bone contusion (arrow). (B) A sagittal proton density-weighted image demonstrates a tear of the anterior cruciate ligament (arrow), which appears somewhat more globular than expected and is deflected away from its usual proximal attachment on the posterior aspect of the femur. F, femur; P, patella; T, tibia.

Sagittal T2-weighted sequences are best for inspecting the anterior and posterior cruciate ligaments for the presence of tears, as well as for detecting the presence of joint effusions. Proton density-weighted sagittals provide optimal assessment of the menisci. T2- (and T1-) weighted images are employed to evaluate the medial and lateral collateral ligaments. Plain films are useful in acute fracture detection and the evaluation of secondary OA, and occasionally reveal abnormalities of the soft tissues (Fig. 8–52).

Foot

The 26 bones of the foot include the tarsals, the metatarsals, and the phalanges (Fig. 8–53). One of the most common injuries is fracture of the calcaneus. While approximately one-quarter of such injuries are avulsions, the remaining three-quarters are secondary to axial loading, as when someone leaps out of a second-story window to escape a fire. One of the most serious injuries of the midfoot is the Lisfranc tarsometatarsal dislocation, named after the surgeon in Napolean's army who used to perform foot amputations at that joint. It is detected as a lack of continuity along the medial aspects of the second cuneiform and the second metatarsal. One of the most prevalent forefoot fractures is the Jones fracture of the base of the fifth metatarsal,

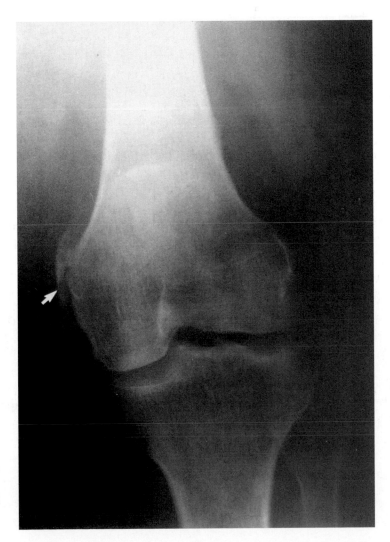

Figure 8–52. This middle-aged man with a remote history of knee injury demonstrates calcification in the medial collateral ligament (arrow), indicative of previous injury to this ligament, a finding referred to as a Pellegrini-Stiede lesion. Note also the presence of mild medial compartment joint space narrowing and osteophyte formation, indicative of secondary osteoarthritis.

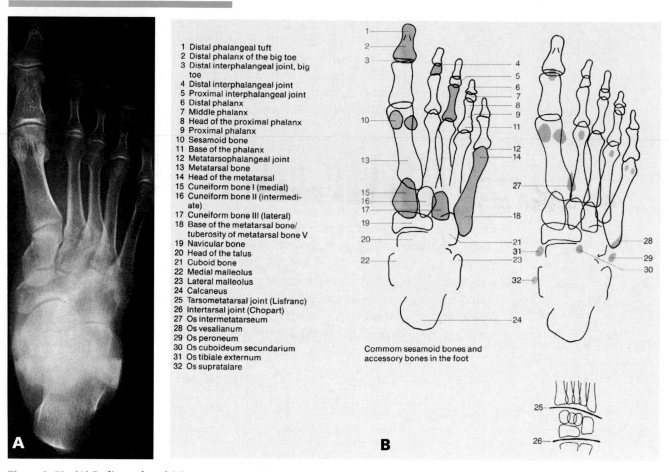

1 Distal phalangeal tuft
2 Distal phalanx of the big toe
3 Distal interphalangeal joint, big toe
4 Distal interphalangeal joint
5 Proximal interphalangeal joint
6 Distal phalanx
7 Middle phalanx
8 Head of the proximal phalanx
9 Proximal phalanx
10 Sesamoid bone
11 Base of the phalanx
12 Metatarsophalangeal joint
13 Metatarsal bone
14 Head of the metatarsal
15 Cuneiform bone I (medial)
16 Cuneiform bone II (intermediate)
17 Cuneiform bone III (lateral)
18 Base of the metatarsal bone/tuberosity of metatarsal bone V
19 Navicular bone
20 Head of the talus
21 Cuboid bone
22 Medial malleolus
23 Lateral malleolus
24 Calcaneus
25 Tarsometatarsal joint (Lisfranc)
26 Intertarsal joint (Chopart)
27 Os intermetatarseum
28 Os vesalianum
29 Os peroneum
30 Os cuboideum secundarium
31 Os tibiale externum
32 Os supratalare

Commom sesamoid bones and accessory bones in the foot

Figure 8–53. (A) Radiograph and (B) accompanying diagrams illustrate the important osseous structures of the foot.

named after the physician who diagnosed his own Jones fracture after a dancing injury. It most often stems from repetitive stress.

Nondisplaced fractures may require no treatment, or if the bone is subject to continued use, may be splinted or casted to ensure immobility at the fracture. Even many displaced fractures will heal well without reduction; however, such outcomes as lower limb length discrepancy, significant rotation, or displacement of articular surfaces (with subsequent secondary OA) must be avoided. Many displaced fractures do require reduction, which may be either closed (nonsurgical) or open (surgical). Aside from assessing the adequacy of reduction, follow-up radiographs are employed to rule out complications (such as fracture and dislocation) and to verify healing. Signs of healing include periosteal reaction, bony callus bridging the fracture, and indistinctness of the fracture line itself.

FRACTURE: CERVICAL SPINE

EPIDEMIOLOGY

The initial imaging study in the multiply traumatized patient typically consists of portable cervical spine radiography (Fig. 8–54). Spinal injuries are a major source of disability and mortality, and rapid evaluation and treatment are critical in preserving spinal cord function.

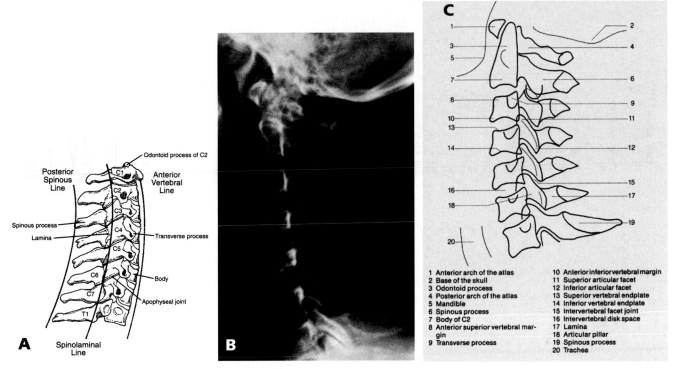

1 Anterior arch of the atlas	10 Anterior inferior vertebral margin
2 Base of the skull	11 Superior articular facet
3 Odontoid process	12 Inferior articular facet
4 Posterior arch of the atlas	13 Superior vertebral endplate
5 Mandible	14 Inferior vertebral endplate
6 Spinous process	15 Intervertebral facet joint
7 Body of C2	16 Intervertebral disk space
8 Anterior superior vertebral mar-	17 Lamina
gin	18 Articular pillar
9 Transverse process	19 Spinous process
	20 Trachea

Figure 8–54. (**A**) The major lines of the cervical spine as seen in the lateral view. (**B**) This lateral view of the cervical spine and (**C**) accompanying diagram illustrate the important anatomical structures of the cervical spine as seen radiographically.

PATHOPHYSIOLOGY

The most common mechanisms of cervical spine fractures are flexion (e.g., sudden deceleration in a forward-moving vehicle) and axial loading (e.g., diving head first into a shallow swimming pool). The levels between C5 and C7 are most commonly involved. A critical distinction is that between stable and unstable fractures. In unstable fractures, the spinal canal is no longer protected by its ligamentous and osseous supports, meaning that any movement of the neck could result in damage to the cord (Fig. 8–55).

Examples of unstable fractures include a flexion teardrop fracture (with ligamentous instability secondary to avulsion) and a hangman's fracture (with fracture of the pars interarticularis of C2 and anterolisthesis of C2 on C3), an extension injury (Fig. 8–56). Fractures that may or may not be stable (possibly unstable), depending on the extent of injury, include a Jefferson fracture (a "burst" fracture of C1 secondary to axial loading, with fractures of the anterior and posterior arches on at least one side), and a unilateral facet lock, seen on the lateral view as a slight anterolisthesis and rotation of one vertebral body on the other. Stable injuries (assuming they are isolated) include a fracture of the posterior arch of C1 and the so-called clay-shoveller's fracture, caused by avulsion by the supraspinatus ligament (Fig. 8–57).

CLINICAL PRESENTATION

In the case of the multiply traumatized patient, acute management decisions may determine whether the patient lives or dies, as well as the level of residual disability.

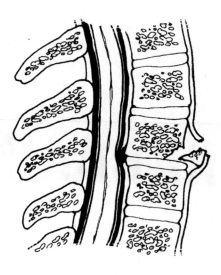

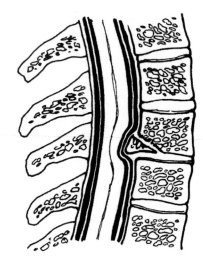

A Flexion teardrop

B Retropulsion of fragment into vertebral canal

Figure 8–55. Typical appearances of unstable fractures of the cervical spine. (A) A flexion teardrop fracture is seen, with a fragment avulsed off of the anterior-inferior portion of a vertebral body and disruption of the supporting ligaments. (B) A fragment of a vertebral body has been retropulsed into the vertebral canal, where it exerts mass effect on the spinal cord.

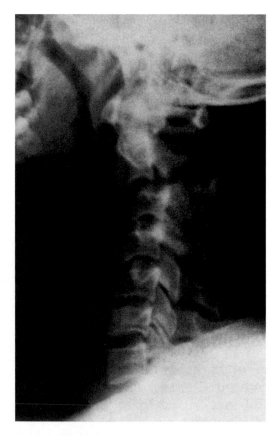

Figure 8–56. This lateral cervical spine radiograph demonstrates anterior displacement of C2 on C3, due to a fracture through the pars interarticularis of C2. This injury is referred to as a "hangman's" fracture.

Figure 8–57. This lateral radiograph of the cervical spine demonstrates classic "clay-shoveller's" fractures of the spinous processes of C6 and C7. These are stable fractures.

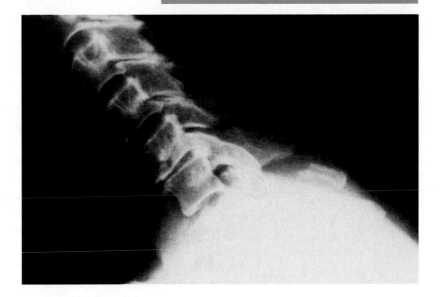

Before any radiologic study is ordered, the presence of life-threatening injuries must be assessed, and the patient must be stabilized. The five steps of acute management consist of the well-known A-B-C-D-E mnemonic: *a*irway management, *b*reathing, *c*irculation (with control of bleeding), *d*isability (neurologic assessment), and *e*xposure (cutting off clothing). A helpful mnemonic in neurologic assessment of deep tendon reflexes is that sacral level 1–2 is responsible for the Achilles tendon reflex, lumbar level 3–4 is responsible for the patellar tendon reflex, cervical level 5–6 is responsible for the biceps tendon reflex, and cervical level 7–8 is responsible for the triceps tendon reflex.

Even once the patient is stabilized, the clinician must continue to balance the need for definitive diagnostic information against the need to monitor and manage the patient. Moving the patient from the emergency room to the radiology suite typically compromises access to the patient by personnel and equipment that would be vital if acute resuscitation becomes necessary. Simply put, the radiology department is not the ideal environment in which to manage a cardiac arrest or a disoriented and combative patient. Despite these caveats, however, diagnostic imaging constitutes a vital ingredient in the acute care of the vast majority of multiply traumatized patients.

Imaging evaluation of the cervical spine is indicated in patients whose mental status is altered (compromising history taking and neurologic evaluation), who complain of neck pain, who are tender to palpation of the cervical spine, whose neurologic examination is abnormal, who are at high risk due to the mechanism of injury (fall from a height greater than 10 feet or high-speed motor vehicle accident), or who suffer severe pain at another site that may distract them from neck pain. Depending on the clinical setting, evaluation of the thoracic and lumbar spine may also warrant consideration.

To properly care for the patient in whom spinal trauma is being assessed, it is essential that the patient be handled as though serious injury were present. The patient with an unstable spinal injury may suffer further serious injury if mishandled, and the possibility of inducing quadriplegia is sufficient justification for always erring on the side of overprotection. The patient should be transported with a cervical collar in place, and immobilized on a long spine board, and the patient and the board are moved as a unit until serious injury is radiographically ruled out.

IMAGING

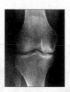

The initial view obtained is generally a cross-table lateral, with the patient lying supine in a cervical collar. Once the cervical spine has been "cleared" by a combination of this view and clinical findings, additional radiographs are necessary to fully exclude injury. These include an additional lateral view, an anteroposterior view, an open-mouth odontoid view, and two supine obliques, making a total of five films in a complete cervical spine series. In some cases, CT examination of the cervical spine may be indicated. Many trauma patients will undergo CT scanning of the head to rule out intracranial injury in any case, and it is simple to add on additional axial images of the cervical spine. This may be especially helpful in patients in whom standard views are unsatisfactory, as when superimposition of shoulder structures compromises views of the lower cervical spine. Moreover, CT is helpful in better delineating equivocal findings on plain films, and in further evaluating the extent of definite injuries detected by plain radiography.

The key to evaluating the cervical spine is to approach the radiograph systematically. Many systems are possible, and the following is but one example. Here is a seven-step checklist to employ in evaluating the cross-table lateral view. Although this list is by no means complete, it suffices to rule out most serious injuries in the acute setting.

1. **Count the number of vertebrae.** A good cross-table lateral view should display all seven cervical vertebrae, as well as the upper portion of the T1 vertebral body. Often the shoulder obscures the lower cervical spine, and a "swimmer's view" must be obtained (the arm closest to the film is extended cranially, as though the patient were reaching to retrieve an object from a high shelf). Just as one would not "clear" a patient's chest after listening to only one lung, one must not "clear" the cervical spine unless the whole cervical spine has been adequately visualized. Although C2 is the single most commonly fractured vertebra in the cervical spine, approximately three-fourths of cervical spine fractures involve the lower levels, and adequate visualization is essential in ruling these out. To assess adequate visualization, begin counting below the base of the skull at C1, and then count downward.

2. **Assess the curvature of the spine.** The normal cervical spine is slightly lordotic (convex anteriorly). If this lordosis is exaggerated or lost, it may indicate ligamentous injury, although poor positioning or muscle spasm occurs more commonly.

3. **Assess vertebral alignment.** Four lines drawn along the axis of the cervical spine should demonstrate smooth, gentle curves (Fig. 8–58). These include the anterior vertebral line, the posterior vertebral line, the spinolaminal line, and the posterior spinal line. Any irregularity in any of these lines should raise suspicion for a fracture or dislocation. Because the spinal cord is housed between the posterior vertebral line and the spinolaminal line, an irregularity in either of these carries the greatest probability of cord injury (Fig. 8–59).

4. **Assess bone integrity.** Different types of vertebral deformity imply different mechanisms of injury. A hyperflexion injury, as in a head-on collision, tends to produce compression of the anterior portions of the vertebral bodies, with tearing of the intraspinous ligaments. Hyperextension injuries, however, tend to fracture the posterior elements and disrupt the anterior longitudinal ligament. So-called burst fractures

Figure 8–58. This normal lateral radiograph of the cervical spine demonstrates the four lines drawn along vertebral structures that should appear as smooth arcs with no abrupt changes in course. From anterior to posterior, these are the anterior vertebral line, the posterior vertebral line, the spinolaminal line, and the posterior spinal line.

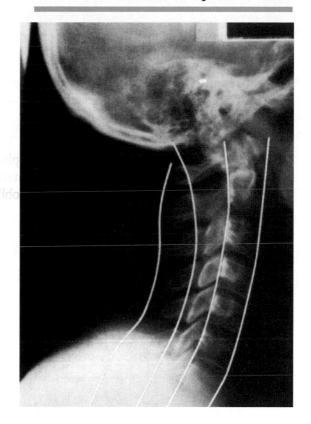

Figure 8–59. A 50% anterolisthesis of one vertebral body on another, with the inferior articular facets of the upper vertebra locked in front of the superior articular facets of the lower vertebra. Naturally, this anterolisthesis tends to compromise the vertebral canal and threatens the cord.

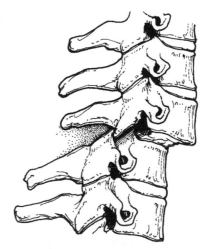

Spondylolisthesis
with locked facets

result from a force directed along the axis of the spine, as when someone dives head first into a shallow pool. These fractures tend to spare the ligamentous components, but fracture fragments may be directed into the vertebral canal, damaging the cord.

5. Assess the intervertebral disk spaces. The space separating the inferior end plate of one vertebral body from the superior endplate of another should be similar at each level. If a single disk space is narrowed, and there are no other signs of long-standing pathology, such as advanced OA of the spine, one must suspect that the disk space narrowing resulted from trauma. This may be associated with ligamentous injury, and there may also be extrusion of disk material into the vertebral canal, compromising the spinal cord. This could be directly imaged by MRI.

6. **Assess the cranium and the first two cervical vertebrae.** To ensure that there is no dissociation of the cranium from the spine, make sure that a line drawn along the clivus intersects the odontoid process of C2 at the junction of its anterior and middle thirds, and that the distance between the anterior arch of C1 and the odontoid does not exceed 3 mm (in adults). In children, this measurement may be as great as 5 mm, due to their greater ligamentous laxity.

7. **Assess the prevertebral soft tissues.** Widening of these tissues may reflect edema or hemorrhage, indirect signs of cervical spine trauma. As a general rule, the soft tissues in front of C2 should not measure more than 4 mm, or measure more than three-fourths of a vertebral body diameter in the lower cervical spine. Prevertebral gas is suspicious for abscess.

Vascular

Circulatory disorders can be divided into two categories, based on whether they involve increased or decreased flow. Increased flow is seen in many conditions discussed previously. The effects of active hyperemia are readily manifest in bone adjacent to fracture lines, which undergoes an initial loss of osteoid and mineral in response to the associated inflammatory response of healing.

Examples of bone disease due to impaired blood flow include AVN and bone infarct. The classic location of AVN is the femoral head, and patients at increased risk for this form of osteonecrosis include alcoholics and patients receiving high-dose steroid therapy. Why? Recent experimental evidence suggests that both conditions promote an increase in the amount of marrow fat, which compromises the capillary bed of the femoral head. Other predisposing conditions include sickle cell anemia, trauma, and collagen vascular diseases.

One of the earliest plain radiographic signs of AVN is mixed areas of sclerotic and lytic change (Fig. 8–60). While it is tempting to suppose that the lytic areas represent

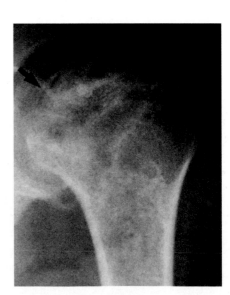

Figure 8–60. This frontal radiograph of the shoulder demonstrates mixed areas of sclerotic and lytic change in the humeral head, with early fragmentation of the joint surface (arrows).

Figure 8–61. A 30-year-old man had a history of chronic steroid use for systemic lupus erythematosus (SLE). A frontal radiograph of the right hip demonstrates evidence of advanced avascular necrosis (AVN), with collapse and deformity of the femoral head and early secondary osteoarthritic changes in the hip joint. This unfortunate patient had two independent risk factors for AVN: SLE and steroid use.

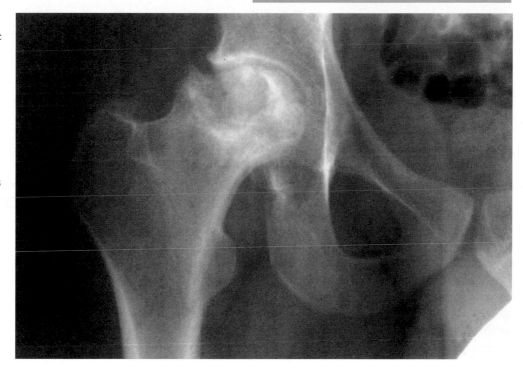

the infarcted tissue, in fact it is the sclerotic areas that have suffered the ischemic insult. These "sclerotic" areas actually represent normally mineralized bone that has died, and which therefore cannot undergo osteoclastic activity. The lytic areas represent inflammation-associated osteoclastic activity in adjacent viable areas of bone. Eventually, the femoral head may collapse, which invariably results in secondary osteoarthritic changes in the hip joint (Fig. 8–61). MRI is far more sensitive than plain film in detecting the early changes of AVN.

The Mathematical Society, 1995

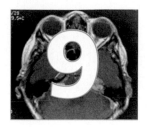

9 Neuroimaging

ANATOMY AND PHYSIOLOGY

The central nervous system (CNS), consisting of the brain and spinal cord, is connected to the peripheral nervous system by afferent (Latin for "to bear toward") and efferent ("to bear away from") neurons. Efferent neurons outnumber afferent neurons by a ratio of 10:1, while interneurons, which function in integration, make up approximately 99% of the 10 billion neurons in the CNS. However, neurons themselves make up only approximately 10% of the cells in the CNS, the rest consisting of glial cells (from the Greek, *gloios*, "glue"). Glial cells guide the growth of neurons during development, support them both structurally and metabolically, and induce changes in blood vessels that are responsible for the blood-brain barrier. Under normal circumstances, adult neurons are incapable of division, and the primary neoplasms of the CNS arise from other cell types, such as glial cells (which give rise to gliomas).

The brain itself may be divided into the brainstem, the cerebellum, and the forebrain (Fig. 9–1). The brainstem, the oldest region of the brain, functions primarily in a

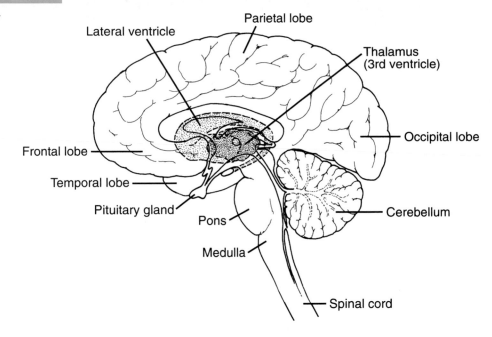

Figure 9–1. The basic anatomy of the brain as seen on a sagittal view of the midline.

variety of vegetative functions, such as the control of heart beat, respiration, and digestion. The cerebellum functions in the coordination of motor activity. The forebrain consists of both the diencephalon (the thalamus and hypothalamus) and the cerebrum, which is most highly developed in human beings, where it constitutes approximately 80% of brain volume. The thalamus is a critical relay station for all synaptic input, while the hypothalamus functions primarily in homeostasis. The cerebrum is divided into the right and left hemispheres, each of which may be divided into an outer shell of gray matter and inner core of white matter. However, there are numerous gray matter nuclei within the inner portions of the hemispheres. Gray matter consists of densely packed neurons and glial cells, while white matter is made up of myelinated fiber tracts connecting parts of the CNS.

The cerebrum may be divided into four lobes. The occipital lobes are responsible for visual processing. The temporal lobes play important roles in hearing, motivation and emotion, and memory. The parietal lobes function in somatosensory and proprioceptive roles, and contain the somatosensory cortex, located immediately posterior to the central sulcus (which divides the frontal and parietal lobes). The frontal lobes contain the motor cortex (immediately anterior to the central sulcus), as well as regions responsible for speech and abstract thought. In addition, there is some division of labor between the two hemispheres, with the right excelling in spatial, artistic, and musical functions, and the left in language and analytical tasks. Hence, a unilateral stroke that leaves a patient mute more likely affects the left hemisphere. Because both sensory and motor tracts generally cross to the contralateral side between the brain and spinal cord, the left half of the brain is connected to the right half of the body, and vice versa.

The brain and spinal cord have a number of special protective structures. The brain is encased in the rigid cranium and the spinal cord by the vertebral column. While the cranium protects the relatively soft brain from mechanical trauma, it also poses special problems when intracranial pressure rises, because the brain has no safe means of decompressing itself. The meninges lie beneath the cranium and vertebral column and consist of the outer dura mater (Latin for "tough mother"), beneath which is the subdural space; the arachnoid (Latin for "spider" because it resembles a cobweb), beneath which is the subarachnoid space, which is accessed during a spinal tap; and the pia mater ("soft mother"), which is attached to the brain and dips down into sulci (Fig. 9–2). Hence a subarachnoid hemorrhage will extend down into cerebral sulci, while a subdural bleed will not (Fig. 9–3).

The brain is cushioned both internally and externally by the cerebrospinal fluid (CSF), which is produced by the choroid plexus of the lateral, third, and fourth ventri-

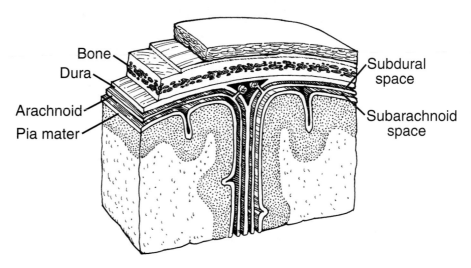

Figure 9–2. The major protective coverings of the brain, which are important in understanding the appearance of processes such as hemorrhage in the subarachnoid, subdural, and epidural spaces.

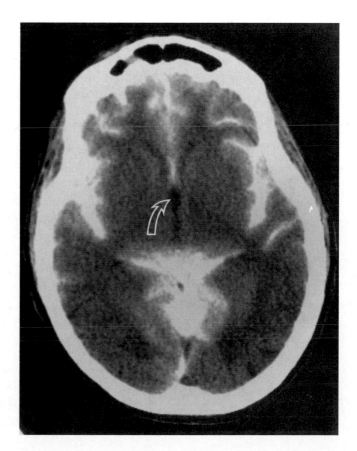

Figure 9–3. An axial computed tomography image of the head of a patient who had received subarachnoid contrast material in the performance of a spinal myelogram. Note that the radio-dense contrast material extends down into the sulci between the pia mater and arachnoid membranes. Neither subdural nor epidural contrast material would exhibit this behavior, due to the barrier of the arachnoid membrane. The arrow is pointing to the third ventricle, which contains no contrast. This illustrates the fact that cerebrospinal fluid (CSF) normally flows from the lateral, third, and fourth ventricles out over the spinal cord and cerebral hemispheres. For this contrast to get from the subarachnoid space around the spinal cord into the third ventricle, abnormal retrograde flow of CSF would be required.

cles, and is absorbed by the arachnoid granulations in the region of the superior sagittal sinus. The normal CSF production and absorption rate is approximately 30 cc per hour. The normal circulation and drainage of CSF can be impeded at a number of critical points, including the foramina of Monro (connecting the lateral ventricles with the third ventricle), the aqueduct of Sylvius (connecting the third and fourth ventricles), and the foramina of Magendie and Luschka, where CSF leaves the ventricular system and circulates in the subarachnoid space around the brain and cord. Obstruction either to flow or resorption may result in hydrocephalus.

The brain's other protective structure is the microscopic blood-brain barrier, which prevents most blood-borne substances from leaving the CNS capillaries and entering surrounding tissues. The blood-brain barrier is made up of glial cell foot processes and tight junctions between capillary endothelial cells. Only simple sugars, oxygen and carbon dioxide, amino acids, and lipid soluble substances such as anesthetic gases can pass. Even alterations in serum potassium ion concentration produce little change in its concentration in CSF. This prevents circulating hormones that can also act as neurotransmitters from wreaking havoc in the brain, and also screens out a variety of foreign chemicals and microorganisms. Unfortunately, the human immunodeficiency virus (HIV) is able to circumvent this defense, probably by entering the CNS in macrophages. Moreover, the blood-brain barrier can prove an obstacle in eradicating certain neoplasms such as lymphoma from the brain, and chemotherapeutic agents often must be administered directly into the CSF. Leakiness in the blood-brain barrier, which may accompany processes such as tumor and infection, is responsible for contrast enhancement, as discussed later.

The brain is critically dependent on a constant blood supply. Because it is incapable of anaerobic metabolism, it requires oxygen to produce adenosine triphosphate (ATP). Moreover, the brain has no glucose stores. Thus, an interruption in the brain's oxygen supply for more than 5 minutes or its glucose supply for more than 15 minutes results in irreparable brain damage. The blood supply of the brain arrives by four principal arteries: the paired internal carotid arteries and the paired vertebral arteries (Fig. 9–4). The internal carotids arise at the carotid bifurcation in the neck and represent the primary supply of the anterior and middle cerebral arteries, while the vertebrals represent the first branches of the subclavian arteries and constitute the primary supply of the posterior circulation. The circle of Willis provides a built-in back up system in the event that one of these vessels should be compromised, with connections between the internal carotid arteries and the posterior circulation via the posterior communicating arteries (Fig. 9–5). However, the circle is complete in only 25% of patients (Fig. 9–6). The venous drainage of the brain is directed toward the occiput, eventually emptying into the internal jugular veins.

IMAGING

CT versus MRI

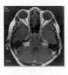
By far the two most important imaging modalities employed in the evaluation of the CNS are computed tomography (CT) and magnetic resonance imaging (MRI) (Fig. 9–7). The widespread clinical application of CT antedated that of MRI by approximately 15 years, and, although MRI

Figure 9–4. The course of the carotid and vertebral arteries in a lateral projection as they course toward the brain.

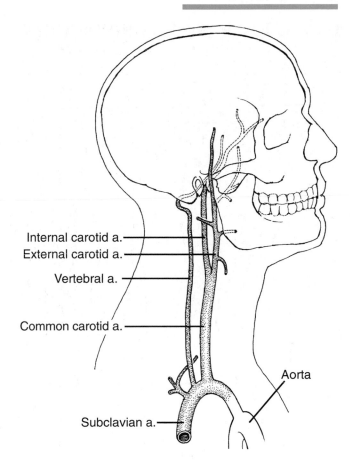

Internal carotid a.
External carotid a.
Vertebral a.
Common carotid a.
Aorta
Subclavian a.

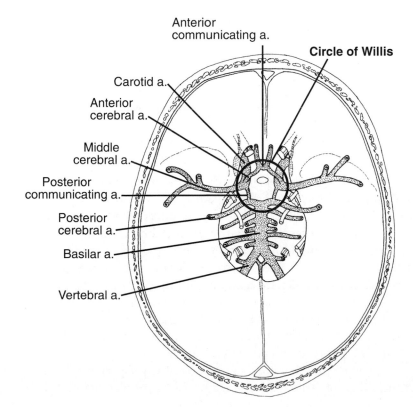

Anterior communicating a.
Circle of Willis
Carotid a.
Anterior cerebral a.
Middle cerebral a.
Posterior communicating a.
Posterior cerebral a.
Basilar a.
Vertebral a.

Figure 9–5. The major vessels of the intracranial circulation, including the circle of Willis.

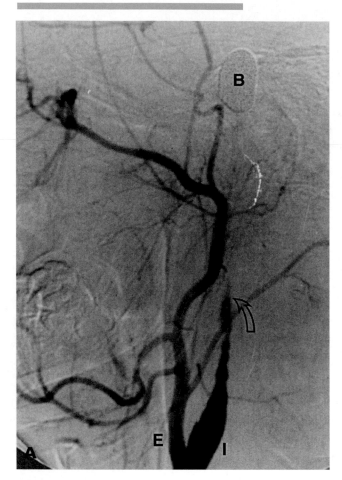 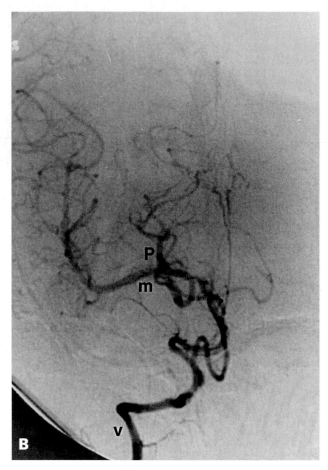

Figure 9–6. A 16-year-old woman was shot in the face by her handgun-wielding (ex-)boyfriend. Images from her digital subtraction cerebral angiogram illustrate the importance of the circle of Willis. (A) The lateral view of a right common carotid artery injection demonstrates a bullet in the region of the cavernous portion of the right internal carotid artery. The proximal internal carotid artery demonstrates a tapered occlusion (arrow), indicating a traumatic dissection. Yet the patient was neurologically intact. How? (B) The frontal view of a right vertebral artery injection demonstrates perfusion of the right middle and anterior cerebral arteries through a patent right posterior communicating artery. This case illustrates the tremendous potential advantage of an intact circle of Willis, which confers the ability to route blood around carotid and vertebral artery occlusions. B, bullet; E, external carotid artery (which gives off multiple branches in the neck); I, internal carotid artery; m, middle cerebral artery; p, posterior cerebral artery; v, vertebral artery.

has supplanted CT in many clinical settings, CT remains the modality of choice in a number of important situations. In general, the advantages of CT over MRI include speed (examinations lasting minutes rather than tens of minutes or even hours), cost, and wide availability. CT is more sensitive than MRI for the detection of small amounts of calcification, which can be important, for example, in determining the likely histology of a tumor, since some tumors often calcify and others rarely or never do so. Moreover, even if all other factors were equal, noninfused CT would be the preferred modality in most acute settings because of its superior ability to detect acute bleeds and because the CT scanner is a much more hospitable environment to the seriously ill patient, whose presence in the radiology department often requires a retinue of monitoring and life support equipment and personnel.

There is, however, one acute situation in which MRI is clearly superior to CT, and this probably constitutes the only true MRI emergency in neuroimaging; namely, a

Figure 9–7. This frontal image from a bilateral internal carotid artery angiogram provides some indication of how far neuroimaging has progressed since the 1970s. This patient suffered from chronic bilateral subdural hematomas, which can be seen displacing the enhancing vessels of the cerebral parenchyma inferiomedially, away from the inner table of the skull. Prior to the advent of computed tomography (CT), angiography represented a primary modality in the diagnosis of such lesions, the presence of which could be inferred by the displacement of normal vessels. Today, however, the diagnosis of a subdural hematoma can be rendered much more rapidly, inexpensively, and with less risk via a CT scan (or MRI).

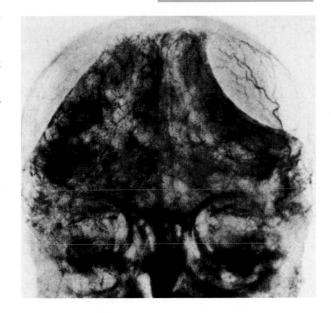

study to evaluate suspected spinal cord compression. The spinal cord responds poorly to lesions exerting mass effect upon it, which occur most often in trauma patients or patients with known metastatic disease likely to involve the spine or its contents. In the case of a patient presenting with the acute onset of neurologic deficits such as lower extremity weakness, paresthesias, or the loss of bowel or bladder control, an MRI is the study of choice to rule out cord compression, and should be performed urgently, before sustained pressure on the cord produces an irreversible neurologic deficit.

In the vast majority of nonacute clinical settings, MRI is superior to CT. While CT is generally confined to imaging in the axial plane (coronal scanning is often used in imaging osseous structures and the paranasal sinuses), MRI is capable of multiplanar imaging (axial, coronal, sagittal, and obliques), and its multiplanar capabilities can be further customized to answer specific questions about the extent of lesions and their impact on adjacent structures. MRI provides greater differentiation of gray and white matter structures, is more sensitive for the detection of subacute and chronic bleeds, and generally provides a more detailed and precise view of anatomic structures. MRI can be used to determine the structure and patency of vascular structures with greater sensitivity than CT, and even without the use of intravascular contrast agents. CT is relatively poor at visualizing soft tissue structures surrounded by or adjacent to large amounts of bone, such as the inferior temporal lobes, which produce so-called streak artifact, while MRI is immune to this problem.

When faced with the decision of which neuroimaging study to order, the clinician should consider consulting a radiologist. However, in the vast majority of cases, the following guidelines should hold. If the process in question began less than 48 hours prior to imaging, noninfused CT is a logical starting point. If the radiological or clinical findings indicate a tumor, consider contrast infusion, which will increase the sensitivity of the examination due to the differences in contrast enhancement between normal and abnormal tissues. If concern for vascular pathology such as stroke is high, contrast should probably be withheld, because extravasated contrast may increase edema in the vicinity of the lesion ("edema" comes from the Greek, *oidema*, meaning "swelling"), exacerbating mass effect on surrounding normal parenchyma and may also exert a chemical irritant effect on the surrounding tissues. If the process is older than 48 hours, begin where possible with MRI. Gadolinium should be given if a primary or metastatic neoplasm is a strong consideration, if the patient suffers seizures, or if the patient has localizing neurologic symptoms. Particularly in the case of MRI, good clinical history is imperative to enable the radiologist to tailor the examination to answer the clinical question at hand.

MRI

MRI of the brain is generally obtained with both T1- and T2-weighted images. T1-weighted images usually provide the greatest anatomic detail, while T2-weighted images are preferred for evaluating pathologic lesions. Why? Most processes that involve inflammation or neoplasia are accompanied by some disturbance of the blood-brain barrier, rendering the capillary endothelium in the region "leakier." This leakiness allows the extravasation of proteins and solutes into the surrounding tissue, with the resultant increase of interstitial osmolality and an accompanying osmotically generated increase in the amount of local water. This increase in water is represented on T2-weighted images as increased brightness. Hence, abnormal "bright" or high-signal regions on T2-weighted images should be regarded with suspicion. In addition to signal abnormality (which, as will be seen, involves more than just abnormal water content), another category of abnormality to look for on MRI is mass effect, the displacement of normal structures from their usual positions by the pathologic lesion.

How does one determine whether an MR image of the CNS is T1- or T2-weighted (Fig. 9–8)? First, it is important to note that not all images are either T1- or T2-weighted. For example, so-called proton density images rely on a technique that minimizes the effects of the T1 and T2 characteristics of tissues and highlights the differences in their proton density. For our purposes, however, T1- and T2-weighted images are most important, and we shall focus on them. One way to determine if an image is T1- or T2-weighted is to determine the TR and TE settings utilized in the scan, by looking at the scan data. TR is a measure of the time protons are given to align with the main magnetic field between radiowave pulses, and TE is a measure of the time allowed for the energy absorbed from the radiowave pulse to be released. T1-weighted images have a short TR (< 800 ms) and short TE (< 30 ms). T2-weighted images have a long TR (> 2000 ms) and long TE (> 60 ms). Proton density images, in contrast, have a long TR and a short TE.

However, even if the scan parameters are not known, T1- and T2-weighted images can be differentiated based on the fact that water (including CSF) appears dark (or low signal) on T1 and bright (or high signal) on T2. Fat, by contrast, appears bright on T1 and dark (compared to water) on T2 (Fig. 9–9). Hence the CSF in the ventricles will appear dark on T1-weighted images and bright on T2-weighted images, and the lipid-rich myelin of the white matter will appear brighter than the gray matter on T1-weighted images and darker than the gray matter on T2-weighted images. In broadest terms, one need only recall that water and fat tend to exhibit opposing signal characteristics and that water is dark on T1 and bright on T2.

CONTRAST ENHANCEMENT

To interpret contrast-enhanced examinations, it is important to possess an understanding of the mechanisms of contrast enhancement in both CT and MRI. As previ-

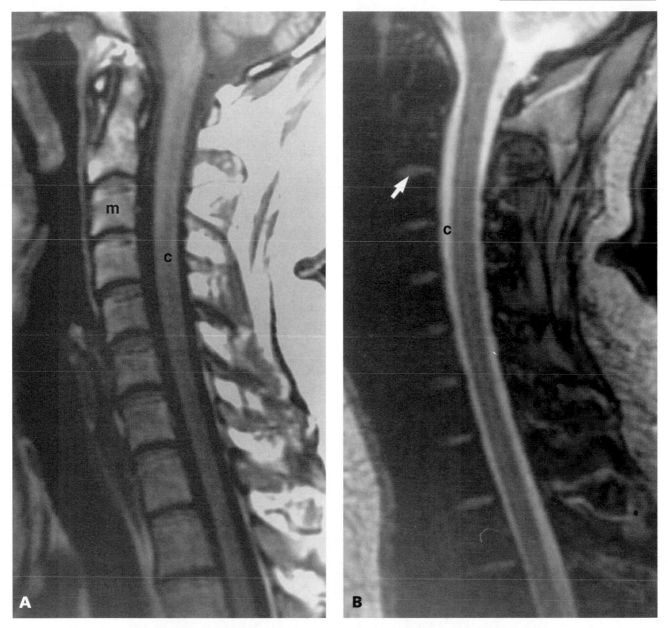

Figure 9–8. These T1- and T2-weighted sagittal images of a normal cervical spine nicely illustrate the differences between the signal intensity of fat and cerebrospinal fluid (CSF) on these sequences. **(A)** On the T1-weighted image, the isointense cervical spinal cord (c) is surrounded by low intensity CSF within the subarachnoid space. The marrow of the cervical vertebral bodies (m) is relatively bright, due to its high fat content, and the subcutaneous fat at the back of the neck is also bright. The intervertebral disks appear relatively dark. **(B)** In contrast, on the T2-weighted image, the CSF (c) surrounding the cord appears bright, as does the nucleus pulposis (arrow) within the intervertebral disks. The subcutaneous fat in the back of the neck is now hypointense to isointense.

ously noted, "enhancement" occurs when an anatomic structure or lesion becomes more conspicuous after the administration of intravascular contrast. CT enhancement occurs on the basis of the attenuation of the X-ray beam by iodine-containing molecules. MRI enhancement relies on the T1-shortening effect of gadolinium-containing molecules. As will be seen, the fact that a structure or lesion does not enhance may be just as important diagnostically as the fact that it does.

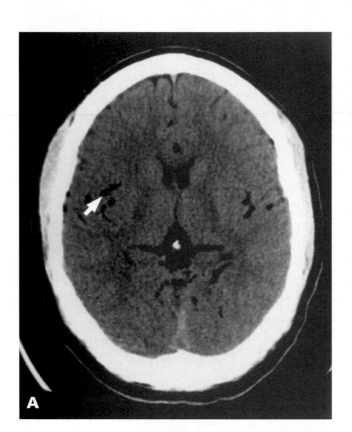
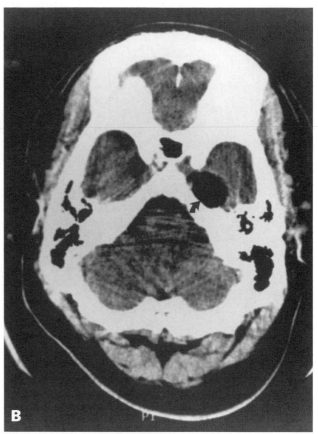
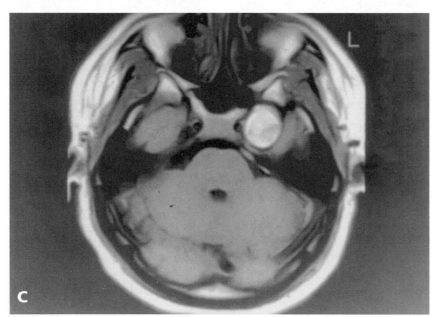

Figure 9–9. This patient presented with the acute onset of meningitic symptoms. (A) An axial image from a noncontrast head computed tomography (CT) scan demonstrates multiple fat-density foci within the subarachnoid space (arrow), which is pathognomonic of a ruptured dermoid tumor. Dermoid tumors contain dermal appendages and often produce lipid material. (B) A second more inferior image demonstrates the primary lesion arising in the region of Meckel's cave (arrow). (C) A T1-weighted axial magnetic resonance (MR) image at the same level demonstrates the T1-hyperintense lesion. Note that a lesion that appears "black" on CT can easily appear "white" on MRI, due to the fact that the modalities image completely different tissue characteristics.

In interpreting an examination, how does one determine whether contrast material was utilized? One means of doing so is to inspect the scan data accompanying the images, looking for such telltale indications as "C+," "postinfusion," or the brand name of the contrast agent. However, a superior method of detecting contrast infusion is to look for increased "brightness" in structures that should normally enhance. In CT, this means inspecting the most highly vascular structures of the head, such as the cerebral vessels and the dura mater. In MRI, the best place to look is the richly vascular erectile tissues of the nasal mucosa, as well as the pituitary gland and the dura mater of the cavernous sinus.

Having said that the cerebral vessels enhance with contrast infusion on CT, why is contrast enhancement of the vessels not visible when contrast is administered in MRI? First, it must be said that MR angiography does permit selective highlighting of the vasculature. However, on standard T1- and T2-weighted imaging the flow of blood (whether or not it contains contrast) within the cerebral arteries and veins is rapid enough that vascular structures are seen as so-called flow voids. (The nasal mucosa, an exception, enhances because it contains a great deal of low-velocity blood.) The reason is that protons in the flowing blood move out of the plane of imaging in the time that elapses between the absorption of the energy of the radiowave pulse and the detection of its release.

The "flow void" phenomenon occurs not only in blood, but in any imaged structure moving at sufficient velocity relative to the imaging apparatus. If the patient's head were moving at sufficient speed, the entire head, too, would appear as a (high-velocity) signal void. Under normal conditions, however, the blood is the only substance moving with sufficient velocity to produce the flow void phenomenon. The flow void principle may be put to excellent clinical use. For example, it aids in the detection of vascular thrombosis, where an expected intravascular flow void is replaced with soft tissue signal, representing stationary thrombus within the vessel.

With respect to CNS imaging, contrast enhancement may be divided into two phases. The first is the intravascular phase, which lasts so long as a sufficient concentration of contrast agent is present within the vascular lumen, whether that of arteries, veins, or capillaries. This is essentially the only phase of enhancement seen on conventional angiography and is also clearly visible on CT (which is why we can inspect the cerebral vasculature to determine if the examination was performed with contrast infusion). Because the gray matter is several times as vascular as the white matter (because it contains cells that are three to four times more active metabolically), the parenchyma of the gray matter will tend to enhance more than the white matter in the intravascular phase. As noted previously, however, intravascular enhancement does not occur on routine T1- and T2-weighted MR images, where instead a flow void is seen.

The second phase, the interstitial phase, is seen with both CT and MRI contrast infusion. To understand how the interstitial phase of contrast enhancement occurs, it is necessary to briefly discuss the blood-brain barrier. The blood-brain barrier is found in 99% of the brain's volume, and, as previously discussed, represents the seal formed by the tight junctions between closely abutting capillary endothelial cells. In addition, there is relatively little pinocytosis across the capillary cells of the brain, with the exception of that involving such metabolic substrates as glucose. Of course, certain areas of the brain are notable for the absence of a blood-brain barrier, such as the pituitary gland, chemoreceptors in areas of the brain connected to the brainstem vomiting center, and the dura, and these areas normally exhibit contrast enhancement (Fig. 9–10). The pituitary gland and the vomiting center do not have a blood-brain

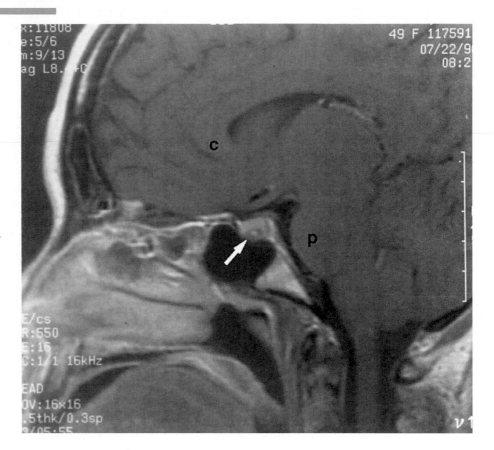

Figure 9–10. A 49-year-old woman presented to her internist complaining of amenorrhea and galactorrhea. A contrast-infused T1-weighted magnetic resonance image of the pituitary gland was performed to locate a suspected prolactin-secreting pituitary microadenoma. This sagittal image demonstrates an area of decreased enhancement within the central aspect of the pituitary gland (arrow), with a punctate area of increased enhancement in its center. Most pituitary adenomas actually appear hypointense on postinfusion images, due to the fact that the normal adenohypophysis (anterior lobe) lacks a blood-brain barrier, and normally enhances. c, corpus callosum; P, pons.

barrier, because in order to perform their functions (regulating the serum concentrations of various hormones and ridding the body of potential poisons, respectively), access of brain cells to the chemical contents of the blood must be preserved. As a result of the blood-brain barrier, the relatively high molecular weight, nonlipophilic contrast agents used in CT and MRI cannot cross normal brain capillaries into the interstitium of the brain parenchyma.

If contrast agents cannot cross the blood-brain barrier, of what use are they in diagnostic imaging? The answer is that, while they cannot cross the blood-brain barrier when it is intact, they can cross it when it is disrupted. Generally speaking, the blood-brain barrier is disrupted by acute inflammation (as in demyelinating diseases such as multiple sclerosis [Fig. 9–11], where chemical mediators increase capillary permeability), neoplasm (where the capillaries formed in conjunction with the growing tumor possess an abnormal endothelium), infection (which produces inflammation), and ischemia (which damages the endothelial cells of capillaries along with the parenchymal cells). In these cases, contrast leaks out of defective vessels into the interstitium, and as a result the immediately surrounding parenchyma demonstrates enhancement. Different types of pathology tend to produce characteristic patterns of enhancement.

SEARCH PATTERN

In order to ensure that common and important abnormalities are not missed, it is helpful to develop an ordered approach to the brain. In MRI, images are usually obtained in sagittal, axial, and coronal dimensions. Beginning with the midline sagittal view, examine the corpus callosum (the major connection between the two cerebral hemispheres, subject to partial or complete agenesis in a number of conditions), the

Figure 9–11. These T1-weighted pre- (left) and postinfusion (right) axial magnetic resonance images of the brain in a patient with multiple sclerosis demonstrate multiple bilateral enhancing plaques, indicating the presence of active inflammation and demyelination.

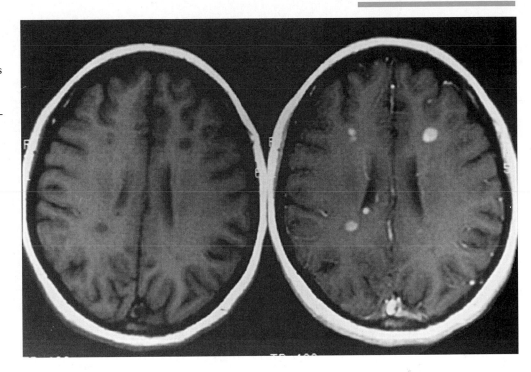

aqueduct of Sylvius (connecting the third and fourth ventricles, and associated with hydrocephalus in aqueductal stenosis), and the optic chiasm and pituitary gland (pituitary tumors may compress the optic chiasm from below, producing bitemporal hemianopsia). Posterior fossa structures to be evaluated include the brainstem, the fourth ventricle, and the position of the cerebellar tonsils, which are inferiorly displaced in an Arnold-Chiari malformation.

On axial images, key structures to assess include the orbits and sinuses, the brainstem, thalamus, basal ganglia, cerebellum, and the frontal, parietal, temporal, and occipital lobes of the brain. Key factors of evaluation include the symmetry of the intracranial structures, with special attention to the presence of asymmetric signal abnormalities (as in hemorrhage or tumor), masses or mass effect (displacement of adjacent structures, such as ventricles), midline shift (such as subfalcine herniation), extra-axial fluid collections (subdural and epidural hematomas), effacement of ventricles and sulci (as in increased intracranial pressure), and the loss of normal demarcation between gray and white matter (diffuse anoxia with edema) (Fig. 9–12). When an abnormal space-occupying lesion is detected, determining its location is critical.

PATHOLOGY

Congenital

Congenital disorders of the CNS are also discussed in the section on obstetrical sonography. There are numerous types of congenital lesions, but three of the most important are neural tube closure defects, migrational anomalies, and the phakomatoses. One of the most common neural tube closure defects is a Chiari II malformation, which is related to the presence of a smaller than normal posterior fossa. These cramped posterior fossa quarters result in herniation of the cerebellar tonsils and ver-

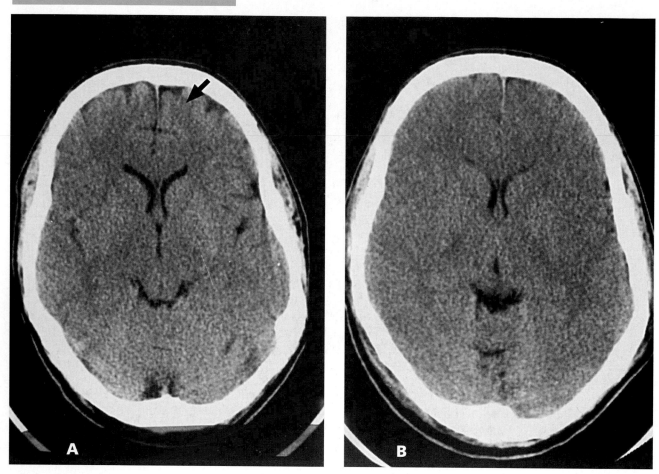

Figure 9–12. A 44-year-old man who had undergone a liver transplant gradually lapsed into a coma. (A) A noncontrast axial computed tomography image obtained prior to his decline in mental status demonstrates a normal-appearing brain with intact gray–white matter junctions (arrow). (B) A corresponding image after his deterioration demonstrates effacement of the frontal horns of the lateral ventricles and the cerebral sulci, as well as loss of the gray–white matter demarcation. These subtle changes resulted from diffuse cerebral edema.

mis through the foramen magnum and compression of the fourth ventricle. Most Chiari II malformations are associated with a myelomeningocele, a failure to close the caudal end of the neural tube. In contrast, the Chiari I malformation is a less severe abnormality involving mere extension of the cerebellar tonsils more than 5 mm below the foramen magnum (Fig. 9–13).

Migrational abnormalities result from the arrested migration of neurons from the subependymal regions outward toward the cortical surface, with gray matter cells ending up where they do not belong. One such migrational abnormality is schizencephaly, in which a cleft of gray matter extends from the cortical surface down to one of the ventricles (Fig. 9–14). Such migrational abnormalities, which are usually associated with abnormal cerebral electrical activity, must be borne in mind when imaging a child who presents with seizures.

PHAKOMATOSES

The phakomatoses are neuroectodermal disorders characterized by coexistent skin and CNS tumors. Among the most common are neurofibromatosis types I and II,

Figure 9–13. A 33-year-old woman presented with lancinating neck pain that radiated to her scalp each time she coughed, sneezed, or performed a Valsalva maneuver. This sagittal T1-weighted magnetic resonance image demonstrates inferior extension of the cerebellar tonsils (curved arrow) more than 5 mm below the foramen magnum (straight arrow), which represents a Chiari I malformation. Symptoms likely relate to a relative obstruction to cerebrospinal fluid flow due to the tonsillar ectopia.

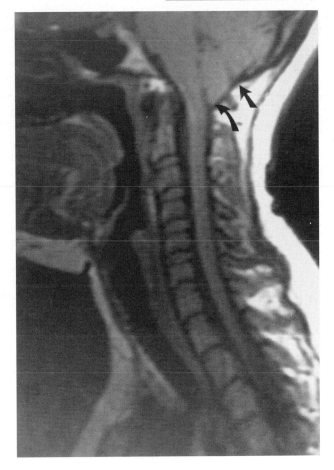

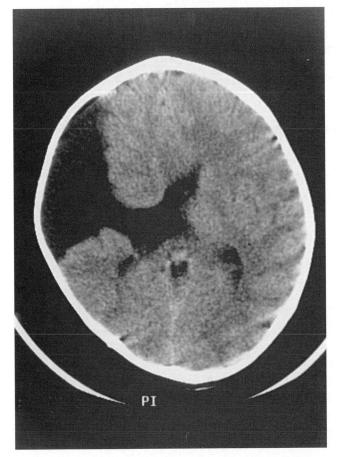

Figure 9–14. This axial image from a head computed tomography scan demonstrates a large, gray matter lined cleft extending from the surface of the right cerebral hemisphere into the right lateral ventricle. This type of schizencephaly is termed *open lip,* because the cleft is filled with cerebrospinal fluid. This infant had suffered seizures and left hemiparesis since birth.

tuberous sclerosis, von Hippel-Lindau disease, and Sturge-Weber syndrome. Neurofibromatosis type I (NF-I) is the most common phakomatosis, found in 1 in 3000 persons, half of whom represent spontaneous mutations and half of whom inherited the disorder via an autosomal dominant route. It is associated with abnormalities of chromosome 17. It is associated clinically with cutaneous café au lait spots and axillary or inguinal freckling, among other findings. Neuroimaging findings include optic nerve gliomas and spinal neurofibromas (Fig. 9–15). Skeletal findings in NF-I related to the presence of neurofibromas include a sharply angled kyphosis of the spine, twisted

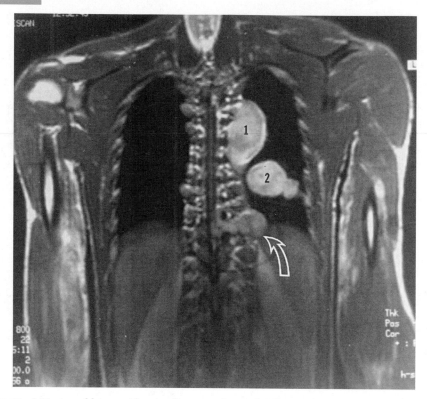

Figure 9–15. A 21-year-old man with neurofibromatosis type I underwent a magnetic resonance imaging examination to evaluate the extent of his disease. This T1-weighted postinfusion coronal image through the chest demonstrates three intrathoracic neurofibromas. The left paraspinal lesion located in the mid-thoracic spine (1) extends along multiple vertebral bodies. A second lesion (2) appears on this image to be within the left lung, but in fact arises from an intercostal nerve. The third lesion (arrow), located in the lower thoracic spine, exhibits a classic "dumbbell" configuration, with paraspinal tumor extending through an expanded neural foramen into the vertebral canal. It does not enhance as intensely as the other two lesions.

ribs, and pseudoarthroses (due to improper healing of a tibial bowing fracture). NF-II is considerably less common, seen in 1 in 50,000 persons, and is associated with chromosome 22 defects. Imaging findings include bilateral acoustic neuromas (actually vestibular schwannomas, discussed later), as well as intracranial meningiomas and cranial nerve schwannomas (Fig. 9–16).

Tuberous sclerosis is characterized by the clinical triad of mental retardation, seizures, and adenoma sebaceum, and is inherited in an autosomal dominant fashion in up to 50% of cases. Imaging findings include multiple CNS tubers (hamartomas), angiomyolipomas in the kidneys, and spontaneous pneumothorax in up to 50% of patients (Fig. 9–17).

Von Hippel-Lindau disease is inherited in autosomal dominant fashion and represents the most life-threatening of the phakomatoses discussed here. It is associated with cerebellar hemangioblastomas and/or renal cell carcinomas in 40% of patients, as well as pheochromocytomas and retinal angiomas.

Sturge-Weber syndrome involves ipsilateral capillary angiomas of the face (portwine nevus of the first division of the trigeminal nerve) and the cerebral hemisphere. Imaging findings include a highly characteristic pattern of unilateral curvilinear calcification that follows the convolutions of the brain, better detected on CT than MRI (Fig. 9–18).

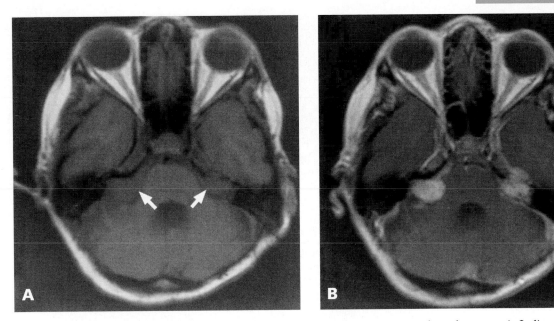

Figure 9–16. A 46-year-old woman with a history of neurofibromatosis type II demonstrates the pathognomonic finding of her disorder, bilateral vestibular schwannomas. (A) A preinfusion axial T1-weighted magnetic resonance image at the level of the internal auditory canals demonstrates bilateral cerebellopontine angle masses (arrows). (B) A postinfusion image at the same level demonstrates strong enhancement of these masses.

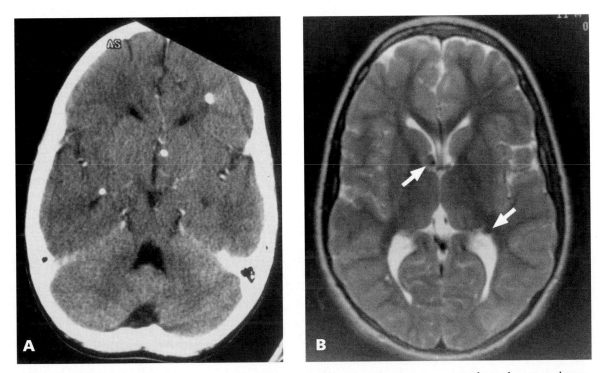

Figure 9–17. A 5-year-old boy with a history of seizures and adenoma sebaceum underwent a contrast-enhanced computed tomography examination to evaluate the intracranial extent of his tuberous sclerosis. (A) An axial image at the level of the third ventricle reveals multiple enhancing parenchymal hamartomas ("tubers"). With time, these lesions tend to calcify, and by the age of 10 years, more than half of patients will have calcified hamartomas. (B) An axial T2-weighted magnetic resonance image in another patient demonstrates tubers adjacent to the posterior aspect of the frontal horn of the right lateral ventricle and the anterior aspect of the atrium of the left lateral ventricle (arrows). The lesions appear predominately low signal due to the presence of calcification.

Figure 9–18. An axial image from a nonenhanced computed tomography (CT) scan of the head of a 12-year-old girl demonstrates classic changes of Sturge-Weber syndrome, including dense linear calcifications following the convolutional pattern of the brain, and ipsilateral hemispheric atrophy. CT is the preferred technique for demonstrating calcifications, which can be mistaken for vascular flow voids on magnetic resonance imaging.

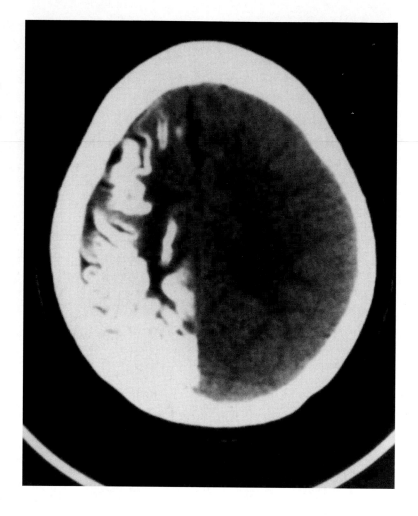

Inflammatory

MULTIPLE SCLEROSIS

EPIDEMIOLOGY

Multiple sclerosis is a relatively common disorder, afflicting approximately 350,000 Americans, two-thirds of whom are women. Each year, approximately 10,000 new cases are diagnosed, most frequently between the ages of 20 and 40 years. Unfortunately, a significant percentage of patients, approximately one-third, eventually develop severe disability, including the loss of ambulation, and two-thirds of patients eventually lose their jobs due to the disease. However, it is not associated with a large increase in mortality, and the average patient lives with the disease for 40 years. Curiously, multiple sclerosis is virtually unknown in arctic and tropical climates, and is most common in the temperate regions of Europe and the United States.

PATHOPHYSIOLOGY

Multiple sclerosis belongs to a major class of neurologic diseases, the demyelinating diseases. In contrast to the dysmyelinating diseases, such as adrenoleukodystrophy, in which the myelin that is produced is abnormal, the demyelinating disorders are associated with the subsequent destruction of initially normal myelin. Normally, the axons of the CNS are enveloped along their course by spiraled layers of the myelin sheath, which are produced by oligodendrogliocytes (while myelin in the peripheral nervous system is the product of Schwann cells). Myelin sheaths with intervening nodes of Ranvier permit saltatory conduction of axonal impulses, which renders conduction through myelinated fibers approximately 50 times faster than that through nonmyelinated ones. Myelin also allows conservation of energy, by permitting sodium-potassium pump action to be largely restricted to the nodes of Ranvier.

At least half of the weight of the white matter of the CNS is made up of myelin, which helps to explain why demyelinating diseases are seen to affect predominately the white matter. In multiple sclerosis, immune-mediated destruction of myelin occurs anywhere in the CNS, producing a protean array of symptoms. The etiology of this attack is unknown, although genetics appears to play a role, as monozygotic twins have an approximately one-third rate of concordance. The disease is defined clinically as multiple CNS lesions separated in time and space, and this correlates pathologically with the presence of multiple sclerotic plaques demonstrating loss of oligodendrogliocytes and myelin with an accumulation of antibody-producing plasma cells.

CLINICAL PRESENTATION

Symptoms are correlated with the function of the affected white matter. Common sites of involvement include the optic nerves, the periventricular cerebral white matter, and the cervical spinal cord. Optic nerve lesions are associated with blurred vision and blindness. On physical examination, patients demonstrate upper motor neuron signs such as hyperreflexia, as well as other long-track signs such as a positive Babinski sign. The clinical course is characterized by alternating periods of remission and relapse, which may or may not eventuate in residual symptoms. Diagnostic tests other than imaging include examination of CSF for so-called oligoclonal bands of IgG, the use of electrophysiologic evoked potentials to measure delayed conduction velocities produced by demyelination, and blood tests to rule out multiple sclerosis mimics.

IMAGING

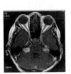
MRI has revolutionized the diagnosis of multiple sclerosis. In clinically confirmed cases, MRI demonstrates lesions over 90% of the time, whereas CT is positive in the minority of cases, and evoked potentials and oligoclonal bands are positive in fewer than 70%. The most sensitive images are heavily T2-weighted sequences, in which plaques typically appear as round or oval lesions of increased signal intensity, especially in the periventricular and deep white matter regions. Often, lesions will be seen to radiate out perpendicularly from the lateral ventricles (Fig. 9–19). Such an appearance is not specific to multiple sclerosis, however, and can be seen in other demyelinating disorders such as Lyme disease. As the disease progresses, global cerebral atrophy, atrophy of the corpus callosum, and increased iron deposition are seen.

Contrast administration does not increase the sensitivity of MRI in lesion detection, but does improve specificity, and the presence of enhancement within plaques (indicating breakdown of the blood-brain barrier) is thought to indicate active demyelination, which is correlated with clinical activity. Therefore, the finding of new areas of enhancement is correlated with a worsening clinical picture. As newer therapies such as interferon-B continue to emerge, MRI is likely to play an increasing role in monitoring treatment response.

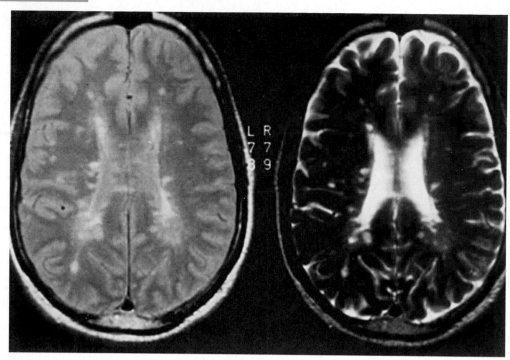

Figure 9–19. Proton-density (left) and T2-weighted (right) axial magnetic resonance images in this 37-year-old woman with a clinical history of multiple sclerosis demonstrate classic changes of multiple sclerosis. Both demonstrate high signal intensity periventricular plaques radiating outward from the lateral ventricles into the deep white matter, so-called Dawson's fingers. This represents the most common location of such plaques, seen in approximately 85% of cases.

Tumorous

EPIDEMIOLOGY

CNS neoplasms are diagnosed in approximately 17,000 patients per year in the United States, and account for approximately 1% of all hospital admissions. Included in these figures are both primary and metastatic lesions.

PATHOPHYSIOLOGY

 Given the fact that metastatic lesions are far more common than primary tumors in such organs as lung, liver, and bone, many physicians would predict that intracranial metastases are a more prevalent form of intracranial neoplasm than primary lesions. In fact, however, metastases from extracranial sources constitute only approximately one-third of intracranial malignancies, with the remaining two-thirds representing primary lesions. The most common tumors to metastasize intracranially in adults include lung and breast carcinomas and malignant melanoma (Fig. 9–20). In children, metastases to the brain are comparatively rare, but skull metastases are not uncommonly seen in neuroblastoma and leukemias. Tumors such as breast and lung cancer may also metastasize to the leptomeninges, where they produce focal or diffuse pial enhancement that may resemble meningitis.

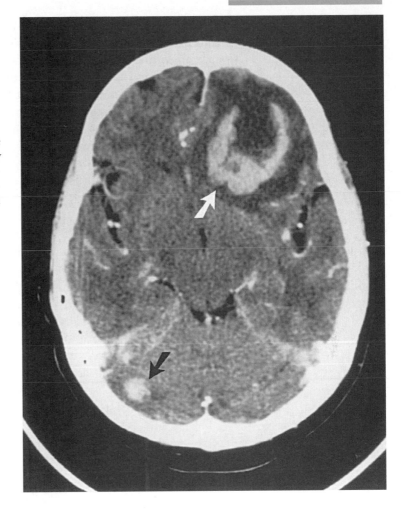

Figure 9–20. A 64-year-old woman with a history of breast cancer presented with gradually worsening headache. An axial image from a contrast-enhanced computed tomography scan demonstrates a 5 cm ring enhancing mass in the left frontal lobe (white arrow), with considerable surrounding vasogenic edema and mass effect on adjacent structures, producing 3 mm of rightward shift of the midline falx cerebri. Also note a second smaller lesion in the right cerebellar hemisphere (black arrow). Metastases are multiple in approximately three-fourths of cases. Corticosteroids are often administered acutely in an effort to reduce the degree of vasogenic edema and mass effect. These lesions were proven at autopsy to represent breast cancer metastases.

Primary brain neoplasms are defined as tumors that arise from the brain or its linings, but typically included in this category are lesions such as craniopharyngiomas and chordomas, which are intracranial and may cause CNS symptoms.

CLINICAL PRESENTATION

Numerous neurologic symptoms may result from intracranial neoplasms, including alterations in consciousness and behavior, cranial nerve palsies, endocrinologic abnormalities, and seizures.

IMAGING

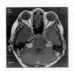 In both CT and MRI, contrast administration is vital to reliably identify and characterize intracranial neoplasms, although preinfusion imaging should be performed first to determine the relatively common presence of hemorrhage. One of the most crucial determinations the radiologist can make regarding an intracranial neoplasm is whether it is intra-axial or extra-axial in location, because the differential diagnosis of intra- and extra-axial lesions is completely different. Some characteristics of intra-axial masses include limited contact with the dura, acute angles between the mass and the dura, white matter expansion,

the absence of a "dural tail," and absence of bone destruction. Extra-axial masses, however, usually exhibit such characteristics as a broad base of contact with the dura, an obtuse angle of dural contact, white matter buckling, medial or central displacement of vessels, a dural tail, and bone destruction (Fig. 9–21). As one would expect, if a mass is extra-axial in origin, a rim of CSF is often interposed between the mass and underlying brain. Because a lesion with an apparently indeterminate point of origin in one plane of imaging may demonstrate a clear origin when imaged in another plane, MRI represents a major advance in brain tumor imaging due to its multiplanar capabilities.

Extra-axial neoplasms

Two of the most common extra-axial neoplasms are meningiomas and schwannomas. Meningiomas constitute 20% of all adult brain tumors, occurring mainly in middle and old age, and are more common in women than in men. They are histologically benign tumors that grow slowly and produce symptoms secondary to compression of adjacent brain. Because of their slow growth and lack of irritation of brain parenchyma, they may be large at the time of diagnosis. They are multiple in up to 10% of cases. Typical locations include the frontal and parietal convexities and the parasagittal region. Approximately one-quarter of meningiomas demonstrate calcification. Another characteristic finding in meningioma, related to its location next to the overlying skull, is hyperostosis. Meningiomas typically demonstrate intense and homogeneous contrast enhancement on both CT and MRI (Fig. 9–22).

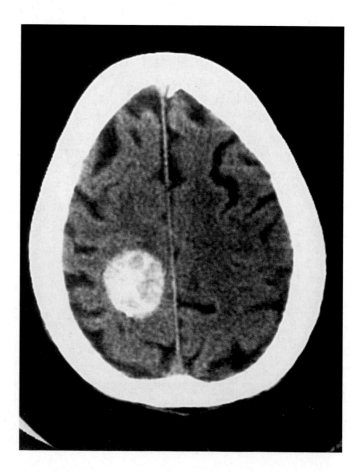

Figure 9–21. This axial image from a noncontrast head computed tomography scan using brain windows demonstrates a round, calcified mass in the right hemispheric high convexity. Is this lesion intra- or extra-axial? At first glance, one might suppose that it is intra-axial, due to the fact that on this image, it is completely surrounded by brain parenchyma. However, this lesion in fact represents a calcified meningioma, which has grown downward from the dural high convexity, radially displacing brain.

The schwannoma is a tumor of the Schwann cells that produce myelin around peripheral nervous system axons—in the case of intracranial tumors, around the axons of the cranial nerves. The vestibular schwannoma is the most common type of intracranial schwannoma, formerly referred to as an acoustic neuroma (however, it is neither acoustic, inasmuch as two-thirds of these tumors involve the vestibular portion of the eighth cranial nerve, nor is it a neuroma, inasmuch as it derives not from

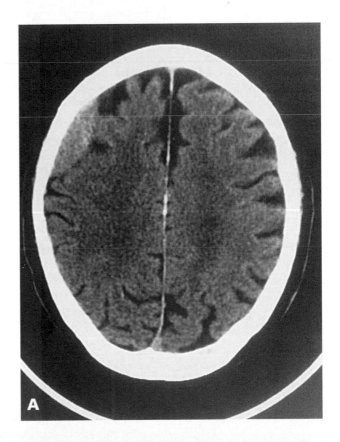

Figure 9–22. (**A**) This axial image from a postinfusion head computed tomography scan demonstrates an extra-axial, enhancing lesion overlying the right frontal lobe, which is displaced medially. We can be confident that the lesion is extra-axial because of its long base along the dura, the fact that it makes obtuse angles with the brain, the distinct plane that separates it from the underlying brain, and the displacement of underlying gray matter and sulci away from the skull. (**B**) Axial pre- (left) and postinfusion (right) T1-weighted magnetic resonance images at a slightly different level demonstrate the typical intense enhancement of these lesions. Meningiomas are the most common extra-axial tumors in adults.

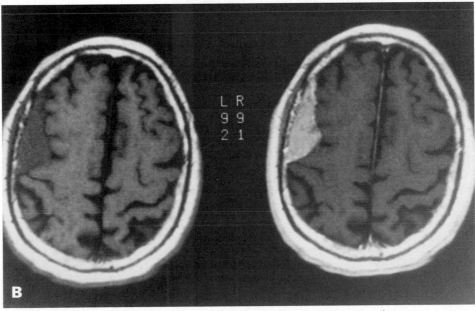

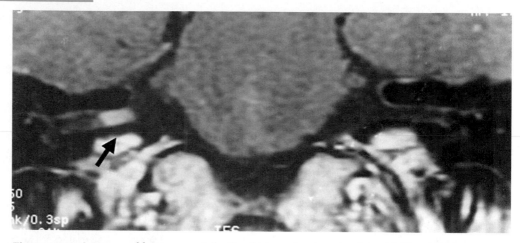

Figure 9–23. A 52-year-old man presented with a history of progressive right-sided hearing loss. A coronal image from a postinfusion T1-weighted magnetic resonance study demonstrates abnormal enhancement of the eighth cranial nerve within the internal auditory canal (arrow), indicating the presence of a vestibular schwannoma. The fact that the tumor is located almost entirely within the canal virtually rules out the possibility of a meningioma.

the neuron, but from the myelin-producing supporting cell). The vestibular schwannoma is the most common mass in the cerebellopontine angle. It can be differentiated from a meningioma in this location by the fact that it typically extends into and expands the internal auditory canal. These benign tumors produce symptoms secondary to their size and location, which may result in compression of the cochlear and vestibular nerves, with progressive neurosensory hearing loss and tinnitus (Fig. 9–23).

Intra-axial neoplasms

Intra-axial primary neoplasms exhibit different profiles in adults and children. In children, two-thirds of lesions are infratentorial; that is, they are located below the tentorium cerebelli, which separates the anterior and middle cranial fossae from the posterior fossa (Fig. 9–24). In adults, the vast majority of lesions are supratentorial.

Approximately 40% of intra-axial primary neoplasms in adults are gliomas, tumors that arise from the glial cells. Gliomas are graded histologically, based on such criteria as the number of mitoses, the presence of necrosis, and nuclear pleomorphism. Grade I astrocytoma is the least aggressive and grade IV represents the highly malignant glioblastoma multiforme. Recent genetic studies have suggested that these various grades in fact represent stages in the evolution of a single tumor, which tends to progress toward higher and more malignant forms. Imaging characteristics on MRI include low signal on T1-weighted images, high signal on T2-weighted images, and enhancement that may be solid or ring-like. Associated findings include surrounding edema and mass effect, which can cause more extensive symptoms than would be predicted based on the size of the tumor alone. Glioblastoma multiforme may exhibit considerable necrosis and hemorrhage. Glioblastoma is one of only two tumors (the other being lymphoma) that can cross the corpus callosum into the opposite hemisphere (Fig. 9–25).

Primary lymphoma of brain is a non-Hodgkin's lymphoma that occurs without evidence of involvement outside the CNS. It is associated with immunodeficiency states such as acquired immunodeficiency syndrome (AIDS) and organ transplanta-

Figure 9–24. An 8-year-old boy presented with severe headaches and deteriorating mentation. (A) Pre- (top) and postcontrast (bottom) infusion sagittal T1-weighted magnetic resonance images in the midline demonstrate a large enhancing mass in the posterior fossa (arrow), which is compressing the fourth ventricle and producing obstructive hydrocephalus, with dramatic dilatation of the third ventricle. (B) Proton density and T2-weighted axial images demonstrate marked transependymal flow of cerebrospinal fluid (CSF) outward from the lateral ventricles. Medulloblastoma belongs to the group of neoplasms referred to as primitive neuroectodermal tumors. It presents most frequently between the ages of 2 and 8 years, and the tumors arise from the roof of the fourth ventricle. Though very radiosensitive, they commonly metastasize early via the CSF.

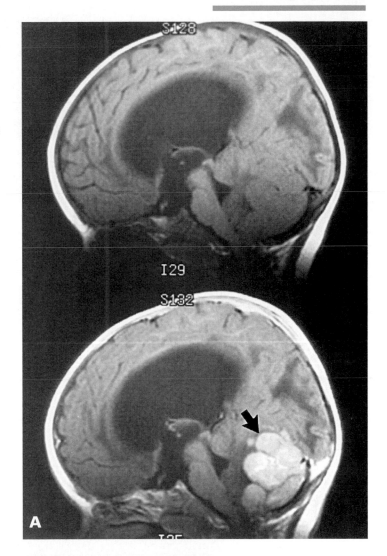

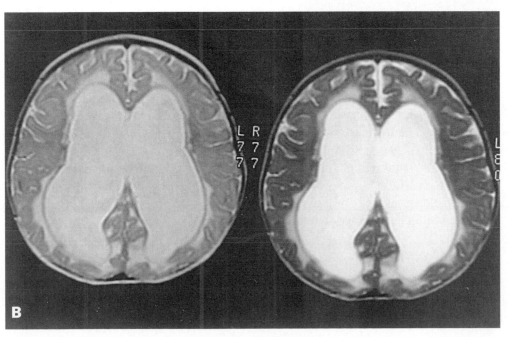

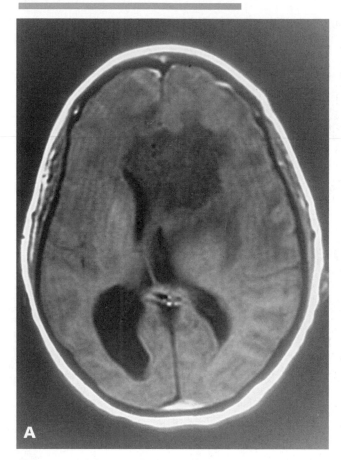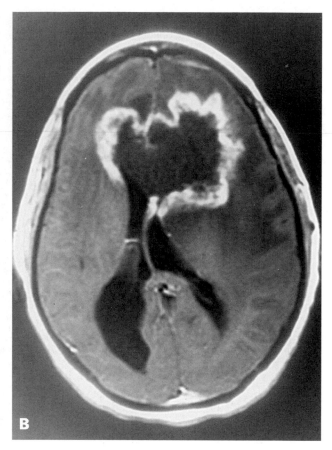

Figure 9–25. (A) Pre- and (B) postinfusion axial magnetic resonance images demonstrate a classic appearance of a glioblastoma multiforme, which unfortunately represents the principal brain tumor of adults. Histologically, the tumors exhibit an aggressive appearance, with cellular pleomorphism, necrosis, and neovascularity. These features are reflected on imaging studies as well, where the tumor demonstrates considerable necrosis, edema, and often hemorrhage. Nodular ring enhancement, as in this case, is also common. Note that this tumor exhibits a relatively specific pattern of spread, traversing the corpus callosum to involve both frontal lobes. Lymphoma is the only other tumor that commonly exhibits this behavior. The prognosis in these tumors is extremely poor, with most patients expiring within 6 to 12 months after diagnosis.

tion, and the increasing incidence of the former condition is likely to render lymphoma the most common primary brain tumor within the next decade or two. The tumors are highly cellular and proliferate rapidly; thus, they tend to exhibit a good response to radiation and steroids, though their behavior is modified for the worse in AIDS patients. Distinguishing imaging characteristics include lack of necrosis, a tendency to cross the midline, mild edema, and a relative lack of mass effect. Multiple lesions are present in as many as one-half of patients (Fig. 9–26). This can confuse the differential diagnosis of primary versus metastatic disease, due to the fact that metastases are multiple in nearly three-fourths of cases.

EPILEPSY

One of the most classic presenting complaints in adult intracranial neoplasms is new-onset seizure. In aggregate, approximately 150,000 new cases of epilepsy, or chronic

Figure 9–26. This coronal postinfusion magnetic resonance image in an acquired immunodeficiency syndrome patient demonstrates multiple bilateral ring enhancing lesions with surrounding edema. The largest is located on the right in a parafalcine location. These lesions represented primary central nervous system lymphoma. Although such tumors are relatively radiosensitive, the overall prognosis is quite poor, with a high rate of recurrence and a median survival of less than 1 year.

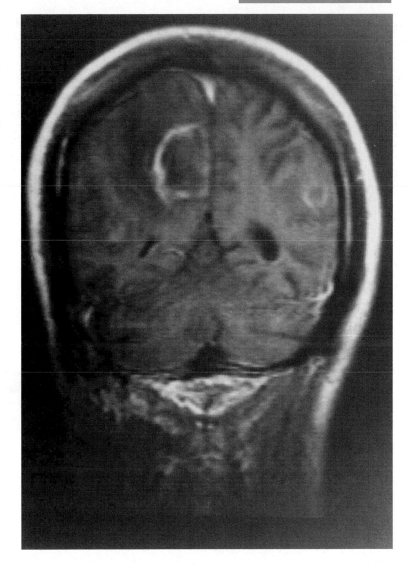

seizure disorder, are diagnosed each year, and there are approximately 2 million patients with epilepsy in the United States. The lifetime risk of developing a seizure disorder is approximately 3%. Numerous causes other than tumor, such as congenital anomalies, trauma, infection, and metabolic disorders, may be responsible. In patients without an underlying neoplasm, medical therapy is effective in controlling seizures two-thirds of the time. Of the remaining one-third, approximately 5000 surgical candidates are identified each year.

Whenever a previously healthy adult develops a new onset seizure disorder, CNS imaging is warranted to rule out the presence of a neoplasm. Because fewer than 5% of strokes present with seizure, one should think twice before attributing a seizure disorder to stroke. Even imaging findings typical for stroke should not eliminate suspicion for an underlying neoplasm. One clue to the presence of an underlying neoplasm is a substantial amount of vasogenic edema, which is typically seen in tumor or abscess. While the surgical objective in many tumor cases is to debulk the lesion, surgery for epilepsy aims for complete removal of the epileptogenic lesion, as even a small lesion residual may result in continued or recurrent seizures.

Infectious

MENINGITIS

EPIDEMIOLOGY

Meningitis is the most common form of CNS infection, and can be divided into three clinical and pathologic categories: acute superative meningitis, usually due to bacterial infection; lymphocytic meningitis, which is usually viral; and chronic meningitis, as seen in tuberculosis and coccidiodomycosis (Fig. 9–27). This discussion focuses on acute meningitis.

PATHOPHYSIOLOGY

 Organisms usually reach the meninges via one of three routes: hematogenously in septic patients, direct invasion in postsurgical or post-traumatic settings, or contiguous spread from the sinuses or middle ear. The infection is spread via the CSF, which circulates between the pia mater and arachnoid layers of the meninges. The infection may disseminate to involve the full extent of the meningeal membranes. Hydrocephalus may be precipitated by a combination of congestion of venous sinuses and postinflammatory fibrosis.

The pneumococcus, the meningococcus, and *Hemophilus influenzae* (or *H. flu*) are the principal etiologic organisms. Pneumococcal meningitis is the most common form in adults, and was uniformly fatal before the introduction of antibiotics. Currently, mortality may range as high as 30%, and many survivors are left with neurologic residua such as seizure disorders and deafness. Meningococcal meningitis may be associated with a characteristic skin rash. *H. flu* is most common in children, who are routinely immunized against more common strains of the organism in an effort to prevent meningitis, a practice that is also affecting the epidemiology of epiglottitis.

CLINICAL PRESENTATION

The patient with meningitis classically presents with severe headache, stiff neck, and fever. The most striking physical examination finding is nuchal rigidity, reflecting the underlying inflammation of the pia and arachnoid membranes, which are stretched when the neck is flexed.

IMAGING

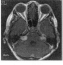 Bacterial meningitis is not an imaging diagnosis. The diagnosis can only be made with confidence through examination of the CSF, usually obtained via lumbar puncture, which is typically performed at or below the L2–3 level, because the spinal cord typically terminates at approximately the level of L1. Characteristic CSF findings include cloudy fluid with increased leukocytes, increased protein, and decreased glucose, secondary to bacterial glycolysis.

Imaging is often obtained to rule out the presence of other conditions that may mimic meningitis, such as a mass lesion, and to detect the presence of increased intracranial pressure, which would preclude lumbar puncture due to the danger of transtentorial herniation. Signs suggestive of meningitis on CT include cerebral edema, manifested as a loss of the usually sharp demarcation between gray and white

Figure 9–27. A 10-month-old boy was brought to the emergency room with new-onset seizures. A head computed tomography examination (not shown) was unremarkable. (**A**) However, pre- (left) and postcontrast (right) infusion T1-weighted axial magnetic resonance (MR) images reveal strong abnormal enhancement of the meninges around the cerebral hemispheres and in the basilar cisterns (arrow). In general, this finding suggests diagnoses such as sarcoidosis and tuberculosis. Note also that these MR images are degraded by motion artifact, as the child was sleeping fitfully during the examination. (**B**) A portable chest radiograph demonstrates an endotracheal tube extending almost to the carina. The most remarkable findings are prominent left hilar adenopathy (arrow) and a diffuse, bilateral pattern of miliary pulmonary opacities, indicative of tuberculosis. The infant was immediately placed on antituberculous therapy.

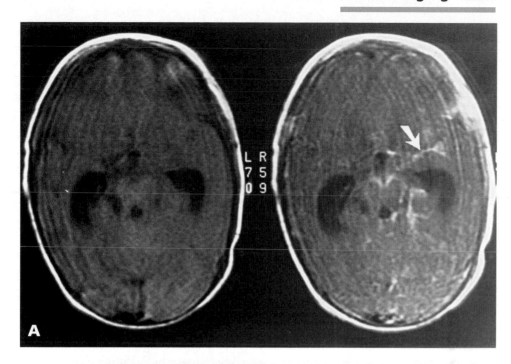

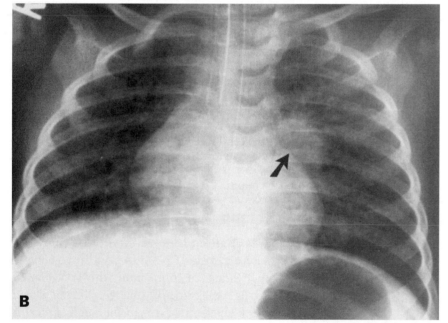

matter, and the presence of communicating hydrocephalus, which appears as enlargement of the ventricles and effacement of the basilar cisterns. Although contrast-enhanced MRI is not routinely obtained, it may demonstrate enhancement of the meninges and ependymal lining of the ventricles.

ABSCESS

Most abscesses result from the contiguous spread of infection from the paranasal sinuses, the mastoid air cells, or the middle ear, although dental and facial sources may also be involved. Some abscesses result from hematogenous spread, most commonly in endocarditis. A brain abscess begins when a portion of the brain is inoculated with a pathogen, which leads to cerebritis. Direct microbial cytotoxicity and host inflammatory response are accompanied by vascular congestion and increased permeability, with the development of edema. If severe enough, capillary perfusion pressure may be overcome by locally increased interstitial pressure, causing necrosis, which appears pathologically as softening and liquefaction. Within a period of days to weeks, the necrotic region becomes encapsulated by a rim of highly vascular granulation tissue, presumably in an attempt to isolate the infection and protect the surrounding tissue. CT findings include a ring-enhancing lesion, reflecting the increased vascularity of the capsule, with a low-density center of necrosis (Fig. 9–28). MRI likewise demonstrates an enhancing rim, the differential for which can include neoplasm and resolving hematoma.

ENCEPHALITIS

The most common and dangerous form of encephalitis is caused by the herpes simplex virus. It is almost always of the type I variety, except in neonates, who may acquire type II (genital) infection during vaginal delivery. The organism exhibits a distinct predilection for the inferior frontal and temporal lobes, producing predictable symptoms such as seizures, personality changes, and confusion, often preceded by a flu-like prodrome of headache and fever. For antiviral therapy (acyclovir) to be effective, it must be instituted within the first several days of the illness, placing a premium on early diagnosis. MRI is more sensitive than CT and demonstrates an increased signal on T2-weighted images, as well as gyral enhancement in the temporal lobes (Fig. 9–29). Immunofluorescent staining and viral cultures from CSF and/or brain biopsy can definitively establish the diagnosis, but often antiviral therapy must be instituted with only a presumptive diagnosis in hand, in order to prevent rapidly irreversible brain damage. While the majority of patients survive the illness, many are left with permanent and devastating neurologic effects, including severe personality and behavioral changes.

PARASITIC INFECTIONS

Although parasitic infections are less common in industrialized nations than in developing countries, they are seen often enough to warrant brief discussion. The most prevalent parasitic CNS infection in the United States may be toxoplasmosis, which is discussed later in connection with HIV disease. In immunocompetent patients, cysticercosis is the principal infection. It results from fecal–oral transmission of the eggs of the pork tapeworm *Taenia solium* and is most frequently encountered in Latin American immigrants. Organisms that reach the parenchyma of the CNS take up residence as viable cysts, often distributed along the gray–white matter junctions. When the organism dies, it incites a local inflammatory reaction that causes both clinical symptoms such as seizures and, on imaging studies, contrast enhancement. The dense scolex of the organism may be visible within the lumen of the cyst (Fig. 9–30).

HUMAN IMMUNODEFICIENCY VIRUS

EPIDEMIOLOGY

Between one-third and two-thirds of patients with HIV infection eventually develop neurologic symptoms, and neurologic complaints represent the presenting symptom

Figure 9–28. This axial image from a contrast-enhanced computed tomography scan demonstrates classic features of a brain abscess, including a ring-enhancing lesion with central low-density necrosis, mass effect on the adjacent brain (note the rightward displacement of the midline falx cerebri), and a considerable amount of surrounding vasogenic edema.

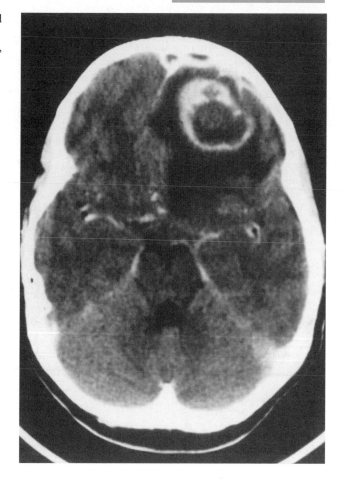

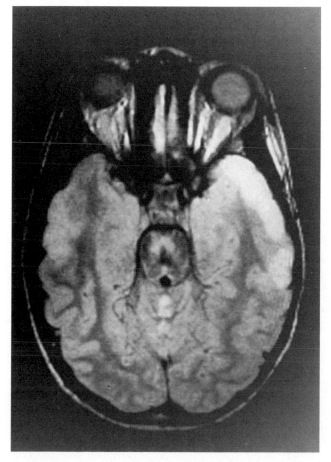

Figure 9–29. This axial proton-density weighted magnetic resonance (MR) image of the brain demonstrates a prominent increase in signal intensity in the left temporal lobe, representing inflammation and edema. This location is characteristic for type I herpes encephalitis. Because herpes can rapidly produce a necrotizing encephalitis with severe long-term neurologic sequelae, prompt institution of antiviral therapy is critical. MR represents the most sensitive imaging modality in the detection of early changes.

Figure 9–30. This young woman recently immigrated from Latin America and presented with new-onset seizures. An axial image from a postinfusion head computed tomography scan demonstrates a ring-enhancing lesion in the left hemisphere. It is located at the gray–white matter junction and demonstrates surrounding low attenuation edema. Note the central nidus of enhancement, giving the lesion a "target" appearance. This central nidus represents the scolex of the organism. Over 90% of patients with central nervous system cysticerosis present with seizures.

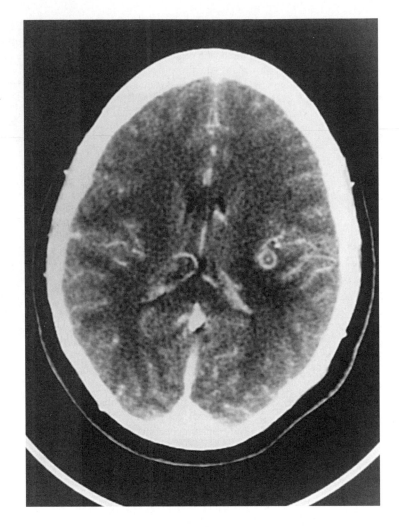

of HIV infection in approximately one-tenth of patients. CNS involvement is found in 75% of AIDS patients at autopsy. In the United States, approximately 50,000 patients per year develop neurologic complications of HIV infection.

PATHOPHYSIOLOGY

 The neurologic manifestations of HIV infection can be traced to one of three etiologies: opportunistic infections related to immunodeficiency, vascular insults, or direct HIV-mediated neurotoxicity. Toxoplasmosis is the principal HIV-related opportunistic infection. Seropositivity to this ubiquitous protozoan is found in up to 70% of the American population, and it causes disease in approximately 10% of AIDS patients, usually as a reactivation of latent infection.

CLINICAL PRESENTATION

The presentation of patients with HIV-associated CNS infection is generally nonspecific, but will vary depending on whether the patient suffers from an opportunistic infection, a vascular insult, or primary HIV encephalopathy. The latter is associated with a progressive subcortical dementia.

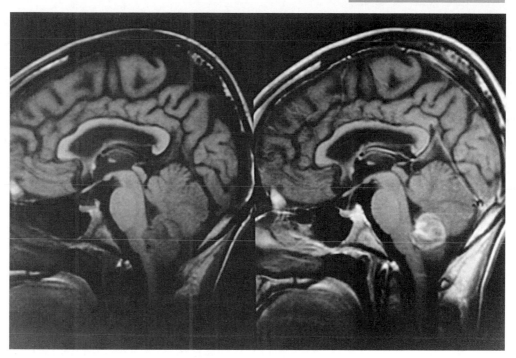

Figure 9–31. A 21-year-old man with acquired immunodeficiency syndrome presented with incoordination and gait abnormalities. Pre- (left) and postinfusion (right) T1-weighted sagittal magnetic resonance images demonstrate an enhancing mass in the inferior aspect of the cerebellum. Principal differential diagnostic considerations included toxoplasmosis and lymphoma. A follow-up scan after 2 weeks of antitoxoplasma treatment (not shown) demonstrated significant improvement, consistent with a diagnosis of toxoplasmosis. Such lesions often heal with calcification.

IMAGING

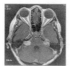 The CNS lesions of toxoplasmosis are usually well-localized, with an abscess-like appearance. A minority may be hemorrhagic. When a mass lesion is detected in an HIV-positive patient with new-onset neurologic symptoms, the most important differential diagnosis is that between toxoplasmosis and lymphoma. The incidence of primary CNS lymphoma in AIDS is as high as 6%. In contrast to toxoplasmosis, lymphoma often exhibits a hyperdense appearance on nonenhanced CT scan. Moreover, lymphoma tends to occur in a periventricular location, while toxoplasmosis is often seen in the basal ganglia. The key distinguishing feature, however, is prompt response to antibiotic therapy, which only toxoplasmosis exhibits (Fig. 9–31).

Traumatic

EPIDEMIOLOGY

Trauma is the leading cause of death in the United States in persons younger than 44 years of age, and approximately one-half of those deaths are the result of brain injury. Only 10% of CNS trauma is fatal, however, and each year, 100,000 patients who survive are left with permanent neurologic sequelae ranging in severity up to paralysis and the persistent vegetative state. The suffering occasioned by CNS trauma is further heightened by the fact that it tends to strike individuals in the "prime of life," with nearly two-thirds of cases occurring in men between the ages of 20 and 30 years.

PATHOPHYSIOLOGY

 Head trauma is categorized in a number of important ways. Closed head trauma refers to injuries in which the dura remains intact, while in open head trauma it is disrupted. Primary brain injury refers to damage occurring at the moment of impact, whether it be an object penetrating the head, a collision between the head and an external object, or a deceleration injury in which the head itself does not collide with any object, but differential inertial properties of gray and white matter result in shearing of tissues. Examples of primary traumatic injuries include contusions and hematomas, vascular injury, and so-called shearing injury, including diffuse axonal injury (Fig. 9–32). Secondary injuries include infarction due to edema, herniation, embolism, and infection due to penetrating trauma.

A key element in the pathophysiology of head trauma is the fact that the brain is a relatively noncompliant tissue within a closed, rigid space. Severe head trauma may initiate a vicious cycle producing inexorably rising increased intracranial pressure. The inciting trauma causes tissue damage, with disruption of blood vessels, inflammation,

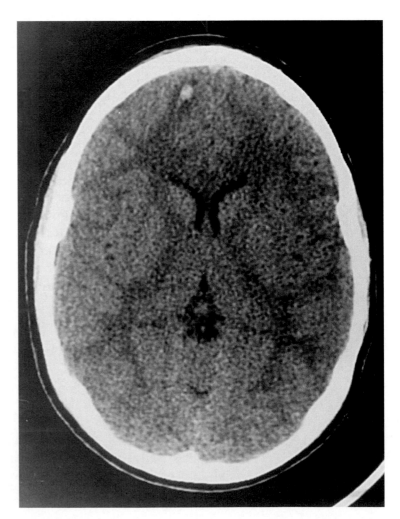

Figure 9–32. This patient suffered a deceleration-rotation injury as a result of a motor vehicle accident, and was brought to the hospital in a coma. An axial image from a noncontrast head computed tomography scan demonstrates an area of increased attenuation at the gray–white matter junction of the right frontal lobe. This represented a hemorrhagic shear injury. The mortality rate of these lesions is as high as 50%, and the long-term neurologic prognosis is often poor.

and resultant edema and swelling. This results in an increase in interstitial pressure outside the capillaries, which has the effect of diminishing blood flow. If autoregulatory compensation is not effective, further tissue damage then results, with further swelling and edema, further increased intracranial pressure, and so on. Hence, one of the principle roles of surgery in head trauma is to reduce intracranial pressure, by decompressing the brain. For example, an acute hematoma may be evacuated through burr holes. Medical measures include mannitol infusion to increase intravascular osmotic pressure, thereby reducing transcapillary flow of fluid into the brain parenchyma, and hyperventilation, which normally results in hypocarbia and an autoregulatory decrease in cerebral perfusion (which may help to reduce hyperemic swelling).

Any force that increases intracranial pressure, whether it be diffuse cerebral swelling from hyperemia or edema, or more focal mass effect from a hematoma, tumor, or infarction, will press brain tissue into the path of least resistance. In a unilateral hematoma along one of the cerebral hemispheres, the brain will tend to shift toward the opposite side, effacing or obliterating the ipsilateral ventricle and causing subfalcine herniation (ipsilateral brain tissue crossing the midline under the falx cerebri into the opposite side). If supratentorial pressure is sufficient, uncal herniation may result, in which the uncus (the medial portion of the temporal lobe) moves medially and inferiorly, compressing the oculomotor nerve (with pupillary dilatation), the posterior cerebral artery, and the midbrain, which may result in death.

CLINICAL PRESENTATION

Fully one-half of cases of CNS trauma result from motor vehicle accidents. A large percentage of cases involve alcohol or drug use, which hampers clinical assessment of the acutely injured patient and renders neuroimaging even more important, because history and physical examination cannot be relied on in the intoxicated patient. When a history cannot be obtained, it is often impossible to be certain whether superficial injuries are the result of a primary traumatic event or if the "trauma" resulted from some other neurologic deficit; for example, a patient who suffered a stroke or a seizure, then fell over and struck his head. Again, neuroimaging is key in diagnosis.

IMAGING

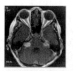 The most important imaging modality in suspected or known acute head trauma is the noncontrast CT. CT is superior to MRI for the detection of acute blood and fractures, and is more readily available, quicker, and more accommodating to the patient requiring close clinical monitoring (Fig. 9–33). MRI is the most sensitive modality for the detection of more subtle regions of parenchymal injury, but these need not be demonstrated emergently, because their detection does not alter therapeutic management. The acute question is simply whether there is a treatable lesion. To answer this question, CT is the modality of choice.

The role of plain skull films is highly limited, for the following reason. Suppose the clinician orders skull films, and a fracture is detected; a CT of the head is indicated to assess for the possibility of intracranial injury. Suppose the clinician orders skull films and no fracture is detected; if there is clinical suspicion of trauma of sufficient force to fracture the skull, a CT is also indicated to rule out intracranial injury, even if no fracture is seen. CT may, however, miss nondisplaced fractures parallel to the plane of imaging, and skull films may still be warranted if the diagnosis of a nondepressed skull fracture would have important medicolegal implications, as in suspected child abuse.

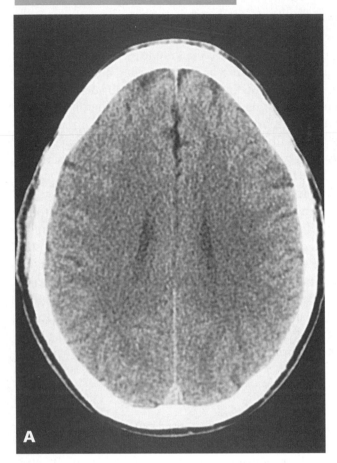
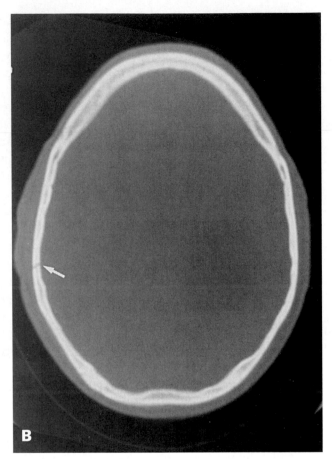

Figure 9–33. A 24-year-old man was referred from the emergency room with the clinical history, "Struck on head with bottle." When a request was made for more clinical information, the clerk in the emergency room sent a second requisition, this time reading, "Struck on head with vodka bottle." Absent further clinical history, the radiologist cannot be certain that the optimal imaging studies were performed; for example, had the patient been struck in the area of the eye, special attention to the orbits might be warranted, or had the patient exhibited hemotympanum, further evaluation of the temporal bone would be indicated. However, the principal point of this case is to show the importance of properly evaluating the osseous structures in traumatic cases. (**A**) A noncontrast axial image with "brain windows" demonstrates mild extracranial soft tissue swelling along the right side, but no other evidence of injury. (**B**) However, the same slice viewed with a "bone window" algorithm clearly demonstrates a nondisplaced frontoparietal skull fracture underlying the soft tissue swelling (arrow). All computed tomography scans obtained for the evaluation of trauma should include bone windows, which are much more sensitive than soft tissue windows for the detection of osseous injury.

The triage of head trauma may be divided into surgical and nonsurgical findings. Nonsurgical findings include contusion, infarction, and mild to moderate edema. Surgical findings, those warranting emergent surgical consultation, would include more severe edema threatening herniation, or subdural or epidural hematomas.

Which trauma patients should receive CNS imaging? The imaging yield will generally be quite low in patients who do not have a clinically apparent neurologic deficit, an obvious injury, a history of loss of consciousness, or severe trauma. When the patient cannot give a history due to age or intoxication, the history is inconsistent or unreliable, or physical examination is deemed unreliable due to factors such as intoxication, seizure, or associated injuries, most clinicians will choose to scan the patient. However, before radiological evaluation takes place, the patient must be stabilized, and at least a single lateral view of the cervical spine should be obtained to rule out spinal instability or injury to the cord. The cervical spine may be further evaluated by CT at the same time the head is scanned. Following is a brief discussion of some of the most frequent and important imaging findings in acute head trauma.

Subdural hematoma

Young patients typically develop subdural hematomas secondary to motor vehicle accidents, while those in older patients typically result from falls. The mortality rate associated with these injuries is high, at least 50%, and only one-fifth of those who survive can expect to recover fully. Subdural hematomas may result from closed or open injury, with tearing of bridging veins and bleeding into the potential space between the dura mater and pia arachnoid membranes. Because this space is interrupted by the falx cerebri, these hematomas do not cross the midline, but they will cross sutures, to which only the overlying dura is adherent. Because they are not bounded by sutures, they tend to spread out over the underlying hemisphere, giving them an elongated, crescentic shape (Fig. 9–34). Because acutely extravasated blood is usually high attenuation (bright) on CT, they are generally easily detected. However, some subdurals may be isodense, and a careful search must be made for midline shift, ventricular distortion, and sulci that do not extend all the way to the apparent brain surface (Fig. 9–35). What could make an acute subdural hematoma isodense? The density of acutely extravasated blood is related to the concentration of red blood cells.

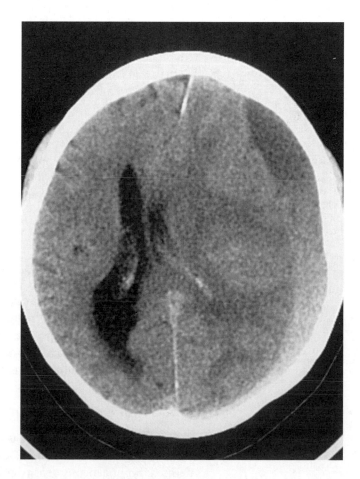

Figure 9–34. A 74-year-old woman developed sudden slurred speech and slowed mentation, and was sent to the radiology department to rule out a cerebrovascular accident. This non-contrast axial computed tomography image demonstrates a large crescent-shaped left subdural hematoma, which involves virtually the entire left hemisphere. It is associated with prominent mass effect on the adjacent brain, with compression of the left lateral ventricle and shift of the calcium-containing falx cerebri to the right. In addition, the hematoma itself contains a hematocrit level, with hyperdense fresher blood inferiorly, and hypodense fluid superiorly. Such a finding constitutes one of the strongest reasons for imaging the central nervous system in patients with neurologic complaints, as a subdural hematoma represents a surgically treatable cause of dementia.

Figure 9–35. A 45-year-old man presented with increasing left leg weakness. An axial image from a nonenhanced computed tomography scan at the level of the high cerebral convexities reveals no abnormal hypodense or hyperdense tissue. However, the cerebral sulci do not extend all the way to the skull on the right side, as they do on the left. This indicates the presence of an isodense subdural hematoma, a potentially curable etiology of the patient's left-sided weakness. It can be helpful to administer contrast, because displacement of the cortical surface vessels away from the skull may become more apparent.

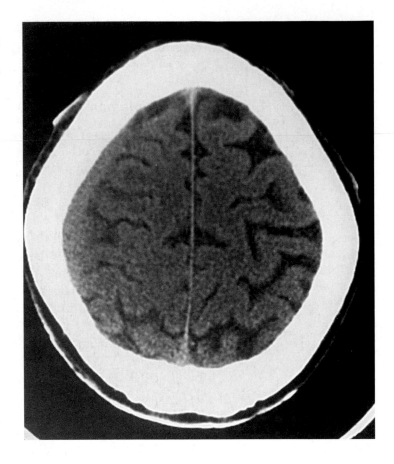

Hence, erythrocyte-poor blood (as in anemia) or dilution of blood (as with CSF if the arachnoid membrane is torn) may render the hematoma isodense.

Epidural hematoma

Approximately 90% of epidural hematomas result from temporal bone fracture, with tearing of the middle meningeal artery or veins. The resultant blood collection strips the dural membranes from the inner table of the skull, hence the name *epidural.* As in subdural hematoma, patients may exhibit a so-called lucid interval after the injury before deteriorating, during which time intracranial pressure has not yet increased sufficiently to impair consciousness. Patients are usually younger than those suffering subdurals, and because many of these bleeds are self-limited and the patients have a greater neurologic resiliency, the prognosis is not as poor. These hematomas cannot cross sutures (unless there is diastasis or "opening up" of the suture secondary to fracture), and for this reason the blood is more tightly contained and tends to assume a "biconvex" or "lens" shape, meaning that, in contrast to the subdural hematoma, the collection bulges inward toward the brain. These lesions can cross the midline, because they separate the falx cerebri and dural sinus from the skull.

Intracerebral contusions and hematomas

Both contusions and hematomas result from regions of parenchymal hemorrhage, with accumulation of blood (Fig. 9–36). The term *hematoma* is used to describe a well-defined, homogeneous density collection of blood, while *contusion* refers to a lesion of

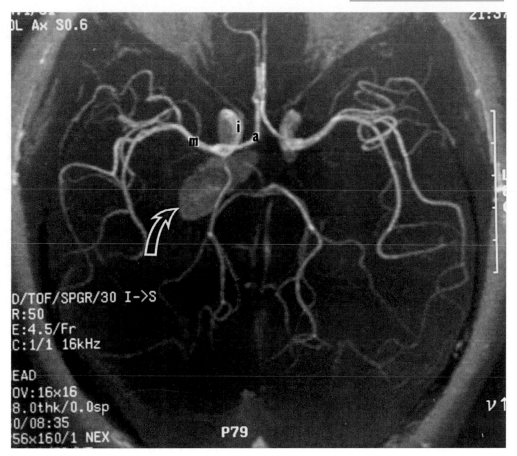

Figure 9–36. A 13-year-old boy with factor IX deficiency presented to the emergency department after minor head trauma with left-sided stroke-like symptoms. This axial magnetic resonance angiogram, which displays flowing blood as "white," demonstrates a large area of hemorrhage surrounding the right posterior communicating artery (arrow), which resulted from the patient's coagulopathy. a, anterior cerebral artery; i, internal carotid artery; m, middle cerebral artery.

mixed density with less clearly defined margins. These lesions are most often found in the anterior frontal and temporal lobes, where the brain is accelerated against bone. A clue to the presence of both is extracranial swelling, which indicates the site of impact. When the bleed is on the same side of the brain as the impact, the lesion is called a *coup* (French for "blow") injury, whereas when it is opposite the impact, it is called a *contrecoup* ("opposite the blow") injury (Fig. 9–37). With time, these lesions become isodense and then hypodense, and are eventually replaced by an area of encephalomalacia.

Diffuse axonal injury

Diffuse axonal injury is the principal cause of persistent coma immediately following trauma and is the primary lesion responsible for poor long-term outcome in head trauma patients. The injury results from disruption of axonal fibers by deceleration forces, typically at gray–white matter interfaces, because the gray matter is more gelatinous in consistency than the firmer white matter. Eventually, wallerian degeneration results, with loss of axons in distal white matter tracts. While CT may detect associated hemorrhage, only MRI can detect nonhemorrhagic lesions, which appear bright on T2-weighted images and are associated with a poorer prognosis.

Figure 9–37. A 55-year-old man with a history of heroin use fell off a park bench and was brought to the emergency department with acute mental status changes. An axial image from a nonenhanced computed tomography scan of the head demonstrates prominent extracranial soft tissue swelling and subcutaneous air (black arrow), the site of a large laceration where the patient's head struck a bottle. However, the intracranial injury is found on the opposite side of the head (white arrow), where an area of mixed high and low density lesions indicates a hemorrhagic cortical contusion with surrounding edema. This represents a contrecoup injury, produced by a "rebound" deceleration of the brain against the skull opposite the direct impact.

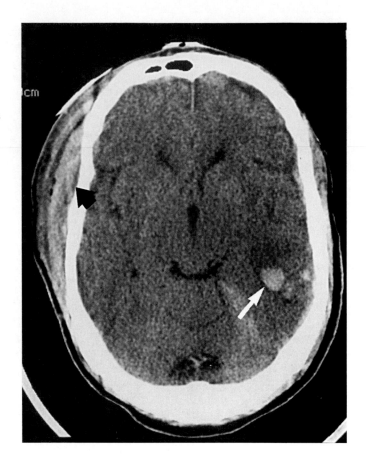

Vascular

STROKE

EPIDEMIOLOGY

Stroke refers to an abrupt neurological deficit stemming from a vascular insult. While the incidence of stroke in the United States has steadily declined over the past few decades, it remains the third or fourth leading cause of death in the United States, and over 500,000 Americans still suffer strokes each year. Perhaps even costlier is the heavy toll it exacts among survivors, many of whom are left with severe neurologic impairment. The principal risk factors for stroke are hypertension and atherogenic factors such as cigarette smoking and hyperlipidemia.

PATHOPHYSIOLOGY

 Because neurons in the adult do not divide, the damage caused by a stroke is irreversible. However, strokes are sometimes preceded clinically by so-called transient ischemic attacks (TIAs), neurologic deficits that completely resolve within 24 hours, and many other strokes pursue a stuttering course. Therefore, while completed strokes are not amenable to therapy (except rehabilitation), preventive measures such as carotid endarterectomy and anticoagulation may be indicated in patients who have suffered a TIA, and therapeutic maneuvers such as heparinization and even thrombolysis may be warranted in some patients whose stroke is not completed.

Clinically, the site of stroke can often be discerned on the basis of the patient's neurologic deficit. The most common location of stroke is in the middle cerebral artery (MCA) distribution, which supplies the bulk of the frontal, temporal, and parietal lobes (Fig. 9–38). Patients with MCA strokes may present with contralateral hemiplegia and hemianesthesia, and when the dominant hemisphere is involved, aphasia. The anterior cerebral artery (ACA) supplies portions of the frontal and parietal lobes, especially along the midline. ACA occlusion may cause contralateral foot and leg weakness. The posterior cerebral artery (PCA), or vertebrobasilar system, supplies the cerebellum, the occipital lobes, the thalamus, and the upper midbrain, through which most of the brain's input and output pass. Even a small infarction in some portions of the PCA territory may produce catastrophic consequences, including apnea, coma, cranial nerve deficits, and major motor and sensory deficits.

IMAGING

Stroke versus another process

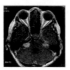 Imaging has several critical roles in stroke, all related to its pathophysiology and therapy. One often underappreciated role of imaging is to determine whether the patient's neurologic deficit may stem from some cause other than stroke. It is not uncommon for patients to be referred for head CT scans with the history of "Stroke—rule out bleed," who turn out to be suffering from nonvasoocclusive processes, such as a subdural hematoma or a tumor. While this occurs in only a minority of patients, all patients with suspected stroke deserve

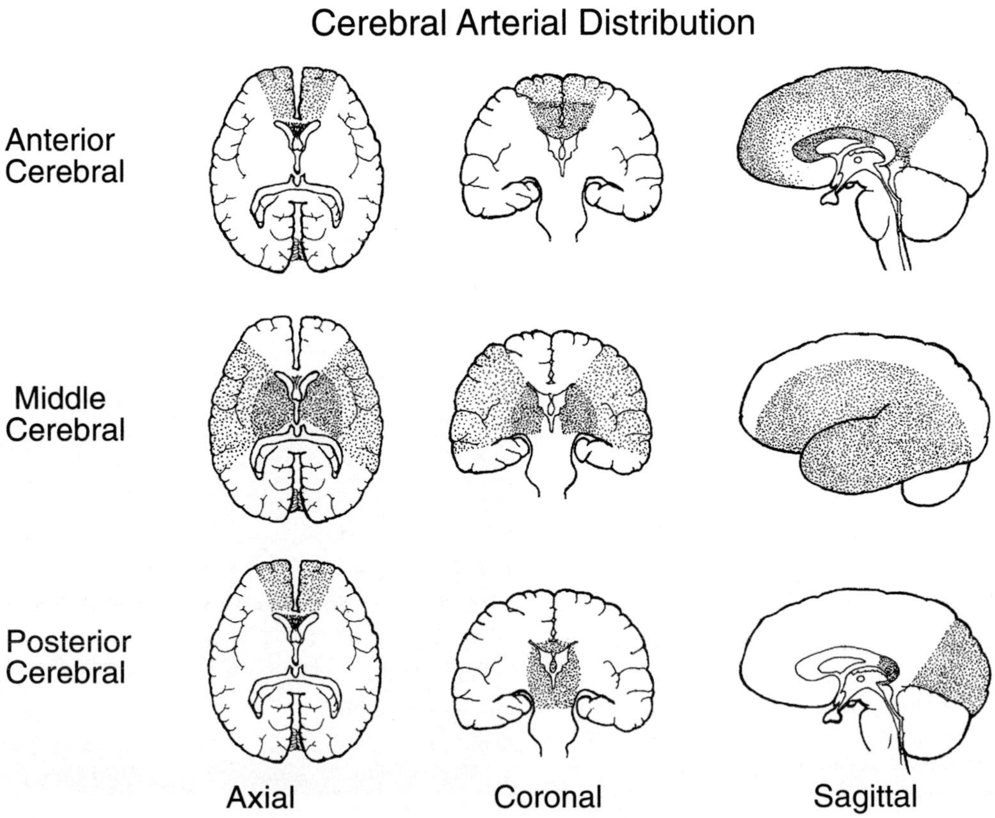

Cerebral Arterial Distribution

Anterior
Cerebral

Middle
Cerebral

Posterior
Cerebral

Axial   Coronal   Sagittal

Figure 9–38. The arterial territories of the brain, as visualized on axial, coronal, and sagittal views.

imaging in order to rule out such mimics, some of which can be highly treatable. Other unusual disease processes that may "mimic" conventional stroke are vasculitis, coagulopathies, and venous occlusion; these are called mimics because, even though they cause cerebral infarction, their management is often quite different from that of the typical thrombotic or embolic arterial occlusion.

One of the key criteria for the diagnosis of stroke is the correspondence between the region of abnormality and a known vascular territory. If the region of altered attenuation and mass effect does not correspond to such distributions as the MCA, ACA, or PCA, some other process should be suspected, such as venous obstruction or global ischemia (Fig. 9–39). In the latter case, edema and subsequent encephalomalacia will be seen bilaterally in so-called "watershed" regions between vascular territories, such as between the MCA and ACA, or the MCA and PCA. Moreover, arterial occlusion should produce a wedge-shaped configuration that extends out to the surface of the brain, involving the gray matter.

Hemorrhagic versus nonhemorrhagic stroke

Broadly speaking, there are three types of stroke: thrombotic, embolic, and hemorrhagic. Approximately two-thirds of strokes are thrombotic in origin, and one-third are embolic. The principal sources of emboli causing stroke are the internal carotid arteries and the left atrium, particularly in patients with atrial fibrillation (in whom the

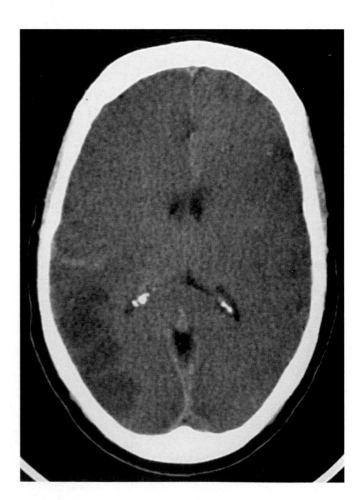

Figure 9–39. A 51-year-old man developed acute left-sided neurologic symptoms, followed by a cardiac arrest. A noncontrast axial computed tomography image demonstrates right parietal low attenuation extending to the cortical surface, corresponding to the distribution of the posterior division of the right middle cerebral artery. In addition, there is evidence of global ischemia, with diffusely decreased parenchymal attenuation, obscuration of the gray–white matter demarcation, and effacement of cerebral ventricles and cortical sulci, findings indicative of diffuse cerebral edema.

combination of chamber dilatation and poor emptying is thrombogenic). Both the internal carotid arteries and the atria can be well-evaluated by ultrasound, which non-invasively demonstrates atherosclerotic plaques and thrombi and can be used to assess the degree of vascular stenosis. MRI is increasingly used for these purposes. However, the gold standard for carotid evaluation remains contrast arteriography (Fig. 9–40).

Even if it were clinically possible to determine with certainty which patients were suffering from stroke, imaging would still play an important role in almost every case. In order to manage patients optimally, it is necessary to know not only that they are suffering a stroke, but what kind of stroke they are suffering. From the standpoint of acute management, the distinction between thrombotic and embolic strokes is rarely critical. The crucial distinction to be drawn is that between hemorrhagic and non-hemorrhagic strokes. Hemorrhagic strokes may result from a hemorrhagic infarction, either thrombotic or embolic, in which the blood vessels themselves are so damaged by ischemia that they rupture, or from anatomic processes, such as aneurysms (Fig. 9–41). It is estimated that approximately 20% of strokes are hemorrhagic, and of these slightly over one-half reflect hemorrhagic infarction. The remainder result from ruptured aneurysms and vascular malformations.

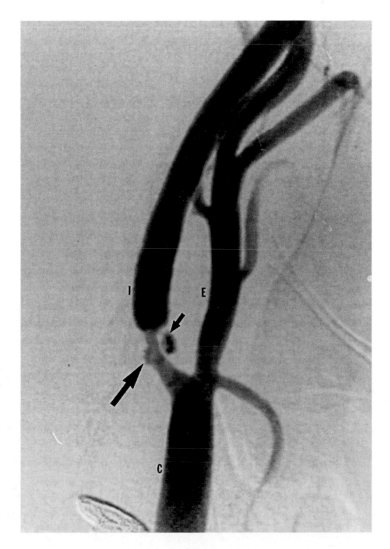

Figure 9–40. A 70-year-old man presented with two transient ischemic attacks (TIAs). Bilateral carotid arteriograms were performed by placing a catheter into the femoral artery, up through the aorta, and into each proximal common carotid artery, followed by injection of iodinated contrast. A lateral view demonstrates opacification of both the external carotid artery (which gives off multiple branches in the neck) and the internal carotid artery. The proximal internal carotid artery demonstrates an approximately 75% atherosclerotic stenosis (large arrow). Moreover, the plaque itself is ulcerated (small arrow), which predisposes to active thrombus formation and embolization. The patient subsequently underwent successful carotid endarterectomy, with no further TIAs. C, common carotid artery; E, external carotid artery; I, internal carotid artery.

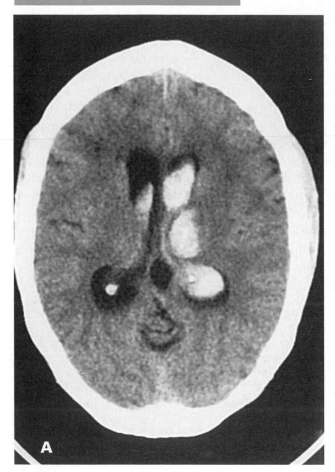
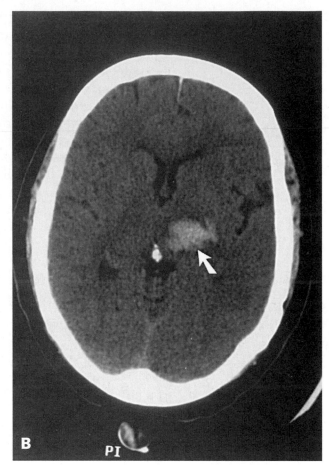

Figure 9–41. A 67-year-old woman with a history of hypertension was brought to the emergency room unconscious. (**A**) An axial image from a noncontrast computed tomography (CT) scan demonstrates a hyperdense focus of acute parenchymal hemorrhage in the region of the left caudate nucleus, with mass effect on adjacent structures and extension of blood into the lateral ventricles. The basal ganglia, including the caudate nucleus, are a common location for hypertensive hemorrhage. This patient should not be anticoagulated. (**B**) An axial CT image in a 65-year-old woman with a history of hypertension demonstrates a hyperdense hemorrhagic infarction centered in the left thalamus (arrow), which is producing mild midline shift. In the days before CT, the presence of a space occupying lesion (tumor, infarction, etc.) in such a case might have been inferred from a frontal plain radiograph of the skull, based on the subtle rightward shift of the calcified pineal gland.

The clinician needs to know if the stroke is hemorrhagic because the standard therapeutic regimen for stroke includes anticoagulation with heparin, which could be catastrophic in a patient with intracranial bleeding. Acute cerebral hemorrhage is best detected by CT scan, which demonstrates fresh blood as high attenuation (bright) material, as compared to the low density CSF and the isodense brain parenchyma (Fig. 9–42). The blood may be confined to a portion of the parenchyma, or may rupture into the subarachnoid, subdural, or ventricular spaces.

Hemorrhagic lesions are of two types: subarachnoid hemorrhage and parenchymal hemorrhage. In the nontraumatic setting, subarachnoid hemorrhage usually results from rupture of an aneurysm, which occurs in approximately 30,000 cases per year. Sudden, severe headache is a common presentation, and patients complaining of the worst headache of their life must be evaluated for this possibility (Fig. 9–43). Most patients have so-called berry aneurysms (saccular aneurysms) around the circle of

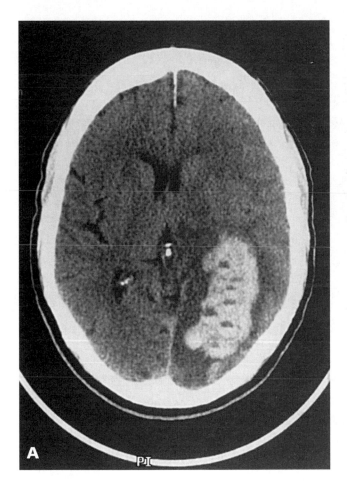 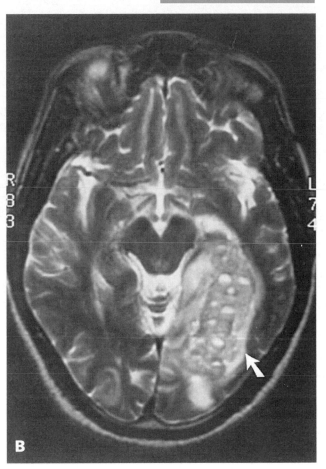

Figure 9–42. (**A**) An axial image from a nonenhanced computed tomography scan of the head demonstrates a large hemorrhagic infarction involving the left occipital lobe and thalamus. Multiple blood-fluid levels are seen, with the more recent (and hence denser and brighter) blood layering out beneath. Note that there is no mass effect on adjacent structures, indicating that much of the surrounding edema has resolved. (**B**) A contemporaneous axial T2-weighted magnetic resonance (MR) image also demonstrates layering of blood within the infarction (arrow), with the higher signal blood (late subacute, approximately 1 week old) layering out above lower signal blood (early subacute, approximately 2 to 3 days). The MR imaging characteristics of hemorrhage is a complex subject.

Willis. Common locations include the anterior communicating artery, the MCA, and the posterior communicating artery. The presence of blood in the subarachnoid space can be confirmed with lumbar puncture. However, it must be borne in mind that blood in the subarachnoid space does not always stem from a ruptured aneurysm and may instead reflect a parenchymal hemorrhage that has extended into the ventricles or subarachnoid space. Patients with suspected aneurysm should be evaluated by cerebral angiography, in part to characterize the exact site and nature of the aneurysm in preparation for neurosurgical correction and in part to rule out the presence of other aneurysms (which are multiple in 20% of patients). Patients at increased risk for cerebral aneurysms include those with polycystic kidney disease (10 to 30% of patients) and family histories of the disorder.

Primary parenchymal hemorrhages are most often seen in patients with a history of chronic hypertension, often with a more immediate acute exacerbation. For example, cocaine and amphetamine abusers are at increased risk, secondary to the acute

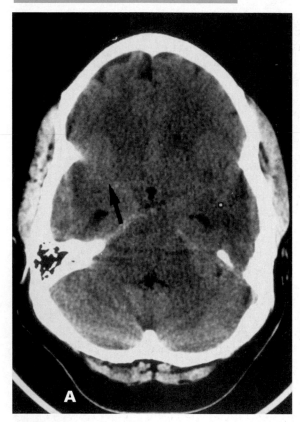
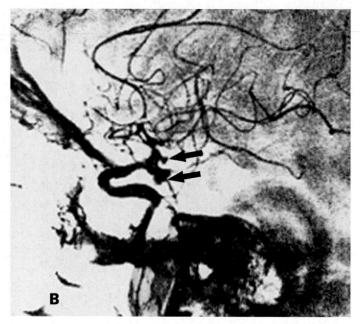

Figure 9–43. A 35-year-old woman presented to the emergency department with the worst headache of her life. A noncontrast computed tomography scan was obtained. (**A**) This axial image demonstrates subtle but definite high-attenuation material within the subarachnoid space, greater on the right than on the left (arrow). A cerebral angiogram (not shown) demonstrated a berry aneurysm of the right posterior cerebral artery (PCA), which had bled. (**B**) This lateral view from an internal carotid artery angiogram obtained with the patient facing to the viewer's left demonstrates aneurysms arising from the anterior choroidal artery (upper arrow) and the PCA (lower arrow).

increase in blood pressure that accompanies the use of these vasoactive drugs. Especially in a young patient, the possibility of an underlying vascular malformation, which may be surgically correctable, must be ruled out, although they account for only 1 in 20 parenchymal hemorrhages (Fig. 9–44). Other risk factors for parenchymal hemorrhage include anticoagulant therapy (which increases the risk 5 to 10 times) and amyloid angiopathy, which is seen in the elderly. Neoplasm also warrants consideration, and the most prevalent primary neoplasm to hemorrhage is glioblastoma. Relatively common hemorrhagic metastases include lung, thyroid, and renal cell carcinomas, as well as melanoma. Factors contributing to tumor hemorrhage include neovascularity, vascular invasion, and tumor necrosis, as the growth of malignant cells outstrips the local blood supply.

Contrast versus noncontrast study

A common question in the imaging of suspected stroke is whether to administer contrast material. In the acute setting, the answer is no. For one thing, the use of contrast infusion in CT may render the detection of small regions of bleeding more difficult,

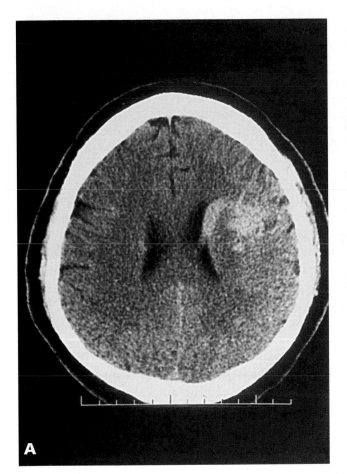
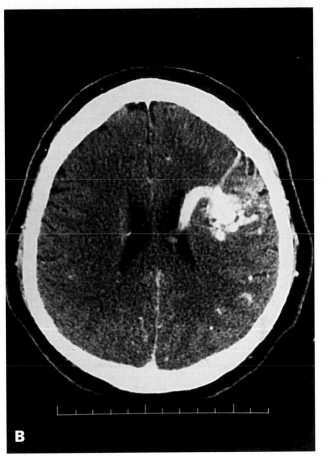

A

B

Figure 9–44. A 54-year-old man presented with his first seizure. (A) An axial image from a noncontrast computed tomography (CT) scan of the brain reveals a region of abnormally high attenuation within the left frontal lobe. The lateral aspect of the lesion is somewhat poorly defined and appears intermingled with normal-appearing brain parenchyma, while there is a more medial projection that is well defined and extends to the lateral ventricle. (B) In order to better characterize the lesion, iodinated contrast material was administered, which confirms that the lesion exhibits no mass effect or edema. This appearance of a large serpiginous tangle of vessels associated with a large draining vein extending to the lateral ventricle is diagnostic of a parenchymal arteriovenous malformation. Despite the fact that these lesions do not displace or "invade" the surrounding normal parenchyma, they often produce symptoms by "stealing" blood from it. Both conventional angiography and magnetic resonance imaging/magnetic resonance angiography are superior to CT at detecting and characterizing such lesions. Fortunately, the vast majority of such lesions are isolated, but they do carry a risk of hemorrhage of several percent per year.

because both acute blood and contrast appear bright. Performing infusion after the nonenhanced study would add to the CT evaluation, but probably only on a case-by-case basis, with the nonenhanced study proving adequate in the vast majority of cases. If the case can be monitored while the patient is in the scanner, the findings on the nonenhanced study will in some cases warrant infusion, such as when the findings are suspicious for underlying tumor or abscess, which will be better characterized with enhancement. There is another at least theoretical basis for withholding iodinated contrast material in patients with typical strokes: contrast that penetrates the disrupted blood-brain barrier may irritate cerebral tissues, increasing the risk of seizures, and produce increased edema and associated mass effect. This does not appear to be a problem with the gadolinium-based contrast agents used in MRI, although contrast infusion is generally unnecessary to characterize a stroke by MRI.

Natural history of stroke

While the brain is exquisitely dependent on a minute-to-minute basis for the oxygen and glucose necessary to sustain its neurons (it contains no myoglobin, glycogen, or fat), the imaging findings of neuronal death do not typically appear for hours or even a full day. The first cells to go are the neurons themselves, which consume three to four times as much energy as the glial cells of the white matter and are therefore more sensitive to a diminution of supply. As cells die, their membranes cease to maintain the usual balance between intra- and extracellular solutes, with the result that water begins to accumulate in the region of infarction. Both CT, which may show no significant change up to 24 hours after infarction, and MRI, which shows changes within 6 hours, typically depend on the local increase in brain water to demonstrate acute stroke. As long as the infarction is nonhemorrhagic and no other mimics of conventional stroke are involved, it does not matter clinically speaking whether the CT scan elucidates the stroke, because the patient's management will remain the same in either case. For this reason, even though MRI is more sensitive to stroke than CT, it offers virtually no significant clinical advantage in the acute situation.

It should be noted, however, that both CT and MRI may demonstrate stroke within minutes of its occurrence. On CT the actual thrombus or embolus may be seen within a vessel, such as the MCA, as a hyperintense area of attenuation within the vessel lumen ("hyperdense MCA sign"). MRI may demonstrate a lack of normal "flow void" within the affected vessel, when normally high-velocity blood is replaced by stationary clot. Another sign appearing within hours is a loss of the usually sharp gray matter–white matter demarcation and effacement of sulci, due to edema (Fig. 9–45A,B).

As the infarction develops, edema begins to produce mass effect. This may range from increasing sulcal effacement to more severe manifestations such as subfalcine or uncal herniation. In general, the larger the region of brain infarcted, the greater the peak mass effect observed during the 3rd through 7th days postevent (Fig. 9–45C). In an effort to combat acute cerebral swelling, mannitol (which increases intravascular oncotic pressure, and therefore tends to draw water back into the intravascular space) and hyperventilation (which causes arteriolar smooth muscle contraction, and therefore decreases intravascular hydrostatic pressure) may be employed. Between approximately 3 to 10 days postevent, the risk of so-called reperfusion hemorrhage is increased (Fig. 9–45D). At about 1 week, the brain begins to soften, producing encephalomalacia. Encephalomalacia is seen as decreased attenuation on CT, and as increased T2-weighted signal on MRI, in both cases secondary to the relative increase in water content. Eventually, the softened brain parenchyma is replaced by CSF, and the adjacent ventricular system dilates to fill the vacated space, a process referred to as *ex vacuo dilatation* (Fig. 9–45E).

One or more lacunar infarcts are frequently found on CNS imaging, especially in hypertensive patients and the elderly. These measure less than 1.5 cm in diameter and are caused by the occlusion of small, penetrating arteries supplying the basal ganglia and internal capsule. Such strokes are suspected when the patient presents with pure motor or pure sensory deficits, or with syndromes such as dysarthria and clumsiness of the hands.

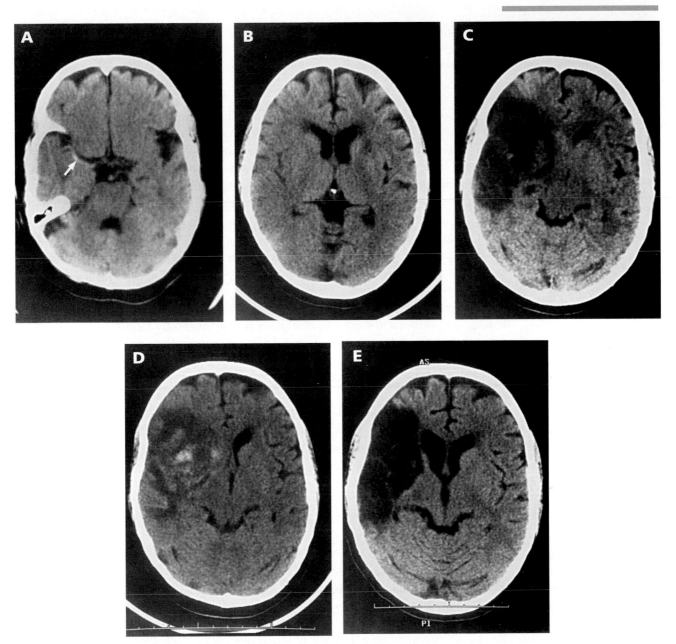

Figure 9–45. A 60-year-old woman presented with an 8-hour history of left hemiparesis and facial droop. (A) An axial image from a non-contrast computed tomography (CT) scan at the level of the basilar cisterns demonstrates a subtle finding sometimes seen in early stroke; namely, a hyperdense cerebral artery—in this case, the right middle cerebral artery (MCA; arrow). This so-called hyperdense artery sign is due to the presence of in situ or embolic thrombus within the vessel lumen. Its analogue on magnetic resonance imaging would be the absence of the expected flow void within the vessel. (B) Another image from the same study, near the level of the foramen of Monro, demonstrates subtle loss of gray–white matter demarcation and effacement of sulci in the right cerebral hemisphere as compared to those on the left. (C) An axial image from a scan several days later demonstrates prominent cerebral edema in the territory of the right MCA. The edema is causing mass effect on the frontal horn of the right lateral ventricle, as well as shift of midline structures such as the third ventricle to the left. (D) An axial CT image obtained 10 days postevent demonstrates continued edema and mass effect in the right MCA distribution, but there has been interval appearance of high-density regions, indicating hemorrhage. (E) An axial CT image 14 weeks postevent reveals that the right-sided edema has completely subsided, and that the infarcted brain parenchyma has been almost completely replaced by cerebrospinal fluid density fluid. The frontal horn of the right lateral ventricle is now larger than its left counterpart, a phenomenon called *ex vacuo dilatation.*

LOW BACK PAIN

EPIDEMIOLOGY

Low back pain is an extremely common problem in the United States, and it is estimated that 80% of Americans suffer from it at some point in their lives. It is second only to the common cold as the condition for which patients most often seek medical care, and it is the single most expensive medical condition afflicting Americans between the ages of 20 and 50 years. At this time, approximately 5 million patients are disabled by low back pain. While symptoms resolve in the majority of patients, they also recur in 60 to 85%. Risk factors for low back pain include obesity, pregnancy, cigarette smoking, and psychosocial factors, such as lower educational status, which is positively correlated with both increased incidence of low back pain and poorer outcome. Imaging reveals the cause of continued pain and functional incapacitation in approximately 20% of cases.

Of conservatively treated patients, 50% experience resolution of symptoms within 1 week, and 90% have complete resolution within 12 weeks. Conservative treatment consists of bed rest and the use of nonsteroidal antiinflammatory drugs. Weight reduction, smoking cessation, and regular exercise are effective long-term strategies to reduce the frequency and severity of recurrence. Surgical therapy is generally reserved for patients with definitive radiological evidence of an anatomical etiology, a corresponding pain syndrome and associated neurologic deficits, and failure to respond to 1 to 2 months of conservative therapy. Approximately 1 to 2% of Americans have undergone lumbar spine surgery to correct low back pain.

PATHOPHYSIOLOGY

 There are several anatomic causes of low back pain, one of the most common being disk herniation (Fig. 9–46). The intervertebral disk is composed of a soft, fibrous center, the nucleus pulposus, surrounded by a tough outer covering, the annulus fibrosus. A disk herniation occurs when a portion of the nucleus pulposus ruptures through a tear in the annulus fibrosus. Beginning in the second decade of life, the intervertebral disks degenerate, exhibiting a decrease in water content and proteoglycans, with an increase in collagen. This is accompanied by a decrease in signal intensity within the disk on T2-weighted images, often referred to as desiccation. With time, there is loss of intervertebral disk height and bulging of the disk material against the annulus fibrosis. If the annulus remains intact, there can be no herniation, but with time, fissures and frank tears may form in the annulus, permitting the disk material to protrude beyond the column of the vertebral bodies, where it may impinge on the spinal cord or nerve roots. The pain of a herniated disk is thought to result from the impingement of the disk material on the receptors of the annulus fibrosus or posterior longitudinal ligament, which runs along the posterior margin of the vertebral bodies.

In the lumbar spine, a disk herniation may impinge on any nerve root still within the neural canal at that level (recalling that the cord itself generally terminates between T11 and L1). In the typical case, a disk herniation will cause symptoms one level below the disk, so that an L4-5 herniation will cause an L5 radiculopathy (from the same Latin root as our word *radical*, meaning "root"). A typical presentation would be a history of back pain with more recent unilateral pain radiating down the leg in the

Figure 9–46. A 57-year-old woman complained of pain radiating from her left buttock down her leg to the lateral aspect of her ankle. (**A**) A T2-weighted sagittal magnetic resonance image through the lumbosacral spine demonstrates low signal, dessicated intervertebral disks in the lower spine. The termination of the spinal cord (small arrow) is seen at the level of the first lumbar vertebra, which is normal. Note, however, the prominent posterior herniation of disk material at the L4-5 level (arrow) and a mild disk bulge at the L5–S1 level. (**B**) A T1-weighted axial image at the L4-5 level demonstrates the slightly higher intensity disk material compressing the thecal sac (white arrows), predominately on the left side, which correlates well with the patient's symptoms. S, articular facet of the more superior vertebral body; I, articular facet of more inferior vertebral body.

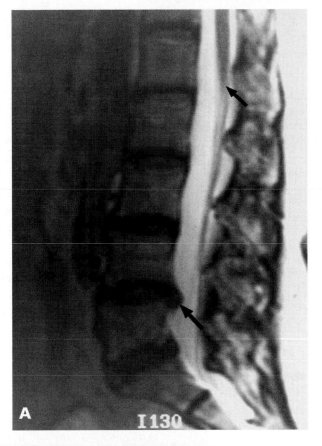

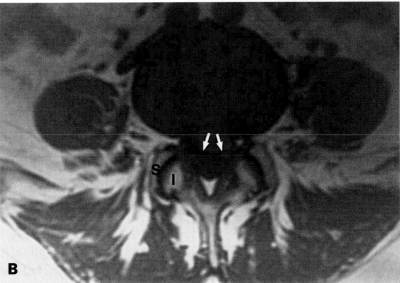

distribution of the sciatic nerve, called sciatica. Physical examination reveals the level, with the L4 root responsible for the knee jerk, while the ankle jerk is at S1. More than 90% of lumbar disk herniations occur at the L4-5 or L5–S1 levels.

The distinction between a posterior disk herniation and a lateral disk herniation is often difficult or impossible to make on purely clinical grounds. Only about 1 in 20 disk herniations is lateral, but failure to diagnose a lateral disk on imaging could cause the surgeon to operate at the wrong level. Consider, for example, a patient with clinical symptoms referable to the L4-5 level. By far the most common etiology of such symptoms would be a posterior disk herniation causing compression of the L5 nerve root. However, a lateral disk at the L5–S1 level could cause identical symptoms, and result in failed back surgery if the surgeon were to operate based on clinical criteria alone. In other words, a lateral L5–S1 disk herniation may produce clinical signs and symptoms identical to a posterior L4-5 herniation.

The second major offender in low back pain is spondylosis, also referred to as degenerative disease or osteoarthritis of the spine (although the latter is a misnomer and should be reserved for degenerative change at the apophyseal joints only). It is more common than herniated disks; while approximately one-third of asymptomatic individuals have at least one herniated disk, virtually every person has some degree of spondylosis by their later years. The back pain of spondylosis is usually of an aching nature and is exacerbated by prolonged standing or walking. Plain films may be used to diagnose lumbar spondylosis, but myelography, CT, or MRI is necessary to assess the degree of spinal stenosis and nerve root compression.

IMAGING

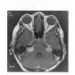 MRI has dramatically enhanced spine imaging, due to its superior tissue resolution, multiplanar imaging capabilities, noninvasive nature, and freedom from the artifact produced by bone in CT. T1-weighted images provide the best information about spinal anatomy, including the cord, while T2-weighted images (in which CSF is bright) provide a myelographic effect that is excellent for assessing both cord and nerve root compression and intrinsic cord lesions. A good search pattern for assessing the spine begins with sagittal sequences. Standard parameters, such as vertebral body and disk space height and vertebral alignment, should be determined, as well as the signal of the bone marrow (which should be bright on T1 due to fat). The cord itself should be inspected for abnormalities in caliber or signal, and to ensure that it ends at or about the usual L1 level. On both sagittal and axial images, the neural foramina should be examined to rule out encroachment by osteophytes or disk material on the nerve roots.

Two types of disk abnormalities are seen on imaging, annular bulges and herniations (Fig. 9–47). An annular bulge is a broad extension of the disk beyond the vertebral end plate. This is a prominent finding in patients older than age 20 years, and is most often asymptomatic. A herniation, on the other hand, is a focal protrusion of the disk material through the annulus fibrosus, which may extend into the vertebral canal, the neural foramen, or even extraforaminally, a so-called far-lateral herniation. When the herniated fragment of disk material becomes detached from the disk, it is referred to as a free fragment, which, if it migrates superiorly or inferiorly, may cause misleading clinical signs at a level above or below the actual herniation (Fig. 9–48).

Spondylosis manifests radiographically as osteophyte formation at the vertebral end plates and facet joints, which may encroach on both the vertebral canal, causing cord impingement, and the neural foramina, causing radiculopathy. Additional factors in a spondylosis syndrome include hypertrophy and ossification of the posterior longitudinal ligament and ligamentum flavum, which tend to compress the thecal sac in an anterior-posterior dimension, and congenital spinal stenosis, or "short pedicle syndrome," which makes the canal narrower to begin with and therefore decreases neurologic tolerance for any degree of compromise. Spinal stenosis is a component of achondroplasia, the most common form of dwarfism.

Figure 9–47. (A) The lumbar spine as seen in a lateral view demonstrates how a posteriorly bulging intervertebral disk might encroach on a neural foramen and compress an exiting lumbar nerve root. (B) A view through the midline of the spine shows how the bulging disk causes posterior displacement of the posterior longitudinal ligament. (C) An axial view shows the typical appearance of a disk bulge or herniation compressing the thecal sac, and potentially the nerve roots it contains.

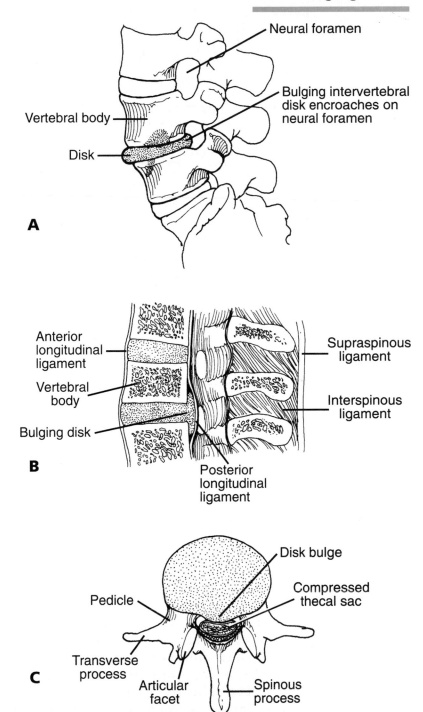

In some cases, low back pain and radiculopathy may be traced to spondylolysis, a congenital or acquired defect in the pars interarticularis of the vertebral body, which appears on oblique radiographs as a break in the neck of the "Scottie dog" discussed below. Spondylolysis is often compounded by spondylolisthesis, which frequently occurs at the L5–S1 level, and represents the displacement of one vertebral body on another (Fig. 9–49). Such slippage tends to compromise the vertebral canal and is usually treated with a combination of posterior decompression laminectomy and posterior vertebral fusion.

Failed back surgery occurs in 10 to 40% of patients. Common causes of failed back

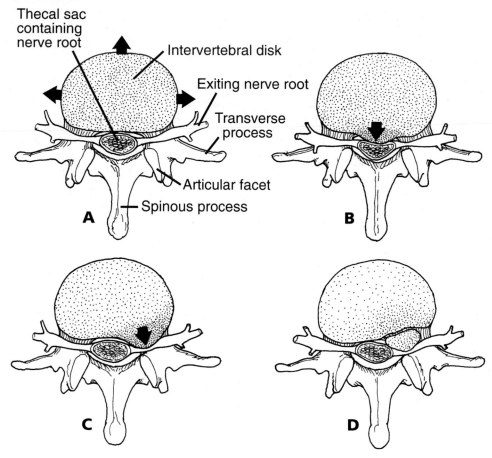

Figure 9–48. Intervertebral disk abnormalities illustrate the variety of ways in which nerve root compression may result. **(A)** There is a diffuse disk bulge extending anteriorly and laterally (arrows), but not affecting the thecal sac or exiting nerve roots. **(B)** A focal posterior disk bulge impinges on the thecal sac (arrow). **(C)** A lateral disk bulge compresses an exiting left nerve root (arrow). **(D)** A free fragment of herniated disk material, which may have migrated from another level, compresses an exiting nerve root.

surgery syndromes include recurrent or residual herniation, arachnoiditis, and spinal stenosis. Postoperative imaging plays an important role in patients with recurrent or residual symptoms. For example, either disk material or scar tissue may impress on the thecal sac or nerve roots. If the compression is due to disk material, the patient is often reoperated. On the other hand, scar is generally not reoperated. The two can be distinguished based on their imaging characteristics: scar, which is vascularized, will enhance with contrast administration; disk material, which is avascular, will not enhance.

CERVICAL DISK DISEASE AND SPONDYLOSIS

Principles similar to those in the low back apply to the neck as well. Patients with herniated cervical disks often complain of a dull, aching pain that radiates to the shoulder. When nerve root compression occurs, radicular symptoms result, including pain

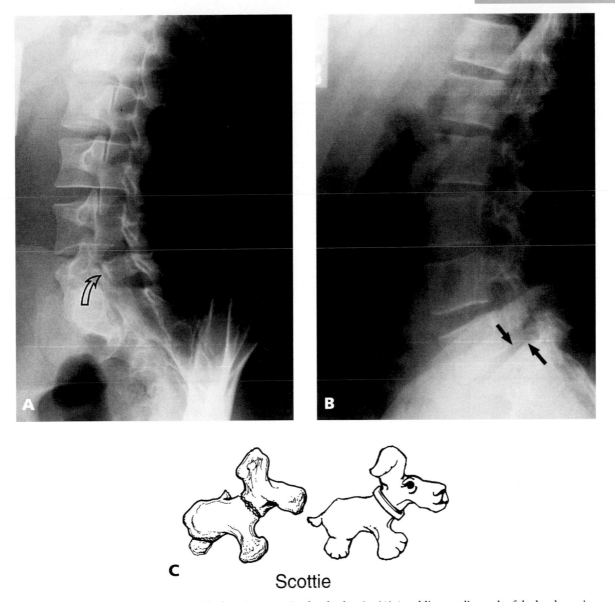

Scottie

Figure 9–49. A 35-year-old man presented with chronic, worsening low back pain. (A) An oblique radiograph of the lumbar spine demonstrates a defect in the left pars interarticularis of the fifth lumbar vertebra (L5), appearing as a break in the neck of the "Scottie dog," known as spondylolysis (arrow). (B) A lateral view of the lumbar spine demonstrates anterior slippage of L5 on S1, called *anterolisthesis* (arrows). (C) The "Scottie dog" appearance of a lumbar vertebra on an oblique view, demonstrating that a fracture through the pars interarticularis appears as a break in Scottie's neck.

radiating into the arm, weakness, and loss of sensation in a specific nerve distribution. A lesion at C5-6 commonly causes loss of the biceps reflex, while the triceps reflex is impaired by lesions at C6-7. The most common level of cervical disk herniation is C6-7, with approximately two-thirds of herniations at this level, and the majority of the remainder at C5-6. Cervical spondylosis occurs most frequently at the C5-6 interspace and presents with a more insidious onset of symptoms than is seen in acute disk herniation. The encroachment of osteophytes on the neural foramina is well-evaluated on oblique views of the cervical spine, although MR is of course much more sensitive for the detection of noncalcified disk material.

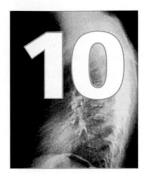

10 Pediatric Radiology

The purpose of this chapter is not to survey all of pediatric radiology, but to explore some of the most common or illustrative pediatric medical and surgical pathologies, and to review some of the principal anatomic, physiologic, and pathologic differences between children and adults. Perhaps the most critical lesson of pediatrics is that children are poorly served if treated as miniature adults—a principle that applies in every area of pediatric imaging.

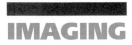

IMAGING

A number of special characteristics of pediatric patients create special challenges and opportunities in pediatric imaging. One of the most important challenges is the need to keep exposure to ionizing radiation to an absolute minimum. Although there is no definite evidence that the low levels of radiation exposure associated with diagnostic imaging produce adverse genetic or somatic effects, both experience with populations exposed to relatively high levels of radiation (Hiroshima and Nagasaki, Japan) and theoretical models of DNA damage would suggest that the hazards of radiation exposure are greater at earlier ages. In practical terms, keeping exposures to a minimum means employing sensitive film-screen combinations, employing intermittent rather than continuous fluoroscopic monitoring, making use of metallic gonadal shields, and whenever possible, employing modalities that do not involve ionizing radiation.

Another challenge faced by pediatric imaging is the frequently encountered need to immobilize the patient. Infants and young children typically cannot understand or comply with instructions to remain still, and may be frightened and upset by the unfamiliar environment of the radiology department and its equipment. Not only lengthier examinations such as nuclear medicine, magnetic resonance imaging (MRI), and computed tomography (CT), but even relatively quick procedures such as chest and bone radiographs require that the patient be still during data acquisition. In the case of a chest radiograph, the exposure may last only a split second, while nuclear medicine and MRI procedures may in some cases require 1 hour or more. When the procedure is brief, the patient's parent can often restrain the child by holding the arms and/or legs. In addition, immobilization devices such as boards or "papoose" wraps may be used. When the examination requires more time, sedation may be necessary. Generally, children younger than several months of age are immobilized, while those between several months and 4 to 5 years require sedation for longer examinations.

An imaging modality particularly well suited to the pediatric patient is ultrasound, which displays a number of important advantages. First, ultrasound involves no ionizing radiation, and there are no known risks to health of the pressure waves employed in diagnostic sonography. Second, infants and young children are often small enough that a surprisingly great extent of the body is accessible to sonographic imaging. Moreover, the fact that the infantile calvarium is not completely closed renders ultrasound a key neuroimaging modality early in life. Third, although patients may occasionally complain that the ultrasound transducer "tickles," sonography involves no pain and can be comfortably performed in real time, thus making patient restraint and sedation generally unnecessary. Of course, a number of structures such as non-consolidated lung and the older child's brain remain inaccessible to ultrasound, as in the adult.

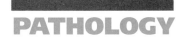

PATHOLOGY

Circulatory System

CONGENITAL HEART DISEASE

EPIDEMIOLOGY

Congenital heart disease is found in 1% of newborns. The two most common forms are bicuspid aortic valve and mitral valve prolapse (discussed in Chapter 2). These are generally asymptomatic in the pediatric patient.

PATHOPHYSIOLOGY

 Fetal circulatory patterns differ markedly from those seen after birth (Fig. 10–1). The principal difference stems from the fact that the fetus is not breathing air, and acquires all of its oxygen and disposes of all of its carbon dioxide through the placenta and the maternal circulation. Two bypasses in the fetal circulation—the foramen ovale, an opening in the interatrial septum, and the ductus arteriosus, which connects the left pulmonary artery to the proximal descending aorta—serve to redirect blood flow away from the fetal lungs. During in utero life, the collapsed lungs manifest a high resistance to flow, and right heart pressures are higher than left heart pressures. As a result, blood is shunted through both these bypasses into the systemic circulation, where it either supplies systemic tissues or enters the umbilical artery and returns to the placenta. Beginning at birth, the combination of lung expansion and ventilation causes pulmonary vascular resistance to fall, and once it falls lower than systemic resistance, shunts resulting from such lesions as a patent ductus arteriosus, atrial septal defect, or ventricular septal defect will shift from right-to-left to left-to-right.

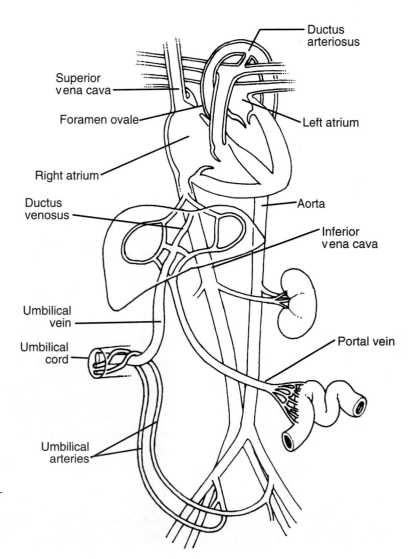

Figure 10–1. The major structures of the fetal circulation. Note that the foramen ovale and the ductus arteriosus represent major routes by which the pulmonary circulation is bypassed.

CLINICAL PRESENTATION

A critical clinical discriminator in congenital heart disease is cyanosis (from the Greek *kyanos*, "blue"). Acyanotic disease implies that there is a left-to-right shunt, with oxygen-saturated blood being shunted back to the lungs. Cyanosis implies a right-to-left shunt or admixture lesion (such as a truncus arteriosus, in which the right and left ventricles empty into a single vessel), in which desaturated blood is entering the systemic circulation. Lesions that commonly present in the first few weeks of life include hypoplastic left heart syndrome and transposition of the great arteries. Hypoplastic left heart syndrome presents within a few days of birth with congestive heart failure (CHF), and closure of the ductus arteriosus during the first week commonly results in cardiogenic shock and death. Transposition of the great arteries consists of origination of the aorta from the right ventricle, and origination of the pulmonary artery from the left ventricle. This situation creates two separate circulations and is incompatible with life unless lesions such as atrial or ventricular septal defects permit mixing. This is the most common lesion to present with cyanosis in the first 24 hours of life.

IMAGING

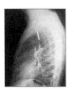 Classically, cardiac catheterization represented the definitive means of diagnosing congenital heart disease. Today noninvasive modalities such as echocardiography and MRI are playing an increasingly important role. A key role of the radiologist is plain film diagnosis. Perhaps the single most important parameter in plain film diagnosis is pulmonary perfusion. Broadly speaking, pulmonary perfusion may be decreased, normal, or increased

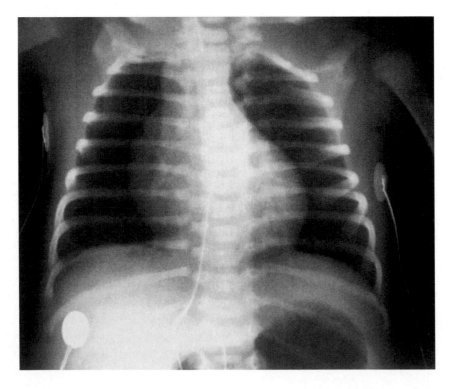

Figure 10–2. This chest radiograph in a cyanotic newborn demonstrates virtual absence of any identifiable pulmonary vessels, as well as an enlarged heart. The etiology in this case was a severe pulmonic stenosis, which was not accompanied by a ventricular septal defect. This child was alive only because of a patent ductus arteriosus and atrial septal defect, which provided some blood flow to the lungs. Note the endotracheal tube and umbilical vein catheter extending up into the right atrium.

(Fig. 10–2). Other important features that can be employed in conjunction with pulmonary perfusion to arrive at a diagnosis include chamber enlargement, the appearance of the aorta and pulmonary vein, and soft tissue and bone changes (such as rib notching).

Decreased pulmonary perfusion, manifested by small pulmonary vessels and radiolucent lungs, generally implies an obstruction to right ventricular outflow (Fig. 10–3). An important etiology is tetralogy of Fallot. This consists of an obstructed right ventricular outflow tract, right ventricular hypertrophy, a ventricular septal defect, and an aorta overriding the interventricular septum. It is associated with a right aortic arch in one-quarter of cases, and the heart often exhibits a boot-shaped appearance, due to right ventricular enlargement (Fig. 10–4).

Normal pulmonary vascularity often implies uncomplicated valvular disease or coarctation of the aorta. Types of valve disease include pulmonic stenosis and congenital aortic stenosis. Pulmonic stenosis may produce right ventricular hypertrophy and prominence of the main pulmonary artery, while aortic stenosis generally causes left ventricular hypertrophy and CHF. Coarctation of the aorta is most often of the juxtaductal type, with narrowing of the aorta at or just below the ductus arteriosus, and generally does not present until later childhood. It is commonly associated with a bicuspid aortic valve. Important radiographic signs include a visible indentation in the aorta at the coarctation and inferior rib notching, which is produced when dilated intercostal arteries providing collaterals around the obstruction produce remodeling in the adjacent ribs (Fig. 10–5).

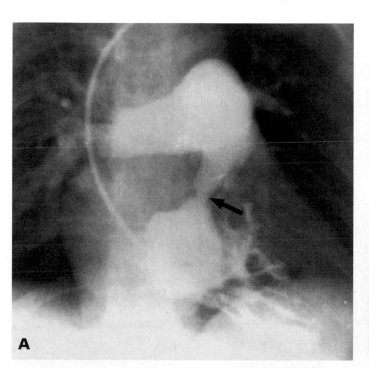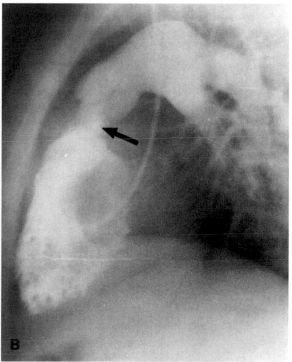

Figure 10–3. (A) Frontal and (B) lateral views of a cardiac catheterization demonstrate a catheter descending through the superior vena cava and into the right atrium. Contrast injection demonstrates an infundibular pulmonic stenosis (arrow), which restricts the right ventricle's outflow. Such stenoses are often associated with right ventricular hypertrophy and may also be accompanied by poststenotic dilatation of the pulmonary artery.

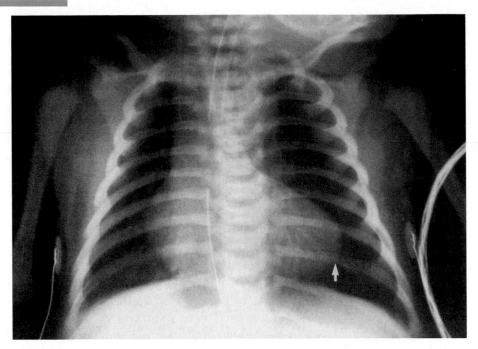

Figure 10–4. This chest radiograph in a neonate demonstrates a classic appearance of tetralogy of Fallot, with a right-sided aortic arch, a small pulmonary artery, decreased pulmonary vascularity, and an upturned cardiac apex (arrow) producing a so-called boot-shaped heart. Tetralogy of Fallot consists of pulmonary stenosis, resultant right ventricular hypertrophy (producing the upturned apex), a ventricular septal defect, and an overriding aorta. It represents the most common form of cyanotic congenital heart disease in children and adults. Note the endotracheal tube extending nearly to the carina and the umbilical artery catheter extending high into the right atrium.

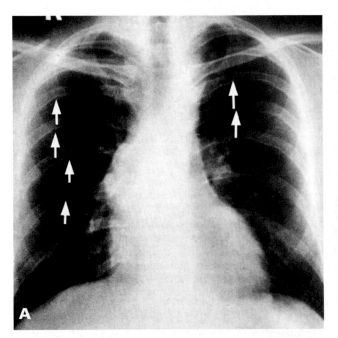
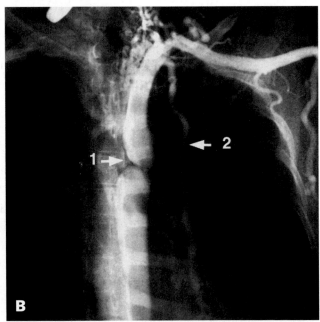

Figure 10–5. (A) A frontal chest radiograph in a 23-year-old patient with upper extremity hypertension demonstrates a rounded left ventricular contour, an inconspicuous aortic arch, and prominent bilateral rib notching (arrows). (B) A frontal view of an aortogram reveals a tight coarctation of the aorta at the isthmus (1), as well as a dilated left internal mammary artery (2), which is supplying collateral flow past the coarctation. This artery is often used in cardiac bypass surgery. It is rare for rib notching to appear before 8 to 10 years of age.

Figure 10–6. This frontal image from a cardiac catheterization was obtained by passing a catheter (arrow) up through the inferior vena cava into the right atrium and through an atrial septal defect into the left atrium. Injection of contrast produces opacification of both the aorta (A) and pulmonary artery (P), which confirms the presence of a left-to-right shunt. Atrial septal defects are usually well tolerated and may present in adulthood, while ventricular septal defects typically present earlier.

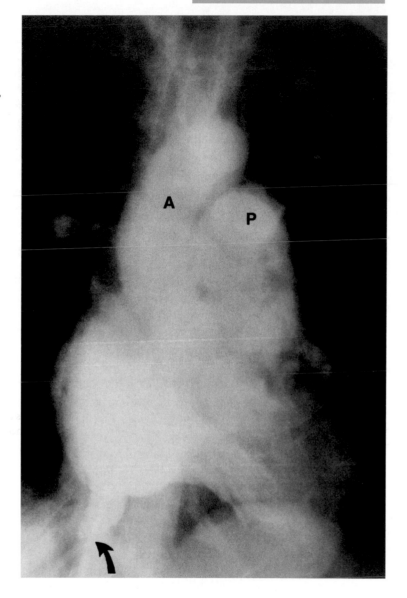

Increased pulmonary perfusion may represent either active or passive pulmonary overcirculation. Active pulmonary overcirculation implies a left-to-right shunt producing a right ventricular output at least two to three times that of the left ventricle. Common causes include atrial septal defect, ventricular septal defect, and patent ductus arteriosus. Atrial septal defect is the most common symptomatic congenital cardiac anomaly. Due to low atrial pressures, it often does not present for decades, and is also the most prevalent congenital cardiac anomaly to present in adulthood (Fig. 10–6). Ventricular septal defect is the second most common congenital cardiac anomaly, and if large may present with CHF in the 2nd or 3rd month of life. Fortunately, three-quarters of these lesions close spontaneously by the age of 10 years. The ductus arteriosus normally closes functionally at 48 hours. In patent ductus arteriosus, the fall in pulmonary vascular resistance with breathing produces a reversal of flow through the ductus, from the aorta and into the pulmonary arteries. Again, large lesions produce CHF at 2 to 3 months.

Respiratory System

The neonatal chest differs from that of the older child and adult in a number of important respects. Anatomic differences include airways that are more flaccid, proportionately smaller peripheral airways, less developed collateral air circulation through the pores of Kohn and channels of Lambert, and greater mucus production. These factors mean that the neonatal and infant lung are more susceptible to obstruction, either from airway collapse or blockage by secretions, than those of the adult. This obstruction, in turn, may result in either atelectasis (due to collapse of unaerated distal airspaces) or air trapping (due to increased residual volume in a check-valve type of airway obstruction). The following discussion concerns common or paradigmatic causes of neonatal respiratory distress.

NEONATAL RESPIRATORY DISTRESS

The neonate in respiratory distress may exhibit a variety of nonspecific findings, including tachypnea, grunting, nasal flaring, chest wall retractions, cyanosis, or blood gas abnormalities. The conditions producing respiratory distress in the neonate may be divided somewhat arbitrarily into medical and surgical conditions. Surgical conditions are those that usually require urgent surgical intervention, while medical conditions usually respond to pharmacologic maneuvers and ventilatory support. Of course, this is not a hard and fast distinction, and in severe cases, conditions classified here as medical may also require surgical therapy, such as extracorporeal membrane oxygenation (ECMO) in patients with very severe pulmonary disease. The chest radiograph plays a crucial role in differentiating between medical and surgical conditions. Moreover, it is vital in distinguishing between different disorders within each of these categories—a distinction that further powerfully influences therapy.

MEDICAL CONDITIONS

Hyaline membrane disease

Epidemiology

Hyaline membrane disease (HMD) is the most common cause of neonatal respiratory distress, seen in 30,000 to 50,000 infants per year in the United States. It nearly always occurs in premature infants, with a positive correlation between the degree of prematurity and the probability of developing HMD.

Pathophysiology

The pathophysiology of HMD centers on a deficiency of pulmonary surfactant, which normally lowers the surface tension of the alveolar air sacs. Alveolar surface tension results from the fact that the water molecules lining the alveolar air sacs (without which the diffusion of gases could not occur) are more strongly attracted to one another than to the air above them in the alveolar sacs. This exerts a double effect: (1) the liquid layer resists any force that tends to increase its surface area, making the alveolus harder to inflate; and (2) the water molecules try to get as close together as possible, which tends to collapse the alveolus. As a result of these forces, the compliance of the lung, which is defined as the change in lung volume produced per unit force of inflation, decreases.

Surfactant is produced by the type II pneumocytes, which can be differentiated microscopically from type I pneumocytes by their cuboidal shape and the fact that they contain lamellar inclusion bodies. Surfactant molecules are normally interposed between water molecules lining the alveoli. They lower the overall cohesive force between these molecules, because the attractive force between water molecules and surfactant molecules is very low. When surfactant supplies are deficient, alveolar surface tension is dramatically increased, with the result that the amount of muscular work required to snap them open at inspiration is considerably greater. Moreover, surfactant deficiency increases the recoil forces of the alveoli and promotes their tendency to collapse at expiration.

Unfortunately, alveolar atelectasis tends to set in motion a vicious cycle of alveolar hypoxia and decreased pulmonary perfusion. Atelectatic airspaces become hypoxic, which in turn leads to acidosis in the affected portion of the lung. This acidosis, in turn, leads to a reflex decrease in local pulmonary perfusion, which then exacerbates hypoxia and initiates another turn of the cycle. Therefore, the short-term keys to maintaining adequate gas exchange are aerating collapsed airspaces and supplying supplementary oxygen.

The clinical result of surfactant deficiency is a neonate who is rapidly exhausted by the work of breathing. The child develops diffuse atelectasis, which in turn tips the balance of the Starling forces in favor of pulmonary edema. Proteinaceous material gradually builds up along the lining of the air sacs (hence the name *hyaline membrane disease*) (Fig. 10–7). Because surfactant production, which is not necessary during in utero life, does not begin

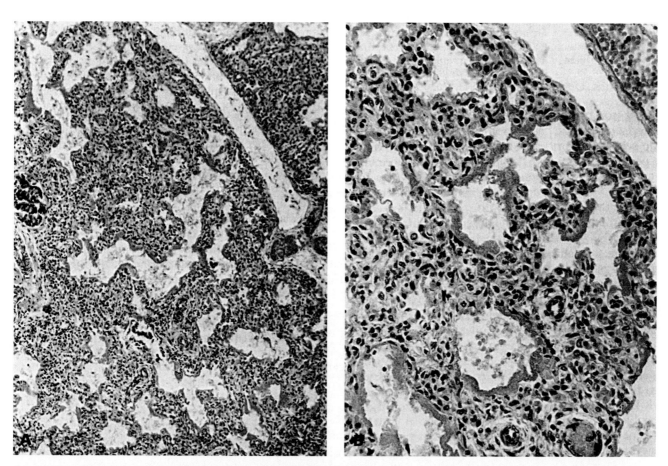

Figure 10–7. These light micrographs demonstrate the typical histologic appearance of hyaline membrane disease. (A) The distal airspaces are collapsed, and both proximal and distal airspaces are lined by hyaline membranes. (B) At higher power, the hyaline membranes lining the airways and larger airspaces are seen to better advantage. These membranes appear pink (eosinophilic) when viewed in color.

until approximately 24 weeks gestation, low birth weight infants are at higher risk, with nearly two-thirds of those below 1000 g developing some degree of HMD. Two-thirds of affected neonates are male, who also are more often severely affected.

Clinical presentation

Clinically, neonates with HMD exhibit chest wall retractions, because the infant recruits accessory muscles of respiration in an effort to generate greater negative intrathoracic pressures; cyanosis, due to lower oxygen saturation; grunting, indicative of the increased work of breathing; tachypnea, which results from the attempt to maintain adequate ventilation in the face of lower tidal volumes; and expiratory grunting, the result of the effort to open up collapsed alveoli. Of course, such findings can be seen in a variety of pulmonary pathologies, and the chest radiograph is crucial in helping to establish the correct diagnosis of HMD. This is especially true in older premature neonates; for example, those weighing 1500 g, whose risk of developing HMD is only 16%. The probability of developing HMD can be assessed based on measurement of the lecithin:sphingomyelin ratio, which is decreased in infants at risk.

Imaging

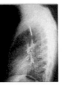 The radiographic findings of HMD are predictable. It is critical that the abnormalities are diffuse and bilateral, because surfactant is homogeneously deficient throughout the pulmonary parenchyma. Characteristic findings include low lung volumes, manifesting as a bell-shaped thorax; a diffuse, fine granular appearance to the lungs, due to accumulation of edema and proteinaceous secretions within the acini; and air bronchograms, because the conducting airways coursing through partially collapsed lung are not only patent but overdistended, due to their high neonatal compliance (Fig. 10–8).

Recent advances in the treatment of HMD now save the lives of many premature infants who would have certainly died only a few decades ago. One such advance is the ability to prevent HMD in many cases of expected premature birth. Maturity of the surfactant system is normally induced by glucocorticoid secretion, and its development can be accelerated in utero by the administration of exogenous glucocorticoids. Another recent advance is the availability of exogenous pulmonary surfactant, which can be administered as an aerosol directly into the airspaces through the endotracheal tube.

However, despite these advances, many neonates still require ventilatory support in order to inflate their stiff airspaces and to provide adequate levels of arterial oxygenation. Especially in this situation, imaging is helpful not only in diagnosing HMD but in assessing response to treatment and the development of complications. Mechanical ventilation involves insertion of an endotracheal tube and the use of positive airway pressures. Higher oxygen concentrations are employed in order to maintain an adequate level of tissue oxygenation. Umbilical vessel catheters may be inserted to administer medications and to monitor blood gases. Diuretics are often administered in an effort to counteract pulmonary edema, which decreases alveolar oxygen diffusion.

Unfortunately, each of these therapeutic maneuvers has potential adverse consequences, which are not peculiar to HMD, but may be seen in any condition requiring intensive monitoring and ventilatory support. Umbilical artery catheters (UACs) and umbilical vein catheters (UVCs) are favored routes of central venous access in neonates, because the vessels are relatively large and easy to cannulate. The UAC tra-

Figure 10–8. A 1-day-old infant's chest radiograph manifests two problems. First, the lungs are small and demonstrate a diffuse granular haziness, which represents hyaline membrane disease. Second, the endotracheal tube is poorly positioned, with its tip extending into the right mainstem bronchus.

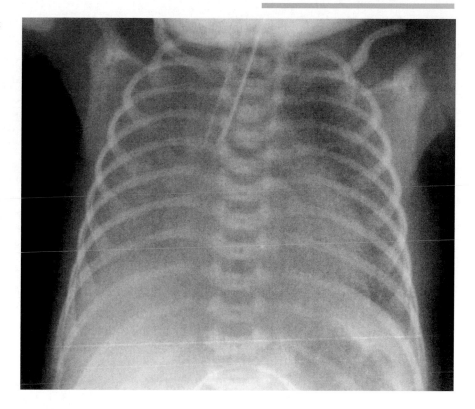

verses the inferior epigastric artery, the internal iliac artery, the common iliac artery, and the abdominal aorta. Its tip should be positioned above or below the renal arteries to prevent the possibility of renal artery occlusion, either at the level of the eighth through twelfth thoracic vertebral bodies or at the second or third lumbar vertebral body. The UVC is used primarily for blood draws (other than arterial blood gases) and for the administration of medications. It traverses the portal sinus (where the portal veins branch), the ductus venosus (which normally closes on the 3rd or 4th day of life), the hepatic veins, and the inferior vena cava, with its tip coming to rest in the right atrium. Misplacement in the left atrium (through a patent foramen ovale) can cause systemic embolization from thrombi that may form on the tip, while placement of the tip into a portal or hepatic venous branch may cause complete vascular occlusion.

Ventilatory support has a number of potential complications. As in the older child and adult, tube malposition may give rise to a number of problems (Fig. 10–9). If the tube is too high in the trachea, the lungs will not be properly ventilated. Alternatively, a tube that is positioned too low, such as in the right mainstem bronchus, may cause only the right lung to be ventilated, with collapse of the left lung.

A complication of HMD more peculiar to the intensive care nursery is pulmonary interstitial emphysema (PIE), which results from overdistention of poorly compliant air sacs, with build up of gas in the pulmonary interstitium (Fig. 10–10). The presence of PIE aggravates the difficulty of adequately ventilating the lungs, because the presence of air within the interstitium stiffens them and reduces pulmonary compliance. The intensivist managing a patient with HMD and PIE may feel caught in a vicious cycle. The increased airway pressures necessary to ventilate the stiff lungs of HMD may themselves result in stiffer lungs through the development of PIE, which in turn may necessitate higher airway pressures to maintain ventilation.

PIE is recognized radiographically when streaks or bubbles of air begin to appear

Figure 10–9. This newborn infant with respiratory distress underwent endotracheal intubation for mechanical ventilatory support. Note that the lungs are quite underinflated, while there is an unusual degree of gaseous distention of the entire visualized alimentary canal. This was due to an esophageal intubation. Note also that the nasogastric tube is positioned much too shallowly, reaching down only into the midesophagus.

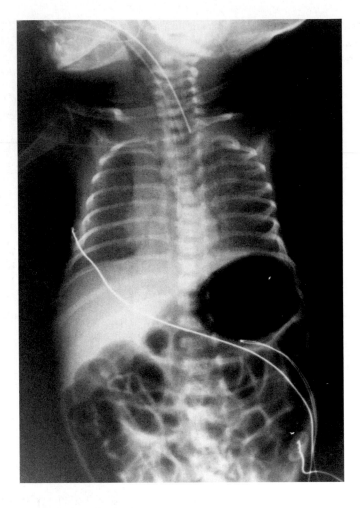

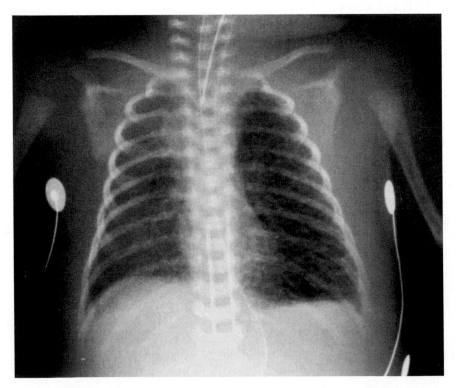

Figure 10–10. This 32-week premature male infant developed neonatal respiratory distress syndrome at birth, requiring mechanical ventilation. The film demonstrates an umbilical vein catheter tip at the level of the T8 vertebral body, an endotracheal tube tip at the level of T2, and a nasogastric tube side port below the level of the gastroesophageal junction. There are multiple tiny cystic lucencies scattered diffusely throughout both lung fields, with greater lucency of the left lung as compared to the right, and a paramediastinal opacity in the right upper lobe. These findings represent pulmonary interstitial emphysema due to ventilatory barotrauma, with accumulation of air in the peribronchovascular spaces. In addition, there is collapse of the right upper lobe, presumably secondary to mucus plugging. Potential complications include pneumothorax, pneumomediastinum, and pneumopericardium.

in the lungs. These may be focal or diffuse, unilateral or bilateral. The principal complications of PIE, which occur when air migrates centrally or peripherally through the lymphatics, are the development of pneumomediastinum or pneumothorax (Fig. 10–11). Air reaches the pleural space through rupture of a subpleural bleb. Findings of barotrauma on chest radiography include not only pneumothorax and pneumomediastinum, but pneumopericardium, pneumoperitoneum, and venous air embolism, the presence of air in the heart and great vessels.

Another complication of HMD is persistent patent ductus arteriosus. This occurs

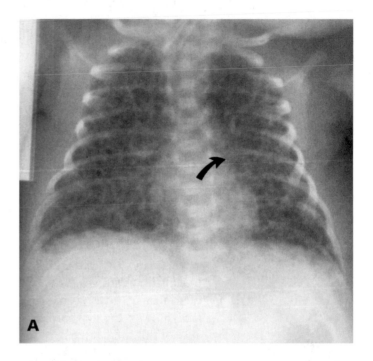

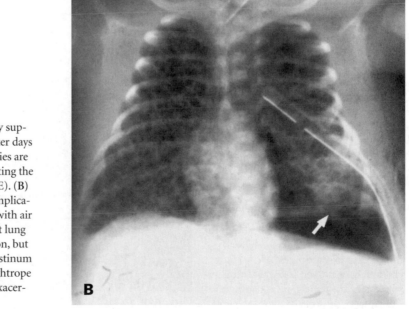

Figure 10–11. This child was placed on ventilatory support at birth for hyaline membrane disease. (**A**) After days of positive airway pressures, extensive cystic lucencies are visible throughout both lung fields (arrow), indicating the presence of pulmonary interstitial emphysema (PIE). (**B**) Shortly thereafter, another film demonstrates a complication of PIE, the development of a pneumothorax, with air in the pleural space surrounding the base of the left lung (arrow). A chest tube has been placed for evacuation, but the pneumothorax persists, with shift of the mediastinum to the right. At this point, the intensivist walks a tightrope between maintaining adequate gas exchange and exacerbating the air leak.

when the ductus remains physiologically open more than the usual 48 hours after birth. It results from the effect of abnormally low arterial oxygen pressure on the ductus itself. The progressive fall in pulmonary vascular resistance that normally occurs after birth allows a left-to-right shunt to develop, manifesting as increased pulmonary vascularity and CHF. Treatment is with indomethacin, which blocks the synthesis of prostaglandin E_1, which otherwise acts as a vasodilator and keeps the duct open. In the 40% of patients in whom indomethacin is not successful, the duct may be surgically ligated via a left thoracotomy.

An important complication of long-term ventilatory support is bronchopulmonary dysplasia (BPD), which occurs secondary to oxygen toxicity (likely mediated by highly chemically reactive superoxides) and barotrauma. Pathologically, BPD is characterized by destruction of type I pneumocytes and interstitial edema, followed by interstitital fibrosis and emphysema. These changes often result in long-term dependence on oxygen support. BPD in its later stages is recognized as bubbly, coarse interstitial opacities, with hyperaeration, and the lung often eventually acquires a honeycomb appearance (Fig. 10–12). BPD is associated with an increased incidence of lower respiratory tract infections and reactive airways disease (asthma), likely because of scarred (and hence lower caliber) airways and less efficient clearance mechanisms. Fortunately, with time many children can "grow out" of their BPD, because the lung continues to manufacture new alveoli through much of childhood. Only approximately 15 to 20% of the adult number of alveoli are present at birth.

Transient tachypnea of the newborn

The fetal lung is filled with fluid that is essential to normal lung development. Recall that oligohydramnios (as seen, for example, in such conditions as renal agenesis and in utero urinary tract obstruction) is associated with pulmonary hypoplasia. Transient tachypnea of the newborn (TTN) occurs when there is inadequate or delayed clearance of this fluid at birth, resulting in a "wet lung." Normally, fetal lung fluid is cleared

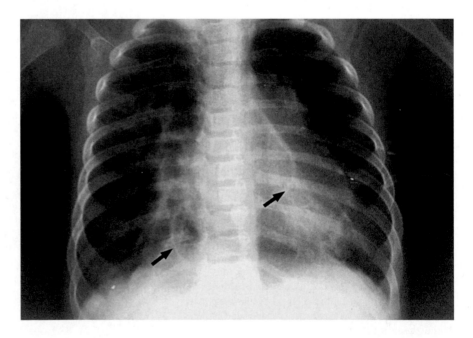

Figure 10–12. A 5-month-old boy with a history of ventilatory and oxygen therapy for hyaline membrane disease demonstrates pulmonary changes of bronchopulmonary dysplasia, with large lung volumes due to emphysema, and streaky linear areas of fibrosis (arrows). Although respiratory function typically improves as new airspaces develop, such children have an increased incidence of respiratory tract infections and asthma.

during parturition by the squeezing action of the birth canal on the fetal thorax and by the resorptive capacity of the fetal lymphatics and pulmonary capillaries. Any condition that interferes with these normal mechanisms, including cesarean section, precipitous delivery, and lymphatic obstruction, predisposes to TTN. The characteristic radiographic appearance includes interstitial edema and hyperinflation (large lung volumes, as opposed to the small lung volumes of HMD) (Fig. 10–13). Some infants will also have small pleural effusions, indicating that the usual lymphatic drainage of the pleural space is, at least temporarily, inadequate. Even many normal newborns will have a TTN-like chest X ray in the first minutes after birth, before clearance mechanisms have had an opportunity to take full effect. The natural history of TTN is complete resolution within 48 hours.

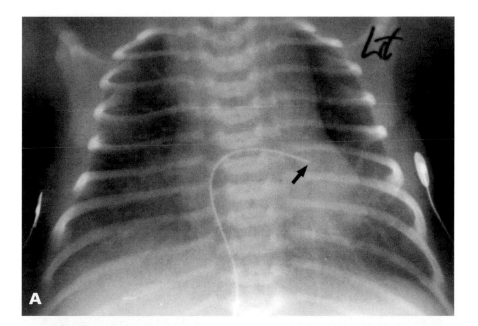

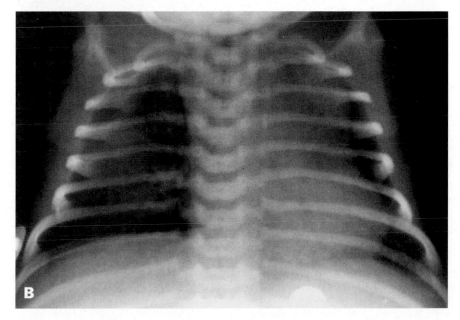

Figure 10–13. This newborn developed respiratory distress over the first few hours after birth. (A) A frontal chest radiograph demonstrates diffuse bilateral interstitial opacities, most prominent in the left base. Note that the lung volumes are large, and also note the position of the umbilical vein catheter (arrow), which has crossed from the right atrium into the left atrium through a patent foramen ovale. This situation should be corrected, because thrombus developing on the catheter tip could embolize to systemic organs such as the brain. (B) One day later, the opacities had entirely cleared, consistent with a diagnosis of transient tachypnea of the newborn.

Meconium aspiration

Meconium is the term for the normal neonatal bowel contents and is composed primarily of desquamated mucosal epithelial cells and bile salts. It usually has a greenish appearance and is evacuated within approximately 6 hours after birth. However, it may be evacuated in utero in response to perinatal stress, most likely as a vagal response. Approximately 20% of pregnancies have meconium-stained fluid, but only about 1 in 20 meconium-stained neonates develops meconium aspiration syndrome. The syndrome arises when meconium is aspirated below the level of the vocal cords, with predictable consequences. Meconium particles can produce mechanical airway obstruction. The tenacious character of meconium renders such airway plugs difficult for the neonate to clear. Bile acids and pancreatic enzymes in meconium can rapidly produce a chemical pneumonitis, due to direct toxicity on the epithelium of the airways and airspaces. Radiographic findings begin with disordered aeration, with areas of atelectasis due to complete airway obstruction and areas of hyperinflation due to a check-valve type of obstruction. Overall, the lungs are usually hyperinflated, with patchy areas of strand-like opacity (Fig. 10–14). Up to one-quarter of patients will demonstrate a pneumothorax, most often as a complication of mechanically assisted ventilation.

Neonatal pneumonia

Pneumonia complicates approximately 1 in 200 births. Risk factors for neonatal pneumonia include maternal sepsis and premature rupture of membranes, reflecting the two routes of infection: transplacental transmission in utero and perinatal transmission via an infected birth canal. The most common organism is beta-hemolytic strep-

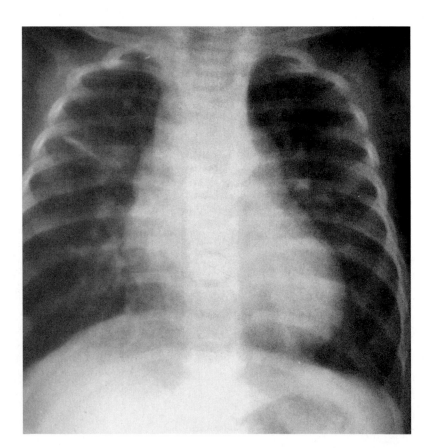

Figure 10–14. This frontal chest radiograph in a newborn demonstrates a typical appearance of meconium aspiration syndrome, with asymmetric nodular and linear appearing opacities scattered throughout both lungs. Note also that the lung volumes are large.

Pediatric Radiology **469**

tococci, acquired via the birth canal. Patients present with respiratory distress and metabolic acidosis that may progress to sepsis and shock. The latter complications make early recognition critical. The radiographic appearance of neonatal pneumonia is variable and may mimic that of HMD, with diffuse granularity, or TTN, with diffuse, streaky opacities. Pleural effusion, present in two-thirds of cases of neonatal pneumonia, can be an important discriminating factor in this regard, as it is never found in pure HMD. It should be noted that the classic lobar infiltrates seen in older children and adults are only rarely seen in the neonate.

SURGICAL CONDITIONS

Diaphragmatic hernia

Congenital diaphragmatic hernia (CDH) occurs in 1 in 2500 live births, with a high mortality rate, especially when the condition is not immediately recognized. In an increasing number of cases, the defect is detected via prenatal ultrasound. CDH-related morbidity stems from the presence of abdominal contents, including bowel or solid organs, within the thorax. The lack of space for lung development results in pulmonary hypoplasia. Hence, respiratory distress in the neonate with CDH has two causes: the presence of a mass within the thorax and a lack of a normal volume of lung tissue. The first cause is remediable through surgical repair, with reposition of the abdominal contents and repair of the hernia; however, the second is not, or at least only marginally so, as not only alveoli but airways and associated vasculature are absent. Radiographic features of CDH include the presence of a soft tissue mass within the thorax and contralateral displacement of the mediastinum (Fig. 10–15). Confirmatory tests include the passage of a nasogastric tube, which may follow an abnormal course into the thorax; injection of air through the nasogastric tube, which will result in the development of cystic-appearing spaces within the intrathoracic soft tissue mass (representing air within bowel); the introduction of a small amount of

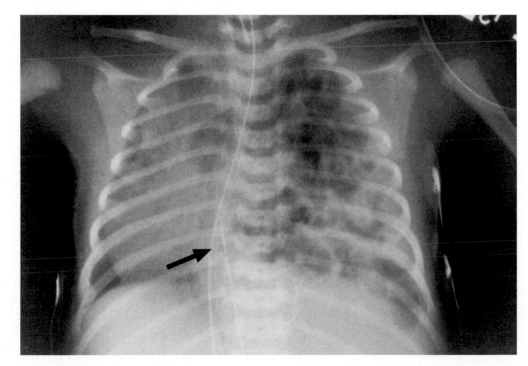

Figure 10–15. This full gestation girl experienced respiratory distress at birth. A chest radiograph demonstrates filling of the left hemithorax with multiple thin-walled, gas-containing structures, with shift of the mediastinum (including the nasogastric tube) to the right (arrow). The left hemidiaphragm is poorly seen. The diagnosis of congenital diaphragmatic hernia was suggested and subsequently confirmed at surgery. Over 90% of these lesions occur on the left, and associated mortality is high, primarily due to associated pulmonary hypoplasia.

contrast material through the nasogastric tube; and ultrasound, which will disclose the diaphragmatic defect and the presence of peristalsing bowel within the thorax. As expected, CDH is associated with other abnormalities, including gut malrotation.

Cystic adenomatoid malformation

A radiographic mimic of CDH is cystic adenomatoid malformation, which may also present with a multicystic appearing mass in the thorax. Abnormal growth of terminal respiratory structures leads to a hamartomatous mass of glandular tissue that may communicate with the airways, exhibiting air or air-fluid levels in the cysts. Surgical resection of the abnormal lobe is curative.

Congenital lobar emphysema

Congenital lobar emphysema results from progressive hyperinflation of one or more of the pulmonary lobes. At least half of cases are idiopathic, but many result from central airway obstruction, with a check-valve mechanism that allows the lobe to fill during inspiration, but prevents emptying at expiration. In decreasing order of frequency, the most commonly affected lobes are the left upper lobe, the right middle lobe, and the right upper lobe. The lesion characteristically presents as an opacity in the first few days of life, due to impaired emptying of lung fluid. Thereafter, it presents as a hyperlucent, hyperexpanded lobe, which causes contralateral shift of the mediastinum (Fig. 10–16).

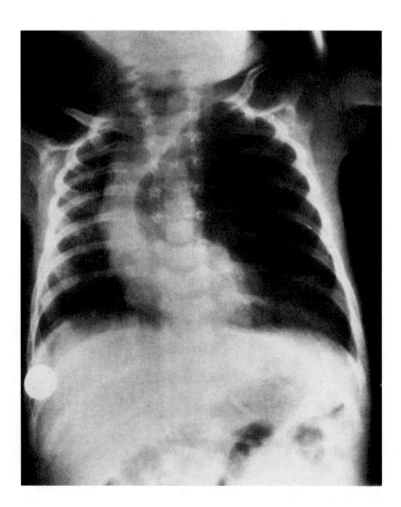

Figure 10–16. This frontal radiograph in a newborn demonstrates marked hyperexpansion of the left upper lobe, with herniation of lung to the right and accompanying shift of mediastinal structures, secondary to congenital lobar emphysema.

Tracheoesophageal fistula

Esophageal atresia (EA) and tracheoesophageal fistula (TEF) both represent anomalies in the development of the primitive foregut, which normally separates during the 5th week of life into the esophagus and trachea. These anomalies occur in approximately 1 in 2500 live births. EA may be suggested by a prenatal ultrasound showing polyhydramnios, secondary to the inability of the fetus to ingest normal quantities of amniotic fluid. EA and TEF are suggested postnatally by the development of coughing, choking, and cyanosis in the first day of life. Most commonly, attempted passage of a nasogastric tube and subsequent chest radiograph reveal the tube ending in a blind pouch in the upper chest (Fig. 10–17). The presence of gas within the bowel proves that there is a distal esophageal–tracheal communication. While many anatomic types are possible, the most common involves a blind esophageal pouch with a more distal fistula between the trachea and esophagus. A gasless abdomen indicates that the second most prevalent anatomic type is likely present, with no communication between the trachea and esophagus (pure EA).

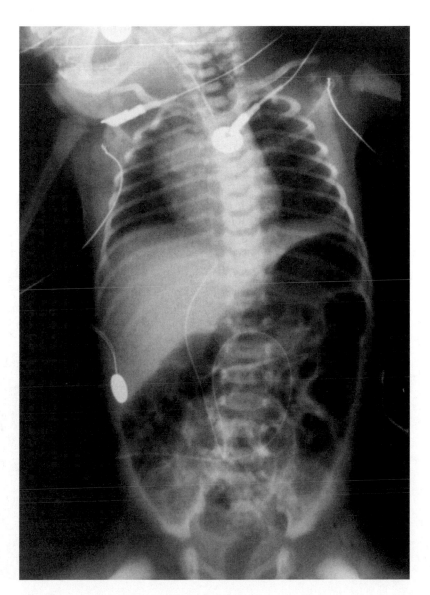

Figure 10–17. The intensive care team had difficulty passing a nasogastric tube in this newborn infant. This "babygram" demonstrates why. The air-filled esophagus ends in a blind pouch in the upper chest, in which the nasogastric tube has coiled back on itself. This infant had the most common form of tracheoesophageal fistula, with the upper esophagus ending in a blind pouch, but the distal portion of the esophagus connecting via a fistula to the trachea. The distal fistula explains how gas found its way into the bowel in a patient with a discontinuous esophagus.

CHILDHOOD RESPIRATORY DISTRESS

Many of the conditions that cause respiratory distress in the adult manifest similarly in children. These include such common disorders as asthma and pneumonia. However, there are three common, community-acquired childhood respiratory conditions that deserve special mention. These are croup, foreign body aspiration, and epiglottitis.

CROUP

Croup, more descriptively referred to as acute laryngotracheobronchitis, represents the most common cause of upper airway obstruction in children. It is most commonly seen in the 6 month to 3 year age group. The principal infectious organisms in croup include parainfluenza virus and respiratory syncytial virus. Although it involves the entire upper airway, the critical zone of airway narrowing is the immediate subglottic region, approximately 1 cm below the larynx, due to the fact that loose mucosal attachment in this region permits excessive edematous narrowing. Patients present with a barky cough and stridor. The classic finding on a frontal radiograph is a tapered narrowing of the trachea in the subglottic region, producing a "V" configuration of airway narrowing. The critical reason for obtaining radiographs is not to diagnose croup, which is generally a self-limited process of several days' duration, but to exclude other more worrisome entities such as foreign body aspiration and epiglottitis.

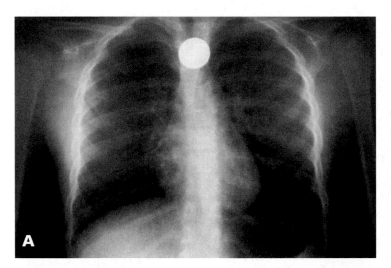

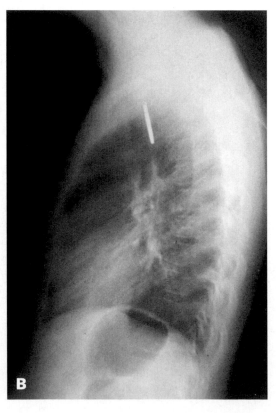

Figure 10–18. This child presented to the emergency room complaining of acute dysphagia. (A) A frontal view of the chest demonstrates a large, round metallic object superimposed over the upper mediastinum. What is this object and where is it located? The object is a quarter, which the child has swallowed. Its location is suggested by its orientation, with the coin lying in a coronal rather than sagittal plane. Because the trachea is wider front to back than side to side, a coin in the trachea would normally be seen on edge on a frontal film. The fact that the coin is seen en face on the frontal view suggests that it is in the esophagus. (B) This is confirmed on the lateral view, which clearly demonstrates that the coin is posterior to the tracheal air column. Such foreign bodies are sometimes removed under fluoroscopy, by passing a balloon catheter beyond the coin, inflating the balloon, and withdrawing the catheter, which pulls the foreign body back as well.

FOREIGN BODY ASPIRATION

Airway foreign bodies represent a common cause of respiratory distress, particularly between ages 6 months and 4 years, when children characteristically put objects in their mouths (Fig. 10–18). In contrast to croup and epiglottitis, there is generally no history of antecedent infectious symptoms, and the child presents with acute stridor, wheezing, and cough. As expected, foreign bodies follow the path of least resistance through the tracheobronchial tree, and most lodge in the right mainstem bronchi or its branches. Foreign bodies that are not removed may result in long-term complications such as recurrent pneumonias, hemoptysis, and bronchial stenosis, and bronchoscopic removal is generally indicated. Most aspirated foreign bodies are not radiopaque. Common radiographic findings include direct visualization of radiopaque foreign bodies on radiography or fluoroscopy, unilateral air trapping and hyperinflation due to a "check-valve" type of obstruction, and less commonly, atelectasis from complete obstruction. By obtaining inspiratory and expiratory films, or by observation of breathing under fluoroscopy, it is possible to increase diagnostic confidence. The nonobstructed lung will be able to empty normally, while the obstructed lung will not. Therefore, on an expiratory film the mediastinum will shift away from the side of the foreign body (Fig. 10–19).

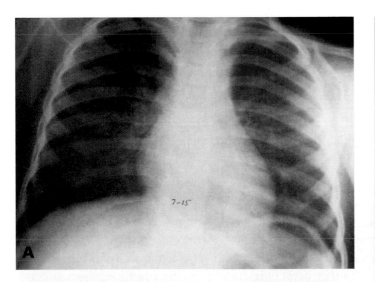

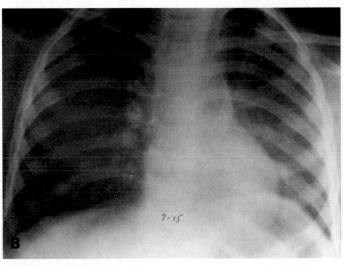

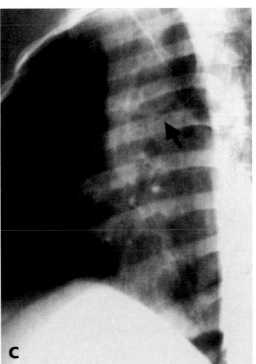

Figure 10–19. A 2½-year-old girl presented with the acute onset of coughing and wheezing. (A) A frontal view of the chest at inspiration demonstrates that the right lung appears somewhat more lucent than the left, but no other abnormality is seen. (B) However, during expiration there is a shift of the heart to the left, because the obstructed right lung is unable to empty due to a check-valve obstruction. (C) A slightly oblique lateral view reveals the foreign body (arrow) within the right mainstem bronchus.

Figure 10–20. This young child presented with severe sore throat and drooling. A lateral view of the soft tissues of the neck demonstrates a classic "thumb sign" of a thickened epiglottis (arrow), as well as thickening of the aryepiglottic folds below. These findings are diagnostic of epiglottitis, a potentially life-threatening condition.

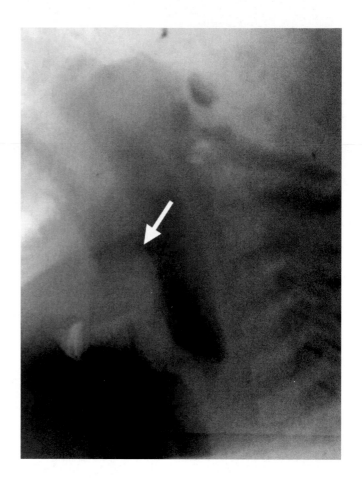

EPIGLOTTITIS

Epiglottitis represents an acutely life-threatening condition, because it may result in sudden and complete airway obstruction with asphyxiation. Children suspected of suffering from this condition should not be moved, and no maneuvers that might compromise breathing should be performed until personnel and equipment capable of airway intervention and management are present. If it is necessary to obtain radiographs, a portable unit should be used. Epiglottitis most commonly occurs between 3 and 6 years of age and is most often due to *Hemophilus influenzae*, although widespread immunization against *H. flu* is likely to alter this. Patients present with a history of fever, dysphagia, drooling, and sore throat. The classic radiographic and pathologic finding is thickening of the aryepiglottic folds, which manifests as a thumb-like thickening of the epiglottis on lateral views of the neck soft tissues (Fig. 10–20).

Nervous System

NEONATAL INTRACRANIAL HEMORRHAGE

EPIDEMIOLOGY

Infants born prior to 32 weeks gestation suffer a markedly increased risk of intracranial hemorrhage and ischemia. Twenty-five percent of infants below 1500 g develop intracranial hemorrhage, and it develops to some degree in up to two-thirds of infants at 28 to 32 weeks gestation. Such events can prove catastrophic, because infants so affected may suffer permanent and severe neurologic sequelae.

The occurrence of intracranial hemorrhage is linked to a number of risk factors. Antepartum factors include the medical condition of the mother, involving such risk factors as toxemia, diabetes, heart disease, and other factors predisposing to premature birth. The most effective medical response to intracranial hemorrhage is the prevention of premature birth. Intrapartum factors include abnormal fetal presentation and prolonged labor. Postpartum events associated with increased risk include respiratory distress, cardiopulmonary abnormalities, infection, and hemolysis.

PATHOPHYSIOLOGY

 To understand why premature infants are at risk for intracranial hemorrhage, it is necessary to understand the special developmental neuroanatomy of neonates. As one would predict, the areas of the brain most vulnerable to ischemic insult are the zones with the highest metabolic rate. In the neonate, these include the zones characterized by the highest rates of neural proliferation, maturation, and myelination, including the cerebellum, the basal ganglia, and the periventricular white matter. An area of special risk is the germinal matrix, located near the head of the caudate nucleus (Fig. 10–21). The germinal matrix is the subventricular and ventricular area of proliferation of neuronal and glial

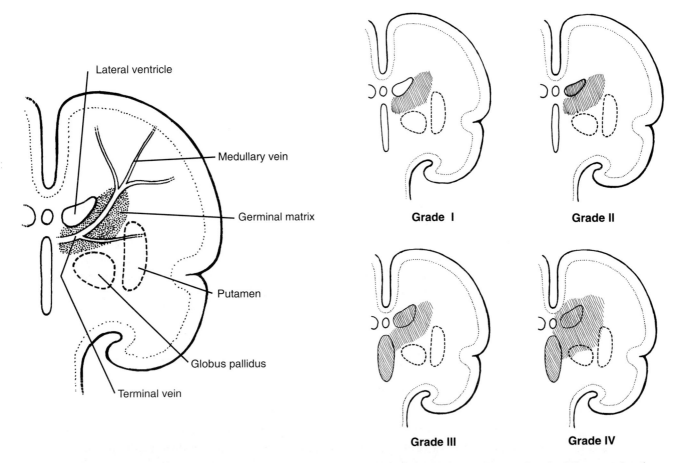

Figure 10–21. The normal position of the germinal matrix adjacent to the head of the caudate nucleus, as well as the different grades of germinal matrix hemorrhage (coronal view).

precursors. Cells migrate from this subependymal location out into the cortex. Of special note is the fact that this area is richly vascularized and has little supporting stroma; thus, any microscopic interruption of vascular integrity would tend not to be well contained and likely to develop into macroscopic hemorrhage. Germinal matrix hemorrhage is more prevalent in very premature infants and rare in those of 40 weeks gestation, because the germinal matrix becomes less and less prominent over the last 12 weeks of gestation and virtually disappears by term.

The pathophysiology of the condition centers on the autoregulation of cerebral blood flow. This autoregulation is disrupted in the premature newborn, who is less adept than a full-term infant at maintaining constant cerebral perfusion pressure in the face of changing arterial pressure. Moderate to severe asphyxia is the disrupting factor, rendering cerebral blood flow pressure-passive. This "pressure passivity" is the key to understanding the apparently paradoxical development of both ischemic and hemorrhagic injury, and in experimental models predicts the later development of ultrasonographically detectable hemorrhage. In normal infants, cerebral blood flow is independent of arterial pressure over a wide pressure range. When arterial pressure is reduced, flow can be maintained by lowering cerebrovascular resistance. When hypertension obtains, arteriolar constriction is induced. In the distressed newborn, small decreases in arterial pressure lead to a significant decrease in cerebral blood flow, which, if sustained, eventuates in ischemic injury. This situation is further aggravated by hypoxemia. In hypertension, increased pressure is transmitted unimpeded to the walls of the capillary bed, with an associated increased risk of hemorrhage (Fig. 10–22). Thus, the key pathophysiologic factor is a change in blood pressure, and management focuses on reducing distress and maintaining stable pressures.

Several other factors are critical to understanding why intracranial hemorrhage constitutes such a thorny problem. The prevention of asphyxia is a key strategy, yet the birth process itself can be likened to an asphyxial insult. Asphyxia normally leads first to hypertension, then later to hypotension, perhaps due to depletion of cardiac carbohydrate stores. Abrupt increases in arterial pressure are a fact of life in the first few days, accompanying even handling, feeding, and other routine activities. A second such factor is arterial $PaCO_2$ (partial pressure of carbon dioxide in arterial blood), which is a major regulator of intracranial vascular resistance at all stages of life. High $PaCO_2$ causes vasodilation and is associated with increased incidence of germinal matrix hemorrhage, while hyperventilation (blowing off carbon dioxide) at birth seems to suppress the development of hemorrhage. A third such factor is the blood-brain barrier, which is compromised in asphyxia through the combined effects of hypertension and vasodilation. This helps to explain why asphyxiated infants are at higher risk for kernicterus (hyperbilirubinemia-mediated brain damage), even with only moderate hyperbilirubinemia. The fourth factor is ischemic injury. Arterial hypoxemia and hypercarbia result from decreased placental and/or alveolar gas exchange. Depletion of myocardial glycogen leads to decreased blood pressure. Cerebral edema (from lactic acid accumulation, tissue injury, and compromised blood-brain barrier) and/or intraventricular hemorrhage may further decrease perfusion pressure. Finally, cerebral ischemia itself predisposes to further injury by delaying the restoration of autoregulation.

CLINICAL PRESENTATION

Intracranial hemorrhage most commonly presents in the first several days of neonatal life. Classic signs include obtundation, hypotonia, and a drop in the hematocrit. It is also associated with intractable metabolic acidosis. However, most cases detected by

Figure 10–22. This premature infant suffered birth anoxia. (A) A coronal head ultrasound image obtained at 1 day demonstrates a prominent echogenic focus adjacent to the right lateral ventricle (arrow). (B) A follow-up examination performed several weeks later demonstrates multiple cystic-appearing spaces adjacent to the lateral ventricles, indicating loss of cerebral parenchyma, characteristic of periventricular leukomalacia. This is a common manifestation of hypoxic ischemic injury, as the periventricular regions represent arterial watershed (border) regions.

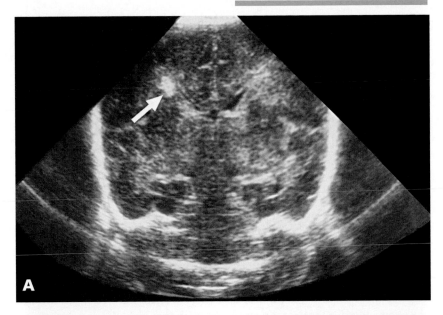

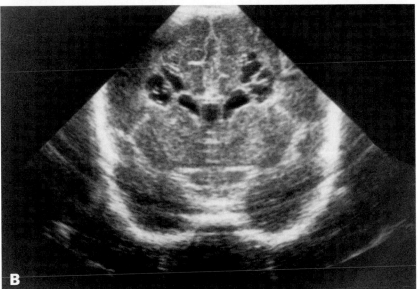

sonography are clinically silent, indicating the importance of sonographic screening in premature neonates at risk.

IMAGING

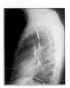
The key imaging modality in this setting is ultrasound, which can be performed quickly and efficiently in the neonatal intensive care unit and involves no exposure to ionizing radiation. Because the anterior fontanelle has not yet closed in these infants, it provides an excellent acoustic window on the brain. Head ultrasound is routinely performed in infants less than 32 weeks gestation, generally around postnatal day 4 to 7, by which time 90% of hemorrhages will have occurred. Clinical indications for earlier screening include an abnormal neurologic examination and a drop in hematocrit with no known source of bleeding. Another important setting is infants who will require anti-

coagulation for ECMO, in whom the presence of intracranial hemorrhage must first be ruled out.

Intracranial hemorrhage is graded on a scale of I to IV. Grade I is confined to the subependymal germinal matrix. The classic ultrasound finding in germinal matrix hemorrhage is echogenic foci immediately posterior to the caudothalamic groove. Grade II adds to this extension of blood into the ventricles, seen as echogenic intraventricular material, without ventriculomegaly. Grade III includes both ventricular extension and ventriculomegaly (Fig. 10–23). Grade IV includes intracerebral hemorrhage as well. Prognosis declines with increasing grade, and grades III and IV are associated with large increases in morbidity and mortality. Between 40 and 50% of infants with grade IV hemorrhage suffer severe neurologic impairment, while more than three-quarters of infants with grades I and II hemorrhage develop only mild or no neurologic impairment.

Periventricular leukomalacia is another common ultrasound finding in ischemic injury, which results from ischemic damage to the deep white matter of the hemispheres. It manifests initially as areas of increased echogenicity, followed eventually by cystic lesions (porencephaly), giving the brain an appearance that has been said to resemble Swiss cheese.

Abdomen

ACUTE ABDOMEN

A number of acute abdominal processes are unique to the pediatric population, or at least occur predominantly in infants and children. To determine which process is involved in a particular patient, several extraradiologic factors are critical. First is the patient's age. Pediatric patients are predisposed to certain conditions at certain points in their development. For example, conditions such as necrotizing enterocolitis (NEC), meconium ileus, and bowel atresias will present in the first few days of extrauterine life, while hypertrophic pyloric stenosis presents around the age of

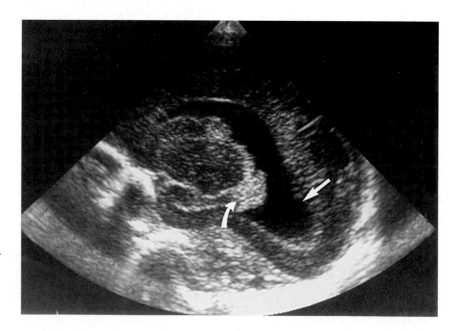

Figure 10–23. This sagittal neonatal head sonogram demonstrates a grade III intracranial hemorrhage, with blood around the choroid plexus in the lateral ventricular atrium (curved arrow), as well as dilatation of the ventricle itself (arrow).

1 month, and it would be somewhat unusual to see intussusception in the first few months of life. Additional factors would include whether the patient is infected (fever, white count), the appearance of the vomitus (bilious vomiting implies obstruction distal to the ampulla of Vater), and history of previous surgery (in which case adhesions constitute one of the most important etiologies of obstruction throughout life).

In terms of radiologic workup, plain films can be used to evaluate for obstruction. If obstruction is proximal within the bowel, there will be relatively little intestinal air, although the stomach and duodenum may be dilated (as in the classic "double bubble" of duodenal atresia, with air in the stomach and duodenal bulb), while more distal obstruction will be accompanied by numerous distended loops (Fig. 10–24). If obstruction is high, upper gastrointestinal (GI) contrast studies will often be indicated, while a pattern of distal obstruction warrants contrast enema. The plain film can also rule out free intraperitoneal air, although a view allowing air to be seen in tangent in the nondependent portion of the abdomen should be used, such as an upright or left-side-down decubitus film. Ultrasound is used primarily to assess for appendicitis and hypertrophic pyloric stenosis, and to rule out masses. CT is seldom necessary in the acute, nontraumatic setting.

It is sometimes said that if a clinician can order only one film in children with

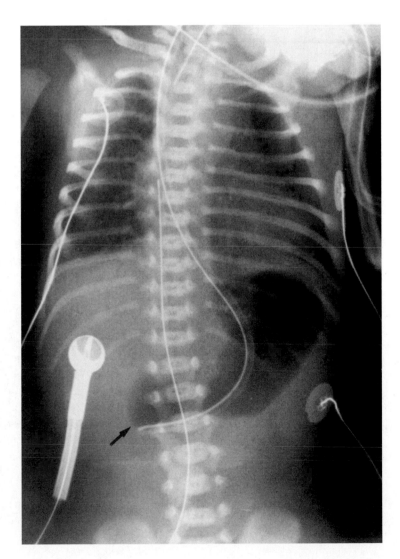

Figure 10–24. This newborn infant's "babygram" demonstrates a classic "double bubble" sign, with a gas-filled, dilated stomach representing the first bubble and the gas-filled duodenal bulb representing the second bubble. The degree of distention would have been greater but for the presence of a nasogastric tube extending to the point of obstruction (arrow). This is a classic appearance of duodenal atresia, which occurs in 1 in 4000 births and is thought to result from a failure of normal gut recanalization, resulting in an atretic segment of duodenum. An additional hint to the diagnosis on the film is the complete absence of gas in the bowel distal to the proximal duodenum. Down syndrome is present in one-third of these patients. Note also an endotracheal tube and an umbilical vein catheter extending into the right atrium.

acute abdominal presentations, it should be the upright chest film. The reasoning behind this dictum is that apparent acute abdominal presentations often turn out to stem from extra-abdominal pathology. A classic example is the child with abdominal pain and fever who is discovered on chest radiography to have a lower lobe pneumonia (Fig. 10–25). Occasionally the pulmonary infiltrate will be detected on the

Figure 10–25. A 4-year-old boy presented to the emergency department febrile and complaining of abdominal pain. (A) An upright frontal chest radiograph reveals vague airspace opacification along the right side of the heart, which does not efface the heart border. (B) The lateral view confirms that the process is located in the superior segment of the right lower lobe. Pneumonia represents an important mimic of acute abdomen, particularly in children.

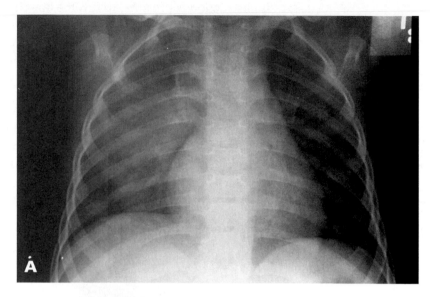

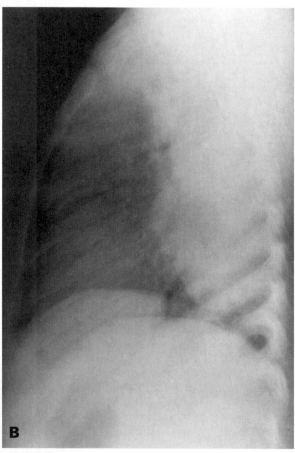

abdominal flat plate as increased opacity in the otherwise overpenetrated lung base, which is only detectable if the physician remembers to look at the corners of the film. Even when an abdominal plain film has been obtained and reveals nothing more than a nonspecific ileus pattern, a chest radiograph will sometimes hold the key to the diagnosis.

The neonate

NEC occurs primarily in premature neonates exposed to hypoxic stress. Such infants have immature guts that exhibit poor peristalsis and impaired immune function, and are therefore at risk for infection. Clinicians note onset of vomiting, blood in the stools, metabolic acidosis, and apneas and bradycardias in the first week of life. It is important to recognize NEC so that feedings may be halted, as the continued introduction of hyperosmolar feeds into the gut markedly exacerbates the mucosal injury and bacterial superinfection. The usual radiologic examination is the plain film, which may demonstrate bowel distention, an abnormally dilated, fixed loop of bowel, and free air within the peritoneal cavity (indicating bowel perforation). Two highly specific findings in the appropriate clinical setting are pneumatosis intestinalis (thin collections of air within the bowel wall, secondary to disruption of the mucosa) and portal venous gas (branching collections of air in the right upper quadrant produced by passage of intraluminal air into the portal venous system) (Fig. 10–26). Once NEC is diagnosed, continued

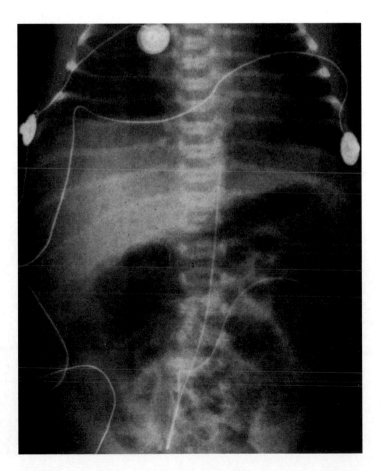

Figure 10–26. Note the multiple linear and bubbly appearing lucencies superimposed over the bowel gas in this neonate with necrotizing enterocolitis. These are due to gas within the bowel wall, which is called *pneumatosis intestinalis.*

radiographic follow-up is important to detect pneumoperitoneum, which suggests that NEC has lead to bowel necrosis and perforation, and warrants surgical intervention.

Midgut volvulus (from the Latin *volvere*, "to roll") may present at any age, but is typically seen in term infants within the first several days of life. It constitutes a surgical emergency, because it may result in infarction and necrosis of bowel. To occur, it requires the presence of malrotation, with an abnormally short mesentery and defective fixation of bowel due to failure of normal intestinal rotation and fixation during the 6th week of intrauterine life. Volvulus occurs when the malrotated proximal small intestine twists around its abnormally short mesentery. This in turn may twist the superior mesenteric artery (SMA), compromising its flow and potentially infarcting all of the bowel supplied by it (extending from the proximal jejunum at the ligament of Treitz to the splenic flexure of the colon). A neonate who develops bilious vomiting, abdominal pain and distention, and blood tinged stools should undergo an upper GI barium study to rule out midgut volvulus. If volvulus is present, there will be obstruction at the duodenal "C" loop, often with a "corkscrew appearance" as the barium traces out the helical pattern of the twisted bowel (Fig. 10–27).

Even if volvulus is not present at the time of examination, malrotation will be evidenced by abnormal location of the duodenal–jejunal junction, which is normally positioned to the left of the spine at the level of the duodenal bulb. Alternatively, if no malrotation is present, the duodenal "C" loop will have a normal appearance, and the duodenal–jejunal junction will be identified to the left of the L1 vertebral body, the expected location of the ligament of Treitz.

Other neonatal conditions merit brief discussion. Bowel atresia, probably reflecting an in utero ischemic insult, involves the distal small bowel more often than proximal and presents in the first few hours of life with vomiting and obstruction. Meconium ileus is seen almost exclusively in newborn patients with cystic fibrosis, whose viscous meconium may "plug up" the bowel, most commonly the ileum, with resultant evidence of obstruction. The radiologist not only diagnoses but may treat this condition, if it is not complicated by an atresia, volvulus, or stenosis. Refluxing contrast

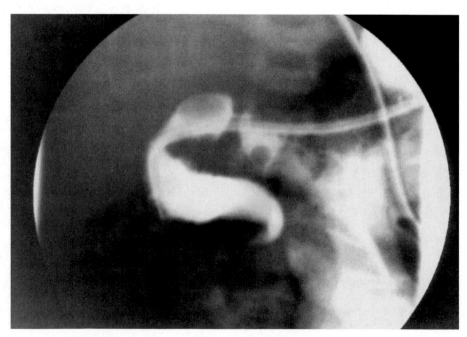

Figure 10–27. A 7-day-old boy with bilious nasogastric tube drainage underwent an upper gastrointestinal examination to rule out malrotation with midgut volvulus. A frontal spot film from that examination demonstrates that the duodenum has assumed a corkscrew-like appearance, indicating the presence of volvulus. This represents a surgical emergency, because the bowel supplied by the superior mesenteric artery, which is involved in the volvulus, may become ischemic and even infarct.

through the colon may loosen the thick viscous meconium in these infants and to relieve the obstruction.

The infant and child

Hypertrophic pyloric stenosis involves idiopathic hypertrophy of the circular muscle surrounding the pyloric channel connecting the stomach and duodenum. It occurs in 1 of every 500 children around the age of 1 month, most frequently in boys. It presents as nonbilious vomiting and dehydration, with laboratory tests indicating a hypochloremic metabolic alkalosis due to the loss of gastric HCl. It is best diagnosed clinically with palpation of an "olive" in the right upper quadrant. In equvocal cases, ultrasound can confirm the diagnosis by revealing increased muscular thickness and length of the pyloric channel (Fig. 10–28). Because the patient can be stabilized via intravenous hydration, it does not constitute a surgical emergency.

The most common cause of intestinal obstruction in infants older than one week of age is inguinal hernia, 90% of which occur in males. Patency of the processus vaginalis, the canal through which the testis descends into the scrotum, allows abdominal contents to slide into the inguinal canal, in some cases extending down into the scrotum, where a mass can be palpated. Eighty percent of inguinal hernias are right sided. The typical patient presents with abdominal distention, vomiting, and irritability. Plain film findings include small bowel obstruction, thickening of the inguinal fold on the affected side, and air-filled bowel in the inguinal canal or scrotum. Ultrasound may show a peristalsing mass in the same regions.

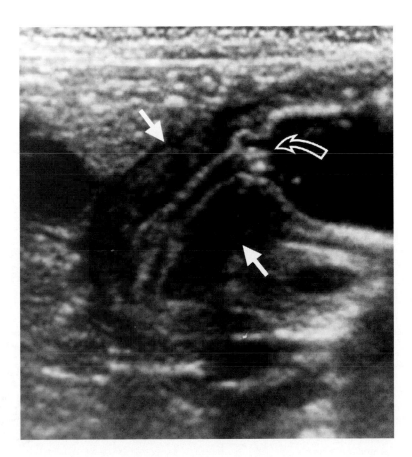

Figure 10–28. A 5-week-old boy developed projectile nonbilious vomiting after feedings. A longitudinal ultrasound image of the pyloric channel demonstrates marked thickening of the pylorus (solid arrows), which measures 4.5 mm in diameter on each side. Note that the gastric antrum contains fluid, which cannot empty due to the marked pyloric hypertrophy and resultant stenosis. The open arrow denotes the opening of the antrum into the pylorus.

Appendicitis is the principal cause of emergency surgery in children. Stasis within the appendix, often caused by an obstructing appendicolith, allows bacterial overgrowth, inflammation, vascular compromise, and eventual perforation, which may result in fatal peritonitis. A calcified appendicolith is visible on plain film in only 15% of patients. Other plain film findings include evidence of small bowel obstruction, a soft tissue mass in the right lower quadrant, focal right lower quadrant ileus, and free intraperitoneal air. Barium enema may demonstrate mass effect on the cecum and failure to fill the entire appendix. However, the appendix may fail to fill in up to 10% of normal patients. Ultrasound has become the imaging modality of choice in suspected appendicitis. Findings include a noncompressible appendix with a total diameter of more than 6 mm, an appendicolith, and a complex fluid collection.

Another condition the radiologist may be called on not only to diagnose but to treat is intussusception, the telescoping of a more proximal segment of bowel into a more distal segment, typically involving the the downstream displacement of a segment of ileum (the intussusceptum) into the right colon (the intussuscepiens) (Fig. 10–29). Ninety percent of cases occur in the first 2 years of life. It is thought that most cases of intussusception in children stem from virally induced intestinal lymphoid hyperplasia, which acts as a lead point. On plain radiography, the abdomen may demonstrate signs of intestinal obstruction, a right-sided soft tissue mass, or even the head of the intussusceptum within air-filled colon. Ultrasound may demonstrate an oval soft tissue mass on longitudinal view, and a round mass on the cross-sectional view, both often demonstrating concentric rings of bowel. Retrograde contrast examination of the bowel will demonstrate the head of the intussusceptum as a filling defect with the intussuscepiens. In addition to diagnosis, gentle pressure from retrograde flow of contrast or air will often reduce the intussusception (Fig. 10–30). There is a

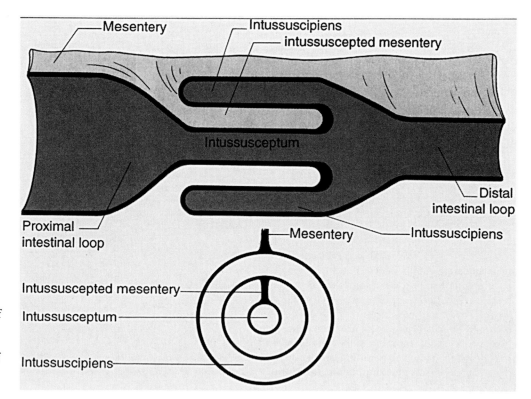

Figure 10–29. Anatomy of intussusception. The lower cross-sectional diagram explains the "target" sign of intussusception by ultrasound.

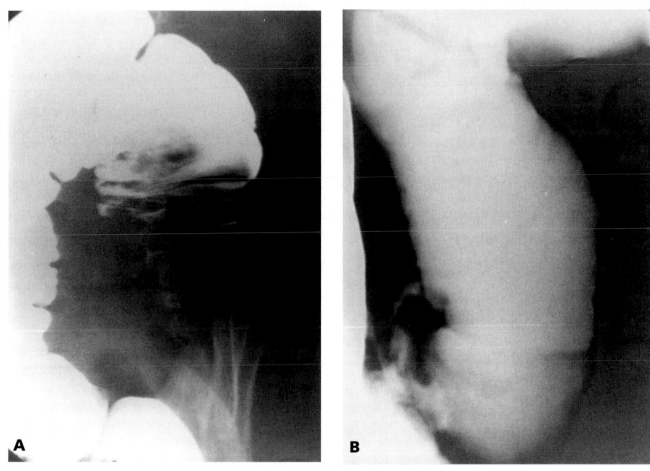

Figure 10–30. (A) This spot film from a barium enema in a patient with abdominal pain, vomiting, and blood per rectum demonstrates the classic radiographic appearance of an ileocolic intussusception, in which a segment of the small bowel has traveled antegrade into the lumen of the ascending colon. Note that the patient is positioned prone at this point, causing the ascending colon to be on the right side of the film. Note the convex filling defect with contrast partially outlining the outer wall of the intussusceptum, the so-called coiled spring appearance. (B) After gentle pressure from an elevated bag of contrast was applied, the intussusception was reduced, and the ascending colon regained its expected appearance. At least 80% of intussusceptions are amenable to radiologic reduction, which in many cases spares the patient an operative procedure.

10% risk of recurrence. The only contraindications to radiologic reduction are evidence of perforation, such as free air or symptoms of peritonitis.

MASSES

WILMS' TUMOR

Epidemiology

The most prevalent solid abdominal mass of childhood, which is also the most common renal cancer, is Wilms' tumor, of which approximately 400 cases per year are reported in the United States. It also represents the fourth most common childhood malignancy, after leukemia, central nervous system neoplasms, and neuroblastoma. The mean age of presentation in Wilms' tumor is 3 years, and 85% of cases present before the age of 6 years.

Pathophysiology

 Also known as nephroblastoma, Wilms' tumor arises from the primitive metanephric blastema, and is typically centered in the renal cortex, sparing the collecting system. Roughly 1 in 10 tumors presents bilaterally, which seems to be associated with a better prognosis. Another important prognostic factor is the histology of the tumor, with 85% of tumors exhibiting a favorable triphasic pattern (consisting of primitive blastema, stroma, and epithelial cells), while 15% of tumors are anaplastic, an unfavorable pattern. Wilms' tumor is associated with a number of syndromes, including aniridia, hemihypertrophy, Beckwith-Wiedemann syndrome (macroglossia, organomegaly, and omphalocele), and Drash's syndrome (pseudohermaphroditism, glomerulonephritis, and nephrotic syndrome). In addition, it appears with increased frequency in horseshoe and fused kidneys.

Clinical presentation

Presenting complaints typically consist of a rapidly enlarging, painless abdominal mass, without systemic symptoms. A minority of patients demonstrate microscopic hematuria.

Imaging

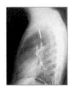 Ultrasound constitutes the first line of imaging, because it provides quick and reliable detection as well as the best assessment of the degree of vascular invasion. Many Wilms' tumors will involve the renal vein and inferior vena cava, some actually extending into the heart. Sonography usually reveals a large mass, with internal areas of necrosis and hemorrhage, arising from the kidney and displacing adjacent abdominal structures (Fig. 10–31). CT typically demonstrates a well-defined, low attenuation mass with heterogenous

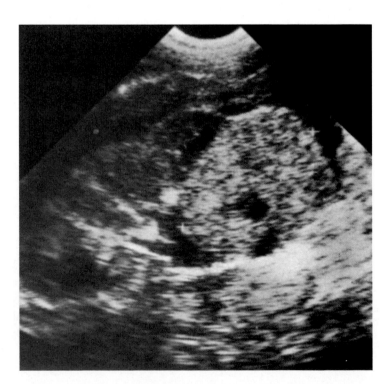

Figure 10–31. This longitudinal ultrasound image of the right flank in a 4-year-old girl demonstrates an echogenic mass occupying the lower half of the right kidney. A Wilms' tumor was found at surgery.

enhancement. Only about 15% of Wilms' tumors demonstrate calcifications. Treatment usually consists of surgery and chemotherapy, with radiation therapy reserved for more advanced tumors that are not totally resectable or have metastasized hematogenously. Despite the rapid growth of Wilms' tumor, the prognosis is generally favorable, with overall survival approaching 90%.

NEUROBLASTOMA

Epidemiology

Neuroblastoma is the second most common intra-abdominal malignancy of childhood. Approximately 70% of neuroblastomas arise in the abdomen, with over 40% originating in the adrenal gland, while the chest, neck, and pelvis represent other sites. At 2 years, the mean age of this neoplasm is slightly lower than that of Wilms' tumor, and three-quarters of patients present before age 5 years.

Pathophysiology

 The tumor arises from neural crest tissue either in the adrenal gland or somewhere along the sympathetic chain. Neuroblastoma is at the malignant end of a spectrum of tumors ranging to the intermediate grade ganglioneuroblastoma and the benign ganglioneuroma. Some neuroblastomas spontaneously differentiate into these more mature forms. They also occasionally exhibit the extraordinary property of undergoing spontaneous regression, even in very advanced disease. In contrast to Wilms' tumor, neuroblastoma has fewer and less syndromic associations. However, it does sometimes exhibit certain clinical constellations of metastatic spread. Orbital ecchymosis and proptosis, so-called raccoon eyes, often occur in combination with a primary adrenal tumor and extensive skeletal involvement, especially the skull, which is called Hutchinson's syndrome. The "blueberry muffin" syndrome is associated with multiple skin metastases.

Clinical presentation

Patients typically present with large abdominal masses and metastatic disease. In addition, 70% will have systemic symptoms, including hypertension, hyperglycemia, tachycardia, and other signs of increased catecholamine production. Hence, laboratory analysis usually reveals increased urine levels of vanillylmandelic acid or homovanillic acid. A minority of patients will present with paraneoplastic effects, including the so-called "dancing eyes and dancing feet" syndrome.

Imaging

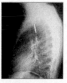 The imaging of neuroblastoma contrasts with that of Wilms' tumor in a number of respects. While Wilms' tumor seldom calcifies, 50% of neuroblastomas demonstrate calcifications on plain radiography, and 90% are calcified on CT. In contrast to Wilms' tumor, neuroblastoma tends to be a poorly marginated mass that insinuates itself around and engulfs other abdominal structures. It often extends across the midline and even into the thorax. Ultrasound usually demonstrates a large mass with heterogeneous and echogenic echotexture. As an extrarenal mass, it often displaces the axis of the kidney

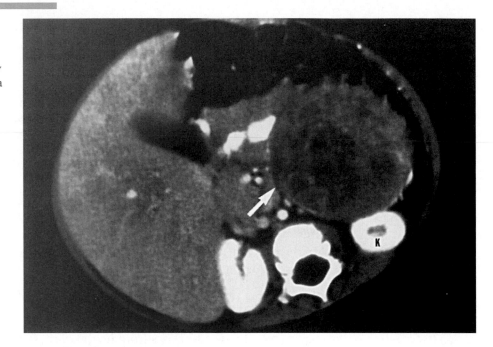

Figure 10–32. A 15-month-old presented with a left-sided abdominal mass. An axial section from a postinfusion computed tomography scan of the abdomen demonstrates a large heterogeneous mass (arrow) displacing an apparently intact left kidney posteriorly. Calcifications were seen within the mass at other levels. At surgery, a neuroblastoma was removed. K, left kidney.

(Fig. 10–32). In addition to demonstrating calcifications, CT is used to detect metastatic disease, which most often involves the liver and lymph nodes. Bone marrow involvement, which is common, is typically assessed by bone scintigraphy. MRI is primarily used in patients with neurologic symptoms, in whom intraspinal involvement must be ruled out. Prognosis is best for younger patients and those with a nonabdominal primary tumor.

Musculoskeletal System

DEVELOPMENTAL DYSPLASIA OF THE HIP

EPIDEMIOLOGY

Once referred to as congenital hip dislocation, developmental dysplasia of the hip (DDH) is seen most frequently in white infants and exhibits a female:male ratio of 5:1. It can also be associated with neuromuscular diseases, such as myelomeningocele. The incidence is estimated at 1 per 1000 births.

PATHOPHYSIOLOGY

 In most cases, DDH is thought to be secondary to hormonally induced laxity of the capsular ligaments, compounded by in utero positions that stress the hip, such as a restricted intrauterine space due to oligohydramnios. It more commonly involves the left hip than the right, which is thought to be due to the fact that fetuses tend to lie with their backs to the maternal left side, with their left hips against the maternal sacrum. If uncorrected, DDH can lead to early secondary osteoarthritic changes, with deformity of both the acetabulum and femoral head. Treatment includes casting in a frog-leg position if the hip is relocatable or surgery in cases of irreducibility or failed conservative therapy.

CLINICAL PRESENTATION

DDH is suspected clinically in newborns with a breech presentation, who have a 25% risk, because the hips are extended during birth. Findings on clinical examination include asymmetry of the normal skin folds around the hip, shortening of the thigh, and a "click" during the Ortolani reduction test (performed by flexing the hip and gently abducting).

IMAGING

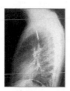 Imaging plays a critical role in the diagnosis of DDH. The essential parameter in the imaging evaluation is the relationship of the femur to the acetabulum. The finding of a well-seated and nondislocatable femoral head on stress views excludes the diagnosis. A variety of measurements have been described that provide quantifiable criteria of dysplasia and dislocation. Formerly, plain films represented the mainstay of imaging diagnosis, but currently ultrasound represents the best modality. Ultrasound shows the cartilaginous femoral head and acetabulum without ionizing radiation or the administration of contrast material, requires no sedation, and can evaluate the dynamic function of the hip joint in real time (Fig. 10–33). However, ultrasound is optimal only up to 10 months of age; after that point, ossification of the hip structures interferes with adequate beam penetration. One of the disadvantages of ultrasound as compared with other modalities such as CT and MRI is the fact that it is extremely operator dependent.

TRAUMA

Musculoskeletal trauma in children differs from that in adults in several important respects. First, children generate smaller forces and are situated closer to the ground

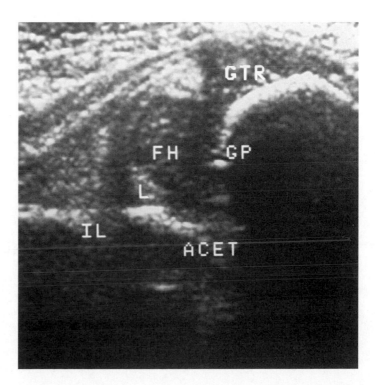

Figure 10–33. This ultrasound image of the left hip in a newborn female demonstrates conclusive evidence of developmental dysplasia of the hip. The femoral head is laterally displaced from the acetabulum. ACET, acetabulum; FH, femoral head; GP, femoral growth plate; GTR, greater trochanter; IL, ilium; L, limbus of the cartilaginous acetabulum.

than adults, which tends to protect their skeletons from fracture. However, the bones of children are different from adult bones in ways that make them more liable to fracture. Pediatric bones are shorter and thinner than those in adults, and they are also less dense, containing proportionately more water. Children's bones are therefore not as resistant to bending, torquing, and axial loading forces. Yet this also means that the bone of a child will often bend to a remarkable degree before it develops the frank fracture one would expect in an adult.

One result of the greater flexibility of children's bones is the occurrence of several types of fractures that do not occur in adults. One such peculiarly pediatric fracture is the so-called greenstick fracture, so named because the injury resembles the effect sometimes produced by bending a green stick until it breaks: one side of the shaft fractures, but the other merely bends. A variant is the bending fracture, in which neither side of the cortex appears to be disrupted, but the bone is clearly bent. It should be noted that in both cases, the apparent bending in fact represents multiple microfractures that are not seen radiographically. However, the distinction is real, because the adult bone would fracture completely through. Another special pediatric type of fracture is the torus fracture, which manifests as a bulge in the cortex on one or both sides, secondary to axial loading forces and buckling of the bone.

A third difference between the pediatric and adult musculoskeletal systems is the differing strength of ligaments and bones in the two groups. The bones of a young adult are typically stronger than the ligaments holding them together, meaning that sprains are quite common. In the later decades of life, osteoporosis tends to weaken the bones and fractures occur more easily. In a child, however, the bones are usually not as strong as the ligaments, and a fracture is more likely than a ligamentous injury to result from trauma to such joints as the ankle, elbow, and wrist. Typically, the apophyses at which ligaments attach to the bone are weaker than the ligaments themselves, hence the increased incidence of avulsion injuries. So common are fractures and avulsion injuries, and so uncommon are the dislocations that often occur in strong-boned adults, that anytime a dislocation is suspected in a child, an additional search should probably be made for an occult fracture.

Perhaps the most important anatomic difference between adult fractures and pediatric fractures is the presence in the child's bones of growth plates (physes) between the epiphyses and metaphyses of the long bones (and elsewhere). The growth plate is the weakest part of the bone and is involved in many pediatric fractures. Approximately 80% of these injuries are due to shearing forces, and 20% to axial loading. The site involved in one-half of growth plate injuries is the distal radius. The Salter-Harris

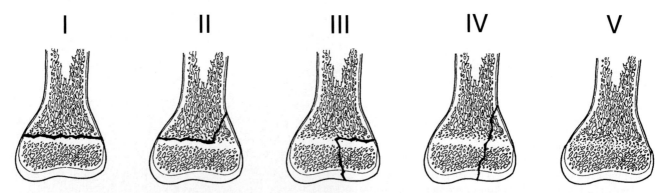

Figure 10–34. The Salter-Harris classification of growth plate injuries, as described in the text.

Figure 10–35. This oblique radiograph of the ankle in a child demonstrates a Salter-Harris I fracture of the distal tibia, after a fall. Note that there is anterior slippage of the metaphysis relative to the epiphysis, causing a "step off" at the physis. Approximately 5% of growth plate fractures are type I, with a very favorable prognosis for complete healing.

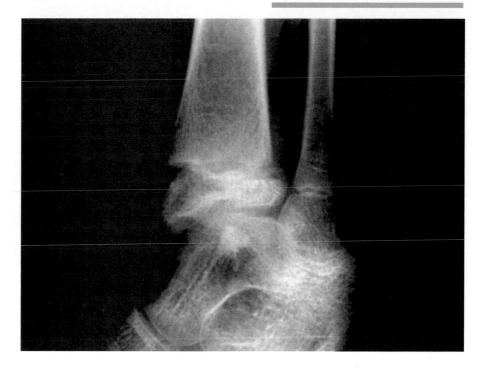

classification is widely used to categorize growth plate injuries (Fig. 10–34). A Salter-Harris type I injury represents a slip of the epiphysis due to shearing forces and hence involves only the growth plate (Fig. 10–35). A type II injury extends at least partially through the growth plate, but with metaphyseal extension. A type III injury involves the growth plate and the epiphysis (Fig. 10–36). A type IV injury extends through the epiphysis, growth plate, and metaphysis. A type V injury represents a crush injury to the growth plate, which often appears radiographically normal. The prognosis for normal growth is good in types I and II injuries, fair for type III injuries, and poor for type IV and particularly type V injuries.

To understand why the prognosis varies according to fracture type, it is necessary to review the structure of the growth plate. At the epiphyseal end are both the germinal zone of proliferating cartilage cells, without which growth cannot occur, as well as the epiphyseal blood vessels that nourish them. On the diaphyseal side, on the other hand, are the centers of ossification and the blood vessels supplying them, which are easily replaced in case of injury. The most serious injuries are those that disrupt the epiphyseal aspect of the growth plate, as the loss of cells in the germinal zone, either through direct trauma or vascular compromise, is irreversible, at least if it involves more than a short segment of the physis. Hence, injury to the epiphyseal side of the growth plate may produce partial or complete growth arrest, most likely when the entire physis has been destroyed in the type V crush injury. The restoration of normal alignment is also critical. If the growth plate is not properly realigned, a bony bar may form across a portion of it, which can cause the bone to become angulated and deformed, as the intact remainder of the growth plate continues to grow. The younger the patient (and the more growth remaining to be completed), the greater the potential damage of a growth plate injury.

Because fracture lines in children may be particularly subtle, one secondary sign of fracture frequently sought by pediatric radiologists is evidence of a joint effusion or hemarthrosis. If of sufficient magnitude, these are frequently manifest by the elevation

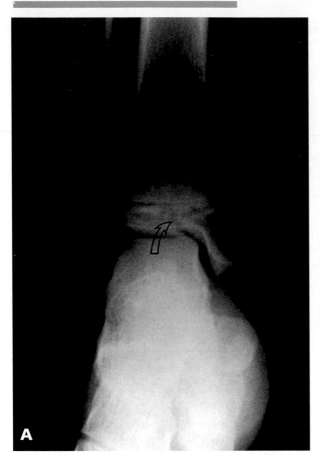

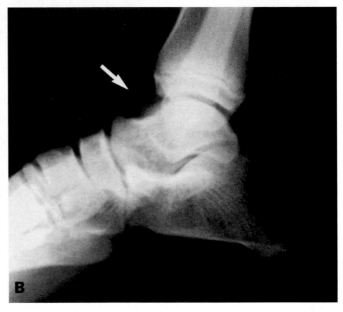

Figure 10–36. (A) This frontal radiograph of the ankle demonstrates a Salter-Harris III fracture of the distal tibia (arrow), with the fracture extending through the tibial epiphysis and into the growth plate. (B) The lateral view demonstrates a prominent tibiotalar hemiarthrosis (arrow), secondary to the involvement of the articular surface.

or even obliteration of fat pads around joints, particularly the elbow on a lateral radiograph. In a child, elevation of the anterior humeral fat pad or appearance of the posterior humeral fat pad (which is not normally visible, being hidden by the olecranon fossa) is considered presumptive evidence of a supracondylar humeral fracture. The patient is usually splinted or casted and brought back in 10 days for repeat imaging, by which time osteoclastic lysis along the fracture line or periosteal reaction should be present.

RICKETS

EPIDEMIOLOGY

Rickets is an example of osteomalacia, the inadequate mineralization of osteoid, which in the immature skeleton of a growing child tends to manifest itself at the physis, or growth plate, of long bones. While the majority of children in many large metropolitan areas appear to have suffered some degree of r ickets at the turn of the century, the disorder is not commonly seen today, due in large part to the supplementation of milk with vitamin D.

PATHOPHYSIOLOGY

To understand the biochemical basis of rickets, it is necessary to understand vitamin D metabolism, which culminates in the production of 1,25-$(OH)_2$-cholecalciferol, or calcitriol, the hormone that actively promotes both calcium absorption in the intestines and the mineralization of bone. Rickets may result from a defect in any one of the three basic stages in vitamin D's metabolic pathway. The first stage is obtaining an adequate amount of vitamin D. This may stem from malnourishment and an inadequate vitamin D intake, from inadequate exposure to sunshine (from 7-dehydrocholesterol, ultraviolet radiation brings about the formation of cholecalciferol), or from impaired GI absorption. Because vitamin D is fat soluble, the latter condition occurs in pancreatitis or biliary tract disease (due to the absence of bile or pancreatic lipase) and in patients with conditions associated with a damaged ileum, as in Crohn's disease.

Once vitamin D is in the body, it must be converted to 25-(OH)-cholecalciferol, the second stage in vitamin D metabolism, which takes place in the liver. Conditions that interfere with this process include a variety of hepatic parenchymal diseases, as well as anticonvulsant therapy. Anticonvulsants induce hepatic microsomal enzymes and thereby hasten the degradation of biologically active vitamin D metabolites.

The third stage in vitamin D metabolism is the conversion of 25-(OH)-vitamin D to 1,25-$(OH)_2$-vitamin D in the kidney. A variety of conditions may interfere with this step, including chronic renal failure and a variety of renal tubular disorders. While a combination of insufficient sun exposure and malnutrition was responsible for most cases of rickets at the turn of the century, renal osteodystrophy is now the most common cause.

Because bone mineralization also requires an adequate supply of phosphate and calcium, a deficiency of either of these may also cause osteomalacia. Lack of calcium may result from insufficient dietary intake or malabsorption. Defective phosphate metabolism has a variety of causes, including simple phosphate deficiency and numerous disorders of renal tubular reabsorption of phosphate, such as Fanconi's syndrome. Hypophosphatasia is a rare disorder associated with low levels of the enzyme alkaline phosphatase, which is required by osteoblasts to create the locally high concentrations of phosphate necessary for bone mineralization, and often presents with many of the radiographic features of rickets.

CLINICAL PRESENTATION

Children with long-standing rickets present with bowing of weight-bearing bones such as the femur and tibia and have an increased incidence of fractures due to weakening of the bones.

IMAGING

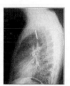

The radiographic findings in rickets stem from the production of defective bone, particularly at the growth plate. As one would predict, the most severely affected bones will be those undergoing the most rapid growth, such as the distal femur, the proximal tibia, the proximal humerus, and the distal radius and ulna. Aside from generalized osteopenia and retarded growth, rickets demonstrates widening of the growth plate, flaring and cupping of the metaphyses, and eventually, bowing and deformity of the bones

Figure 10–37. A knee film in a 1-year-old boy demonstrates a number of classic findings of infantile rickets. There is widening of the growth plate, cupping of the metaphyses, and a somewhat frayed, indistinct appearance to the metaphyseal margins. In addition, there is a hint of bowing of the distal femur and the proximal tibia. This child suffered from nutritional rickets, the most common form.

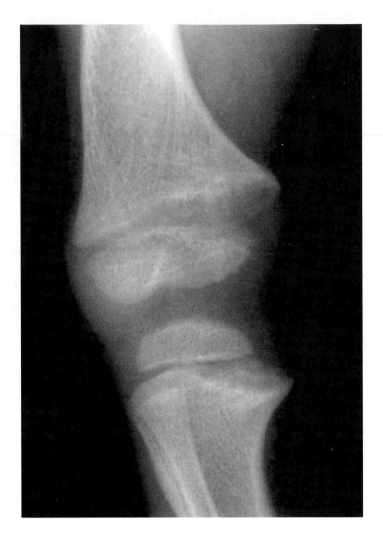

due to bone softening (Fig. 10–37). Once skeletal deformity results, surgical correction may be required. Although rickets is not as common as in years past, it is a disease the radiologist cannot afford to miss, because simple vitamin supplementation may prevent the development of severe skeletal deformity.

LEAD POISONING

A radiographic counterpart to rickets, which demonstrates metaphyseal lucencies, is plumbism, or lead poisoning, the radiographic hallmark of which is dense metaphyseal bands (Fig. 10–38). Another difference between the two disorders is that fact that while the most serious effect of vitamin D deficiency is seen in the skeleton, the bone changes of lead poisoning are merely a harbinger of more serious pathology elsewhere in the body. Lead toxicity's most serious effects are seen in the central nervous system, where it may result in irreversible mental retardation. Children suffering from lead intoxication may exhibit loss of appetite, vomiting, and abdominal cramps.

So-called lead lines or dense metaphyseal bands result from the toxic effect of lead on the growth plate. It is commonly thought that these dense lines result from the actual accumulation of lead, although this is not the case. Rather, the lead causes fail-

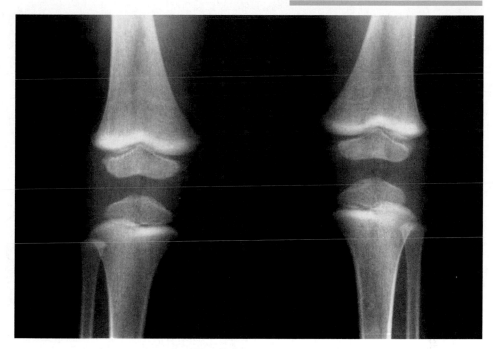

Figure 10–38. A 2½-year-old boy presented with leg pain. The frontal radiographs of both knees reveal dense transverse metaphyseal bands involving the femurs and tibias, which are highly suggestive of lead poisoning. These so-called lead lines do not represent an accumulation of lead in the metaphysis, but rather poisoning of cells in the zone of provisional calcification, with resultant failure of removal of calcified cartilaginous trabeculae. Once the radiologic diagnosis was suggested, serum lead levels were measured, which were elevated, and treatment was initiated. If left untreated, plumbism can result in increased intracranial pressure and irreversible mental retardation.

ure of the removal of calcified cartilaginous trabeculae in the zone of provisional calcification, with the result that an extradense line of calcification is seen along the metaphyseal side of the growth plate. Since the removal of lead from gasoline, the most common source of exposure is lead from paints, which children may ingest in the form of dust or paint chips. In cases of suspected lead ingestion, a plain film of the abdomen sometimes reveals radiopaque flecks within the GI tract (Fig. 10–39).

CHILD ABUSE

EPIDEMIOLOGY

The term *abuse* is subject to variable interpretation and may encompass intentional physical injury, sexual assault, neglect, and varying degrees of psychological trauma. Between 1 and 2 million cases of abuse occur every year in the United States.

PATHOPHYSIOLOGY

Children who have suffered one episode of undetected abuse have a 15% risk of repeat abuse, which carries a mortality rate of up to 10%. In other words, 1 to 2% of children who suffer undetected abuse will die as a result. Many others will suffer permanent disability. A failure to detect child abuse therefore carries a high risk of mortality. For this reason, mandatory

Figure 10–39. This abdominal plain film demonstrates multiple radiopaque chips scattered throughout the bowel, best seen in the right lateral abdomen. These chips represented lead that the child had been ingesting in the form of paint.

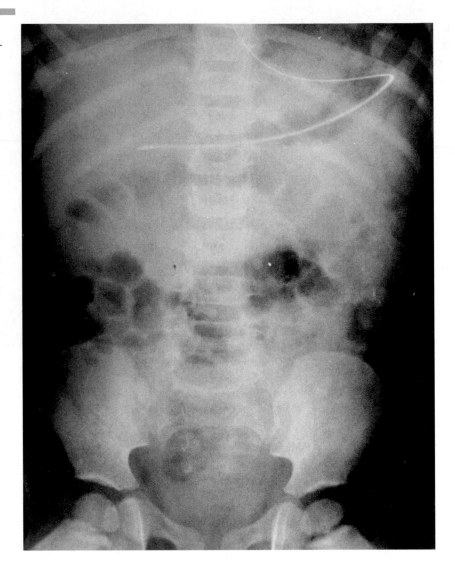

reporting statutes have been adopted in 50 states, and health care providers have been granted immunity for reports made in good faith.

CLINICAL PRESENTATION

Two-thirds of abuse takes place before the age of 6 years, at which stage it may be difficult for children to provide a history. However, a host of clinical clues applicable even at these young ages should increase suspicion of abuse. These include a history that does not correspond to the child's injury, an inconsistent or conflicting history, inappropriate parental concern, failure to seek parental sympathy and support, evidence of poor hygiene or nutrition, and an unreasonable delay in seeking care. Examples would include a 2-month-old who supposedly rolled off the changing table and fell onto the floor (the ability to roll over is acquired around the age of 5 months) or a child who supposedly sat down in scalding water (pain in the feet would prevent the child from sitting down). As a general rule, no child who is too young to move independently can cause itself significant injury.

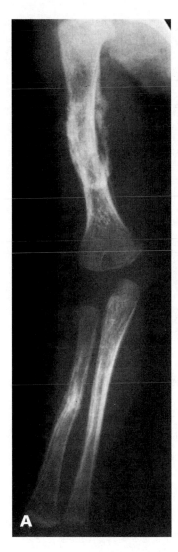

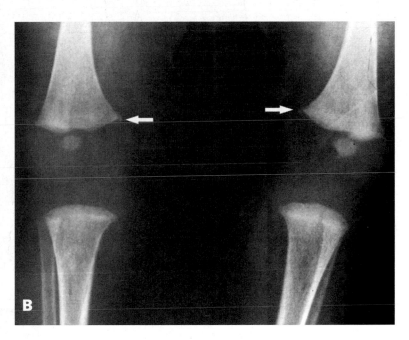

Figure 10–40. (A) This frontal radiograph of the arm reveals healing fractures of the humerus and radius. (B) This frontal radiograph of the knees demonstrates bilateral metaphyseal corner fractures (arrows), a highly specific finding of child abuse. For their own safety such children should be immediately removed from the environment in which the abuse is occurring.

IMAGING

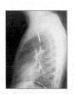 If the definition of abuse is restricted to physical injury, it is estimated that up to two-thirds of cases are radiologically detectable, meaning that radiologists play a critical role in making the diagnosis of abuse. Often, the radiologist detects evidence of abuse in a child in whom the diagnosis was not even suspected. Findings of child abuse on radiologic examination include skeletal injuries, intracranial injuries, and injuries to the abdominal viscera. While any form of skeletal injury may result, certain patterns of injury are relatively specific for abuse. These include metaphyseal fractures, such as the so-called corner or bucket-handle fractures at the chondro-osseous junction, which are commonly bilateral and involve the tibia, femur, and humerus (Fig. 10–40). When the child is squeezed in the anteroposterior axis, posterior rib fractures near the costovertebral junction may result. The finding of multiple fractures of various ages should set off alarm bells, although other disorders such as osteogenesis imperfecta must be considered. A classic sign of fracture is periosteal reaction secondary to subperiosteal

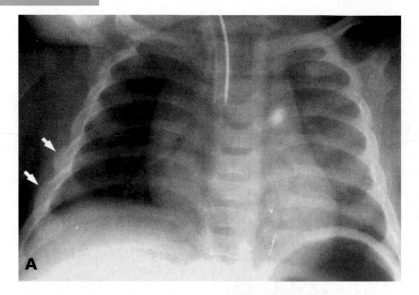

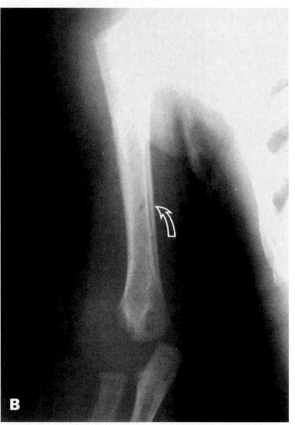

Figure 10–41. This infant was brought to the emergency department in severe respiratory distress. (A) A frontal chest radiograph obtained after intubation demonstrates clear lungs, but a very significant skeletal finding—at least two right-sided rib fractures (arrows). The child's parent provided no history of trauma, and the possibility of abuse arose. A radiographic skeletal survey was ordered. (B) A frontal view of the right humerus demonstrates prominent periosteal reaction along the humeral diaphysis (arrow), indicating post-traumatic subperiosteal hemorrhage. When added to the more acute rib fractures, this provides very strong evidence of abuse.

hemorrhage, which lifts the infant's loosely bound periosteum off the shaft and is followed by subperiosteal mineralization within 1 to 2 weeks (Fig. 10–41).

Intracranial injury carries a high risk of mortality and developmental delay. The most specific finding is an interhemispheric subdural hematoma, usually as part of the "shaken baby" syndrome, although skull fractures, subarachnoid hemorrhage, cerebral edema, and atrophy may also be seen (Fig. 10–42). The retinas should be closely inspected in every case, because the vast majority of "shaken babies" will

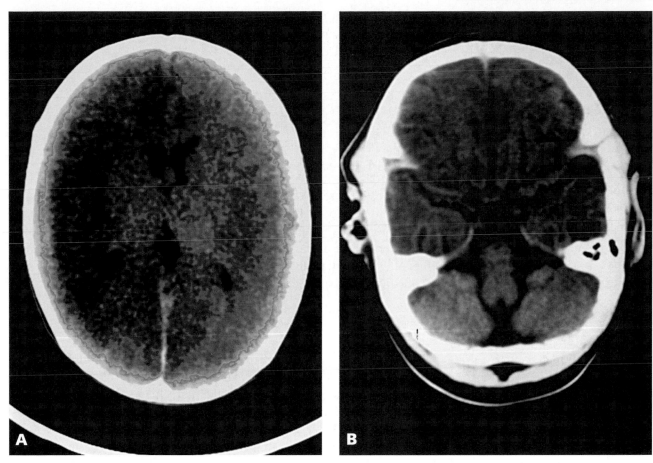

Figure 10–42. A 2-year-old boy was the victim of a strangulation injury. (A) An axial image from a noncontrast head computed tomography scan through the frontal horns demonstrates global cerebral swelling with obliteration of sulci, diminution in the size of the ventricles, and complete loss of the normal demarcation between gray and white matter. These findings indicate diffuse edema from hypoxia. (B) An image at the level of the suprasellar cistern demonstrates diffuse hypoattenuation in the inferior aspects of the frontal and temporal lobes, although the posterior fossa structures remain relatively bright. This represents the so-called white cerebellum sign, which reflects the relatively privileged status of the posterior fossa circulation. The prognosis in these types of injuries is poor.

exhibit retinal hemorrhages. Visceral injuries typically involve the liver, spleen, or kidneys, and the presence of visceral trauma in children younger than 5 years old (absent a history of motor vehicle accident or the like) should raise high suspicion of abuse.

What constitutes an appropriate imaging strategy for the suspected abuse victim? The mainstay of diagnosis is a plain radiographic skeletal survey, with tightly coned views of each anatomic region. Clinicians and radiologists must resist the temptation to reduce the child's radiation dose by obtaining as few radiographs as necessary to image the whole skeleton. The findings of abuse are often subtle, and can only be detected with tightly coned views of each anatomic region (anterioposterior and lateral skull, anteroposterior and lateral chest with bone technique, humeri, forearms, femurs, tibias, and perhaps the hands and feet). Some investigators suggest the use of bone scintigraphy as a screening procedure, due to its high sensitivity and ability to encompass the entire skeleton. If neurologic findings are present, a noninfused head CT is warranted, which should be followed up with MRI if the CT is negative and clinical suspicion is high. Body CT is indicated only in the presence of clinical findings such as abdominal distention and tenderness.

Urinary Tract

INFECTION

EPIDEMIOLOGY

Urinary tract infections are a relatively common problem in children, constituting the second most prevalent infection in the pediatric age group (after respiratory tract infections) and the most common problem of the urinary tract. It is estimated that up to 10% of girls experience a urinary tract infection. In children with urinary tract infections, reflux of urine from the bladder into the ureters and/or renal collecting systems is seen in one-quarter to one-half of patients.

PATHOPHYSIOLOGY

Pathophysiologically, most urinary tract infections are thought to stem from the ascent of bacteria from the perineum up through the urethra. Girls are thought to be at especially high risk, due to their relatively short urethras. The close proximity of the female urethral orifice and the anus may be another factor. This latter suggestion is supported by the fact that the most common organism, responsible for up to three-quarters of cases, is the enteric commensal, *Escherichia coli*. There are several normal barriers to bacterial growth and migration. First, the low pH of the vagina and perineum exerts a bacteriostatic effect. Second, any bacteria that reach the bladder are normally flushed out with voiding. Third, the ureterovesical junction exhibits an antireflux valve flap action. Factors that interfere with these protective mechanisms include an alteration in normal vaginal/perineal flora, urinary stasis, and immaturity or deformity of the ureterovesical junction.

Vesicoureteral reflux tends to resolve spontaneously with time, as the distance traveled by the distal ureter in the submucosa of the bladder increases with age. The longer the submucosal ureter, the more effective the ureterovesical junction's intrinsic antireflux mechanism. Contraction of the smooth muscle within the bladder wall at voiding increases intravesical pressure and tends to produce reflux if the ureterovesical junction valve mechanism is incompetent. Aside from primary valve incompetence, other structural lesions that predispose to vesicoureteral reflux include a periureteral diverticulum (an outpouching of the bladder wall), a ureterocele (protrusion of the distal ureter into the bladder lumen), and a ureteral duplication. Moreover, any form of bladder outlet obstruction will lead to abnormally increased intravesical pressures during voiding, with a further increase in the probability of reflux. Complications of ascending infection due to reflux include pyelonephritis, renal scarring, hypertension, and renal failure.

CLINICAL PRESENTATION

A urinary tract infection is defined as the presence of more than 100,000 organisms in a clean-catch urine specimen. The presence of any bacteria in a specimen obtained by catheterization or suprapubic puncture is also abnormal. The younger the child, the less likely that the clinical presentation will be specific. Anorexia, fever, lethargy, and failure to thrive are the most frequently noted findings in the young patient. More classic symptoms of frequency, dysuria, flank pain, and fever are seen in older children.

IMAGING

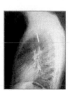

The imaging of urinary tract infection in children is focused on answering two critical questions. First, is there a structural abnormality of the urinary tract that would predispose to infection, such as a urethral outlet obstruction or a bladder diverticulum producing urinary stasis (Fig 10–43)? Second, is there vesicoureteral reflux? While a first urinary tract infection in a girl may be treated empirically, it is generally agreed that any recurrent urinary tract infection in a girl or the first urinary tract infection in a boy warrants imaging evaluation. Some clinicians recommend that any child younger than 4 years of age with a urinary tract infection undergo imaging.

Key studies include the voiding cystourethrogram, the nuclear medicine cystogram, and ultrasound of the upper urinary tract. The voiding cystourethrogram provides the best anatomic evaluation of the bladder and urethra, and is also quite sensitive in the detection of vesicoureteral reflux (Fig. 10–44). It is performed by the transurethral insertion of a bladder catheter, followed by the instillation of iodinated contrast under fluoroscopic monitoring. The nuclear medicine cystogram involves the

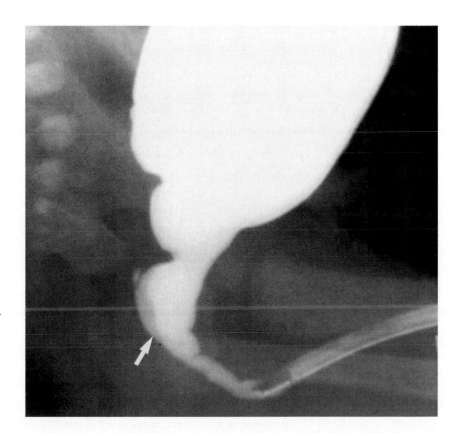

Figure 10–43. This voiding cystourethrogram was performed in an infant boy with a weak urinary stream and urinary tract infection. A lateral spot film demonstrates marked dilatation of the posterior urethra (arrow), caused by obstructing posterior uretheral valves. This condition is seen in 1 in 5000 males. Note the catheter extending into the more distal urethra. Such valves are commonly lyzed by electrode fulguration.

Figure 10–44. (A) This oblique view from a voiding cystourethrogam demonstrates bilateral vesicoureteral reflux, with grade II reflux on the right and a combination of reflux and a ureteropelvic junction (UPJ) obstruction on the left. R, right renal collecting system; B, bladder. (B) A delayed frontal film demonstrates marked dilatation of the left renal collecting system, which still contains contrast, due to the UPJ obstruction. L, left renal collecting system.

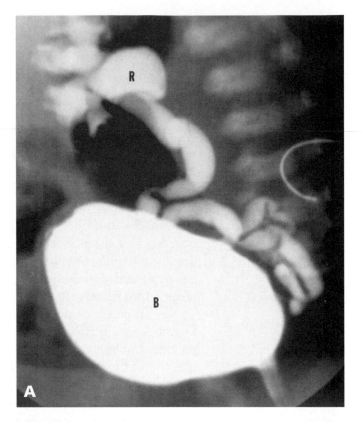

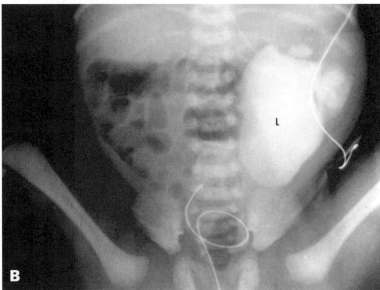

transurethral introduction of a radiotracer into the bladder. While radionuclide cystography provides a poorer anatomic evaluation of the urinary tract than voiding cystourethrogram, it possesses the advantage that its radiation dose is lower and it is equally sensitive in the detection of reflux (Fig. 10–45). Ultrasound is employed primarily to evaluate for renal size, the presence of renal parenchymal scarring, and hydronephrosis. The imaging study with the best sensitivity in the diagnosis of pyelonephritis is renal cortical scintigraphy, which can also be used to evaluate function and parenchymal scarring.

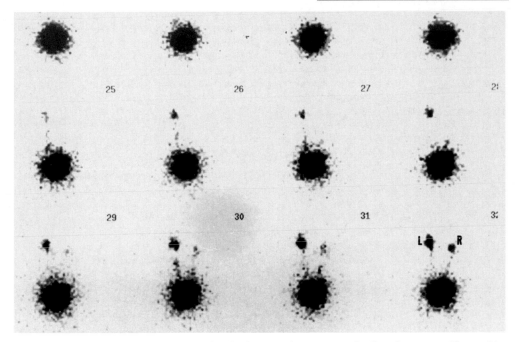

Figure 10–45. A 2-year-old girl presented with a history of vesicoureteral reflux, documented by a voiding cystourethrogram. A nuclear medicine study employing the transurethral administration of technetium-99m-sulfur colloid was performed a year later to determine if reflux was still present. Sequential posterior images demonstrate filling of the bladder with radiotracer solution. Before voiding, prominent reflux of contrast into the left ureter and renal pelvis are seen. As the patient begins to void, there is additional reflux on the right, indicating continued incompetence of both ureterovesical junctions.

Medical management is generally employed for more mild degrees of vesicoureteral reflux, the theory being that if the urine can be kept sterile, no complications of reflux are likely to arise, and meantime, most children will outgrow their reflux. When reflux is more severe and associated with dilatation of the upper urinary tract (hydronephrosis), surgical intervention may be indicated.

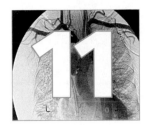

Self-Assessment

CASE 1

This plain abdominal radiograph reveals the presence of multiple oblong opacities within the air-filled colon. What might these represent and how did they get there? Can you tell if this patient is male or female?

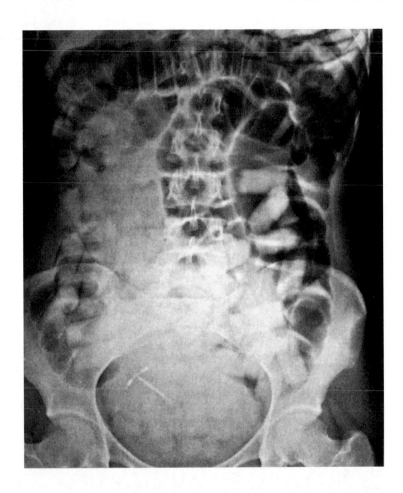

CASE 2

This 59-year-old woman with a history of vulvar cancer presented with right hip pain. What abnormalities do you see on this frontal radiograph of the hip?

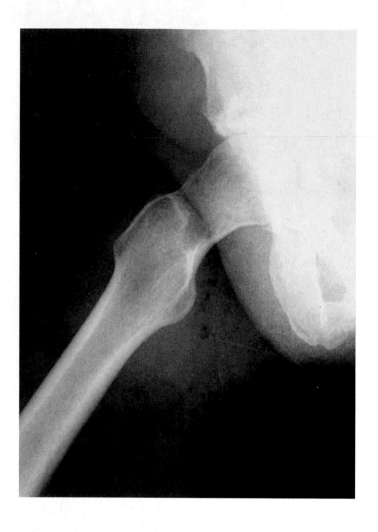

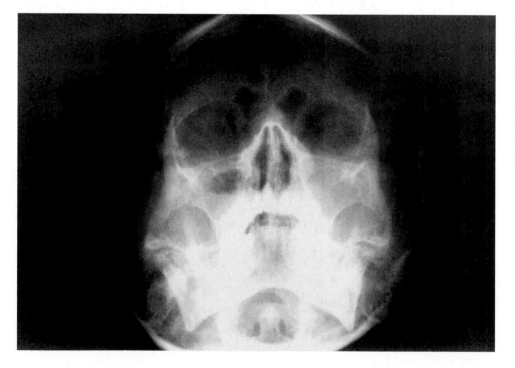

CASE 3

This 39-year-old man presented with the acute onset of right facial pain. Does the frontal radiograph demonstrate any explanation for the patient's symptoms?

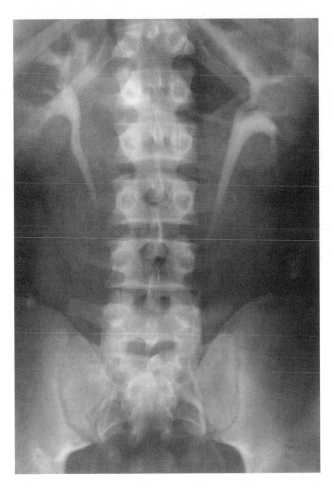

CASE 4

This young adult who presented with right flank pain underwent an intravenous urogram. A single overhead radiograph reveals the source of the patient's symptoms. What is it? (Note: The patient's urinalysis demonstrated no hematuria.)

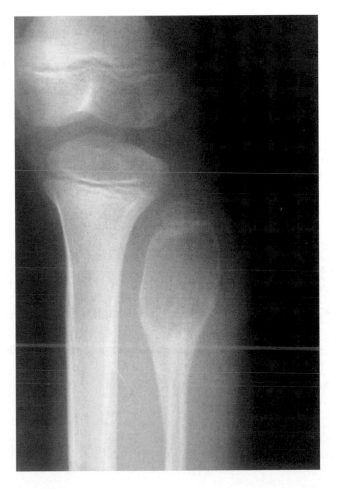

CASE 5

This 7-year-old boy presented with a painful left-sided limp. What do you see in his radiograph?

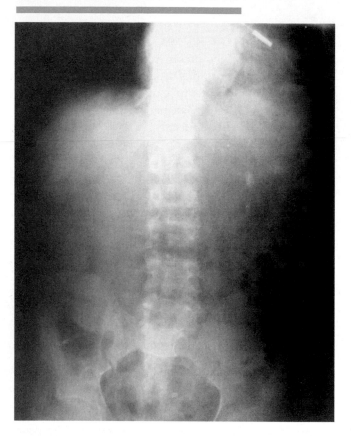

CASE 6

This 50-year-old patient with a history of alcoholism was admitted to the hospital with a suspected stroke. A portable plain radiograph of the abdomen was obtained on the second day after admission to rule out obstruction, because the patient had developed vague abdominal tenderness. What does the radiograph reveal?

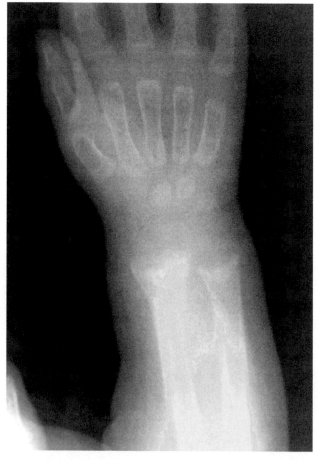

CASE 7

This 2-year-old boy presented with refusal to use the right wrist, and a radiograph was obtained to rule out fracture. Is there a fracture? What abnormality does the radiograph demonstrate and what are its major causes?

CASE 8

This 10-year-old boy presented with symptoms of an acute stroke. What abnormality do you detect on these T1-weighted sagittal magnetic resonance images, and what could account for it?

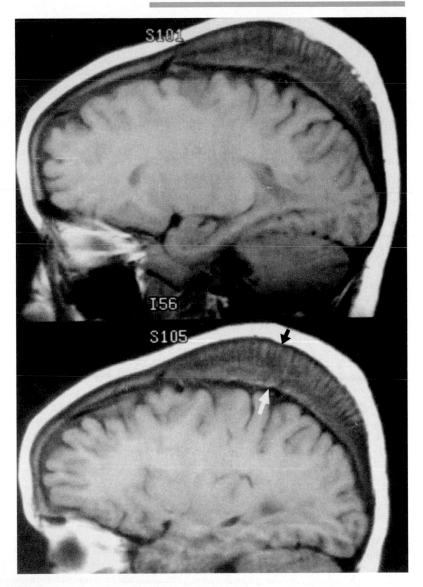

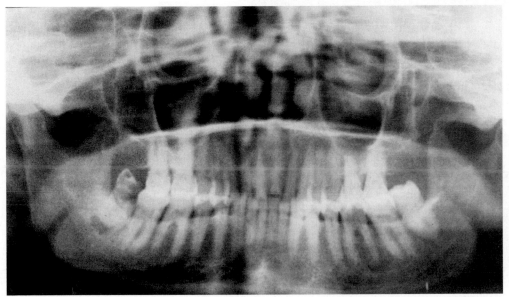

CASE 9

This 69-year-old hospitalized patient complained of a toothache. A panorex view of the maxilla and mandible was ordered. A panorex is performed using a special apparatus in which both the tube and the film pivot around the patient's face. Do you see any explanation for the patient's toothache?

CASE 10

This 51-year-old obese woman presented with a history of vomiting and abdominal distention. What do you see in this supine radiograph? What is the most likely etiology of these findings?

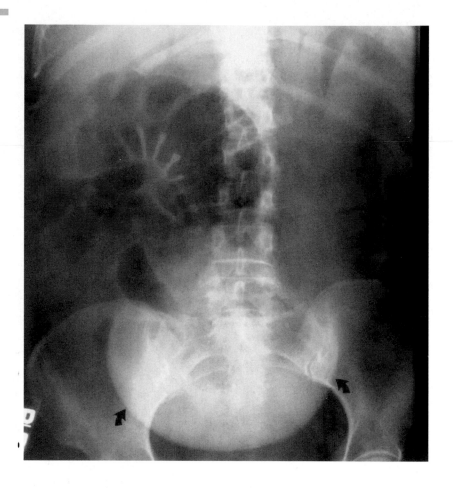

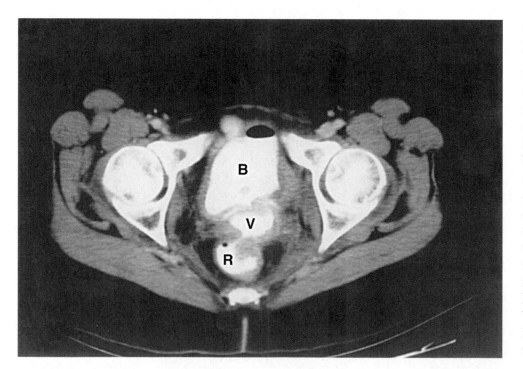

CASE 11

This 43-year-old woman with a history of treated squamous cell carcinoma of the cervix presented with a history of vaginal bleeding and a foul-smelling vaginal discharge. A contrast-enhanced computed tomography examination was performed, from which an axial image through the lower pelvis is shown. What does it show? How do you explain this finding?

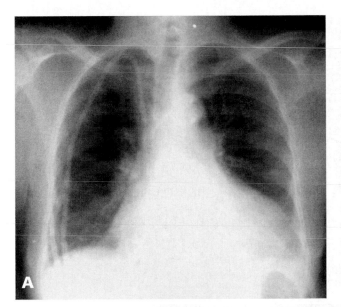

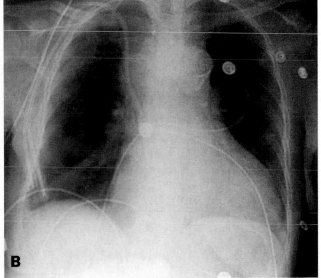

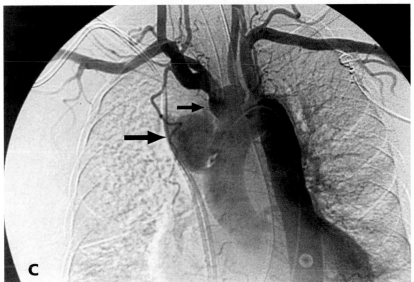

CASE 12

This 60-year-old woman with a history of end-stage renal disease recently underwent replacement of her double-lumen central venous catheter for hemodialysis. (A) A portable chest radiograph demonstrates the catheter, inserted via the right internal jugular vein. Is there any evidence of pneumothorax or other complication of line placement? (B) Some weeks later, the patient was admitted to the intensive care unit with a septic picture. A portable chest radiograph obtained at that time demonstrates an important change. What has changed, and how would you account for it? (C) The cause of this unusual configuration was found in the patient's aorta. In this digital subtraction aortogram, a pigtail catheter has been advanced into the ascending aorta via a femoral artery approach. What does the contrast injection reveal?

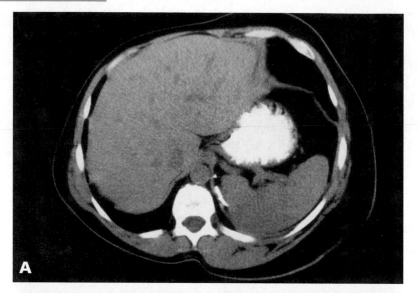

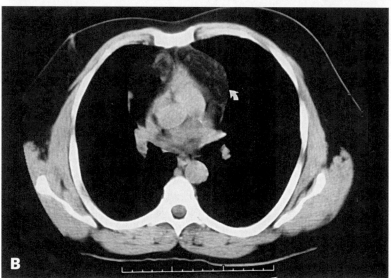

CASE 13

This 39-year-old male presented for a surveillance computed tomography scan 1 year after undergoing a left nephrectomy and adrenalectomy for renal cell carcinoma. (**A**) An axial section at the expected level of the upper kidneys reveals empty renal fossae. What else do you notice? (**B**) An image of the thorax at the level of the proximal great vessels reveals no evidence of thoracic asymmetry, although there is a striking amount of anterior mediastinal lipomatosis (arrow). How can we account for these peculiar findings?

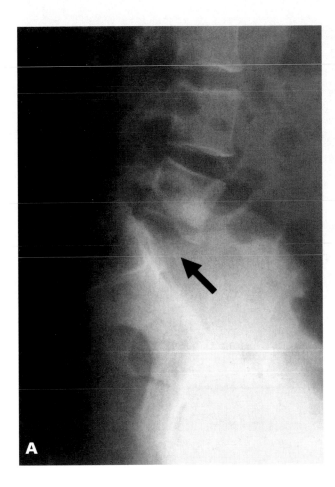

CASE 14

This 41-year-old human immunodeficiency virus-positive woman presented with a history of staphylococcus bacteremia 3 weeks previously. She now complains of severe low back pain. (A) What does the lateral radiograph of the lumbar spine reveal? (B) What does this contrast-enhanced T1-weighted magnetic resonance image (in which the patient appears to be facing the opposite direction) reveal?

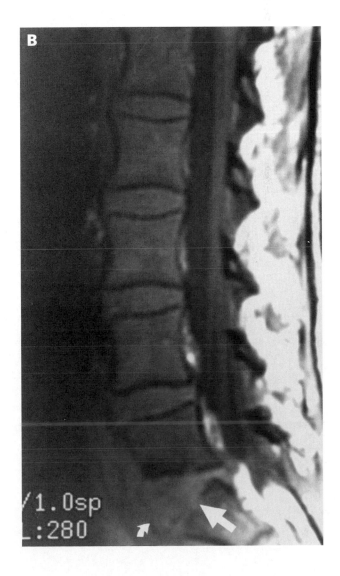

CASE 15

This 45-year-old hospitalized patient complained of the recent onset of abdominal pain and underwent portable abdominal radiography to rule out an intestinal obstruction. This film, exposed with the patient lying supine, demonstrates a large, lobulated, calcific mass in the right side of the pelvis (arrow). What is the differential diagnosis of this finding? Could it be a laterally displaced uterine fibroid? Could it be a primary musculoskeletal tumor, such as an osteosarcoma or chondrosarcoma? Does the shape of the mass or its location offer any clue?

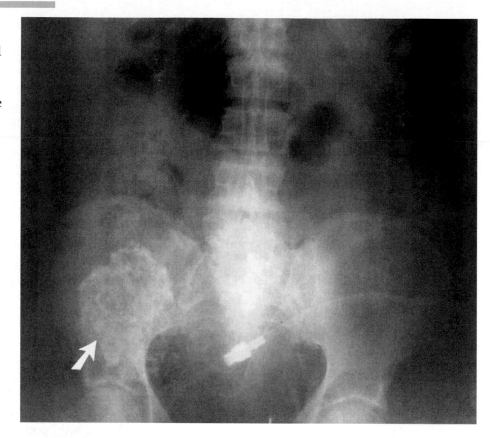

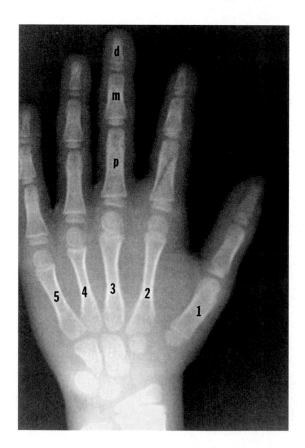

CASE 16

This patient presented complaining of pain. A single frontal radiograph of the hand was obtained. Is this a skeletally mature or immature patient? Do you see an explanation for the patient's pain? How would you describe the abnormality? How might you further evaluate this patient? d, distal phalanx; m, middle phalanx; p, proximal phalanx; 1 to 5, first to fifth metacarpals.

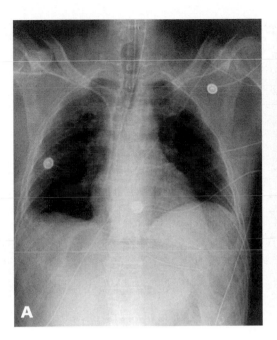

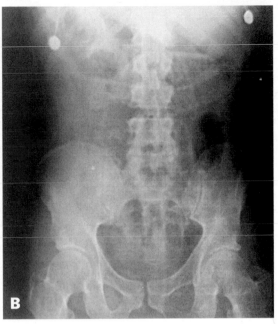

CASE 17

This 53-year-old male suffered a cardiac arrest 2 days previously. (A) At the time this portable chest radiograph was obtained, the patient was in the intensive care unit. How would you describe the position of the lines and tubes? Do you see any abnormalities? If you were not sure about your finding, what would you do next? (B) A portable abdominal radiograph was obtained at the same time as the chest film. What is the finding?

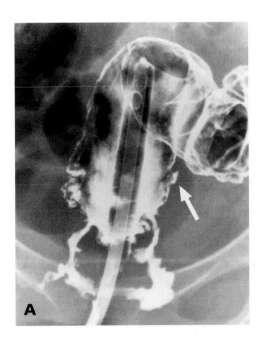

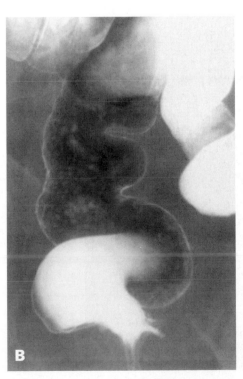

CASE 18

(A) This spot film from a double-contrast study of the anorectal region was performed after insertion of a soft catheter into the rectum. What are the findings on this image, and what diagnosis do they suggest? (B) What would be your diagnosis of this spot film from the rectum of another patient?

CASE 19

Is this anteroposterior chest radiograph normal? What syndrome could account for any constellation of findings you may seen?

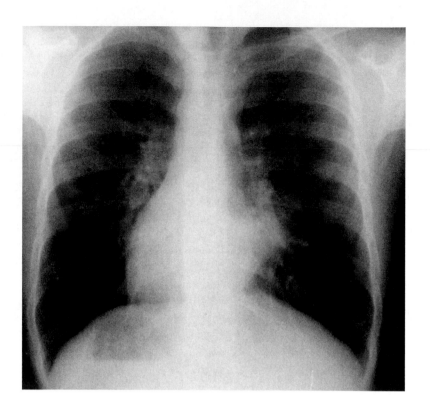

CASE 20

Is this hand radiograph normal? How would you describe the abnormality?

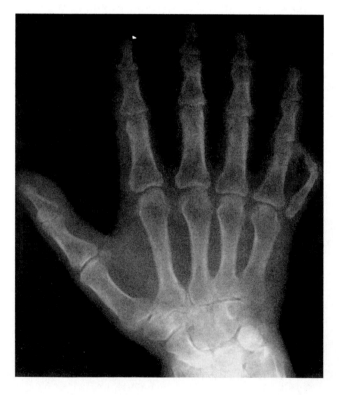

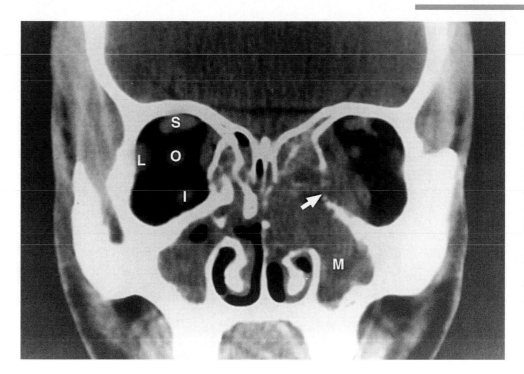

CASE 21

This 26-year-old acquired immunodeficiency syndrome patient presented with left-sided sinus pain and associated facial swelling. A coronal image from a computed tomography scan of the paranasal sinuses reveals the etiology of his symptoms. Comparing the two sides, what abnormalities can you discern?

CASE 22

This 22-month-old child developed severe dysphagia, neck stiffness, and fever. Physical examination demonstrated prominent bilateral cervical lymphadenopathy. Differential diagnostic considerations included neuroblastoma, foreign body, traumatic instrumentation, and retropharyngeal abscess, with the infectious presentation favoring the latter. A contrast-infused computed tomography scan of the neck was obtained. What are the findings on this axial image, and what would be the most probable diagnosis?

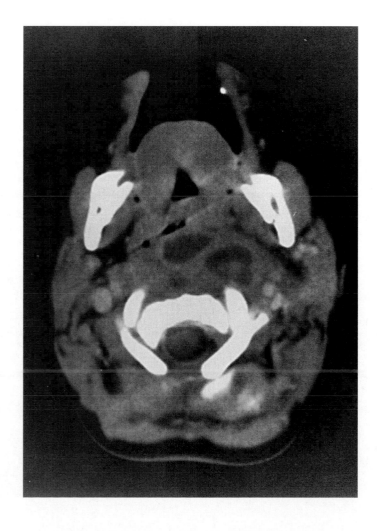

CASE 23

This young woman with systemic lupus erythematosus on chronic corticosteroid therapy developed severe right hip pain. Plain films of the hip (not shown) were normal. The patient manifested no signs of infection, although these could be masked by her immunosuppressive therapy. What diagnoses would you consider in this patient? Based on this preinfusion T1-weighted coronal image of the right hip, what is your diagnosis? A, acetabulum; N, femoral neck; T, greater trochanter.

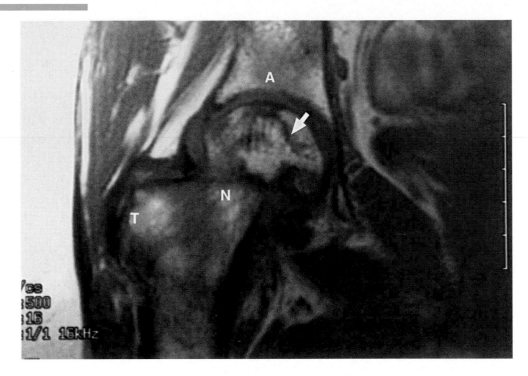

CASE 24

This 60-year-old man with a history of "arthritis" presented with an acute attack of severe right knee pain. What diagnosis would you make based on this frontal radiograph of the knee? Support your diagnosis.

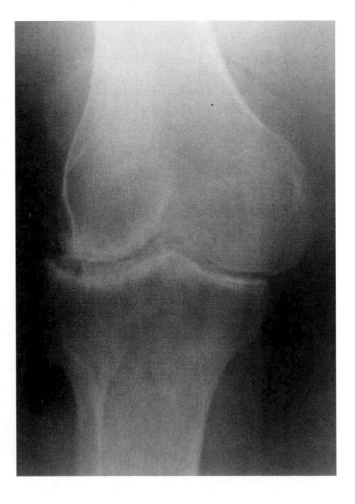

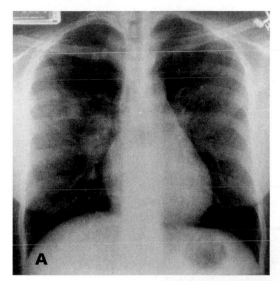

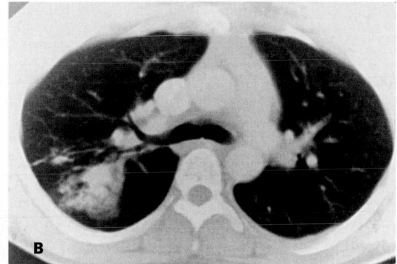

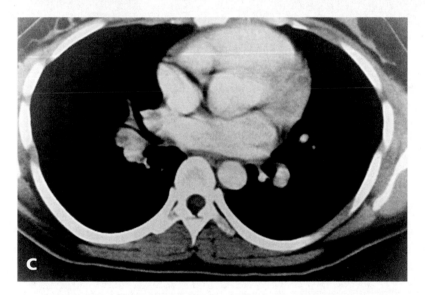

CASE 25

This 23-year-old postpartum woman presented to the emergency department with the abrupt onset of hemoptysis. She reported no prodromal symptoms to suggest an infectious process. (**A**) A posteroanterior chest radiograph was obtained. How would you report this case; in particular, what differential diagnosis would you offer? (**B**) A contrast-infused thoracic computed tomography examination was obtained. What does it show? (**C**) An axial image with mediastinal windows at the level of the left atrium demonstrates a prominent filling defect in one of the right upper lobe pulmonary artery branches. What is your diagnosis?

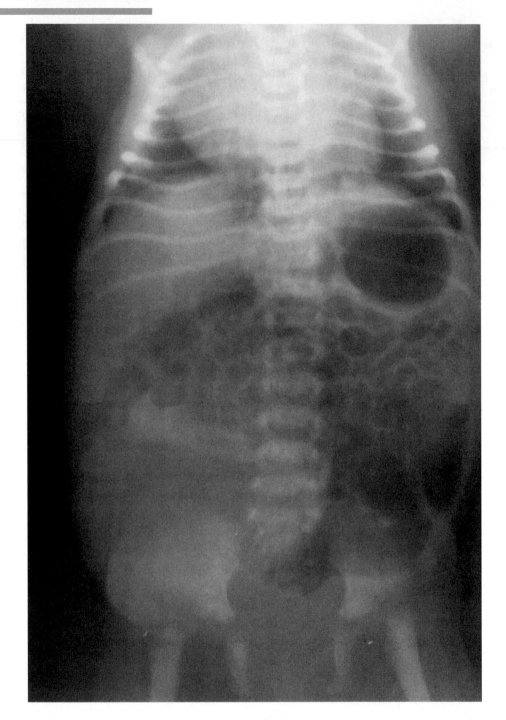

CASE 26

A single frontal "babygram" radiograph is provided. How old is this child? What are the findings on this film? What pathologic condition would you invoke to explain this constellation of findings?

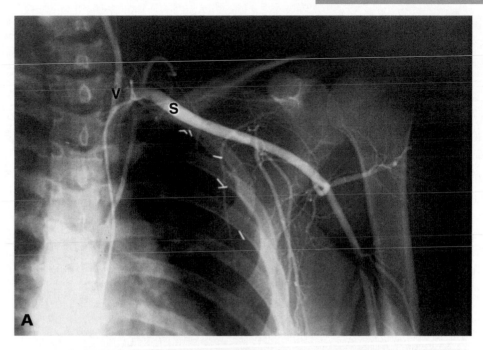

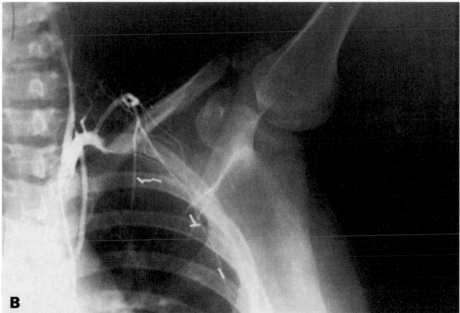

CASE 27

This young adult complained of intermittent left arm weakness and numbness. On physical examination, the patient's symptoms were reproducible with abduction of the shoulder (raising the arm above the head). What diagnoses should be considered with such a presentation? (A) An upper extremity arteriogram was requested for further evaluation. What do you notice in this frontal view of a selective left subclavian artery injection with the left arm at the patient's side? s, left subclavian artery; v, left vertebral artery. (B) When the arm was abducted, a repeat injection was given. What does it show?

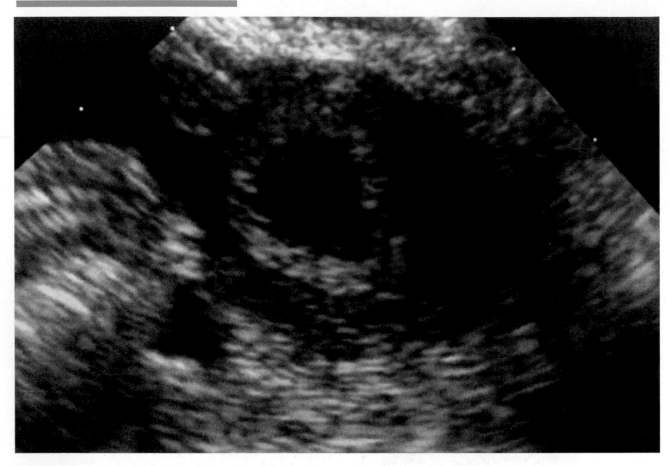

CASE 28

This 19-year-old woman presented to the emergency department complaining of cramping pelvic pain and mild vaginal bleeding. What crucial question must be answered in such a case to properly evaluate the patient? What diagnosis must be excluded, what test would you perform to exclude such a diagnosis, and what would you look for? What does this image reveal and what are the risk factors for this diagnosis?

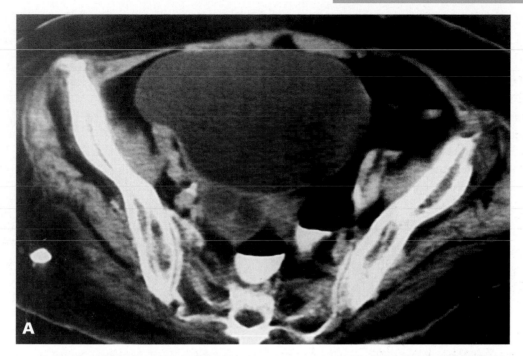

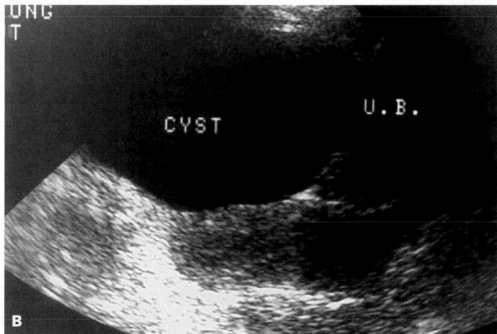

CASE 29

This 60-year-old woman presented with a large pelvic mass. At the referring clinician's request, a computed tomography scan of the abdomen and pelvis was performed. (A) What are your findings on this axial image through the pelvis at the level of the sacrum? What might these findings represent? (B) What do you notice on this ultrasound of the same patient?

CASE 30

This elderly woman presented with complaints of severe left flank pain and pyuria. A contrast-infused abdomen and pelvis computed tomography scan was performed, from which an axial image at the level of the kidneys is presented. What abnormality do you detect?

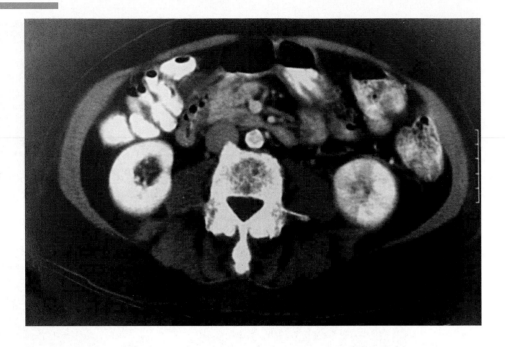

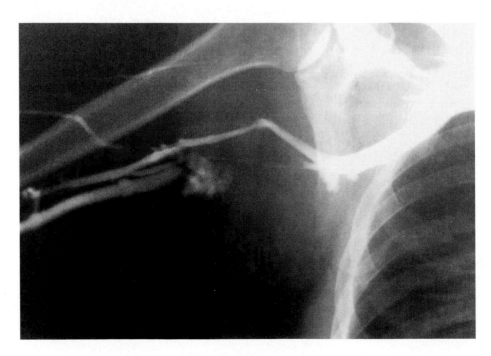

CASE 31

This young man suffered a bullet wound to the right axilla. Peripheral pulses and neurologic function were intact, but there was an expanding subcutaneous mass at the site, and an angiogram was requested to further evaluate the injury. Examine this frontal image from the angiogram. Note that there is an area of extravasation, which is surrounded by tiny metallic densities representing bullet fragments. Can you estimate the amount of blood loss from the site? Is this an arteriogram or a venogram? What is the diagnosis?

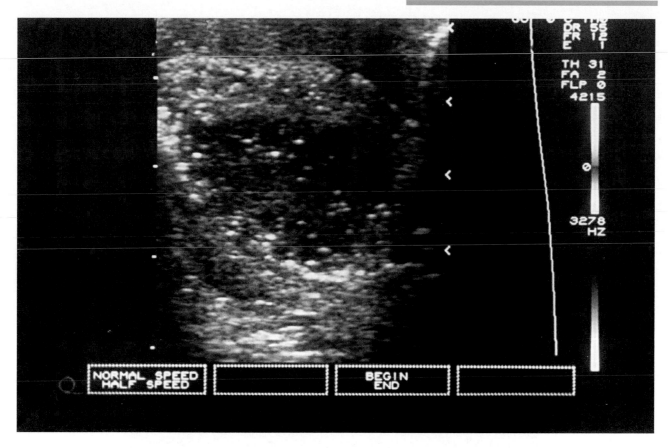

CASE 32

This 35-year-old man presented with a right scrotal mass. What are the most common causes of a solid testicular mass? What are the findings on this axial sonogram of the right testis?

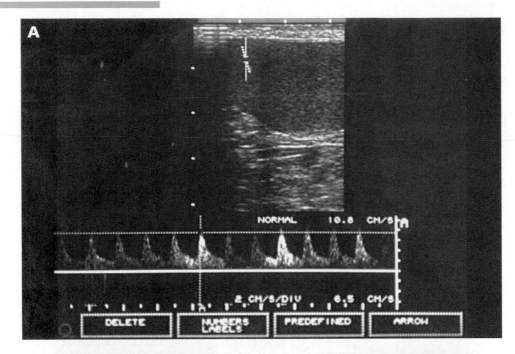

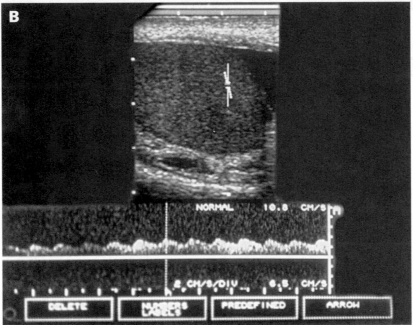

CASE 33

This 22-year-old man presented with the acute onset of right scrotal pain and tenderness. The urinalysis was normal. Without the aid of radiologic studies, what would be your differential diagnosis for this patient? A scrotal ultrasound examination was performed. (**A**) The normal left testis was imaged first. What does this longitudinal image demonstrate? (**B**) What does the examination of the right testis demonstrate? What is the diagnosis?

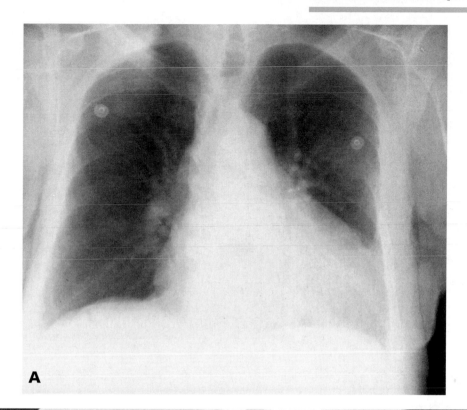

A

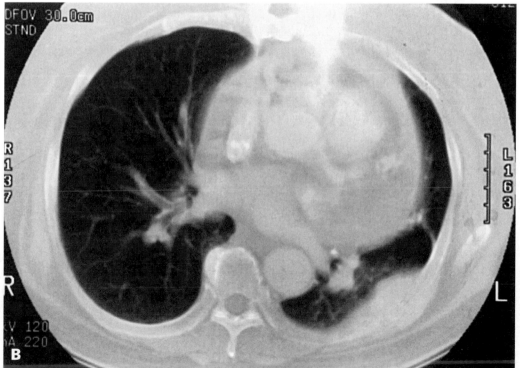

B

CASE 34

This 60-year-old woman presented with a several month history of worsening left-sided chest pain. (A) Do you see any explanation for the patient's pain on this posteroanterior chest radiograph? (B) An axial image from a postinfusion computed tomography scan of the chest was performed. What does this show?

CASE 35

This elderly man received a radiograph of the pelvis in the emergency department. What abnormality can you identify?

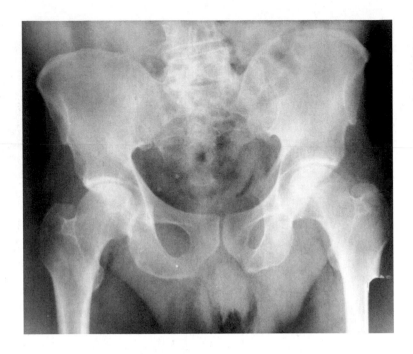

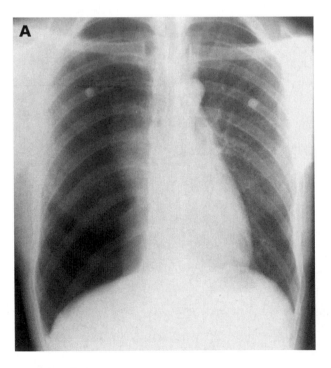

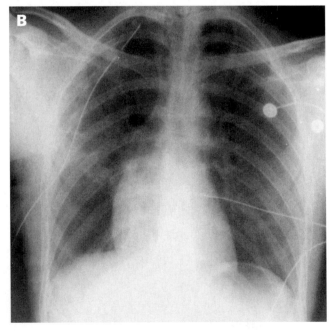

CASE 36

This 24-year-old man presented to the emergency department with acute shortness of breath. (A) A portable chest radiograph was obtained. What is the etiology of this patient's dyspnea, and what therapy would you recommend? (B) What are the significant findings on the follow-up film?

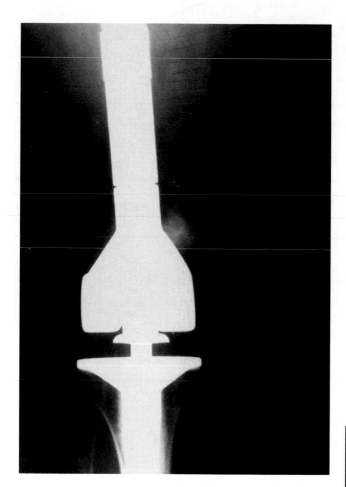

CASE 37

This young woman had undergone limb-sparing surgery for an osteogenic sarcoma of her left femur. She presented with knee pain. A frontal radiograph of the left knee demonstrates a metallic left knee prosthesis. Do you see any worrisome finding?

CASE 38

This lateral chest radiograph in a patient with a history of mitral valve disease demonstrates enlargement of a cardiac chamber. Which chamber is enlarged?

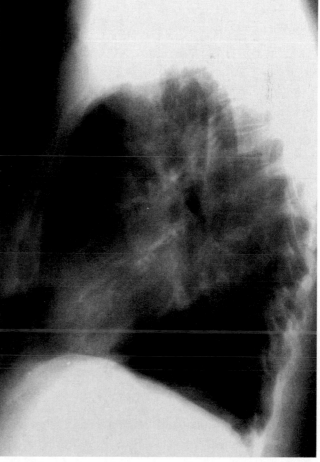

CASE 39

This elderly woman was admitted with symptoms of a urinary tract infection. A contrast-infused abdominal computed tomography scan was obtained to rule out complicated pyelonephritis. What abnormalities do you detect on this film? What is this likely to represent?

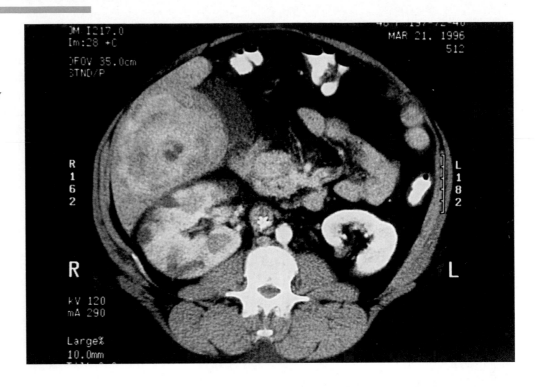

CASE 40

This is an axial image from a postinfusion abdominal computed tomography examination. Was intravenous contrast administered? How can you tell?

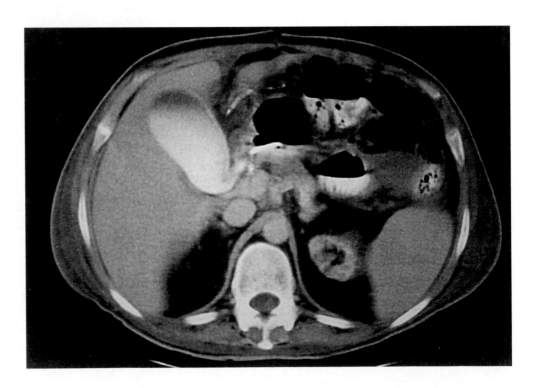

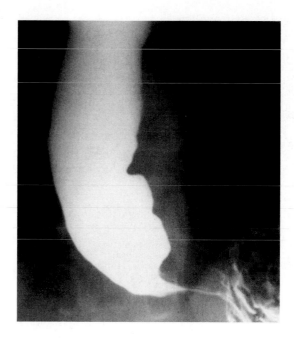

CASE 41

This middle-aged patient complained of chronic dysphagia. A single contrast esophagogram was performed. What abnormality do you note on this spot film of the distal esophagus and gastroesophageal junction? What is your diagnosis?

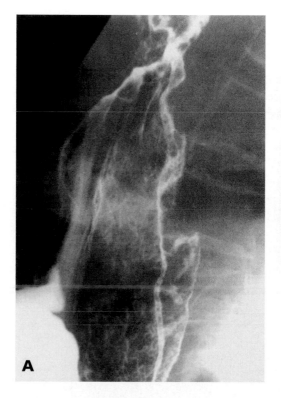

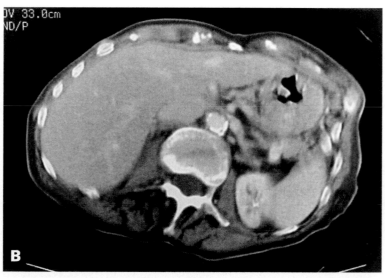

CASE 42

(A) This lateral spot film from a barium upper gastrointestinal examination demonstrates an abnormality in the posterior wall of the gastric cardia and gastroesophageal junction. How would you describe it? What is the differential diagnosis? How would you verify your diagnosis? (B) An axial image from a staging computed tomography scan. What does this image demonstrate?

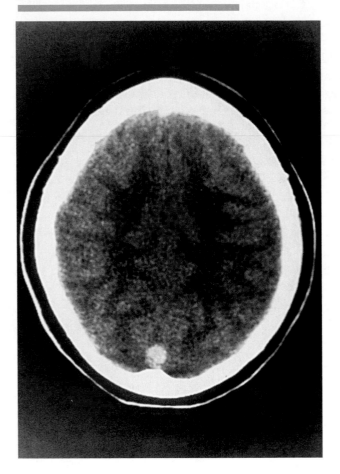

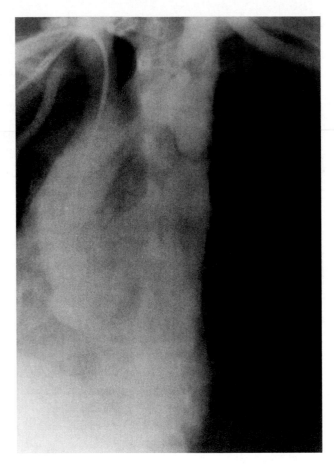

CASE 43

This infant presented with lethargy progressing to obtundation. A noncontrast head computed tomography examination was obtained to rule out an intracranial bleed. What abnormality do you detect on this axial image, and what would you include in your differential diagnosis? What types of processes could be responsible for these findings? Is there a normal structure in this location? What is your diagnosis?

CASE 44

This film from an aortogram in the left anterior oblique projection demonstrates an important congenital abnormality. What is it? What sign could be detected on chest radiography, and what is the diagnosis?

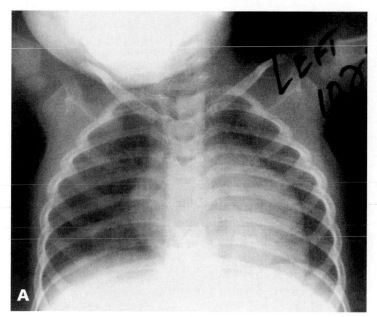

CASE 45

This 1-year-old child presented with the abrupt onset of dysphagia and coughing. (A) A frontal chest radiograph demonstrates clear lungs. Do you detect any abnormality? What study might you consider performing next? (B) On the lateral view, a foreign body (arrow) is easily identified in the mediastinum. Is it in the trachea or the esophagus?

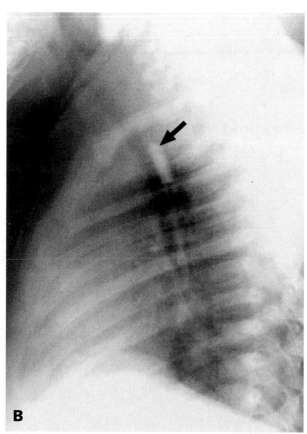

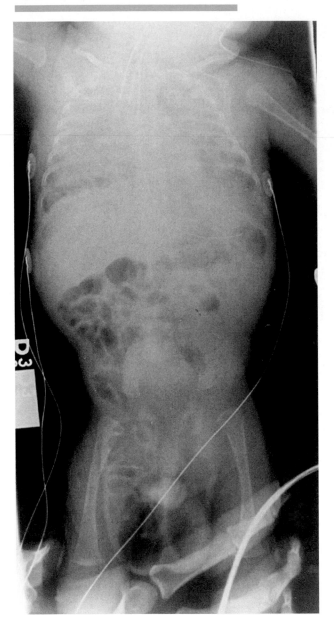

CASE 46

This 7-week-old infant in the neonatal intensive care unit displayed symptoms and signs of intermittent bowel obstruction. Can you find an etiology on this "babygram?" (Note at the bottom of the image the hand bones of the technician who was holding the infant's legs.)

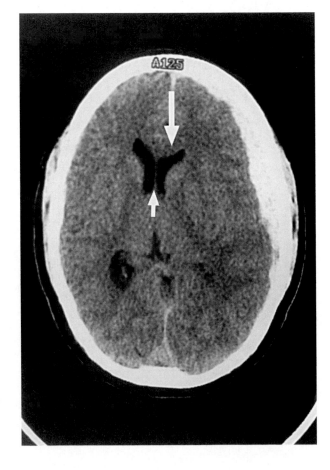

CASE 47

This 30-year-old man was beaten up and presented with obtundation. What abnormality do you detect on this axial image from his noncontrast head computed tomography scan? What is your diagnosis?

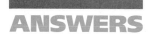

ANSWERS

Case 1 While there are many possible explanations, in this case these opacities represent narcotic-filled condoms in a drug courier. The opacity of the narcotic itself may be due to talc, which is often used to "cut" the drug. In this case, the presence of a "T"-shaped intrauterine contraceptive device within the pelvis indicates that the subject is a woman.

Case 2 The film demonstrates tiny collections of gas within the soft tissues of the proximal thigh. Subsequent aspiration of an associated fluid collection grew out *Staphylococcus aureus.* One of the critical findings to be sought out on every study in a patient with suspected infection is an abnormal collection of air, which may be the only plain radiographic indication of an abscess.

Case 3 There is complete opacification of the left maxillary sinus, with an air-fluid level in the right maxillary sinus. (Note that the maxillary sinuses are projected just below the orbits on this view.) The finding of an air-fluid level usually indicates acute sinusitis. If the patient failed to respond to standard antibiotic therapy, a thin-section computed tomography examination of the paranasal sinuses in the coronal projection might be warranted to rule out an obstruction to normal drainage.

Case 4 The renal collecting systems and proximal ureters exhibit an unremarkable appearance, demonstrating no filling defects or dilation. The real culprit is seen superimposed over the right sacrum—a round, calcific structure that was proved at surgery to represent an appendicolith in an inflamed appendix.

Case 5 The frontal radiograph of the proximal lower leg demonstrates an expansile, cystic-appearing lesion in the proximal left fibula, which is surrounded by a very thin but intact layer of cortex. The lesion's margins are relatively distinct, the epiphyseal plate is intact, and there is no associated periosteal reaction or soft tissue mass. At surgery the lesion proved to be an aneurysmal bone cyst, a benign, non-neoplastic lesion of blood-filled cystic spaces most commonly seen before the age of 20 years. The most common complication of these lesions is pathologic fracture, and for that reason, the lesion was curettaged and packed with bone chips.

Case 6 This patient's radiograph demonstrates no evidence of obstruction, with scattered gas and debris throughout much of the colon, and no dilated segments of bowel. A possible etiology for the patient's abdominal pain is revealed in the left upper quadrant, where course calcifications in the expected location of the pancreatic tail suggest chronic pancreatitis. More significantly, an enteric feeding tube overlies the left side of the heart and had been inadvertently placed in a left lower lobe bronchus. This finding mandates urgent notification of the clinical service, because administration of an enteric feeding through the tube could produce severe chemical pneumonitis. Also note the tiny bone island in the left aspect of the sacrum.

Case 7 No fracture is visible in this case. The distal radial and ulnar metaphyses are cupped and frayed, indicating rickets. Major etiologies include an inadequate dietary supply of vitamin D, a failure to absorb ingested vitamin D due to a gastrointestinal tract abnormality, liver disease (with failure to hydroxylate vitamin D), and renal disease (with failure to hydroxylate 25-OH vitamin D). The most common is nutritional deficiency. In this case, appropriate dietary treatment resulted in complete resolution.

Case 8 Sagittal T1-weighted images from a magnetic resonance imaging examination demonstrate tremendous expansion of the cranial marrow cavity (arrows). Note the multiple verticle striations throughout the expanded marrow, producing a so-called "hair on end" appearance that can also be seen on plain radiography (not shown). What could be responsible for such tremendous marrow cavity expansion, especially in a 10-year-old being evaluated for stroke? The two principal differential diagnoses are sickle-cell anemia and thalassemia. Since vascular occlusion is more common in sickle-cell disease, it represents the most likely possibility, and was in fact the correct diagnosis here. Seen in approximately 1% of the black population, sickle-cell disease results from a point mutation on the hemoglobin molecule, rendering erythrocytes more rigid and subject to increased hemolysis. While the normal lifespan of an erythrocyte is 120 days, the erythrocytes of a sickle-cell patient may survive for as little as 10 days, which is responsible for clinical findings such as anemia and jaundice, as well as radiographic findings such as marrow expansion throughout the body and avascular necrosis of the hips and shoulders.

Case 9 There is destruction of the anterior aspect of the right lower third molar, indicating a large cavity. In addition, there is resorption of bone around the root of that tooth, suggesting an abscess.

Case 10 A supine radiograph of the abdomen demonstrates a large round soft tissue mass superimposed over the lower abdomen, with smooth borders (arrows). Note that its inferolateral borders are extremely well demarcated, suggesting that it is surrounded by air. In addition, there is mild dilation of the hepatic flexure and proximal transverse portions of the colon, as well as some mildly dilated, gas-filled segments of small bowel on the right. No definite bowel gas is seen distal to that point. At surgery, a large ventral hernia containing collapsed bowel was found.

Case 11 There are three contrast-filled structures visible on this computed tomograph. The most anterior is the bladder (B), which contains renally excreted intravenous contrast material. Note that the bladder lumen also contains gas in its anterior aspect, which in the absence of recent instrumentation (such as bladder catheterization) suggests infection or fistula. The most posterior of the contrast-containing structures is the rectum (R), which contains a combination of barium swallowed by the patient and additional rectally administered barium. The contrast-filled structure in the middle is the vagina (V), in which no contrast should be present. A fistula is clearly seen to connect the vagina and the rectum, a so-called rectovaginal fistula. In addition, there is a strong suggestion of a fistula connecting the bladder and the vagina, a vesicovaginal fistula. The most common cause of a rectovaginal fistula is diverticular disease, while the most common causes of vesicovaginal fistulae are surgery, malignancy, and radiation. In this case, radiation therapy for cervical cancer was thought to be responsible for both. The soft tissue infiltration in the fat around the vagina was shown at biopsy to represent recurrent cervical carcinoma.

Case 12 This image shows no evidence of pneumothorax or complication of line placement. (**A**) Note the prominent calcifications within the wall of the aortic arch.

The prominent cardiomegaly likely results from two factors: myocardial ischemia and chronic volume overload from renal failure. (**B**) Look carefully at the position of the central venous catheter. It is now displaced laterally from the mediastinum. One cause of the catheter's displacement could be a mediastinal hematoma, especially if the catheter was recently replaced. (**C**) Contrast injection reveals the presence of two large mycotic aneurysms (arrows), the more proximal of which is responsible for the lateral displacement of the catheter in the superior vena cava. The patient expired shortly after this angiogram. At autopsy, *Staphylococcus aureus* was cultured from the patient's central line. The term *mycotic,* derived from the Greek for "fungus," was coined by William Osler to describe such aneurysms, not because they are necessarily fungal in etiology, but because they resemble mushrooms in their morphology. In fact, most of these lesions are best described as saccular pseudoaneurysms.

Case 13 (**A**) There is a remarkable asymmetry to the abdomen, with the left hemi-abdomen appearing larger than the right. For example, note the greater amount of subcutaneous and intra-abdominal fat on the left. (**B**) Further history revealed that the patient had undergone a right nephrectomy and adrenalectomy at a young age for a Wilms' tumor. The right hemiatrophy is accounted for by the fact that the patient also underwent radiation therapy to the right side of the abdomen. Since the patient had no adrenal gland for the past year, he had been receiving exogenous corticosteroids, which accounted for the lipomatosis.

Case 14 (**A**) There is loss of the normally sharp margins of the inferior end plate of the L5 vertebral body, as well as the superior end plate of S1 (arrow). (**B**) This image reveals end-plate destruction, as well as a mildly enhancing soft tissue mass replacing the L5–S1 intervertebral disk (arrows). The destruction of a vertebral body makes one think of a tumor, but tumors rarely cross a disk space to involve adjacent vertebral bodies. Given the clinical history, a more likely process is infection, often referred to as diskitis. In fact, diskitis actually usually represents hematogenous seeding of organisms to a vertebral end plate, with subsequent extension of the process into and across the intervertebral disk to involve the adjacent vertebral end plate. The culprit in this case was *Staphylococcus aureus.*

Case 15 The clinician should consider a diagnosis of a tumor in this case. The appearance of the calcifications is not quite typical, but a laterally displaced uterine fibroid would be a possibility if the patient were female. It is possible that this is a musculoskeletal tumor, but the portion of the osseous pelvis we can see well does not appear abnormal and shows no evidence of periosteal reaction or expansion. We might describe the contour of this mass as reniform, and furthermore, it is located in the right iliac fossa. Moreover, the patient has an indwelling peritoneal dialysis catheter coiled in the pelvis. In fact, this mass represents a failed renal transplant, which has calcified over the years since it failed. This case illustrates the importance of correlating the morphology and location of findings with other clinical information discernable from the film.

Case 16 The patient is skeletally immature, meaning that the growth plates are not yet closed. Note, for example, the distal radial physis and the physes of the proximal phalanges. There is a nondisplaced oblique fracture through the diaphysis of the second proximal phalanx, which does not appear to extend either proximally to the physis or distally into the proximal interphalangeal joint. A logical next step would be to obtain dedicated radiographs of the second finger, which would provide superior detail of the fracture.

Case 17 (A) The tip of the endotracheal tube is approximately 5 cm above the carina, a right subclavian central line tip is at the level of the right atrium, and a nasogastric tube sideport is just below the level of the gastroesophageal junction. The left hemidiaphragm is elevated (it is normally inferior to the level of the right hemidiaphragm), and there appears to be a right pleural effusion. Far more significant, however, is the presence of a large lucency in the central upper abdomen, which is very suspicious for pneumoperitoneum. If you were unsure about your findings, and if the patient could sit or stand up, an upright portable radiograph could be obtained, and air would be seen under the hemidiaphragms. If the patient could not tolerate one of these views, a left-side down decubitus view could be obtained, which would show the air along the lateral margin of the liver. (B) Note that the walls of several segments of small bowel in the upper abdomen are outlined on both sides by air. This finding's eponym is *Rigler's sign.* In this case, a perforated duodenal ulcer was found at surgery.

Case 18 (A) Note the ragged appearance of the rectal mucosa on the right, and the discrete ulceration seen along the left side. Note also the presence of at least two fistulae extending from the distal lumen down to the perianal region. When inflammatory lesions are seen in the rectum, inflammatory bowel disease immediately comes to mind. The rectum is involved in nearly all cases of ulcerative colitis, but perhaps only half of cases of Crohn's disease. However, ulcerative colitis characteristically spares the anus, while Crohn's disease commonly produces perianal fistulae. The asymmetry of involvement also favors Crohn's disease. In this case, the diagnosis is Crohn's disease. (B) This spot film shows classic diffuse, symmetrical granularity of the rectal mucosa, characteristic of an early inflammatory stage of ulcerative colitis.

Case 19 This radiograph exhibits a striking anatomic abnormality. The cardiac apex is right sided, the gastric bubble is right sided, and changes of bronchiectasis are seen in the medial lung bases, especially on the left side. The patient also exhibited radiographic evidence of sinusitis on other films (not shown). This is a classic case of Kartagener's syndrome, which results from a deficiency of the dynein arms of cilia, rendering them immotile. This deficiency also renders male patients infertile and can cause deafness.

Case 20 This is not a normal radiograph: the patient has a supernumerary sixth digit.

Case 21 First note the normal anatomy of the right orbit; note the superior (S), lateral (L), and inferior (I) rectus muscles, as well as the optic nerve (O). While both maxillary sinuses are opacified, the right contains a bubble of air. The soft tissue mass in the left maxillary sinus (M) has produced destruction of portions of the turbinate and ethmoid bones, and appears to be eroding through the inferomedial wall of the left orbit (arrow), with bone destruction and a soft tissue mass within the orbit. Differential diagnostic considerations in this immunocompromised patient would include opportunistic infections such as pseudomonas and mucormycosis, as well as neoplastic processes such as lymphoma. At biopsy, an aggressive non-Hodgkin's lymphoma was diagnosed.

Case 22 There are at least two cystic lesions in the retropharyngeal soft tissues anterior to the spine. Each demonstrates a mild degree of ring enhancement. These lesions compress and anteriorly displace the esophagus, which explains the patient's severe dysphagia. Such abscesses generally require surgical drainage.

Case 23 The primary diagnostic considerations would be septic arthritis and avascular necrosis (AVN), both of which are easily detected by magnetic resonance imaging at an early treatable stage. This patient's preinfusion T1-weighted coronal image of the right hip demonstrates classic changes of AVN, with linear and crescentic areas of decreased signal within the femoral head (arrow). Common causes of AVN include trauma, steroids, collagen vascular diseases (such as systemic lupus erythematosus), alcoholism, and hemoglobinopathies such as sickle cell disease. AVN may progress to collapse of the femoral head, secondary osteoarthritis, and severe joint deformity and loss of function. Joint-preserving surgical interventions include osteotomy and core decompression in an effort to decrease pressure within the femoral head and thereby restore perfusion.

Case 24 First, note that there is narrowing of the medial and lateral joint compartments. (Which side of the radiograph is medial? The fibula is on the viewer's left, indicating that the medial aspect of the knee joint is on the viewer's right.) In addition, osteophyte formation is seen about the lateral aspects of the femoral condyle and tibial plateau, sclerosis and subchondral cyst formation are seen in the epiphyses of the femur and tibia, and there is slight medial translation of the femur on the tibia. All of these findings are frequently seen in routine osteoarthritis. There is one additional finding on this radiograph that suggests another etiology: prominent chondrocalcinosis, or calcification of the articular cartilage within the knee joint. This indicates calcium pyrophosphate deposition disease. The numerous subchondral cysts are also more characteristic of this disorder. The patient's acute attack of knee pain would qualify for a diagnosis of pseudogout.

Case 25 (A) The film demonstrates an ill-defined, somewhat lobular airspace opacity in the right upper lobe. The differential diagnosis would include an early lobar pneumonia, such as pneumococcal pneumonia, a neoplastic process (which was considered unlikely), and pulmonary embolism (PE), among other possibilities. The lack of fever and leukocytosis argued strongly against infection. If the concern for PE were paramount, a nuclear medicine ventilation/perfusion lung scan would have likely been the next choice. (B) There is a wedge-shaped area of airspace opacity in the right upper lobe, which extends nearly to the pleural surface. (C) In the absence of a tumor in this region, the filling defect in the pulmonary artery is essentially diagnostic of PE, presumably related to the patient's postpartum status, perhaps reflecting thromboembolism involving the pelvic or deep leg veins.

Case 26 The size of the infant and the presence of an umbilical cord clip overlying the right side of the abdomen indicate that the child is probably at most several days old. The key finding is the small size of the thorax relative to the abdomen and the presence of bilateral pneumothoraces. Note the rim of air in the pleural space outlining the lateral aspect of the right lung, as well as the presence of unusual lucency in the costophrenic angle (inferolateral-most portion) of the left hemithorax. We must consider the possibility that some in utero condition has produced bilateral pulmonary hypoplasia, which has resulted in a small thorax and fragile lungs. The diagnosis in this case is the so-called Potter sequence, which results from severe bilateral renal insufficiency, which may be derived from renal agenesis, multicystic dysplastic kidneys, or a bilateral obstruction to urine outflow, such as posterior urethral valves. Decreased or absent urine output results in oligohydramnios (too little amniotic fluid), which interferes with normal lung development. The abnormal appearance of the face (Potter facies) and limb contractures seen in these infants are thought to result from excessive pressure on the fetus, which is not "buffered" by a sufficient quantity of amniotic fluid. Note also the presence of bilateral hip dysplasia, presumably secondary to the cramped quarters in which the fetus was housed.

Case 27 In this case, the suspected diagnosis would be thoracic outlet syndrome. This disorder most often results from compression of the brachial plexus, with resultant upper extremity neurologic symptoms. Another possible etiology is compression of the subclavian artery, which may produce claudication or emboli. Often, the chest radiograph demonstrates a tiny cervical rib arising from the seventh cervical vertebra. (A) The selective left subclavian artery injection demonstrates unremarkable opacification of the left vertebral and left subclavian arteries. Also visible are multiple surgical clips overlying the left upper chest. (B) The repeat injection reveals compression and occlusion of the left subclavian artery where it crosses the clavicle. This is diagnostic of thoracic outlet syndrome.

Case 28 Aside from asking the patient whether she could possibly be pregnant, a human chorionic gonadotropin test must be performed to determine whether she is pregnant. In this case, a urine pregnancy test was positive. In a pregnant patient with symptoms such as pelvic pain and bleeding, the possibility of an ectopic pregnancy must be excluded, because it represents a potentially life-threatening condition. Ultrasound nearly always represents the modality of first choice in evaluating the female pelvis, especially when the patient is pregnant. The crucial finding to be sought is an intrauterine pregnancy, because its presence virtually excludes the possibility of an ectopic pregnancy. Transvaginal imaging is more sensitive than a transabdominal approach. In this case, the uterus was well imaged both transvaginally and transabdominally (not shown), and no evidence of an intrauterine pregnancy was found. This finding alone significantly increases the probability of ectopic pregnancy. However, a sonographic image of the left adnexal region (shown) provided even further diagnostic confidence. There is an echogenic ring-like structure that contains fluid and a smaller, more delicate echogenic ring within its inferior aspect. This represents a yoke sac within an enlarged hypervascular fallopian tube, the so-called tubal ring sign. This finding is at least 95% specific for ectopic pregnancy. Some of the most important risk factors for ectopic pregnancy are previous ectopic pregnancy, previous tubal reconstructive surgery, a history of pelvic inflammatory disease, and the presence of an intrauterine contraceptive device.

Case 29 (A) A very large fluid-filled structure occupies much of the pelvis, displacing adjacent bowel loops. This finding could represent a very distended urinary bladder, which in fact is one of the most common pelvic masses encountered in hospitalized patients. The possibility that this structure represented the bladder was ruled out on two grounds: First, the bladder could be seen on lower images (not shown) to be separate from this structure, which has displaced it anteriorly and inferiorly. Second, delayed images of the pelvis clearly demonstrated no filling of this structure with contrast-opacified urine, while the bladder opacified normally. Note also the presence of two smaller cyst-like lesions behind this larger lesion. The most likely explanation for these findings in this postmenopausal patient receiving no hormonal therapy is a cystic neoplasm arising from the right ovary. (B) The ultrasound also demonstrates a large cyst, clearly separate from the urinary bladder (UB), which contains no internal echoes. While the lack of echogenicity is somewhat comforting, such a large cyst generally mandates surgical evaluation. At surgery, a benign serous cystadenoma was found.

Case 30 Note the appearance of linear areas of low attenuation radiating outward from the pelvis of the left kidney, producing a so-called striated nephrogram, a finding associated with pyelonephritis. Key findings to be ruled out on such a study include abscess, emphysematous pyelonephritis, and signs of chronic infection such as cortical scarring and papillary necrosis.

Case 31 The amount of blood loss cannot be estimated because the apparently small amount of extravasated contrast at the time of the injection may have been preceded by massive blood loss. Two features indicate that this is a venogram. First, there is contrast in the vessel distal to the area of extravasation, but not proximally, which is not characteristic of an artery. Second, there is a prominent valve in the vessel distal to the site of extravasation; only veins contain valves. The diagnosis here is transection of the axillary vein. Note the cephalic vein above, connecting to the more proximal subclavian vein.

Case 32 Common causes of solid testicular masses include infections such as epididymitis or orchitis and tumors, including primary neoplasms and metastatic lesions such as leukemia and lymphoma. On this image, a central hypoechoic mass replaces much of the central testicular parenchyma. Note also the presence of multiple tiny hyperechoic foci throughout the testis. This represents a case of seminoma arising in the setting of testicular microlithiasis, which is associated with an increased risk of neoplasm. Approximately 3000 primary testicular neoplasms are diagnosed each year in the United States, and they represent one of the most common malignancies in men in the second and third decades. Seminomas, which are radiosensitive and have a good prognosis, are the most common type.

Case 33 Typically, the differential diagnosis of a young man with the acute onset of unilateral scrotal pain and no history of trauma includes testicular torsion and epididymoorchitis. The key diagnosis to exclude is testicular torsion, because testicular viability is lost after 4 to 6 hours of ischemia. (A) The longitudinal image of the left testis demonstrates homogeneous parenchymal echogenicity, with a spectral Doppler tracing demonstrating a normal arterial waveform and velocity of 7.5 cm/s. Note that the peak systolic velocity, represented by the highest points of the tracing, is significantly higher than the peak diastolic velocity (the lowest points of the tracing), although both remain above the baseline. (B) In contrast, examination of the right testis demonstrates a significantly reduced peak systolic velocity, which is barely above peak diastolic velocity, which indicates the presence of a partial torsion, with diminution but not complete interruption of arterial flow to the testis. This is a prognostically favorable finding and suggests that the testis is viable and can be surgically detorsed without loss of function.

Case 34 (A) There is a vague opacity overlying much of the lateral aspect of the left midlung. Does this represent an intrapulmonary or extrapulmonary process? Compare the ribs from side to side. Note that the posterior aspect of the left sixth rib is indistinct or missing. This suggests the possibility of a pleural-based process that has destroyed the bone or perhaps a primary destructive rib lesion. (B) The axial image demonstrates a large expansile, destructive lesion within the posterior rib. On biopsy, this proved to be a metastatic adenocarcinoma, the source of which was never identified. Such a case illustrates the importance of examining the entire chest radiograph, not just the heart and lungs, because the crucial abnormality sometimes lies in the bones and soft tissues.

Case 35 First, note the presence of two probable phleboliths in the right hemipelvis, likely of no clinical significance. The crucial finding lies outside the pelvis, at the bottom of the film. Note the presence of gas within the soft tissues of the penis and scrotum. This represents a condition known as Fournier's gangrene, or necrotizing fasciitis of the scrotum. Although the dermis and epidermis may appear intact, the subcutaneous tissues are diffusely infiltrated by a polymicrobial infection, which requires prompt and aggressive surgical debridement and antibiotic therapy. This case emphasizes the importance of inspecting the entire film, including the edges and corners.

Case 36 (A) This case illustrates a potentially life-threatening abnormality that no physician can afford to miss. Note that the right lung is completely collapsed, and the large amount of air accumulating in the right pleural space has produced a condition known as tension pneumothorax, with shift of the heart toward the left. The treatment in such cases is emergent chest tube placement. (B) After chest tube insertion, the follow-up film demonstrates reexpansion of the right lung, with at least one bulla in the right upper lobe. Rupture of such a bulla was the presumed etiology of this patient's pneumothorax, and prophylactic bullectomy may warrant consideration in such a young patient with a history of episodes of pneumothorax.

Case 37 There is a round area of cloud-like ossification immediately lateral to the distal femoral prosthesis. Unfortunately, this represented a recurrence of the patient's tumor.

Case 38 The posterosuperior border of the heart bulges far posteriorly, indicating the presence of left atriomegaly. This was secondary to rheumatic mitral valve disease, producing a combination of stenosis and regurgitation.

Case 39 First, there is a metallic density with a spoke-wheel type pattern in the inferior vena cava. This was an inferior vena cava filter, which had been placed due to a history of pulmonary embolism and failed anticoagulation. Second, there is a heterogeneously enhancing mass in the inferior aspect of the right lobe of the liver. A differential diagnosis of this lesion would include hepatocellular carcinoma, metastasis, adenoma, and focal nodular hyperplasia. Biopsy demonstrated a hepatic adenoma. The third abnormality is multiple wedge-shaped areas of perfusion defect in the right kidney, which represented areas of infarction due to pyelonephritis. Such cases illustrate the importance of not ending the search for abnormalities when a finding is made, but continuing to examine the entire film.

Case 40 Two findings are key regarding the use of intravenous contrast. First, the native left kidney is tiny and contains multiple cysts. The same finding was noted in the right kidney on more caudal images. This indicates the presence of chronic medical renal disease and argues for a patient with little or no renal function. Second, note the prominent enhancement of the bile within the gallbladder. This represents a phenomenon known as vicarious excretion of contrast. Although the hepatocytes are not the primary route of excretion of iodinated contrast material, given time (as in renal failure) they can excrete enough contrast to opacify the bile, as in this case. This study was obtained approximately 24 hours after contrast injection, during which time the patient did not undergo hemodialysis.

Case 41 The esophagus is diffusely dilated and demonstrated a complete absence of peristalsis on fluoroscopic monitoring. Moreover, the distal esophagus tapers down to a "bird's beak" like configuration. This is a classic appearance of achalasia, a condition that results from Wallerian degeneration of Auerbach's plexus. This in turn produces an absence of esophageal peristalsis and failure of the lower esophageal sphincter to relax with swallowing. As expected, patients do a better job of emptying the esophagus in the upright position, which also decreases the risk of aspiration.

Case 42 (A) There is a lobulated filling defect that extends from the proximal stomach up to the gastroesophageal junction, where it exhibits a particularly fungating appearance. The most likely differential diagnostic possibilities include either an esophageal squamous cell carcinoma that has extended into the stomach or a gastric adenocarcinoma that has grown exophytically up into the esophagus. Statistically, the latter is the most likely possibility. Endoscopic biopsy verified a gastric adenocarcinoma. (B) The axial computed tomography image demonstrates prominent thickening of the gastric wall, with a component of the mass protruding exophytically into the lumen. Risk factors for gastric carcinoma include pernicious anemia, a previous Billroth gastrectomy, and chronic atrophic gastritis.

Case 43 There is a round area of increased attenuation in the midline posteriorly. The midline location and the lack of surrounding edema and mass effect argue against a parenchymal hemorrhage. In fact, this appearance is fairly classic for another pathologic entity. Other than blood, two etiologies that could result in increased attenuation are calcification and thrombus. This is the site of the superior sagittal sinus, one of the important dural sinuses that provides venous drainage from the brain. While a dural venous sinus could calcify, thrombosis is more likely, especially in view of the clinical presentation. This is a case of superior sagittal sinus thrombosis, which may occur in association with pregnancy, infection, dehydration, and hypercoagulable states.

Case 44 Note a stenotic region in the descending aorta just distal to the takeoff of the left subclavian artery. This patient presented with upper extremity hypertension.

The diagnosis is aortic coarctation. If the patient were older than 8 years, inferior rib notching may be detectable on the chest radiograph. Today magnetic resonance imaging has replaced angiography as the diagnostic study of choice in coarctation.

Case 45 (A) The tracheal air column has a somewhat atypical contour, appearing unusually straight along its left side. While airway fluoroscopic monitoring would warrant consideration, a lateral chest radiograph would probably represent the best alternative. (B) The tracheal air column is readily visualized anterior to this opacity, indicating that the foreign body is located in the esophagus.

Case 46 Loops of gas-filled bowel descend into the scrotum on both sides, indicating the presence of bilateral inguinal hernias.

Case 47 A rim of high attenuation is visible between the left cerebral hemisphere and the calvarium, which is concave toward the brain. In addition, there is a prominent rightward shift of the septum pellucidum (small arrow) relative to the midline (large arrow). This is a classic appearance of an acute subdural hematoma. A subdural collection of blood lies between the dura and arachnoid. These commonly result from tearing of the bridging veins and often occur in the absence of a skull fracture.

Normal Cross-sectional Anatomy

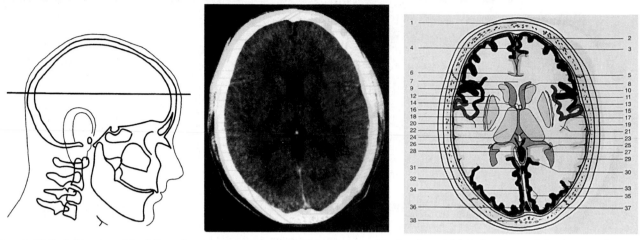

Figure 1. Axial brain CT anatomy. 1, frontal bone; 2, superior frontal gyrus; 3, middle frontal gyrus; 4, falx of cerebrum; 5, inferior frontal gyrus; 6, cingulate gyrus; 7, corpus callosum; 8, lateral ventricle (anterior horn); 9, caudate nucleus (head); 10, insular lobe; 11, precentral gyrus; 12, internal capsule (anterior crus); 13, central sulcus; 14, fornix; 15, postcentral gyrus; 16, interventricular foramen (of Monro); 17, lateral sulcus; 18, claustrum; 19, superior temporal gyrus; 20, putamen; 21, transverse temporal gyri (Heschl's convolutions); 22, internal capsule (posterior crus); 23, pineal body; 24, thalamus; 25, hippocampus; 26, caudate nucleus (tail); 27, lateral ventricle (posterior horn); 28, vermis of cerebellum; 29, middle temporal gyrus; 30, parietooccipital sulcus; 31, straight sinus; 32, parietal bone; 33, occipital gyri; 34, falx of cerebrum; 35, striate cortex; 36, superior sagittal sinus; 37, occipital pole; 38, occipital bone.

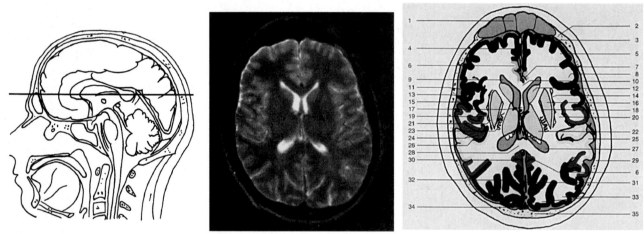

Figure 2. Axial brain MRI anatomy. 1, frontal sinus; 2, frontal bone; 3, superior frontal gyrus; 4, falx of cerebrum (interhemispheric fissure); 5, middle frontal gyrus; 6, cingulate gyrus; 7, pericallosal artery; 8, inferior frontal gyrus; 9, lateral ventricle (anterior horn); 10, corpus callosum (genu); 11, precentral gyrus; 12, caudate nucleus (head); 13, central sulcus; 14, claustrum; 15, postcentral gyrus; 16, putamen; 17, pellucid septum; 18, globus pallidus; 19, extreme capsule; 20, insular lobe; 21, external capsule; 22, thalamus; 23, internal capsule; 24, transverse temporal gyri (Heschl's convolutions); 25, superior temporal gyrus; 26, lateral sulcus; 27, lateral ventricle (posterior horn); 28, corpus callosum (splenium); 29, parietal bone; 30, parietooccipital sulcus; 31, straight sinus; 32, cuneus; 33, occipital gyri; 34, superior sagittal sinus; 35, occipital bone.

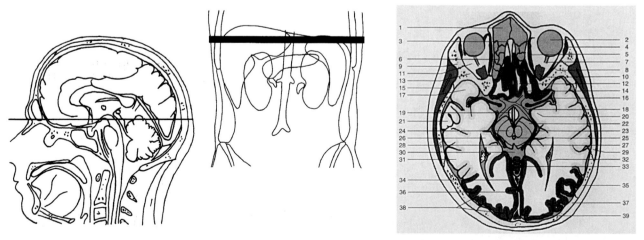

Figure 3. Axial brain MRI anatomy. 1, frontal sinus; 2, ocular bulb; 3, crista galli; 4, lacrimal gland; 5, superior oblique muscle; 6, ethmoid labyrinth; 7, optic nerve; 8, lateral rectus muscle; 9, zygomatic bone; 10, superior rectus muscle; 11, orbit; 12, straight gyrus; 13, sphenoid bone; 14, anterior cerebral artery; 15, temporal muscle; 16, middle cerebral artery; 17, superior temporal gyrus; 18, optic chiasm; 19, hypothalamus; 20, uncus; 21, middle temporal gyrus; 22, cerebral peduncle; 23, posterior cerebral artery; 24, red nucleus; 25, aqueduct; 26, hippocampus; 27, cranial colliculus; 28, ambient cistern; 29, temporal bone; 30, Bichat's canal (cisterna venae magnae cerebri); 31, inferior temporal gyrus; 32, lateral ventricle (temporal horn); 33, cranial lobe of cerebellum; 34, straight sinus; 35, parietal bone; 36, calcarine sulcus; 37, occipital bone; 38, superior sagittal sinus.

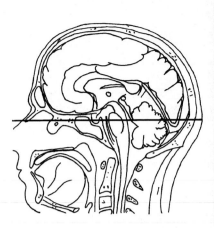
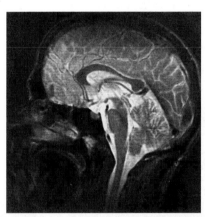
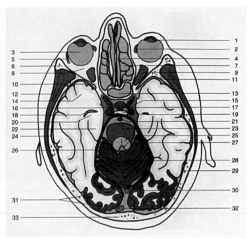

Figure 4. Axial brain MRI anatomy. 1, lens; 2, medial rectus muscle; 3, ocular bulb; 4, nasal septum; 5, lateral rectus muscle; 6, zygomatic bone; 7, ethmoid labyrinth; 8, orbit; 9, inferior rectus muscle; 10, superior orbital fissure; 11, sphenoid bone; 12, temporal muscle; 13, sphenoid sinus 14, temporal lobe; 15, cavernous sinus; 16, internal carotid artery; 17, pituitary gland; 18, lateral ventricle (temporal horn); 19, dorsum sellae; 20, hippocampus; 21, basilar artery; 22, parahippocampal gyrus; 23, pons; 24, temporal bone; 25, reticular formation; 26, tentorium of cerebellum; 27, fourth ventricle; 28, cranial lobe of cerebellum; 29, parietal bone; 30, straight sinus; 31, occipital gyri; 32, superior sagittal sinus; 33, occipital bone.

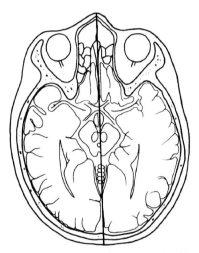
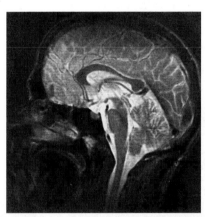
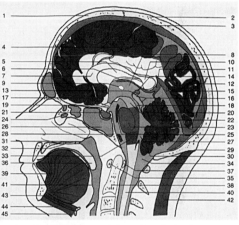

Figure 5. Sagittal MRI brain anatomy. 1, frontal bone; 2, parietal bone; 3, superior sagittal sinus; 4, cingulate sulcus; 5, pellucid septum; 6, internal cerebral vein; 7, corpus callosum (genu); 8, third ventricle; 9, intermediate mass; 10, corpus callosum (splenium); 11, great vein of Galen; 12, parietooccipital sulcus; 13, anterior and posterior commissures; 14, pineal body; 15, straight sinus; 16, cranial and caudal colliculi; 17, optic nerve; 18, aqueduct; 19, infundibulum; 20, mesencephalic tegmentum; 21, pituitary gland; 22, cerebellum; 23, pons; 24, ethmoid labyrinth; 25, basilar artery; 26, sphenoid sinus; 27, fourth ventricle; 28, clivus; 29, occipital bone (external occipital protuberance); 30, uvula vermis; 31, nasopharynx; 32, hard palate; 33, medulla oblongata; 34, cerebellomedullary cistern; 35, atlas (arch); 36, uvula; 37, transverse ligament of atlas; 38, Odontoid process of axis; 39, genioglossus muscle; 40, spinal cord; 41, oropharynx; 42, semispinalis capitis muscle; 43, geniohyoid muscle; 44, mylohyoid muscle; 45, hyoid bone.

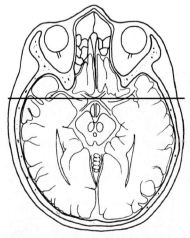
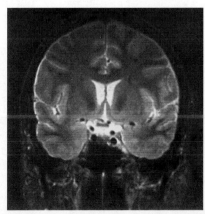
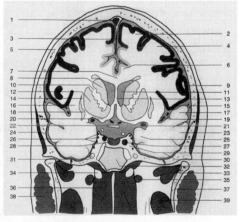

Figure 6. Coronal MRI brain anatomy. 1, superior sagittal sinus; 2, superior frontal gyrus; 3, falx of cerebrum; 4, middle frontal gyrus; 5, parietal bone; 6, cingulate sulcus; 7, corpus callosum (body); 8, caudate nucleus (head); 9, inferior frontal gyrus; 10, internal capsule (anterior crus); 11, lateral ventricle (anterior horn); 12, putamen; 13, pellucid septum; 14, external capsule; 15, lateral sulcus; 16, extreme capsule; 17, superior temporal gyrus; 18, claustrum; 19, insular lobe and insular cistern; 20, roof of chiasmatic cistern; 21, middle cerebral artery; 22, optic chiasm; 23, middle temporal gyrus; 24, temporal bone; 25, parahippocampal gyrus; 26, oculomotor (CN II), trochlear (CN IV), and abducens (CN VI) nerves; 27, internal carotid artery; 28, pituitary gland; 29, cavernous sinus; 30, lateral occipitotemporal gyrus; 31, trigeminal ganglion; 32, sphenoid sinus; 33, lateral pterygoid muscle; 34, auditory tube; 35, levator veli palatini muscle; 36, nasopharynx (constrictor muscle); 37, mandible (ramus); 38, parotid gland; 39, medial pterygoid muscle.

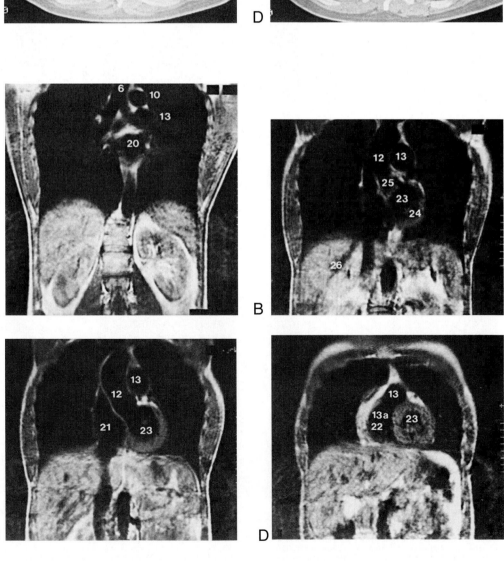

Figure 7. Axial thoracic CT anatomy. 2, carotid artery; 4, subclavian artery; 5, vertebra; 6, trachea; 7, subclavian vein; 8, esophagus; 9, brachiocephalic artery; 10, aorta; 11, vena cava; 13, main pulmonary artery; 16, ascending aorta; 19, lower lobe artery and vein; 20 left atrium; 21, right atrium; 22, right ventricle; 23, left ventricle.

Figure 8. Coronal thoracic MRI anatomy. 6, trachea; 10, aorta; 12, ascending aorta; 13, main pulmonary artery; 13a, pulmonic valve; 20, left atrium; 21, right atrium; 22, right ventricle; 23, left ventricle; 24, papillary muscle; 25, aortic valve; 26, hepatic vein.

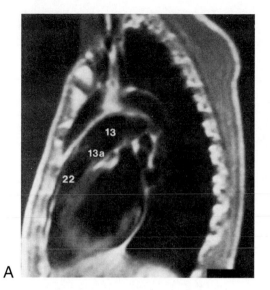

A

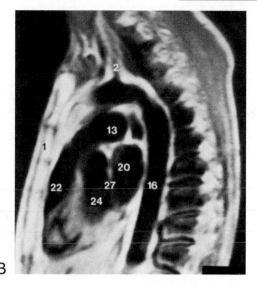

B

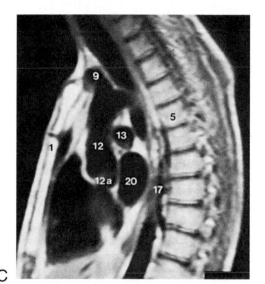

C

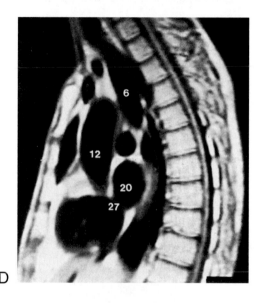

D

Figure 9. Sagittal thoracic MRI anatomy. 2, carotid artery; 5, vertebra; 6, trachea; 9, brachiocephalic artery; 12, ascending aorta; 12a, aortic valve; 13, main pulmonary artery; 13a, pulmonic valve; 16, descending aorta; 17, azygos vein; 20, left atrium; 22, right ventricle; 24, papillary muscle; 27, mitral valve.

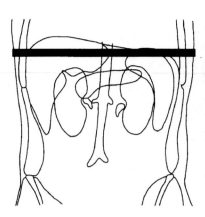
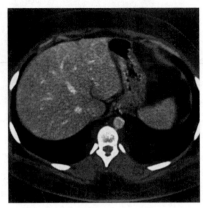
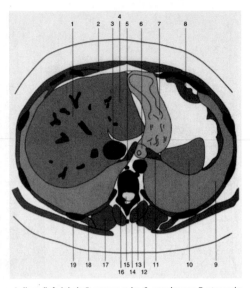

Figure 10. Axial abdomen and pelvis CT anatomy. 1, liver; 2, rectus abdominis muscle; 3, inferior vena cava; 4, liver (left lobe); 5, azygos vein; 6, esophagus; 7, stomach; 8, diaphragm; 9, left lung; 10, spleen; 11, diaphragm (lumbar part); 12, abdominal aorta; 13, hemiazygos vein; 14, spinalis muscle; 15, spinal canal; 16, thoracic vertebra 9; 17, longissimus thoracis muscle; 18, iliocostalis lumborum muscle; 19, latissimus dorsi muscle.

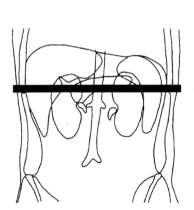
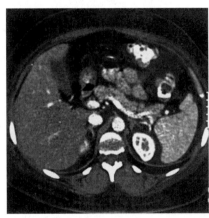
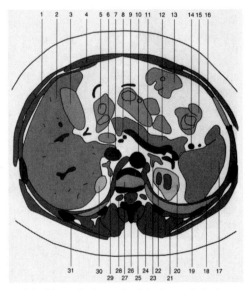

Figure 11. Axial abdomen and pelvis CT anatomy. 1, external oblique muscle; 2, liver; 3, gall bladder; 4, rectus abdominis muscle; 5, ampulla of duodenum; 6, duodenum; 7, inferior vena cava; 8, left gastric artery and vein; 9, jejunum; 10, abdominal aorta; 11, splenic vein; 12, pancreas; 13, transverse colon; 14, splenic artery; 15, descending colon; 16, internal oblique muscle; 17, spleen; 18, left lung (costodiaphragmatic recess); 19, inferior posterior serratus anterior muscle; 20, left renal cortex; 21, iliocostalis thoracis muscle; 22, renal medulla; 23, left adrenal gland; 24, longissimus thoracis muscle; 25, spinalis muscle; 26, spinal canal; 27, thoracic vertebra 11; 28, spinal nerve root T 11; 29, right adrenal gland; 30, right kidney; 31, latissimus dorsi muscle.

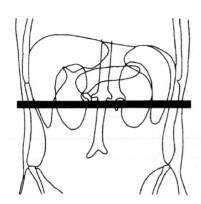
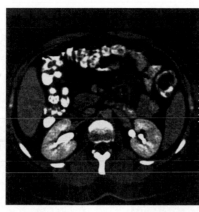
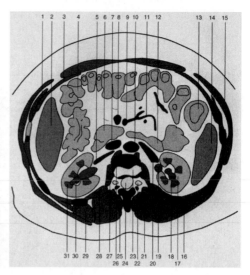

Figure 12. Axial abdomen and pelvis CT anatomy. 1, internal oblique muscle; 2, liver; 3, transversus abdominis muscle; 4, transverse colon; 5, right renal artery; 6, duodenum; 7, inferior vena cava; 8, superior mesenteric vein; 9, superior mesenteric artery; 10, abdominal aorta; 11, middle colic artery; 12, duodenum (inferior horizontal part); 13, descending colon; 14, spleen; 15, external oblique muscle; 16, inferior posterior serratus anterior muscle; 17, left kidney; 18, renal calix; 19, ureter; 20, left renal vein; 21, longissimus thoracis muscle; 22, spinal nerve root; 23, lumbar vertebra 1; 24, spinal canal; 25, spinalis muscle; 26, diaphragm; 27, psoas muscle; 28, quadratus lumborum muscle; 29, iliocostalis lumborum muscle; 30, renal pelvis; 31, renal pyramid.

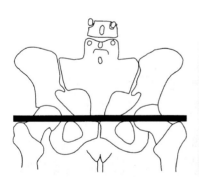
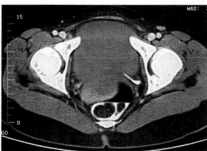
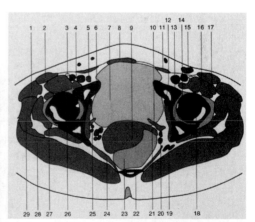

Figure 13. Axial abdomen and pelvis CT anatomy. 1, tensor fasciae latae muscle; 2, sartorius muscle; 3, femoral nerve; 4, external iliac artery and vein; 5, medial external iliac lymph node; 6, pubic bone; 7, urinary bladder; 8, rectus abdominis muscle; 9, uterus; 10, ureter; 11, internal oblique muscle; 12, obturator artery; 13, internal obturator muscle; 14, fovea of head of femur; 15, superficial inguinal lymph nodes; 16, iliopsoas muscle; 17, rectus femoris muscle; 18, head of femur; 19, inferior gluteal artery and vein; 20, inferior vesical artery and vein; 21, fallopian tube; 22, coccyx; 23, rectum; 24, sacrospinal ligament; 25, internal pudendal artery and vein; 26, ischium; 27, gluteus minimus muscle; 28, gluteus maximus muscle; 29, gluteus medius muscle.

Normal Chest Radiograph

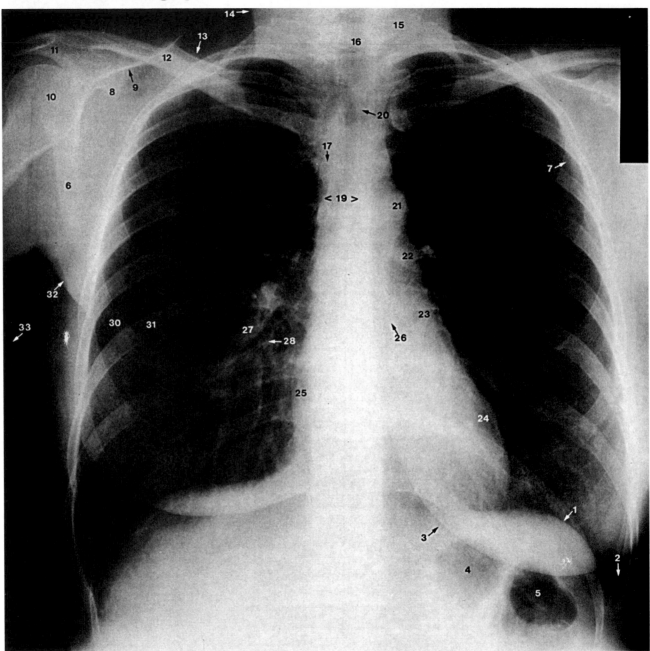

Figure 14. **Frontal chest radiograph.** Diaphragm (1), costophrenic sulcus (2), breast shadow (3), stomach bubble (4), colonic gas in splenic flexure (5), scapula, lateral border (6), scapula, medial border (7), coracoid process (8), spine of scapula (9), humeral head (10), acromioclavicular joint (11), clavicular shaft (12), companion shadow of clavicle (13), sternocleidomastoid muscle (14), transverse process, cervical spine (15), spinous process, cervical spine (16), pedicle (17), head of rib (18), trachea (19), posterior-superior junction line (20), aortic arch (21), main pulmonary artery segment (22), left atrial appendage (23), left ventricular border (24), right atrial border (25), descending thoracic aorta (26), interlobar pulmonary artery (27), bronchus intermedius (28), anterior segmental bronchus of left upper lobe seen on end (29), anterior rib (30), posterior rib (31), anterior axillary fold (32), posterior axillary fold (33).

Suggested Readings

HISTORY OF RADIOLOGY

Doby T, Alker G. Origins and Development of Diagnostic Imaging. Southern Illinois University Press, 1997.

Gagliardi R, McClennan R. A History of the Radiological Sciences: Diagnosis. Roentgen Centennial, Inc., 1996.

GENERAL RADIOLOGY

Noveline R. Squire's Fundamentals of Radiology. Harvard, 1997.

Putnam C, Ravin C. Textbook of Diagnostic Imaging. WB Saunders, 1994.

Taveras J, Ferrucci J. Radiology: Diagnosis, Imaging, Intervention. Lippincott-Raven Publishers, annual updates.

The Requisites Series, Mosby.

THIEME PUBLICATIONS

(books from which figures have been reproduced in this publication)

Allen EA. Tuberculosis and other myobacterial infections of the lung. In Thurlbeck WM, Churg A (eds): Pathology of the Lung, 2nd ed. Thieme, New York, 1995. (Figure 3–50)

Barbaric ZL: Principles of Genitourinary Radiology, 2nd ed. Thieme, New York, 1994. (Figures 1–8,10,14,18,24,33; 5–3,6,7,8,9,10(A,B),14,16,17,20,23,26)

Bischof TP. Vomiting. In Krestin GP, Choyke PL (eds): Acute Abdomen: Diagnostic Imaging in the Clinical Context. Thieme, New York, 1996. (Figure 6–28)

Burgener FA, Kormano M: Differential Diagnosis in Conventional Radiology, 2nd ed. Thieme, New York, 1991. (Figures 5–11; 6–30; 8–2,12,20,21,22,31,35,36,41,47,60; 10–26,40; 11–20)

Cagle PT. Tumors of the lung (excluding lymphoid tumors). In Thurlbeck WM, Churg A (eds): Pathology of the Lung, 2nd ed. Thieme, New York, 1995. (Figure 3–60)

Chung A. Diseases of the pleura. In Thurlbeck WM, Churg A (eds): Pathology of the Lung, 2nd ed. Thieme, New York, 1995. (Figure 3–21)

Dihlmann W: Radiologic Atlas of Rheumatic Diseases. Thieme, New York, 186. (Figures 8–29,34,38)

Hagspiel KD, Krestin GP. In Krestin GP, Choyke PL (eds): Acute Abdomen: Diagnostic Imaging in the Clinical Context. Thieme, New York, 1996. (Figure 6–4)

Haldemann-Heusler R, Pippert H. Left lower quadrant abdominal pain. In Krestin GP, Choyke PL (eds): Acute Abdomen: Diagnostic Imaging in the Clinical Context. Thieme, New York, 1996. (Figure 6–18)

Haublod-Reuter B. Abdominal Trauma. In Krestin GP, Choyke PL (eds): Acute Abdomen: Diagnostic Imaging in the Clinical Context. Thieme, New York, 1996. (Figure 4–53)

Heywang-Köbrunner SH, Schreer I, Dershaw DD: Diagnostic Breast Imaging. Thieme, New York, 1997. (Figures 7–2,4,7)

Hogg JC. Pulmonary edema. In Thurlbeck WM, Churg A (eds): Pathology of the Lung, 2nd ed. Thieme, New York, 1995. (Figure 3–7)

Huber P: Cerebral Angiography. Thieme, New York, 1982. (Figures 9–7,43)

Hüpscher DN: Radiology of the Esophagus. Thieme, New York, 1988. (Figure 4–28)

Jacob A. Right upper quadrant abdominal pain. In Krestin GP, Choyke PL (eds): Diagnostic Imaging in the Clinical Context. Thieme, New York, 1996. (Figures 6–5,13)

Krestin GP, Choyke PL: Acute Abdomen. Thieme, New York, 1996. (Figure 11–1)

Kuhn C III. Bacterial infections. In Thurlbeck WM, Churg A (eds): Pathology of the Lung, 2nd ed. Thieme, New York, 1995. (Figures 3–15,43)

Kurdziel JC, Dondelinger RF. Intraperitoneal fluid collections. In Dondelinger RF, Rossi P, Kurdziel JC, Wallace S (eds): Interventional Radiology. Thieme, New York, 1990. (Figure 1–38)

Lange S, Stark P: Teaching Atlas of Thoracic Radiology. Thieme, New York, 1993. (Figures 3–67,68;10–5,16)

Leucht D, Madjar H: Teaching Atlas of Breast Ultrasound, 2nd ed. Thieme, New York, 1996. (Figure 7–9)

Matsumo AH, Barth KH. Peripheral angioplasty balloon technology. In Mayner-Moliner M, Castañeda-Zuñiga WR, Joffre F, Zollikofer CL (eds): Percutaneous Revascularization Techniques. Thieme, New York, 1993. (Figures 1–35,36)

McSwain ME, Martinez JA, Timberlake GA: Cervical Spine Trauma: Evaluation and Acute Management. Thieme, New York, 1989. (Figures 8–43,56,57,58)

Merz E: Ultrasound in Gynecology and Obstetrics. Thieme, New York, 1991. (Figures 7–13,15,16,19,21,22,23,24,27,28,29,30)

Miller RR. Pulmonary disease in the immunocompromised host. In Thurlbeck WM, Churg A (eds): Pathology of the Lung, 2nd ed. Thieme, New York, 1995. (Figure 3–53C)

Möller TB, Reif E, Stark P: Pocket Atlas of Radiographic Anatomy. Thieme, New York, 1993. (Figures 4–6,15;8–8,46,53,54)

Reeders JWAJ, Rosenbusch G: Clinical Radiology and Endoscopy of the Colon. Thieme, New York, 1994. (Figures 1–4;4–12,13,14,47;10–29)

Reeders JWAJ: Diagnostic Imaging of AIDS. Thieme, New York, 1992. (Figures 1–41;3–55)

Savader SJ. Angiographic, venographic, and hemodynamic evaluation of portal hypertension. In Savader SJ, Trerotola SL (eds): Venous Interventional Radiology with Clinical Perspectives. Thieme, New York, 1996. (Figures 1–37,43)

Schulz RD, Willi UV: Atlas of Pediatric Ultrasound. Thieme, New York, 1992. (Figure 10–31)

Shannon M, Tonino P: MRI of the Shoulder. Thieme, New York, 1992. (Figure 1–29)

Tabár L, Dean PB: Teaching Atlas of Mammography. Thieme, New York, 1985. (Figures 7–3,5,8)

Thurlbeck WM. Chronic airflow obstruction. In Thurlbeck WM, Churg A (eds): Pathology of the Lung, 2nd ed. Thieme, New York, 1995. (Figures 3–41B,C; 10–7)

Venbrux AC. Transjugular intrahepatic portosytemic shunts (TIPS). In: Venous Interventional Radiology with Clinical Perspectives. Thieme, New York, 1996 (Figure 1–40)

Wolf KJ, Fobbe F: Color Duplex Sonography. Thieme, New York, 1993. (Figures 1–22,25)

Index